LOCAL ANESTHESIA
FOR DENTAL PROFESSIONALS

Kathy B. Bassett RDH, BSDH, MEd
Professor, Clinical Coordinator
Dental Hygiene Program
Pierce College
Lakewood, Washington

Arthur C. DiMarco, DMD
Director, RIDE Program
Associate Professor
Department of Dental Hygiene
Eastern Washington University
Spokane, Washington

Affiliate Faculty
School of Dentistry
University of Washington
Seattle, Washington

Doreen K. Naughton, RDH, BSDH
Affiliate Instructor
Department of Dental Public Health Sciences
School of Dentistry
University of Washington

Pearson
Boston   Columbus   Indianapolis   New York   San Francisco   Upper Saddle River
Amsterdam   Cape Town   Dubai   London   Madrid   Milan   Munich   Paris   Montreal   Toronto
Delhi   Mexico City   Sao Paulo   Sydney   Hong Kong   Seoul   Singapore   Taipei   Tokyo

Library of Congress Cataloging-in-Publication Data

Bassett, Kathy.
   Local anesthesia for dental professionals/Kathy Bassett, Arthur DiMarco,
Doreen Naughton.
      p. ; cm.
   Includes bibliographical references and index.
   ISBN-13: 978-0-13-158930-8
   ISBN-10: 0-13-158930-X
   1. Anesthesia in dentistry. 2. Local anesthesia. I. DiMarco, Arthur.
   II. Naughton, Doreen. III. Title.
      [DNLM: 1. Anesthesia, Dental—methods. 2. Anesthesia, Local—
   methods. 3. Dentistry—methods. 4. Injections.   WO 460 B319L 2010]

      RK510.B367 2010
      617.9'676—dc22

                                                      2009024124

Publisher: Julie Levin Alexander
Assistant to Publisher: Regina Bruno
Editor-in-Chief: Mark Cohen
Development Editor: Melissa Kerian
Assistant Editor: Nicole Ragonese
Media Editor: Amy Peltier
Managing Production Editor: Patrick Walsh
Production Liaison: Christina Zingone
Production Editor: Lynn Steines,
   S4Carlisle Publishing Services
Manufacturing Manager: Ilene Sanford
Manufacturing Buyer: Pat Brown
Design Director: Jayne Conte
Cover Designer: Axell Designs

Director of Marketing: Karen Allman
Marketing Manager: Katrin Beacom
Marketing Specialist: Michael Sirinides
Marketing Assistant: Judy Noh
Media Project Manager: Lorena Cerisano
IRC Manager, Rights and Permissions: Zina Arabia
Manager, Visual Research: Beth Brenzel
Manager, Cover Visual Research & Permissions: Karen Sanatar
Image Permission Coordinator: Angelique Sharps
Composition: S4Carlisle Publishing Services
Printer/Binder: Courier/Kendallville
Cover Printer: Lehigh Phoenix/Hagerstown
Cover Image: Corbis/Somos Images

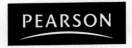

www.pearsonhighered.com

10 9 8 7 6 5 4 3 2
ISBN 10: 0-13-158930-X
ISBN 13: 978-0-13-158930-8

Contents

SECTION I

Pain Control Concepts   1

SECTION II

Pharmacology of Local Anesthetic Pain Control   37

SECTION III

Injection Fundamentals   129

Foreword

Contemporary pain control strategies are largely responsible for lessening and even removing many of the fears experienced in dental visits of the past. The use of local anesthesia has become a standard method of pain control in dentistry. All branches of specialized, clinical oral health care have been advanced through the use of local anesthesia.

Dentists have administered local anesthetic agents since their introduction. Dental and dental hygiene professionals continue to rely on them to provide comfortable and effective pain control for patients of all ages. Dental hygienists in the United States were first licensed to administer local anesthesia in Washington State (1971). Since that time, dental hygienists in most states and provinces in North America and designated oral health professionals in many other countries have been credentialed to administer local anesthetic agents. This ability has increased efficiency in oral healthcare and improved patient and clinician comfort during instrumentation, as well as the quality of outcomes.

For those dental hygienists who graduated prior to the licensure of local anesthesia in their jurisdictions, courses have been developed to enable them to acquire local anesthesia licenses and endorsements. Others, who were previously licensed and are returning to practice after extended absences, are taking advantage of continuing education courses and reviews to update their skills. With appropriate updating, these clinicians are able to provide effective pain control.

In order for clinicians to maintain and improve their knowledge and skills, updated pain control texts and related materials are assuming more importance than ever. Teaching and learning methods have changed over the years as well, accommodating an abundance of evidence-based information. New and revised texts, of necessity, can address this reality by providing students and educators with current research, case studies, clear-cut outlines and objectives, easy reference tables, review questions, PowerPoint™ templates, test banks, and a variety of time-saving, self-directed learning materials, all of which enhance teaching and learning.

Local Anesthesia for Dental Professionals provides teaching materials prepared with contemporary educational methods. This text meets the ever-growing need of educators to interact with an increasing diversity of students. *Local Anesthesia for Dental Professionals* aims to prepare current dental and dental hygiene professionals for licensure examination and clinical practice by helping them assimilate the abundance of relevant information emerging through ongoing research and technology in the oral healthcare arena.

Esther M. Wilkins, RDH, BS, DMD

Preface

Several years ago, a group of educators gathered to discuss the possibility of creating a new text in local anesthesia, united in their frustration with otherwise excellent texts that have only scant ancillary teaching resources. During the evening, a vision emerged of a clinically useful, comprehensive text with multiple student and teacher materials and supplements. In order to address diverse pedagogical methods and learning styles, it was decided that the information would be presented with chapter objectives, photographs, figures, tables, opinion boxes, case studies, and review questions. Supplemental student materials would include workbook exercises, word games, figure identifications, multiple quick-reference appendices, and an anatomy review tool.

We have worked diligently to create a resource that is close to this vision. In addition to the text, an accompanying companion website provides an online study guide to help guide individual study and laboratory experiences. Instructors will be provided an editable PowerPoint™ lecture outline with text figures and video clips of injection techniques, structured to follow the text outline in order to facilitate classroom instruction. A test bank with a variety of question and answer formats, and injection skill evaluation forms are also provided.

Perspectives and opinions on current controversies and less familiar techniques and pharmaceuticals have been addressed in a multitude of boxes. Tabulated pharmacological interactions can be found along with suggested modifications and concerns when considering specific medical conditions and illegal drug use. A separate chapter on dose calculations provides alternate methods for calculating safe drug doses.

Chapters on troubleshooting inadequate anesthesia, treating fearful patients, pediatric considerations, and supplemental techniques are included to assure a broad range of clinical skills and knowledge, especially as they address the predictable and frustrating failures that occur from time to time when administering local anesthesia.

Finally, our purpose in writing this text has been and shall continue to be to enhance the learning and clinical decision-making experience for students and clinicians of local anesthesia. In the words of the renowned Canadian physician, Sir William Osler, "the value of experience is not in seeing much, but in seeing wisely."

Acknowledgments

Many individuals helped in the preparation of this text. Without their hard work, dedication, and patience it would not have been possible. We wish to thank our eyes through the lens, photographer Ron Oyama, who stretched and contorted until he "got the shot" on each and every occasion. We also wish to thank our original illustrator, University of Washington Class of 2012 dental student Blake Davis, who created the concepts for the line artwork and several Pierce College graphic design student interns. Foremost among them is Brian Loke, a quick learner who toiled with us on many occasions to portray structures whose images were, at the very least, unfamiliar to him and, in some cases, downright obscure. His ability to pull the best from each image amazed us time after time. In addition to Mr. Loke, graphic design students Rachael Scholl and Jimmy Lu deserve our deep appreciation for their contributions to the capture and production of the supplemental video clips, as does Albert (Heath) Kaneen for his invaluable assistance with the PowerPoint outlines.

We wish to thank a number of Pierce College dental hygiene students for their excitement and participation as both "human subjects" and clinicians. Special thanks are extended to Amanda Caffey and Sarah McNeil for their invaluable assistance, to clinical subjects Megan Gibons, Mike Thierbach, Bill Bassett, Keavin McIntosh, and Grace (Hollywood) Wood for their patience through long photographic and video sessions and to Sheila Norton, RDH, and Keavin McIntosh, DMD, for their time and contributions as clinical support during these sessions. Additionally, we thank Katy Graham, RDH, MS for sharing a *career's worth* of resources and ideas.

This project could not have come together without the assistance of the companies who provide the local anesthesia drugs and devices that are central to these discussions. For their time, information, photographs and review contributions we thank: Certol International, Dental Systems Group/Carestream Health Inc., Dentsply Pharmaceuticals, LED Dental Inc (Velscope), Milestone Scientific, Miltex Inc., Novalar Pharmaceuticals, Septodont USA, and Sybron Dental.

We lovingly acknowledge the generous gift of time away from family and friends, who allowed us to hole away for days at a time only to emerge from our seclusion with discussions of needles and injections. Thanks are extended to our unwavering champions Karen DiMarco, Ron Oyama, and Jack Naughton for their patience, faith, and support as we guided this project to completion.

We extend our thanks to: Editor-in-Chief Mark Cohen, Development Editor Melissa Kerian, Production Liaison Christina Zingone, and the team at Prentice Hall for their invaluable assistance and support; Production Editor Lynn Steines and the team at S4Carlisle Publishing Services for their expertise and attention to detail; and to our publisher, Pearson Education. Without their interest and guidance, this work might have remained only a vision. We would also like to acknowledge Pearson Field Representative Roy Shaw, who started this project rolling when he asked if there were any books we *wished* we could have.

To the many educators, researchers, and clinicians who have so generously shared with us their insight and intelligence in the spirit of eliminating needless dental suffering, we extend our heartfelt thanks. Finally, we wish to thank Stanley Malamed, DDS, and John Yagiela, DDS, PhD, without whose wisdom and dedication this world would surely be a more painful place.

Contributors

Ann Eshenaur Spolarich, RDH, PhD
Clinical Associate Professor
USC School of Dentistry
Los Angeles, California

Course Director of Clinical Medicine
and Pharmacology
Arizona School of Dentistry and Oral Health
Mesa, Arizona

Clinical Instructor, Dean's Faculty
University of Maryland Dental School
Baltimore, Maryland
Chapter 2—*Fundamentals of Pain Management*

Albert (Ace) Goerig, DDS, MS
Specialist in Endodontics
Olympia, Washington
Chapter 20—*Insights from Specialties (Endodontics)*

Nikki Honey, DDS, MS
Professor of Dental Hygiene, Dental Hygiene Program
Shoreline Community College
Shoreline, Washington
Chapter 10—*Patient Assessment for Local Anesthesia*

Melanie Lang, DDS, MD
Specialist in Oral Surgery
Spokane, Washington
Chapter 20—*Insights from Specialties (Oral Surgery)*

William C. Lubken, DMD
Specialist in Periodontics
Gig Harbor, Washington
Chapter 20—*Insights from Specialties (Periodontics)*

Gregory L. Psaltis, DDS
Specialist in Pedodontics
Olympia, Washington
Chapter 19—*Insights from Pedodontics*

Marilynn Rothen, RDH, BS
Manager, Regional Clinical Dental Research Center
  and Dental Fears Research Clinic
School of Dentistry
University of Washington
Seattle, Washington
Chapter 18—*Insights for the Fearful Patient*

Agnes Spadafora, RDH, BS
Retired, Dental Public Health Sciences and Dental
  Fears Research Clinic
School of Dentistry
University of Washington
Seattle, Washington
Chapter 18—*Insights for the Fearful Patient*

Kimberly Stabbe, RDH, MS
Professor of Dental Hygiene, Dental Hygiene Program
Johnson County Community College
Overland Park, Kansas
Chapter 11—*Fundamentals for Administration
  of Local Anesthetic Agents*

Reviewers

Sheryl Armstrong RDH, BSDH, MEd
Clinical Coordinator, Dental Hygiene
Mohave Community College
Bullhead City, Arizona

Lynn Austin, RDH, MPH
Department Head/Associate Professor, Allied Health
Western Kentucky University
Bowling Green, Kentucky

Sandra N. Beebe, RDH, PhD
Senior Lecturer, Dental Hygiene
Southern Illinois University Carbondale
Carbondale, Illinois

Jacqueline P. Borja, BSDH, MEd
Dental Hygiene
Waukesha County Technical College
Pewaukee, Wisconsin

Eric D. Dixon, DMD
Coordinator/Assistant Professor, Dental Hygiene
Big Sandy Community and Technical College
Prestonsburg, Kentucky

Stephanie Harrison, RDH, MA
Director, Dental Hygiene
Community College of Denver
Denver, Colorado

Linda Jorgenson, RDH, BS, RF
Director, Dental Hygiene
Century College
White Bear Lake, Minnesota

Marilyn Kalal, RDH, MS
Professor, Dental Hygiene
Quinsigamond Community College
Worcester, Massachusetts

Liz Kaz, RDH, MS
Director, Dental Hygiene
Rio Salado College
Phoenix, Arizona

Kristi Morehead
University of Alaska Anchorage
Anchorage, Alaska

Linda Munro, RDH, BS
Instructor, Dental Hygiene
Portland Community College
Portland, Oregon

Dana Parker, DMD, MED
Associate Dean, Dental Programs
Greenville Technical College
Greenville, South Carolina

Terri Poulos, RDH, MEd
Professor, Dental Hygiene
Southwestern College
National City, California

Jennifer S. Sherry, RDH, MSEd
Assistant Professor, Dental Hygiene
Southern Illinois University
Carbondale, Illinois

Debra J. Sidd, RDH, RF, MEd
Instructor/Program Co-Chair, Dental Hygiene
Normandale Community College
Bloomington, Minnesota

Rebecca L. Stolberg, RDH, MS
Associate Professor/Department Chair, Dental Hygiene
Eastern Washington University
Spokane, Washington

About the Authors

Kathy Bassett, RDH, BSDH, MEd, is a professor and the clinic coordinator in the Dental Hygiene Program at Pierce College, Lakewood, Washington. With nearly thirty years of experience in local anesthesia and restorative expanded functions she is the course lead for Local Anesthesia curriculum at Pierce College. She has more than twenty years experience teaching local anesthesia fundamentals and techniques to dental healthcare professionals in basic introductory and continuing education courses, as well as numerous "train-the-trainer" courses for dental hygiene faculty as they have integrated local anesthesia into their individual curriculums. Kathy began her local anesthesia teaching experience with co-author Doreen Naughton as an instructor for the University of Washington's Continuing Dental Education, dental hygiene pre-license examination courses in local anesthesia and restorative functions, and continues to teach those courses through the Pacific Northwest Dental Hygiene Institute at Pierce College.

Arthur DiMarco, DMD, is the director of the University of Washington, School of Dentistry RIDE Program for Eastern Washington University (EWU) and associate professor in the Department of Dental Hygiene at EWU in Spokane, Washington. He has presented at numerous regional and international meetings, including the American Dental Education Association, the Inland Northwest Dental Meeting, and the American Dental Hygiene Association's Center for Lifelong Learning. A veteran of nearly thirty years of clinical practice and more than fifteen years in dental, dental hygiene, and dental assisting education, he is author of the *Local Anesthesia Laboratory Manual* at EWU and course director for the Pain Control curriculum, where he also teaches an elective course in local anesthesia for first year dental students. He recently completed research on the value of the anterior middle superior alveolar nerve block.

Doreen Naughton, RDH, BSDH, has twenty-eight years of clinical practice. She has been the sole proprietor of Dental Hygiene Health Services for twenty years. She has been an affiliate faculty at the University of Washington, Dental Public Health, Degree Completion Program for Dental Hygienists since 1992 and was administrator and instructor for the University of Washington's Continuing Dental Education, dental hygiene pre-license examination courses in local anesthesia and restorative functions for dental hygienists for six years.

Ms. Bassett, Dr. DiMarco, and Ms. Naughton have given hundreds of education courses on many topics, including didactic and clinical courses in local anesthesia for dental professionals and educators and for corporate clinical educators.

Section I

Pain Control Concepts

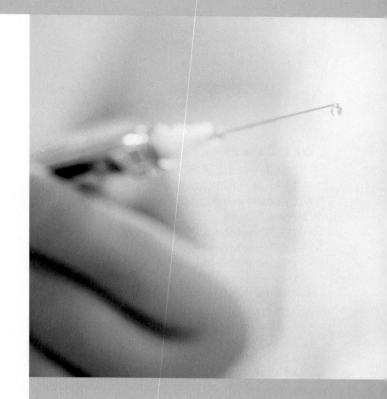

Chapter 1

Local Anesthesia in Dentistry: Past, Present, and Future

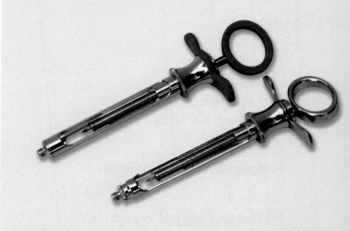

OBJECTIVES

- Define and discuss the key terms in this chapter.
- List early pharmacological agents used for pain.
- List early nonpharmacological methods of controlling pain.
- Discuss problems with the use of cocaine as a local anesthetic drug.
- Discuss the benefit of using epinephrine with local anesthetic drugs.
- Discuss the significance of the local anesthetic agent procaine.
- List the names and dates of development of the five common local anesthetic drugs in dentistry.
- Discuss the evolution of syringes for delivery of local anesthetic drugs.
- Discuss future advances in dental local anesthesia.

KEY TERMS

articaine **4**
breech-loading, cartridge-type syringe **6**
bupivacaine **4**
cocaine **3**
epinephrine **3**
harpoon-type aspirating syringe **6**
intravascular administration **6**

lidocaine **4**
mepivacaine **4**
nerve block anesthesia **4**
novocaine **3**
prilocaine **4**
procaine **3**
self-aspirating syringe **7**

INTRODUCTION

This chapter will provide a brief history of pain control in dentistry. It will discuss the origins of pain control and the individuals who made significant contributions to the practice of dental local anesthesia.

ORIGINS OF PAIN CONTROL FOR DENTISRY

Early civilizations experienced the effects of oral disease, including pain. Evidence points to primitive methods having been used to alleviate dental pain. In the ancient Middle East, for example, root canals were performed using malleable gold and poultices made of figs to replace diseased pulps. The Incas, Egyptians, and Chinese used a variety of obtundants to control dental pain, including coca leaves, henbane, mandrake, arsenic, and opium. Centuries later, nerve compression devices, exposure to cold, and hypnosis were all used to control pain (Wilwerding, 2001). While some aspects of these remedies were successful and a few are still used, most have been replaced with more effective drugs and techniques.

The current practice of local anesthesia owes its existence to the pioneers of modern techniques and drugs, including Niemann, Koller, Hall, Halsted, Freud, Braun, Einhorn, Takamine, Cook, Lofgren, and Lundquist. Their combined contributions span more than two centuries.

Cocaine was the precursor to modern dental anesthetics. In 1860, **cocaine** extracts from the coca leaf were observed to cause a numbing effect on the tongue, leaving it nearly without sensation. The local therapeutic effects of cocaine were explored for dental applications at the same time that Sigmund Freud was studying its effects on the central nervous system (CNS). His research uncovered cocaine's toxic and highly addictive properties. In papers to Dr. Carl Koller, Freud also reported "immediate unpleasant side effects such as nausea, vomiting, and collapse" (Jastak & Yagiela, 1981). These significant adverse effects stimulated the search for more acceptable drugs (Brunton, Laxo, & Parker, 2006; Holroyd, Wynn, & Requa-Clark, 1988; Wilwerding, 2001).

In 1884, cocaine's potent local anesthetic effects on the eye and its benefit in eye surgery were identified. That same year, local anesthetics were introduced in dentistry. Of parallel interest, in 1885, the original formula for Coca-Cola (which contained cocaine) was developed (Jastak & Yagiela, 1981).

Several years later, in 1901, a Japanese researcher, Jokichi Takamine, isolated **epinephrine** for pharmaceutical use, which was followed by Heinrich Braun's observation that adding epinephrine to cocaine solutions decreased its systemic absorption (reducing toxicity) while increasing its anesthetic duration. Braun described this effect as a "chemical tourniquet," which allowed lower doses of cocaine to be administered while achieving similar or better therapeutic effects (Jacobsohn, 1992). The euphoric and addictive properties of cocaine continued to trouble both researchers and clinicians, and the search for a non-addictive alternative eventually lead to the development of the local anesthetic drug **procaine,** in 1904.

Procaine was first synthesized in Germany and was marketed in the United States in 1905 as **novocaine.** Lacking the addictive properties of cocaine, procaine represented an important improvement in safety. Despite its replacement in dentistry in the latter part of the twentieth century by more effective and less problematic drugs, procaine is recognized as the prototype of modern local anesthetic agents. Procaine's almost universal acceptance in dental anesthesia is demonstrated by the observation that many patients still refer to the local anesthetic they receive as Novocaine, regardless of the actual drug administered (see Figure 1–1 ■).

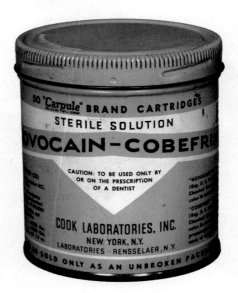

■ **FIGURE 1–1** Novocaine with Neo-Cobefrin Local Anesthetic Can, circa 1940s.
Source: Used with permission. Dr. Samuel D. Harris National Museum of Dentistry, University of Maryland.

In order to overcome procaine's somewhat unpredictable anesthetic effects and a disturbing incidence of allergic responses, **lidocaine** was developed and approved for use in the United States in 1948, followed by **mepivacaine** (1960), **prilocaine** (1965), **bupivacaine** (1983), and **articaine** (2000) (Malamed, 2004).

INJECTION TECHNIQUES IN DENTISTRY

Despite advances in armamentarium and drugs, the fundamentals of local anesthesia, including relevant anatomy and basic injection techniques, have not changed significantly over the past century. When comparing techniques developed in the early 1800s, for example, to instructional materials published more than sixty years ago and to those in circulation today, close similarities can be observed (see Figure 1–2 ■ and Figure 1–3 ■).

Many scientists, including a number of dental experts, have played key roles in the advancement of local anesthesia. Their contributions include improvements in both the practice and science of dental local anesthetics. More recent pioneers have developed improved delivery options and technique guidelines. In the 1940s, for example, with the lead of Dr. Harvey Cook, Cook-Waite Laboratories published the "Manual of Local Anesthesia" (see Figure 1–2, Figure 1–3, and Figure 1–4 ■).

William Halsted, an early pioneer, developed **nerve block anesthesia** techniques including the inferior alveolar nerve block. Additional techniques have been introduced in the twentieth century, including the Gow-Gates (1973), Vazirani-Akinosi (1977), P-ASA, and AMSA nerve blocks (Friedman and Hochman, mid to late 1990s) (Jastak, Yagiela, & Donaldson, 1995).

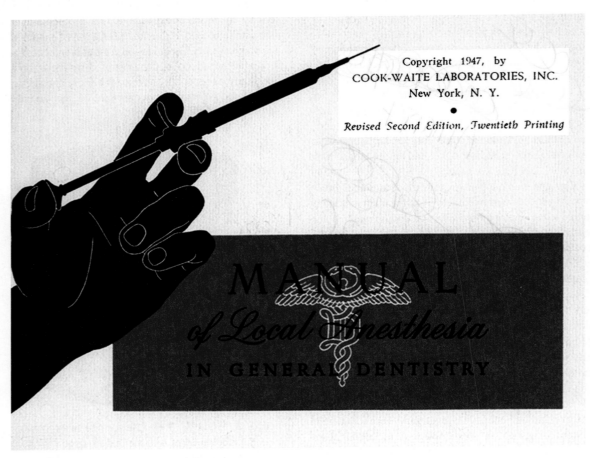

Copyright 1947, by
COOK-WAITE LABORATORIES, INC.
New York, N. Y.

Revised Second Edition, Twentieth Printing

■ **FIGURE 1–2** Manual of Local Anesthesia in Dentistry 1947.
Source: Courtesy of Cook-Waite, Carestream Health, Inc., Kodak Dental Systems.

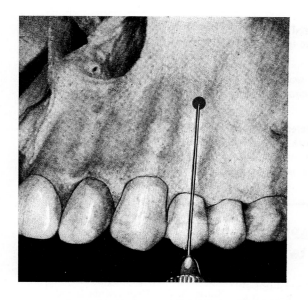

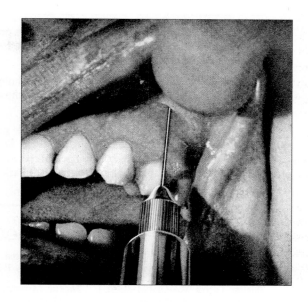

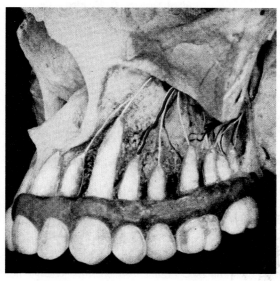

SUPRAPERIOSTEAL
INJECTION
★

To anesthetize the

MAXILLARY
FIRST
BICUSPID TOOTH

★

Needle:

No. 4-25 gauge-Long hub, **or**
No. 2-25 gauge-Short hub, **or**
No. 2-27 gauge-Short hub

Amount of Solution

one to two cc.

■ **FIGURE 1–3**   Manual of Local Anesthesia in Dentistry 1947. Instruction for Supraperiosteal Injection closely resembles today's instruction.
Source: Courtesy of Cook-Waite, Carestream Health, Inc., Kodak Dental Systems.

To The Profession — This Manual has been prepared by the Professional Division of Cook-Waite Laboratories in the belief that a compact guide for the use of local anesthesia will be instrumental in encouraging the practice of better dentistry.

It is recognized that there are variations in technique, many of which produce satisfactory results, but an attempt has been made to set forth here only those techniques which are employed most commonly in general dental practice.

The Professional Division endeavors to provide competent information on the various phases of local anesthesia and allied subjects through lectures, literature and correspondence. Members of the Dental Profession wishing to avail themselves of this service are invited to direct their inquiries to the Professional Division, Cook-Waite Laboratories, Inc., 90 Park Avenue, New York, N.Y. 10016.

BIBLIOGRAPHY

Braun—Local Anesthesia, Lea & Febiger, Philadelphia, 1914

Burket, Lester W.—Oral Medicine, J. D. Lippincott Co., Philadelphia, 1946

Cryer—Internal Anatomy of the Face, Lea & Febiger, Philadelphia, 1914

Fischer-Riethmuller—Local Anesthesia in Dentistry, Lea & Febiger, Philadelphia, 1914

Freeman, Charles W.—A study of the Structure of the Maxilla and Mandible as related to the Application of Local Anesthesia. (An Abstract.) Northwestern University Bulletin, Vol. 36, No. 34, May 4, 1936

Gray, Henry—Anatomy of The Human Body, 23rd edition. Revised by

Lewis, Warren H., Lea & Febiger, Philadelphia, 1936

Hickey, Maurice J.—Local Anesthesia in Oral Surgery, Journal of the A.D.A., Dec. 1946

Hill, R. T.—Anatomy of the Head and Neck, Lea & Febiger, Philadelphia, 1946

McCullogh, Ernest C.—Disinfection and Sterilization, 2nd edition, Lea & Febiger, Philadelphia, 1945

Posner, John J.—Local Anesthesia Simplified, Pattman & White Co., Philadelphia, 1928

Schmitt, Eugene — Intraseptal Anesthesia, Dental Cosmos, Vol. 78, No. 11, Nov., 1936

Sicher, Harry—The Anatomy of Mandibular Anesthesia, Journal of the A.D.A., Dec., 1946

Smith, A. E.—Block Anesthesia and Allied Subjects, C. V. Mosby Co., St. Louis, 1921

Waite, Sheridan C. — Infiltration & Nerve Blocking, 5th edition, Antidolor Mfg. Co., Springville, N. Y.

Ward, Marcus L. — The American Textbook of Operative Dentistry, 7th edition, Lea & Febiger, Philadelphia, 1940

Winter, Leo—Textbook of Exodontia, 5th edition, C. V. Mosby Co., St. Louis, 1943

Winter, Leo—Operative Oral Surgery, 2nd edition, C. V. Mosby Co., St. Louis, 1943

■ **FIGURE 1–4** Early Leaders and Resources in Dental Local Anesthesia.
Source: Courtesy of Cook-Waite, Carestream Health, Inc., Kodak Dental Systems.

DEVICES FOR PAIN CONTROL IN DENTISTRY

In addition to the drugs themselves, their method of delivery to the body has also undergone extensive improvement over the years. The development of hypodermic syringes in the 1850s simplified the delivery of cocaine and other drug solutions (Jastak & Yagiela, 1981). During World War I, Dr. Cook, who was an army surgeon, developed a **breech-loading, cartridge-type syringe** that functioned similarly to a breech-loading rifle (see Figure 1–5 ■). Replacing more cumbersome early designs (see Figure 1–6 ■), this syringe held a glass cartridge containing a local anesthetic drug. Both the syringe and cartridge were introduced in 1921 by Dr. Cook's newly formed company, Cook Laboratories.

In 1947, the Novocol Company developed the first aspirating syringe, which reduced the risk of injection into blood vessels, known as **intravascular administration.** Unlike the syringes used today, it made use of a screw-based technology for securing cartridges. The **harpoon-type aspirating syringe** in current use was developed by Cook-Waite Laboratories in 1957 (originally Cook Laboratories). Today, products are sold under

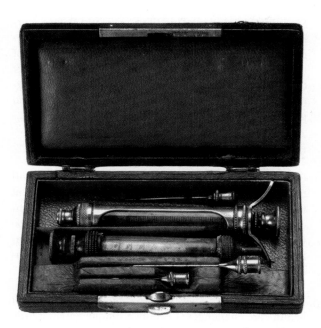

■ **FIGURE 1–5**   Local Anesthetic Syringe and Needle Set, circa late nineteenth century.
Source: Used with permission. Dr. Samuel D. Harris National Museum of Dentistry, University of Maryland.

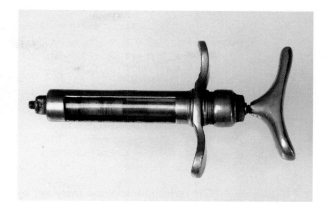

■ **FIGURE 1–6**   Local Anesthetic Syringe, circa mid-1930s.
Source: Used with permission. Dr. Samuel D. Harris National Museum of Dentistry, University of Maryland.

the Cook-Waite label as part of Carestream Health Inc., Kodak Dental Systems.

Due to reports of hepatitis transmission through contaminated needles, disposable, stainless steel needles were introduced in 1959, which effectively eliminated the need for the sterilization and reuse of needles (Jastak, Yagiela, & Donaldson, 1995). The **self-aspirating syringe** was developed in 1970 to provide an easy way of determining whether or not the tips of needles are located within blood vessels.

Computer-controlled local anesthetic delivery (CCLAD) devices were introduced in 1997. The first of these, the Wand (made by Milestone Scientific), is sold today as the CompuDent. Other CCLAD devices include the Comfort Control Syringe (made by Dentsply International in New Jersey), the QuickSleeper (made by Dental Hi Tech in France), the Anaeject (made by J Morita Nashika Line in Japan and distributed by Septodont), and the most recent device, the STA (also made by Milestone). See Chapter 9, "Local Anesthetic Delivery Devices," for further discussion on these devices.

LOCAL ANESTHESIA SCOPE OF PRACTICE

Local anesthetics have been available in dentistry since 1884. Dentists have been able to deliver local anesthetic drugs in cartridge form since 1921. Dental hygienists were first licensed to deliver local anesthetics in the state of Washington in 1971. As of 2009, forty-four states include local anesthesia within their dental hygiene scope of practice. Several of the remaining states are in the process of amending their dental and dental hygiene practice acts to allow dental hygienists to practice local anesthesia.

A summary of the specific requirements for dental hygienists by state is available from the American Dental Hygienists' Association (www.adha.org). These requirements vary regarding the type and degree or extent of injections, as well as the required extent of supervision, education, and examination. Clinicians must be knowledgeable regarding the specifics of the practice acts governing their particular practice locations.

ADVANCES IN PHARMACOLOGY AND TECHNOLOGY
Developments in Pharmacology

Current developments of interest in pharmacology include the use of phentolamine mesylate as a local anesthesia reversal agent, and centbucridine as a local anesthetic drug.

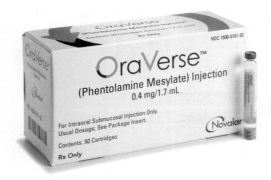

■ **FIGURE 1–7** OraVerse (phentolamine mesylate) by Novalar Pharmaceuticals.

Source: Courtesy of Novalar Pharmaceuticals.

Phentolamine mesylate, an injectable formulation by Novalar Pharmaceuticals under the trade name OraVerse® (see Figure 1–7 ■), is the first pharmaceutical agent available for the reversal of *soft-tissue* anesthesia (which can interfere with speaking, eating, and drinking for prolonged periods). OraVerse was approved by the FDA on May 9, 2008 (Novalar, 2008). For further discussion, see Chapter 17, "Local Anesthesia Complications and Management."

Centbucridine, which has been in use since 1984 in India, has been reported to have advantages over current FDA-approved, local anesthetic drugs. While there are reported therapeutic advantages, including greater potency with far less risk of toxicity to the central nervous and cardiovascular systems, there remain concerns over possible long-term health risks with centbucridine (Dasgupta, Tendulkar, Paul, & Satoskar, 1984; Gupta, Mishra, & Dhawan, 1989; Vacharajani, Parikh, Paul, & Satoskar, 1983).

Developments in Armamentarium

Among the most recent advances in local anesthetic devices is the previously mentioned STA Single Tooth Anesthesia System Instrument CCLAD released by Milestone Scientific in 2007. This device integrates advanced pressure sensing technology for guidance with specific single tooth injection techniques (Hochman, 2007; Wand).

A technology with perhaps significant future implications for dentistry is the SonoPrep by Sontra Medical Corporation. This FDA-approved device, currently available only in medicine, uses ultrasonic technology to provide reversible molecular disruptions of tissue barriers ("skin permeation") in order to deliver topical anesthetics. SonoPrep technology may offer significant benefits in dentistry, including faster onset and greater depth of topical anesthesia.

SOCIAL CONTRIBUTIONS

Future developments in local anesthesia delivery will rely on new technologies, improvements in current technologies, new drugs, and advancements from collaborations with medicine and other cross-disciplines. Clinicians are encouraged to explore advances in technology and to expand their skills and techniques whenever possible in order to enhance patient comfort.

In addition to scientific contributions, corporate leaders have initiated programs to support current health care challenges. Leading a unique collaboration of dental product manufacturers, the Sullivan-Schein Company launched the "Think Pink, Practice Pink" program in the fall of 2007 to benefit the American Cancer Society's (ACS) breast cancer research through the sale of pink dental-related products (Knott, 2008). In response to this initiative, the Septodont Company provided a pink version of its petite local anesthetic syringe (see Figure 1–8 ■).

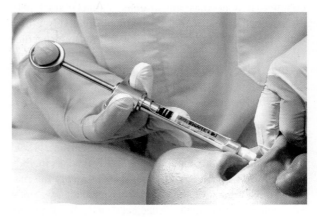

■ **FIGURE 1–8** 2007 "Think Pink, Practice Pink" Cancer Awareness Program. Pink local anesthetic syringes by Septodont were sold to benefit American Cancer Society.

CHAPTER QUESTIONS

1. Which groups of pharmacological agents were used for early pain control?
   a. Coca leaves, henbane, mandrake, opium
   b. Coca leaves, cocaine, lidocaine
   c. Henbane, opium, morphine, methadone
   d. Mandrake, opium, morphine, lidocaine

2. Cocaine is not appropriate for use as a dental anesthetic agent because it:
   a. Is not readily available.
   b. Has a high potential for inducing allergies.
   c. Has addictive properties.
   d. Can not be synthesized in solution.

3. Which *one* of the following is commonly used in dentistry today?
   a. Procaine
   b. Screw-type aspirating cartridge
   c. Harpoon-type aspirating syringe
   d. Ultrasonic anesthetic delivery

4. Which *one* of the following was the first local anesthetic drug developed following the use of procaine?
   a. Lidocaine
   b. Mepivacaine
   c. Articaine
   d. Bupivacaine

5. Phentolamine mesylate (OraVerse) is a new pharmacological agent that can:
   a. Prolong anesthetic effects.
   b. Reverse soft tissue anesthesia.
   c. Allow lower drug doses to be used.
   d. Decrease allergic reactions to local anesthetic drugs.

6. Which *one* of the following was the first CCLAD device marketed?
   a. QuickSleeper
   b. Wand
   c. Comfort Control Syringe
   d. Anaeject

REFERENCES

Anaeject: J Morita Nashika Line, Japan; product information available from Septodont Inc., www.septodontinc.com.

Brunton, L., Lazo, J., & Parker, K. (Eds.) (2006). *Goodman and Gilman's the pharmacological basis of therapeutics* (11th ed.). New York: McGraw-Hill.

Comfort Control Syringe: Product information available at Dentsply International, York, PA 17405; www.dentsply.com.

Dasgupta, D. D., Tendulkar, B. A., Paul, T. T., & Satoskar, R. S. (1984). Comparative study of centbucridine and lignocaine for subarachnoid block. *Journal of Postgraduate Medicine, 30*(4), 207–209.

Gupta, P. P., Mishra, Y. C., & Dhawan, B. N. (1989, June). Comparison of centbucridine and lignocaine in dental surgery. *Indian Journal of Anaesthesia, 37*(3), 106–11.

Hochman, M. N. (2007, April). Intraligamentary anesthesia pressure-sensing technology provides innovative advancement in the field of dental local anesthesia. *Compendium, 28*(4), 186–193.

Holroyd, S. V., Wynn, R. L., & Requa-Clark, B. (1988). *Clinical pharmacology in dental practice* (4th ed.). St. Louis: Mosby.

Jacobsohn, P. H. (1992, Winter). Victory over pain: A historical perspective. *Anesthesia & Pain Control in Dentistry, 1*(1), 49–52.

Jastak, J. T., & Yagiela, J. A. (1981). *Regional anesthesia of the oral cavity.* St. Louis: Mosby.

Jastak, J. T., Yagiela, J. A., & Donaldson, D. (1995). *Local anesthesia of the oral cavity.* Philadelphia: Saunders.

Knott, Maureen, marketing director, Sullivan-Schein Dental (personal communication, June 2008).

Malamed, S. F. (2004). *Handbook of local anesthesia* (5th ed.). St. Louis: Mosby.

Novalar press release (2008, May 12); http://www.novalarpharm.com.

QuickSleeper: Product information available from Dental Hi Tech, France; www.dentalhitech.com.

Vacharajani, G. N., Parikh, N., Paul, T., & Satoskar, R. S. (1983). A comparative study of centbucridine and lidocaine in dental extraction. *International Journal of Clinical Pharmacology Research, 3*(4), 251–255.

Wand: Product information available from CompuDent, STA: Milestone Scientific Inc., Livingston, NJ, 07039; www.milestonescientific.com.

Wilwerding, T. (2001). *History of dentistry,* http://cudental.creighton.edu/htm/history2001.pdf. (Last accessed July 2008).

Chapter 2

Fundamentals of Pain Management

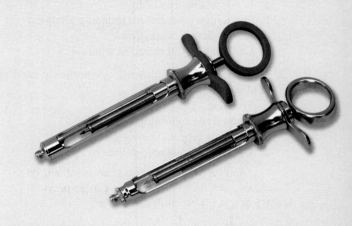

OBJECTIVES

- Define and discuss the key terms in this chapter.
- Discuss the value of pain as a protective response.
- Discuss factors that can contribute to an individual's response to a painful experience.
- Discuss the three general types of pain.
- Differentiate between acute and chronic pain.
- Explain the differences between pain perception and nociception.
- Discuss the physiological reactions of the sympathetic nervous system related to pain.
- Discuss anxiety and fear as they relate to successful anesthesia.
- Give examples of strategies that can help patients cope with fear and anxiety.
- Discuss the influence of previous pain experiences on the ability to administer local anesthetic injections.

KEY TERMS

acute pain **12**
chronic pain **12**
debriefing **16**
fight or flight **15**
neuropathic pain **14**
nociceptive pain **14**
nociceptors **12**
pain **11**
pain disorders **15**
pain threshold **11**
pain tolerance **12**
polymodal **12**

PREP **16**
protective response **11**
psychogenic factors **15**
sensory modality **12**
somatic pain **14**
sympathetic nervous system **15**
visceral pain **14**

INTRODUCTION

Pain control in dentistry requires the study of local anesthesia and an understanding of the science of pain. This chapter will provide an introduction to the fundamentals of pain. It will focus on pain as having both physiological and psychological aspects. Categories of pain and factors that have an effect on the ability to tolerate pain will also be discussed.

PAIN PERSPECTIVES

Pain Experience

Pain is unique and is reported subjectively. Even within an individual's unique experience, the perception of pain on a given day at a given time is not necessarily identical to a previous or future perception of pain in response to an identical stimulus. Pain perception (and reactions to the perceptions of pain) cannot be described as necessarily proportional to the intensity of physical injury or to the degree of harm.

An individual's pain experience is influenced by a number of variables. For example, gender provides both genetic and hormonal influences. Gender also may add many complex components, including socially constructed roles and relationships, personality traits, attitudes, behaviors, values, and degrees of power and influence. Other variables, such as age, physical health, mental health, emotional status, expectations, previous experiences, learned responses, and ethnic and cultural norms, also impact the experience of pain and individual reactions to it.

The definition of pain provided by the International Association for the Study of Pain describes it as a negative experience (see Box 2–1). While the experience of pain is accurately described in negative terms, the rapid sequences of perception and response that make up the experience also serve to protect the body from harm, a decidedly positive benefit.

Avoidance of pain is a strong, innate trait. In dentistry, painful experiences can lead to a strategy of avoiding pain, and therefore treatment. Pain can lead to anxiety and fear, which may result in heightened perceptions of pain, which in turn may cause further avoidance of dental care. The ability to identify factors that can contribute to painful experiences and proactive strategies to avoid unnecessary pain can ensure patient comfort during treatment (Howard, 2007; International Association for the Study of Pain; Pappagallo & Chapman, 2005; Spitzer, 2004).

> Box 2–1 The Definition of Pain
>
> The International Association for the Study of Pain defines pain as "an unpleasant sensory and emotional experience associated with actual or potential tissue damage, or described in terms of such damage" (International Association for the Study of Pain).

PROTECTIVE RESPONSE

As a physiological reaction to the environment, pain is a **protective response,** protecting the body from harm. This protection is rapid, reflexive, and subconscious.

An example of a protective response to pain is known as the withdrawal reflex. This reflex prevents damage by removing tissues from harm when harm is sensed or is imminent. When a hot stove is touched, for example, the hand quickly withdraws from the harmful stimulus (heat). Without the protective reflex, the ability to maintain a healthy body would be seriously compromised. This is the case when an individual with a spinal cord injury is not able to feel sensations or initiate movement below the level of the injury. The normal protective neuronal activity and subsequent muscular reaction is absent and there is a constant need for monitoring and repositioning in order to avoid pressure sore injuries or injuries caused by thermal stimuli.

The protective response is also linked to behavior. If an individual has been stung by a wasp in the past, the mere sight of a wasp might cause the individual to react in order to avoid a sting. This withdrawal is governed by memory (Howard, 2007; International Association for the Study of Pain).

PAIN THRESHOLD VERSUS PAIN TOLERANCE

The terms *pain threshold* and *pain tolerance* are not synonymous. **Pain threshold** may be defined as the point at which a stimulus first produces a sensation of pain (*Taber's Cyclopedic Medical Dictionary* [*Taber's*], 1997). Pain thresholds are innate and are highly reproducible in individuals. They do not usually change appreciably over time. An individual's pain threshold is a function of the physiological reaction to painful stimuli. For example, in dentistry a dental pulp tester is used to determine the viability of teeth. Patients will respond when set levels of stimulation are perceived. This identifies the threshold of pain.

Pain tolerance may be defined as an individual's reaction to painful stimuli. It indicates the amount of pain an individual is willing or able to endure. Tolerance can vary from day to day and from appointment to appointment, and may be influenced by current events and stresses. It can also be altered by environment, experience, and social attitudes. Research has shown that gender and genetics also play key roles in understanding individual variations in pain perception and stimulus processing (Dionne, Phero, & Becker, 2002).

Common pain stimuli produce highly variable reactions from individual to individual. In the example of a pulp tester, the device will elicit pain at reproducible levels but individuals may react to the electric current in markedly different ways. Both emotional and psychological factors influence their reactions. These factors are modified by the significance an individual places on the present circumstance.

It is interesting to note that the terms *pain tolerance* and *pain threshold* are often used interchangeably despite these distinct differences. Patients may state that they have very low pain thresholds. They are actually relating that they are not able to tolerate a lot of pain.

Preappointment medications such as anti-anxiety and anti-inflammatory agents and local anesthesia administered during appointments are used to modify a patient's tolerance to treatment. It is also important to recognize that an individual who suffers from long-term pain may have altered responses to pain of any nature. Preappointment assessment in this area can improve clinical experiences (American Psychiatric Association, 2000; Pappagallo & Chapman, 2005).

PAIN DURATION

Pain may be categorized in a variety of ways. A common classification categorizes pain according to its duration, as either acute or chronic. **Acute pain** may last from a few seconds to no more than six months depending on causative factors. It is generally caused by tissue damage from injury or disease. Individuals suffering from acute pain expect to get better and adopt behaviors that remove or ease the cause or causes of the pain. For example, a patient experiencing postoperative dental pain may rely on pain relievers or ice packs to stop the pain. Pain is often a strong motivator

for seeking treatment, regardless of a patient's level of dental anxiety and fear.

Chronic pain may be defined as pain that persists for more than six months with or without an identifiable cause. The longer acute pain continues, the more likely it is to become chronic. Occasionally, patients who suffer from chronic pain tend to lose hope of getting better, providing an unfortunate pathway to depression.

Individuals suffering from chronic pain may be referred to specialized clinics with experience in managing long-term patterns of pain. Pain clinics provide a wide variety of services, including evaluation, education, and treatment (physical therapy, massage, and acupuncture). They also teach coping skills that can influence the reaction to pain, and they modify behavior through the use of appropriate medications and techniques such as biofeedback (Howard, 2007; *Taber's*, 1997).

PAIN AND NOCICEPTION

Sensory receptors detect a variety of stimuli that are then relayed to the central nervous system (CNS) for interpretation. Specific receptors are associated with each type of sensory input. For example, there are specific taste receptors on the tongue that detect sweet, sour, bitter and salt. In the eye there are two types of photoreceptors, cones and rods.

The ability of a stimulus to be detected by a specific receptor is known as a **sensory modality.** Sensory modalities include hearing, sight, touch, taste, and sound. Changes in temperature are detected by thermoreceptors. Changes in pressure are detected by mechanoreceptors. Alterations in body chemicals are detected by chemoreceptors (Howard, 2007; Pappagallo & Chapman, 2005).

Sensory receptors that detect injury are called **nociceptors** (see Figure 2–1 ▪). Unlike other sensory receptors, nociceptors are activated by injury and relay sensory input whether or not the individual is aware that injury has occurred. This process is influenced by an individual's age, general health, and genetics (Nani, Mellow, & Getz, 1999).

Nociceptors differ in another important way from other sensory receptors in that they are **polymodal,** responding to all types of stimuli. In addition to activating receptors specific for them, thermal, mechanical, and chemical stimuli can all activate nociceptors, which relay pain information to the CNS. Despite the obvious

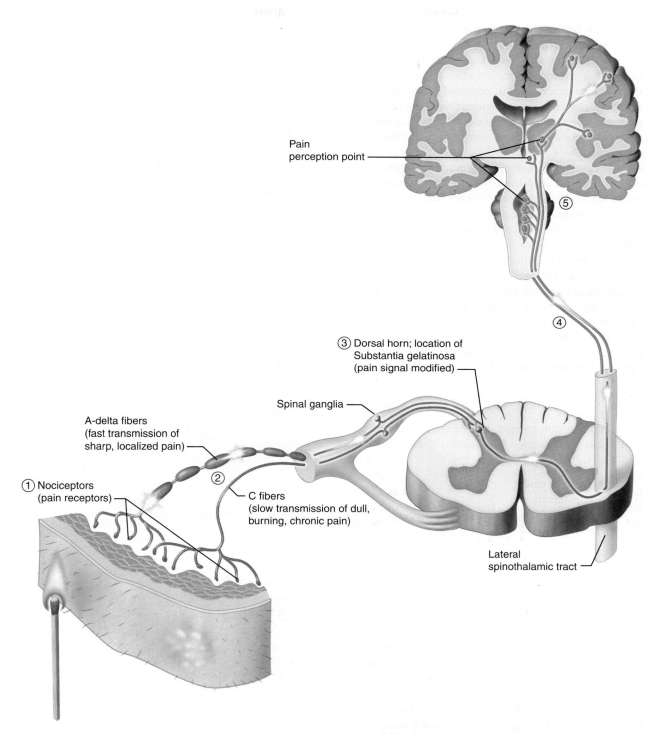

Pain perception point

⑤

③ Dorsal horn; location of Substantia gelatinosa (pain signal modified)

④

Spinal ganglia

A-delta fibers (fast transmission of sharp, localized pain)

② C fibers (slow transmission of dull, burning, chronic pain)

① Nociceptors (pain receptors)

Lateral spinothalamic tract

■ **FIGURE 2–1**   Nociceptors. Nociceptors are sensory receptors that detect when a body tissue has been injured.

Source: Figure 15–1, page 471 [Nociceptors] from Ball, J. W., Bindler, R. C., *Pediatric Nursing: Caring for Children, Nociceptors,* 4th ed. Prentice Hall, 2008.

differences between these stimuli, all can be perceived by nociceptors as painful.

Nociceptors also differ from other sensory receptors in that nociceptors never adapt to stimulation. In the presence of constant stimulation, nociceptors will always respond to the stimulation. This is a key aspect of the protective response to pain. The body is constantly providing sensory warnings when injury is pending or occurring.

As previously noted, the experience or perception of pain does not lend itself well to objective measurement. While this is an accurate statement, pain intensity rating scales nevertheless can be useful for both patients and clinicians. They provide patients with a means of communicating the degree of pain experienced and they provide clinicians with an opportunity to respond appropriately. An example of a subjective pain intensity measurement tool is the Wong-Baker FACES Pain Rating Scale. This simple numeric scale (with associated facial expressions) uses "0" to represent no pain (very happy face) and "5" to represent severe pain (crying face) (see Figure 2–2 ■). Other scales use similar graduated numbers to report the degree of pain experienced.

PAIN CLASSIFICATION BY ETIOLOGY

Pain may be categorized according to its etiology (American Psychiatric Association, 2000; Howard, 2007), as follows:

1. nociceptive pain
2. neuropathic pain
3. pain disorders associated with psychogenic factors

In addition, in response to nociceptive input, fear and other physical conditions can alter the body's ability to receive, transmit, interpret, and respond to pain.

Nociceptive Pain

Nociceptive pain is caused by injury or disease in body tissues. This pain may be constant or intermittent and often escalates with movement. Nociceptive pain can be further subdivided into **somatic** and **visceral pain.** Somatic nociceptive pain occurs on superficial structures such as skin and muscles and is caused by traumatic injuries. The resulting pain may be sharp, aching, or throbbing. Visceral nociceptive pain occurs in internal body cavities and is caused by compression, expansion, stretching, and infiltration. It usually produces squeezing or gnawing sensations (Howard, 2007; Pappagallo & Chapman, 2005).

Neuropathic Pain

Neuropathic pain is caused by nerve injury or dysfunction of the sensory nerves in the central or peripheral nervous systems (Howard, 2007; Pappagallo & Chapman, 2005). There are numerous types of neuropathic pain, most of which are complex and frequently chronic in nature. They may have inflammatory, noninflammatory, and/or immune system components. Pain may be generated in the CNS such as phantom pain from a missing limb or tooth or it may occur due to what is referred to as peripherally generated polyneuropathy, as seen in diabetes. Mononeuropathy is usually associated with a

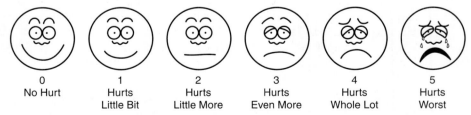

| 0 | 1 | 2 | 3 | 4 | 5 |
| No Hurt | Hurts Little Bit | Hurts Little More | Hurts Even More | Hurts Whole Lot | Hurts Worst |

■ **FIGURE 2–2**   Wong-Baker FACES Pain Rating Scale. **Instructions:** Point to each face using the words to describe the pain intensity. Ask the child to choose face that best describes own pain and record the appropriate number.

Source: Hockenberry, MJ, Wilson, D, Winkelstein, ML: *Wong's Essentials of Pediatric Nursing,* ed. 7, St. Louis, 2005, p. 1259. Used with permission. Copyright Mosby.

single nerve injury or compression, which is seen in trigeminal neuralgia, carpal tunnel syndrome, and post-herpetic neuralgia.

Pain Disorders Associated with Psychogenic Factors

Pain disorders associated with **psychogenic factors** are related to mental or emotional problems that affect the experience of pain. They are diagnosed only after other causes of pain have been eliminated. They are also diagnosed far less frequently than nociceptive and neuropathic pain. While not attributable to specific injuries or pathology, the pain is nonetheless real and can occur at any age, manifesting as head, stomach, chest, or muscle discomfort, or it may occur in any other location or combination of locations. Individuals with depressive or anxiety disorders may experience complications with any type of pain. These individuals may report pain beyond typical intensities and durations. In some instances, previously diagnosed physical pain from known pathogenic origins can be increased or prolonged by psychogenic factors.

Pain is multidimensional and often requires more than one treatment modality. These may include psychotherapy, biofeedback, hypnosis, and antidepressant and nonnarcotic analgesic medications. Patients with pain disorders may respond differently to dental pain (American Psychiatric Association, 2000; Howard, 2007; Pappagallo & Chapman, 2005).

SYMPATHETIC NERVOUS SYSTEM AND PAIN

In response to pain, the CNS simultaneously directs activation of the **sympathetic nervous system.** The sympathetic nervous system stimulates the adrenal medulla, resulting in the release of norepinephrine and epinephrine (see Chapter 6, "Vasoconstrictors in Dentistry"). These neurotransmitters mediate so-called **"fight or flight"** mechanisms, resulting in a host of potential reactions, including: increased heart rate and blood pressure; dilation of the pupils and of the bronchial and skeletal muscle vasculature; and constriction of mesenteric vessels. Both the anticipation of pain and the actual perception of pain stimulate this response.

If these reactions occur, they can be exacerbated by the psychological state of a patient during a dental appointment. Fearful patients often demonstrate similar sympathetic nervous defense reactions before, during, and after injections. While the physical manifestations are similar and are typically of short duration, all adverse reactions to dental anesthesia require prompt and appropriate management, regardless of their etiology (Dionne et al., 2002; Howard, 2007; Pappagallo & Chapman, 2005).

PAIN MANAGEMENT IMPLICATIONS FOR DENTISTRY

The majority of patients willingly schedule and attend their dental appointments. Previous dental experiences have been generally positive. Some avoid dental treatment, primarily due to fears surrounding the administration of local anesthesia. Their experiences have been negative and they are convinced there is little reason to expect better. In other words, fears override the need for dental treatment. In order to develop positive treatment interactions, it is important for clinicians to understand the etiology of the fear and pain experience. Both physiological and psychological factors contribute to difficulties related to treatment.

It has been reported that the main reason individuals avoid dental appointments is fear (Naini et al., 1999). About 40 percent of patients report some level of anxiety related to dental treatment, and roughly 5 percent avoid dentistry due to fear of injections. Patients experience fear on a continuum ranging from mild anxiety to phobia.

Fear can be a barrier to obtaining adequate anesthesia. Fearful patients are typically no less concerned than others about their need for dental treatment but fear can prevent them from experiencing successful treatment. Some patients are fearful only of injections and report their anxiety and fear subsides following the injection. Assessing and addressing fear prior to injections can improve the results of anesthesia. Clinicians need to be aware of strategies associated with treating anxious and fearful patients (Dionne et al., 2002; Fiset, Milgrom, & Weinstein, 1985; Milgrom, Weinstein, & Getz, 1995).

PATIENT MANAGEMENT PERSPECTIVES

Everyone working in the dental setting can offer support to anxious or fearful patients. Dental personnel can identify fearful patients at the time of initial contact whether by telephone or in person. As with nondental-related fears, it may not be easy for fearful patients to acknowledge their dental fears or the degree of their fears. Deliberate behavior on the part of clinicians can be helpful in developing successful patient experiences and can create an environment that encourages discussions of fear. For example, using controlled, calm speech and positive demeanor conveys comfort and instills confidence. Signs of impatience or disapproval should be avoided.

A protocol that can be considered standard for all patients including those with specific fears will incorporate the following:

1. Asking about previous dental experiences and being attentive to the responses
2. Assuring that difficulties during past experiences can be managed and overcome
3. Involving patients when identifying strategies to help manage anxiety and fear

Some strategies to help patients cope with anxiety and fear include an additional sequence of steps that can be referred to as **PREP** (Prepare, Rehearse, Empower, and Praise). Applying the PREP strategy can build trust and provide reassurance. These steps can be found in Box 2–2, and when used along with a process known as **debriefing** can further build trust and reassurance. Clinicians may find the use of these stress-reducing techniques helpful for themselves as well.

The debriefing process can be useful when managing fearful patients. This process allows for discussion periods at the end of appointments to give patients opportunities to relate which aspects of treatment went well and which aspects did not go well. Discussions of treatment to be accomplished at the next appointment can be quite helpful, particularly if they rely heavily on patient input when determining how ambitious the next appointment should be. Plans for modifying aspects that were identified as not going well can be discussed and then applied to subsequent appointments. By proceeding in this manner, the patient not only agrees to go to the next step but has had an active role in determining the content of the step.

It is important that adequate time is scheduled for the debriefing process. Rushing through the discussion does little to reassure patients that recommendations will be heeded.

For some patients, pharmacological intervention may be helpful and necessary. Nitrous-oxide-oxygen sedation, oral conscious sedation, intravenous sedation, and general anesthesia should be discussed with patients as the situation warrants. Pharmacological solutions are especially helpful for anxious patients who avoid dental treatment and present only for emergent care. In these situations, pharmacological agents may be incorporated into treatment. For some patients, medical consultation may be necessary. These individuals often must resort to emergent care due to their intense fear and avoidance of routine dental care, and pharmacologic agents can be incorporated into treatment when indicated.

The phenomena of anxiety and pain related to dental injections are not limited to the experiences of the patient. Clinicians should also consider personal past experiences and perceptions of pain. Learning to give injections can be unsettling for clinicians, especially those who are fearful of receiving injections. Previous experiences and perceptions can interfere with the learning process and limit confidence building. On the other hand, a painful past experience can also provide a positive motivation to provide comfortable injection experiences for others. If necessary, psychological therapy may be helpful in recognizing personal inhibitions that may delay learning and can undermine clinical success in the delivery of injections.

In some cases, it may be appropriate to recommend intervention with a professional psychologist. More in-depth strategies for management of patient fear and phobia are discussed in Chapter 18, "Insights for the Fearful Patient."

Box 2–2   PREP to Minimize Patient Anxiety and Fear

To help patients cope with anxiety and fear:

1. *Prepare* by utilizing relaxation techniques such as deep breathing, distraction such as music or visualization, and muscle relaxation.
2. *Rehearse* procedures allowing patients to practice control and self-calming techniques.
3. *Empower* patients with strategies that give them control during procedures such as raising a hand to ask the clinician to stop.
4. *Praise* patients for using specific coping techniques that are helpful to them.

CHAPTER QUESTIONS

1. Which statement *best* describes pain as a protective response?
   - a. Pain is a physiological, conscious reaction.
   - b. Pain is a psychological reaction based on blood flow to the injured site.
   - c. Pain is a rapid, reflexive, subconscious reaction.
   - d. Pain is a slow, deliberate reaction to avoid further tissue injury.

2. Which of these groups of variables does not affect the experience of pain?
   - a. Sex, genetics, mental health
   - b. Personality, age, hormones
   - c. Attitudes, learned responses
   - d. Body weight, height

3. Which *one* of the following statements regarding nociception is true?
   - a. Nociception is polymodal.
   - b. Nociceptive receptors can distinguish between chemical and thermal stimuli.
   - c. Nociception is a physiological and psychological process.
   - d. Nociceptive pain is identical in somatic and visceral structures.

4. Which *one* of the following is an example of neuropathic pain?
   - a. Fractured bone
   - b. Psychological disorder
   - c. Postsurgery pain
   - d. Trigeminal neuralgia

5. Which one of the following will help patients cope with anxiety and fear?
   - a. avoid discussions about anxiety and fear
   - b. only the dentist should ask about anxiety and fear to avoid patient embarrassment
   - c. assure the patient that difficulties during past dental visits could not have been avoided
   - d. prepare, rehearse, empower, and praise patients to reduce anxiety and fear

6. In the process of debriefing, which *one* of the following is *not* useful when managing fearful patients?
   - a. Patient and clinician discussion period at the end of each appointment
   - b. Patient gives input on the duration and plan for the next appointment
   - c. Future appoints are modified based on the insights from the patient/clinician discussion
   - d. Clinicians select strategies for the patient for his or her next appointment

REFERENCES

American Psychiatric Association (2000). *Diagnostic and statistical manual of mental disorders* (4th ed.). Washington, DC: Author.

Dionne, R., Phero, J., & Becker, D. (2002). *Management of pain and anxiety in the dental office* (Chapters 1, 5). Philadelphia: Saunders.

Fiset, L., Milgrom, P., & Weinstein, P. (1985). Psychophysiological Responses to Dental Injections. *Journal of the American Dental Association, III,* 578–583.

Howard, M. (2007). *Chronic Pain, Institute for Natural Resources Educational Program.* Seattle, WA.

International Association for the Study of Pain; www.iasp-pain.org.

Naini, F. B., Mellow, A. C., & Getz, T. (1999). Treatment of dental fears: Pharmacology or psychology? *Dental Update, 26,* 270–276.

Pappagallo, M., & Chapman, C. R. (2005). *The neurological basis of pain* (Chapters 1, 11). New York: McGraw-Hill.

Spitzer, D. (2004). *Gender and sex-based analysis in health research: A guide for CIHR peer review committee, final report.* Canadian Institutes of Health Research; http://www.cihr-irsc.gc.ca/e/25131.html.

Taber's Cyclopedic Medical Dictionary (1997). Philadelphia: F.A. Davis.

Milgrom, P., Weinstein, P., & Getz, T. (1995). *Treating fearful dental patients: A patient management handbook.* Reston, VA.

Chapter 3

The Neuroanatomy and Neurophysiology of Pain Control

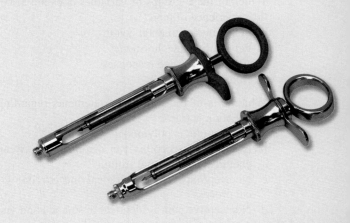

OBJECTIVES

- Define and discuss the key terms in this chapter.
- Explain the normal mechanisms of nerve impulse generation and conduction.
- Define the events in successful nerve impulse generation, including the *resting state, slow depolarization, firing threshold, rapid depolarization,* and *recovery.*
- Describe and explain the significance of Schwann cell sheaths and nodes of Ranvier on the ability of local anesthetic agents to work.
- Describe the significance of the anatomical differences between sensory and motor neurons.
- Identify and discuss the different types of nerve fibers, the differences in how they relate to pain perception, and be familiar with those that normally transmit pain sensations from dental and periodontal structures.
- Differentiate anatomically and functionally between myelinated and unmyelinated nerves.
- Discuss what is meant by *anatomic barriers to the diffusion of anesthetic solutions* and those that present the greatest challenges to diffusion.
- Define the term *dental plexus* and describe where these structures are located.
- Discuss the actions and effects of local anesthetic drugs on neural membranes.

KEY TERMS

absolute refractory **28**
action potential **24**
axon **19**
axolemmas **21**
axoplasm **25**
cell body **19**
concentration
  gradient **28**
core bundles **24**
dendritic zone **19**
dental neural
  plexus **24**
depolarize **30**
durable blockade **32**
electrical potential **25**
endoneurium **23**
epineural sheath **24**

epineurium **23**
extracellular **25**
fasciculi **23**
firing threshold **27**
ganglia **19**
hydrophilic **20**
impulses **19**
impulse extinction **32**
intracellular **25**
ion channels **25**
lipophilic **20**
local anesthesia **33**
motor nerves **33**
myelinated **21**
nerve fibers **21**
neurolemma **20**

INTRODUCTION

Reliable patient comfort is essential to successful therapy in dentistry. The absence of effective pain control on the other hand may frustrate and compromise effective treatment. Successful pain control outcomes may be defined as those in which profound local anesthesia is achieved in a safe manner. These outcomes are not only dependent on a thorough knowledge of the pharmacological actions of local anesthetic drugs but also on the neurophysiology of sensory and motor nerves.

The mechanisms of the normal generation and conduction of pain signals to the central nervous system (CNS) will be discussed in this chapter as a foundation for understanding the effects of local anesthetic drugs upon them. In addition, it is important to understand the anatomy and physiology of nerves prior to administering local anesthetics (Daniel, Harfst, & Wilder, 2008).

NEUROANATOMY

Understanding the mechanisms involved in peripheral nerve anesthesia requires a sound knowledge of anatomy (Jastak, Yigiela, & Donaldson, 1995; Seeley, Tate, & Stephens, 2008). It has been suggested that the most important aspect of delivering profound and reliable local anesthesia comes from a solid understanding of neuroanatomy (Blanton & Jeske, 2003).

Nerve Cell Anatomy

Nerve cells, called **neurons,** are the basic units of nerves. All neurons have four structural areas, their **dendritic zones, axons, cell bodies,** and **terminal arborizations** (see Figure 3–1 ■). While similar in some respects, sensory and motor neurons differ in both structure and function. A primary distinction is that sensory neurons carry in-coming signals, referred to as **impulses,** from the body to the CNS for processing while motor neurons carry impulses away from the CNS to effector cells, tissues, and organs.

Nerve impulses are initiated in dendritic zones of sensory neurons in response to stimulation of tissue. The terminal zones of nerve axons, known as junctions, or **synapses,** contain numerous organelles. These organelles, when stimulated by impulses, release neurotransmitters that convey information to excitable tissues, including other neurons. In the terminal arborization zones of sensory neurons, impulses or signals are transmitted to processing nuclei called **ganglia.**

Nerve Axons, Cell Bodies, and Membranes

Following their initiation, impulses travel along axons, the processes or fibers of individual nerve cells that transmit signals to the central nervous system. Neuronal processes may span considerable lengths. In the case of sensory nerves that innervate oral tissues, all cell bodies are located within trigeminal ganglia.

Regardless of the type of neuron, sensory or motor, the cell body provides metabolic support. In motor neurons, the cell body is closely associated with the axon and conducts nerve impulses. In sensory neurons, the cell bodies are farther away from the axon and do not participate in impulse transmission (see Figure 3–1).

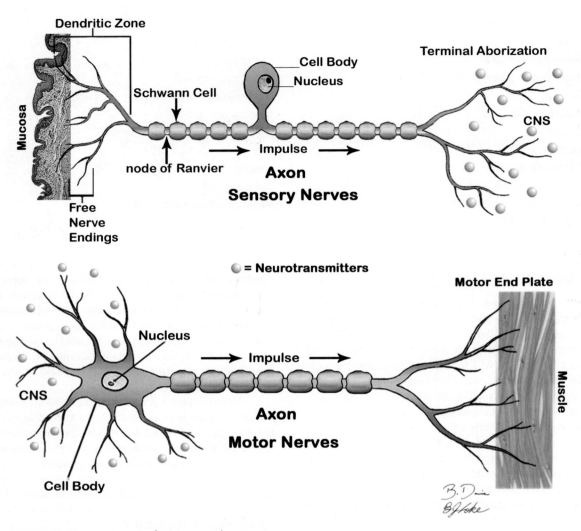

■ **FIGURE 3–1**   Anatomy of Sensory and Motor Neurons.

Nerve membranes, called **neurolemmas,** are bilayered phospholipid membranes. The function of a bilayered membrane is to act as a barrier. Lipid membranes are composed of phospholipids having both **lipophilic** ("fat-loving") and **hydrophilic** ("water-loving") ends. The membranes are held together by the attraction of the lipophilic ends at their centers.

The hydrophilic ends face outward along a membrane and the lipophilic ends face inward to create a fatty core at the center (see Figure 3–2 ■). This fatty core allows small lipophilic molecules, such as local anesthetic molecules called neutral bases, to pass through freely, while water soluble substances, such as sodium

ions, are able to pass through the membrane only by means of designated channels (Disalvo & Simon, 1995). Other hydrophilic local anesthetic molecules, known as cations, are unable to pass through either the membranes or their channels. These lipophilic and hydrophilic local anesthetic molecules will be explained in more detail in Chapter 4, "Pharmacology Basics."

Nerve Myelination

Nerves are classified as *myelinated* or *nonmyelinated* according to the extent of the connective tissue (myelin) enclosing them (see Box 3–1). **Schwann cells,**

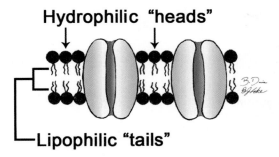

■ **FIGURE 3–2** Anatomy of Neurolemma Hydrophilic and Lipophilic Components of Nerve Membranes.

which produce myelin, are specialized connective tissue cells that surround and protect peripheral nerves (cells that perform this function in the central nervous system are known as *oligodendrocytes*). By producing myelin and forming extensive myelin sheaths around axons, Schwann cells insulate and protect nerve membranes from their surrounding environments. Axons and their associated Schwann cells are collectively referred to as **nerve fibers** (Pogrel, Schmidt, Sambajon, & Jordan, 2003).

Box 3–1   Myelination

Myelin is a protective covering for nerves. It is approximately 80 percent lipid, 20 percent protein, and a very minor percentage carbohydrate in nature (Bennett, 1978). Myelin is responsible for what is known as the "white" matter of the brain and has a primary function of providing electrical insulation to nerves to increase their conduction efficiency, much as the insulation around electrical wires increases their efficiency.

In addition to providing insulation, Schwann cells isolate neurons from changes in their environment, minimizing exposure to injury and, in the event of injury, facilitating healing. While these protective features are important to proper nerve function and health, they are also responsible for significant obstacles to the diffusion of local anesthetic solutions. These solutions cannot diffuse through myelinated nerves except in the areas where they come into direct contact with the membrane at the nodes of Ranvier.

Box 3–2   Demyelination and Disease

In certain diseases, such as multiple sclerosis (MS), signs and symptoms are thought to be a result of an unexplained demyelination of oligodendrocytes that occurs in certain locations in the central nervous system. Without their myelin protection, these nerves cannot function or heal properly, typically transmitting impulses at greatly reduced speeds (*The Merck Manual of Diagnosis and Therapy,* 2006).

Nonmyelinated neurons, also known as unmyelinated neurons, have thin or single layers of Schwann cells covering them. **Myelinated** neurons are enclosed by multiple spiral layers of Schwann cells. These spiral layers wrap around myelinated neurons as many as 300 times creating what is known as a **Schwann cell sheath** providing some of the most efficient cellular protection in the body (Jastak et al., 1995; Tetzlaff, 2000). Nonmyelinated nerves are less isolated from extracellular environments. They are more vulnerable to injury and less able to heal if injured (see Box 3–2).

In myelinated nerves, there are minute gaps consisting of unprotected nerve membranes between adjacent Schwann cells called **nodes of Ranvier** (see Figure 3–3 ■). The outer membrane of a neuron underlying its sheath is referred to as its **axolemma** or neurolemma.

Saltatory Conduction

Nerve impulses in nonmyelinated nerves, which actually do have very thin myelin sheaths, are described as "creeping" along their membranes. While by no means a slow process, this requires activity over the entire surface of the membrane of the axon from the point of stimulation to the point of registration in the central nervous system. The incremental passage of impulses can be visualized as multiple rows of falling dominos, each transferring its energy to the next in order to propagate the impulse (Figure 3–4 ■).

Saltatory conduction refers to the process whereby impulses are more rapidly conducted along myelinated nerves (Jastak et al., 1995; Narhi, Yamamoto, Ngassapa, & Hirvonen, 1994; Seeley et al., 2008). In saltatory conduction, impulses have been characterized as "jumping" over Schwann cells from one node of Ranvier to another, at times having enough energy to

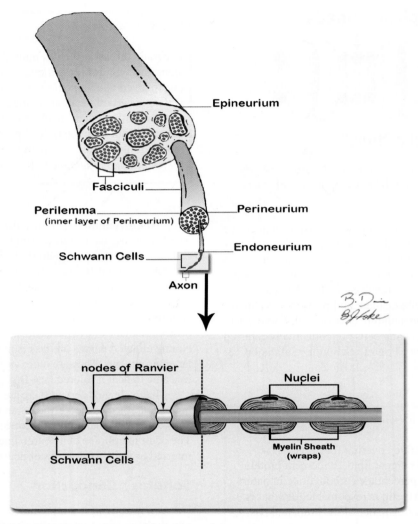

■ FIGURE 3–3   Anatomy of Myelinated Axons.

jump over several nodes at once. While skipping nodes has been demonstrated, particularly in larger, more heavily myelinated nerves, the impulses do not accomplish this by actually "jumping" over Schwann cells. Instead, they have enough energy to travel through one or more internode region (the portion of an axon covered by a Schwann cell) before another impulse is generated. With increasing degrees of myelination there is often enough energy to bypass the next node and travel directly to a subsequent node (up to 8–10 mm) increasing conduction speeds (Malamed, 2004). In general, larger, more heavily myeli-nated nerves transmit impulses more rapidly than smaller, nonmyelinated nerves (see Figure 3–4 ■).

Nerve Fiber Types

Nerve fibers are typed as A, B, or C, with numerous subcategories falling within these classifications (see Table 3–1 ■). By far the most numerous fiber type of the peripheral nervous system is the C fiber. C fibers, which are nonmyelinated, conduct more slowly, providing the sensation of dull and aching pain. Some A fibers, known as A *delta* fibers (Aδ), are lightly myelinated and bear primary responsibility for the experience of sharp pain. Note the difference in Table 3–1 between the conduction speeds of the Aδ fibers, which convey sharp, stabbing pain information rapidly, versus the C fibers, which

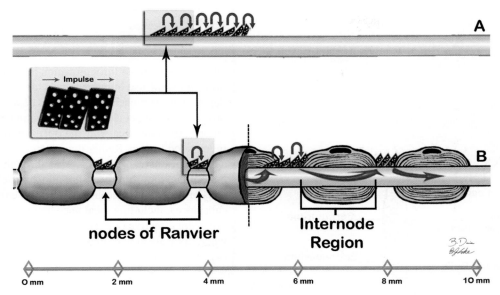

FIGURE 3–4   Impulse Conduction and nodes of Ranvier.
A–Nonmyelinated nerve; B–Myelinated nerve

Table 3–1	Nerve Fiber Types		
Fiber Type	**Function**	**Diameter (mu)**	**Conduction Velocity (meters/second = m/s)**
Aα	Proprioception, body movements	12–20	100
Aβ	Touch, pressure	5–12	30–70
Aγ	Motor to stretch receptors	3–6	15–30
Aδ	*Pain, especially cold, touch*	*2–5*	*12–30*
B	Preganglionic autonomic	<3	3–15
C	*Thermal pain, tension, pressure, displacement receptors*	*0.4–1.2*	*0.5–2*
C	Postganglionic autonomic	0.3–1.3	0.7–2.3

Source: Current Concepts in the Assessment and Treatment of Breakthrough Pain, Gary H. Wright, MD (www.medscape.com).

convey dull, aching information slowly. Both A and C fibers have been found in dental pulps with a greater distribution of C fibers than A (Narhi et al., 1994; Pashley, 1990; Seeley et al., 2008).

Peripheral Nerve Anatomy

Peripheral nerves are made up of many axons that are bundled, protected, and provided with metabolic support by layers of connective tissue. The anatomy from the deep to the superficial aspect of a peripheral nerve starts with individual nerve fibers separated from one another by an **endoneurium,** a structure that insulates the electrical activity of individual nerve fibers (see Figure 3–5 ■). The **perineurium** bundles these fibers into what are known as **fasciculi.** The inner layer of the perineurium is referred to as its **perilemma.** A very loose connective tissue layer, the **epineurium,** surrounds all of the fasciculi, their associated supporting connective tissue including blood vessels and lymphatics, and the perineuria. The

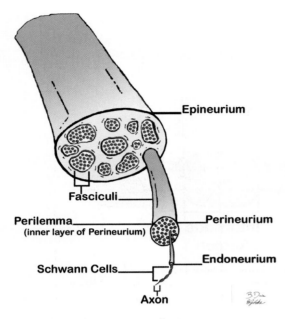

■ **FIGURE 3–5**   Anatomy of a Neuron.

epineurium has its own sheath on its superficial circumference that surrounds the entire nerve called the **epineural sheath.** Of these layers, the two most significant barriers to the diffusion of anesthetic solutions and the development of anesthesia are (in order) the perilemma and the perineurium (see Box 3–3). The larger the nerve, the greater the significance of these barriers (Jastak et al., 1995; Noback & Demarest, 1981).

   The outer region of a nerve is referred to as its mantle and the central region is its core. Fasciculi located in the mantle region are called **mantle bundles.** The fasciculi in the central region are referred to as **core bundles.** The arrangement of bundles into outer (mantle) and inner (core) segments in larger nerves has an impact on the order in which anesthesia develops when exposed to local anesthetic drugs (see Figure 3–6 ■). The significance of core and mantle bundles on local anesthesia will be discussed later in this chapter.

Dental Neural Plexus

A **dental neural plexus** is an interwoven, interconnecting network of nerves supplying the teeth and their supporting structures (Bennett, 1978) (see Figure 3–7 ■). The superior (maxillary) dental plexus derives from terminal branches of the second division of the trigeminal nerve and includes dental, interdental, and interradicular divisions. The inferior (mandibular) dental plexus derives from terminal branches of the third division of the trigeminal nerve. These extensive networks of nerves innervate the maxillary and mandibular teeth and their supporting structures.

NEUROPHYSIOLOGY

Nerve impulses are electrical in nature and depend entirely upon changes in ionic activity along nerve membranes for their generation and conduction. Specific thresholds must be achieved before transmission of impulses to the CNS occurs. In **sensory nerves,** energy from an impulse is duplicated and transferred to succeeding impulses along the axon in the direction of the CNS. These successive impulses are identical in size and nature to the original impulses (also known as **action potentials**). Impulses do not lose any of their strength in the transfer of energy from one section of membrane to the next; in fact, it has been demonstrated that the current flow at successive areas of nerve membranes actually exceeds that which is necessary to fire nerve impulses (Malamed, 2004). The process of sequential impulse generation to the processing areas in the CNS (ganglia and relevant centers in the brain) is referred to as **propagation.**

   When a nerve is receiving little to no stimulation its membrane is said to be in a **resting state.** In reality, nerves respond to some degree of stimulation almost

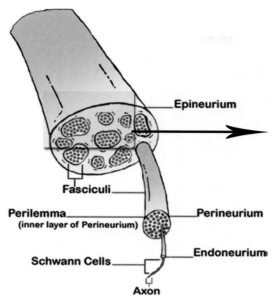

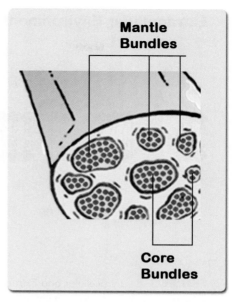

■ **FIGURE 3–6**   Mantle and Core Bundles.

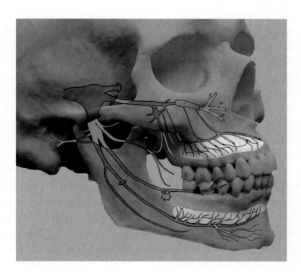

■ **FIGURE 3–7**   Dental Neural Plexus.

constantly and seldom if ever rest even when providing little more than sensory feedback (Jastak et al., 1995). This is accomplished by ion exchange through nerve membranes via designated pathways or **ion channels**

through which ions selectively pass on a continuous basis (Tetzlaff, 2000).

The inner environment of a nerve is known as its **intracellular** environment or **axoplasm,** while the outer environment is designated the **extracellular** environment (see Figure 3–8 ■). The axoplasm of a nerve at rest is maintained in an electrically negative state relative to the more positively charged extracellular environment. It has been determined that the resting state of the axoplasm averages −70 mV (millivolts). This resting state **electrical potential** represents the difference in the electrical charge across the membrane. An imbalance of electrolytes on either side of the membrane, primarily sodium (Na^+) and potassium (K^+) ions, is responsible for this difference.

GENERATION AND CONDUCTION OF NERVE IMPULSES

The generation and conduction of nerve impulses occur over a series of phases or "states." In the resting state, gates in the Na^+ ion channels remain closed. This prevents significant influx of Na^+ ions, either via

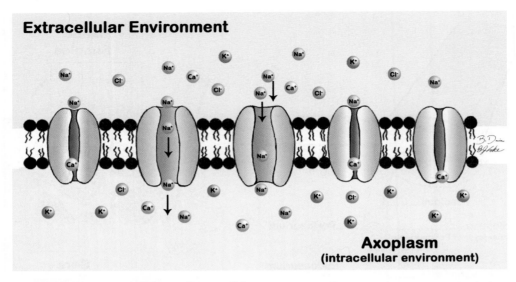

Extracellular Environment

Axoplasm
(intracellular environment)

■ **FIGURE 3–8** Intracellular and Extracellular Environment of Nerve. In response to stimulation, Ca^{+2} ions are released. Na^+ ion channels open, allowing Na^+ influx into the axoplasm.

sodium ion pumps or along their concentration gradient or electrical attraction.

In response to stimulation, Ca^{+2} ions release and open the channels to Na^+ ion influx into the axoplasm, slowly at first. Once there are sufficient Na^+ ions in the axoplasm to reduce the electrical potential by approximately 15–20 mV, the firing threshold for impulse generation is reached and Na^+ ions flood the axoplasm. In sensory nerves, successive impulses propagate to processing centers in the CNS.

Upon successful impulse propagation to an adjacent site, the previous site is known as refractory or unresponsive and is unable to generate an impulse. This pattern continues along the length of the membrane, which forces all subsequent impulses to be generated in one direction only. While the impulses that are propagated toward the CNS eventually prompt efferent responses, impulses are also generated from sites of stimulation in a direction away from the CNS. Unlike the impulses propagated in the direction of the CNS, these impulses extinguish once they arrive at peripheral destinations that have no ability to respond. Since the refractory period lasts only about one millisecond, the membrane in the area may be stimulated again quickly.

These stages are discussed in more detail in the next section and are presented as a group in Appendix 3–1.

Resting State

The electrical potential of nerve axoplasm in the resting state is approximately −70 mV, although the range can extend from −40 to −95 mV for some cells (Jastak et al., 1995). This potential is maintained relative to the extracellular environment primarily by Na^+ and K^+ ions, which can enter the axoplasm only through selective channels in the nerve membrane called ion channels (see Figure 3–9 ■). Chloride ions participate in a more minor way by concentrating in the extracellular fluid with the sodium ions, helping to maintain the resting membrane potential.

Ion channels are closed or *gated* by Ca^{+2} ions binding to **specific protein receptor sites** within the channels in the resting state (see Box 3–4). There are numerous electrolytes in both intra- and extra-cellular environments of nerve membranes. An imbalance is the result of differences in the concentrations of these electrolytes, primarily Na^+ and K^+ ions on either side of the membrane. Na^+ ions are small enough to pass freely through ion channels; however, due to Na^+ high affinity for water, the majority of the Na^+ ions hydrate and are too large to pass through. Even though somewhat larger than Na^+ ions, K^+ ions have a lower affinity for water and the majority easily pass through the

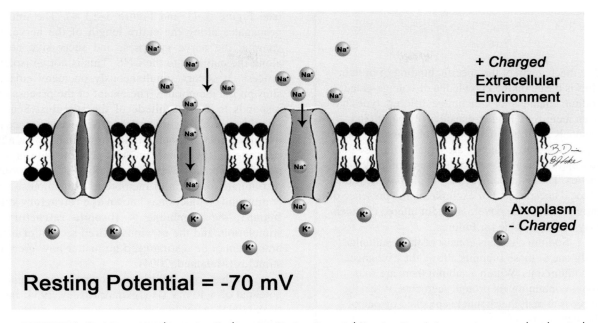

Resting Potential = -70 mV

■ **FIGURE 3–9**   Nerve Membrane Ion Exchange—Resting Potential (Resting State). In a resting state, the electrical potential of nerve axoplasm is approximately −70 mV. This potential is maintained primarily by K⁺ and Na⁺ ions.

channels unhydrated. The negative electrical charge of the axoplasm, however, prevents potassium ions from leaving the axoplasm in significant numbers despite their smaller size and the substantially larger numbers of K^+ ions in the axoplasm. The net result is an excess of extracellular Na^+ and an excess of intracellular K^+. Along with the contribution of Cl^-, this ionic imbalance maintains the resting electrical potential of nerves.

It is the imbalance between K^+ and Na^+ ions on either side of a membrane that largely accounts for the uninterrupted maintenance of the resting potential. This is aided by protein pumps in the membrane, which actively pump ions both in and out of the axoplasm against resistance. If undisturbed, the resting state ionic imbalance will continue indefinitely.

Slow Depolarization and Firing Thresholds

Once a nerve is stimulated, the ion channels respond by opening their gates (Jastak et al., 1995). This is accomplished by the release of calcium (Ca^{+2}) ions from receptor sites on the gates (Malamed, 2004). Ca^{+2} ions may be thought of as the gatekeepers of the resting state. Once the gates are open, the channels are now wide enough for the positively charged and hydrated Na^+ ions to enter the negatively charged axoplasm. **Slow depolarization** occurs until the axoplasm has depolarized approximately 15 to 20 mV, from −70 to somewhere between −55 to −50 mV, which is the threshold for impulse generation. This is known as the nerve's **firing threshold** (see Figure 3–10 ■ and Figure 3–11 ■).

As long as this threshold is not achieved, the nerve is said to be slowly depolarizing and no impulses will be generated. If stimulation proves insufficient to depolarize a membrane, no impulse will be generated (see Figure 3–12 ■).

An example of "failure of impulse generation" occurs when someone tries to tickle an individual's ear with a feather. If the action is insufficient to gain the individual's attention, the nerve is not receiving a strong enough stimulation to raise the threshold to conduct an impulse to the CNS. In this case, this is insufficient Na^+ ion influx to depolarize the membrane 15 to 20 mV to its firing threshold (see Figure 3–12).

Box 3–4   Specific Protein Binding Theory Mechanism

The mechanism of the specific binding of protein sites is based on the knowledge of voltage-gated sodium channels, of which nine different types have been identified. Higher densities of sodium ion channels are found in the nodes of Ranvier. Not all types of sodium channels are equal. Some are more susceptible than others to the actions of local anesthetics. These differences may explain some failures of local anesthesia. For example, in the presence of inflammation, the development of altered channels may be responsible for failures.

Sodium channels consist of three subunits. Only one of these subunits allows the exchange of sodium ions. Within a subunit there are four zones containing six protein segments. When the nerve is at rest, the channel is blocked by one of these proteins.

Once the threshold is reached, rapid depolarization begins and sodium ions flood the channel. During this phase, these protein segments twist into the body of the pore by an action known as a "sliding helix."

After depolarization, when the refractory phase begins, a protein loop extends into the channel and continues to block sodium ion entry. Local anesthetics further block the entry of sodium ions by maintaining the position of the protein loop in the channel during the refractory phase.

Understanding this mechanism and identifying the nature of the binding sites may lead to the development of drugs that target critical sodium channel pathways as well as drugs that are able to function better in the presence of inflammation. It may also reduce the unwanted effects of the current local anesthetic drugs.

Source: Beers & Berkow, 1999; Tetzlaff, 2000.

Rapid Depolarization

Once the firing threshold has been achieved, the nerve quickly depolarizes at the site of stimulation due to the flood of positively charged Na^+ ions into its axoplasm in a process known as **rapid depolarization**

(see Figure 3–11 and Figure 3–13 ■). The impulse propagates along the entire length of the nerve, the ganglia, the nerve synapses, and successive nerves along the pathway to the CNS. This is not an isolated process. It occurs simultaneously on many adjacent sites on the membrane. The extent of the process corresponds to the magnitude of the stimulus. Sensory impulses travel only toward the CNS, because once the impulse or action potential has transferred to an adjacent site on the membrane, the previous site is temporarily unresponsive. The inability to successfully restimulate a section of membrane after impulse generation and conduction is known as a **refractory state.** Initially, the membrane is **absolute refractory** to stimulation, and the previously fired section of membrane cannot be restimulated no matter how great the stimulus (Malamed, 2004).

At this point, the nerve axoplasm has attained a potential of +40 mV (Hodgkin & Husley, 1954; Jastak et al., 1995). After impulse generation and conduction, additional Na^+ ion influx is prevented. Instead, Na^+ ions are actively transported out by **sodium ion pumps,** which enhance the outward movement of Na^+ ions now in greater excess in the axoplasm along their **concentration gradient.** This is also facilitated by the vigorous extracellular movement of Na^+ due to repulsive forces of the now positively charged axoplasm. As ions are transported or move out, the axoplasm returns closer to its resting state of −70 mV.

During this return to the resting state but prior to its complete reestablishment, stimulation may once again be successful. With the resting state only partially attained, a larger stimulus is required to achieve a successful firing. This is known as the **relative refractory state.**

Repolarization

Once a nerve has attained a potential of approximately +40 mV, the process begins to reverse. The reversal of ion concentrations in this recovery phase is called **repolarization.** The axoplasm has an excess of positive charge and an excess concentration of Na^+ ions. As previously stated, Na^+ ions exit the nerve by passive diffusion through the ion channels along their concentration gradient, by repulsion due to the positive electrical charge of the axoplasm, and through active transport of the Na^+ ion pumps. As the passive forces of Na^+ ion movement out of the axoplasm weaken, further movement is assisted by the ion pumps which continue to remove Na^+ and K^+ ions until a potential of −70 mV is

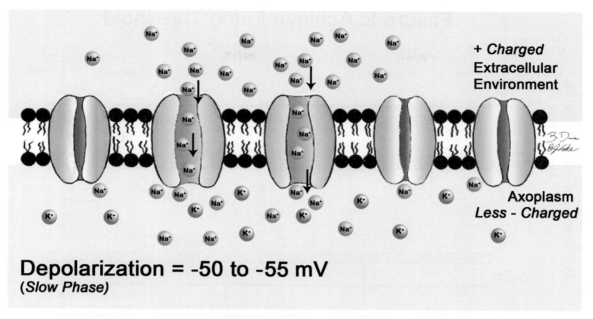

Depolarization = -50 to -55 mV
(Slow Phase)

■ **FIGURE 3–10**   Nerve Membrane Ion Exchange—Depolarization (Slow Phase). Once a nerve is stimulated, the ion channels open their gates in response to the release of calcium (Ca^{+2}) ions. Slow depolarization occurs until the axoplasm has depolarized, approximately 15 to 20 mV, to -50 to -55 mV (firing threshold).

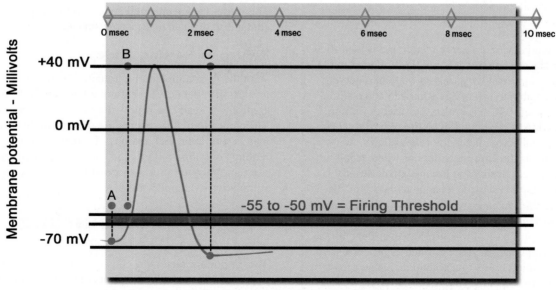

■ **FIGURE 3–11**   Impulse Generation Firing Threshold. The firing threshold is reached once the axoplasm has depolarized to -50 to -55 mV.

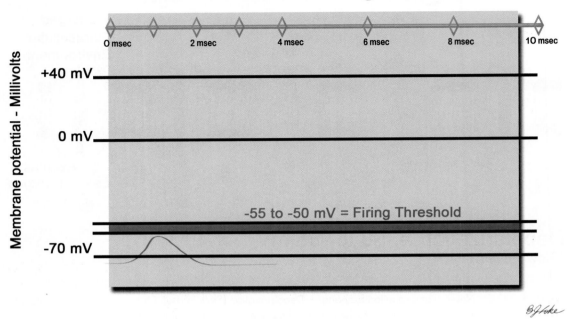

Failure to Achieve Firing Threshold

-55 to -50 mV = Firing Threshold

■ **FIGURE 3–12** Impulse Generation Failure. When Na$^+$ ion influx is not sufficient to depolarize the membrane 15 to 20 mV, no impulse is generated.

Box 3–5 **Depolarization
and Repolarization—
A Terminology Discussion**

The potential across a nerve membrane is identified as **polarized** whenever it is not 0 mV. For example, the normal physiological resting state of a nerve averaging about −70 mV is polarized and a stimulated state of +40 mV is also, by strict definition, polarized. A nerve is said to be **depolarized** when the potential across the membrane is 0 mV.

This is the case regardless of whether it is becoming less positive or less negative. Strictly speaking for a nerve, any change toward 0 mV is a *depolarization* and any change away from 0 mV is a *polarization*.

For purposes of this text however depolarization and repolarization are defined as processes. Depolarization refers to a potential change across the membrane from −70 mV to +40 mV. Repolarization refers to a return to a resting state from +40 mV to −70 mV.

reestablished. Na$^+$ ion movement is then limited to resting state levels by the rebinding of Ca^{+2} ions to receptor sites. This closes the ion channels and assures that Na$^+$ will not continue to depolarize the axoplasm (see Figure 3–14 ■).

Return to Resting State

With the re-attainment of a potential between −60 mV to −90 mV, the nerve membrane has now fully recovered and is ready to repeat the process when another sufficient stimulation occurs. As described, this process may seem long and tedious. In reality, however, it requires only one millisecond for a nerve membrane to react and recover after a successful impulse-generating stimulation (Malamed, 2004).

ACTIONS OF LOCAL ANESTHETICS ON NERVE IMPULSES

Two important factors to consider when discussing the impact of local anesthetics on nerve impulses are the interruptions of those impulses (impulse extinction) and the diminishing effects of the drugs on the nerve bundles (core and mantle bundles).

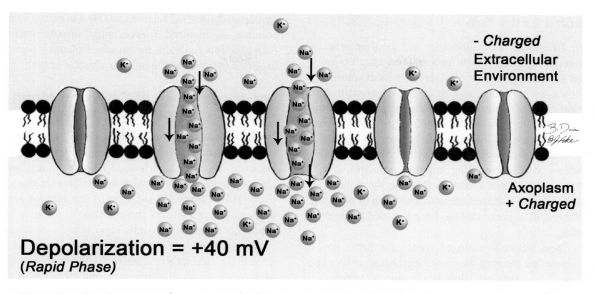

Depolarization = +40 mV
(Rapid Phase)

■ **FIGURE 3–13** Nerve Membrane Ion Exchange—Depolarization (Rapid Phase). Once enough Na⁺ ions have flooded the axoplasm, the firing threshold is achieved and the nerve quickly depolarizes, generating an impulse.

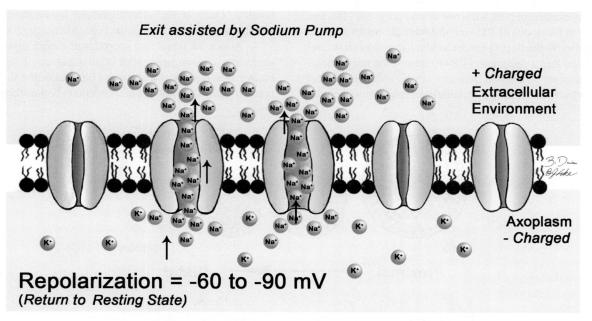

Repolarization = -60 to -90 mV
(Return to Resting State)

■ **FIGURE 3–14** Nerve Membrane Ion Exchange—Repolarization (Return to Resting State). The reversal of ion concentrations in this recovery phase is called repolarization. Once a nerve has attained a potential of approximately +40 mV, Na⁺ ions exit the nerve by passive diffusion through ion channels and through active transport of Na⁺ ion pumps. This phase is complete when the potential returns between −60 mV to −90 mV.

Impulse Extinction

When discussing nerve impulses and local anesthesia, the likelihood that impulse propagation may be interrupted at a particular area of a nerve by local anesthesia is known as nontransmission, or **impulse extinction** (Tetzlaff, 2000). This is somewhat analogous to crimping a hose to stop the flow of water (extinction); uncrimping the hose will reestablish the flow (propagation). Local anesthesia is a deliberate method to achieve impulse extinction. When discussing impulse extinction due to local anesthetics, it is directly related to the volume of local anesthetic delivered, the concentration of the drug, and the length of nerve that has been exposed to the drug (Tetzlaff, 2000).

Upon administration of local anesthetic drugs, Na^+ ion influx through the nerve membrane is blocked and sodium-dependent depolarization is prevented. Both the generation and conduction of nerve impulses can be inhibited by local anesthetic drugs. Decreased responsiveness to stimuli and the failure to transmit an impulse toward the CNS are direct consequences of impulse extinction due to local anesthetic drugs.

Impulse extinction is also related to the presence or absence of myelin (Tetzlaff, 2000). As previously noted, in myelinated nerves, local anesthetic drugs are effective only at the nodes of Ranvier and multiple nodes must be exposed to the drugs in order to block impulses. It is considered that a minimum of 8–10 mm of the nerve membrane must be flooded by an anesthetic solution in order to achieve anesthesia particularly in larger more heavily myelinated nerves (Malamed, 2004). Greater volumes of solution are required to accomplish impulse extinction (**durable blockade**) in the presence of these nerves, an example of which is the inferior alveolar nerve.

The Significance of Core and Mantle Bundles on Local Anesthesia

Nerve fibers housed in mantle (outer) bundles tend to innervate structures in close proximity to them (see Figure 3–15 ■). Fibers housed in core (inner) bundles tend to innervate structures at some distance away from them. For example, in the case of the inferior alveolar nerve at a location near the entrance to the mandibular canal, fibers from the mantle layer tend to innervate the molar region while fibers from the core layer tend to innervate the anterior mandible including the chin and lips. Molar regions anesthetize earlier and more easily in this example, while the lips, chin, and anterior dentition and supporting structures anesthetize later and with more difficulty. This is due to the fact that anesthetic solution reaches the core only after the solution has penetrated through the mantle layer. It takes longer to reach the core and the solution does so in a diluted form due to the binding of drug molecules to receptor sites in the mantle bundles. Once at the core, there are fewer molecules remaining to bind to sites in the core (Malamed, 2004).

A lack of labial and mental soft tissue signs and symptoms of anesthesia after administration of what is known as an inferior alveolar nerve block indicates that the core bundles have not yet been adequately anesthetized.

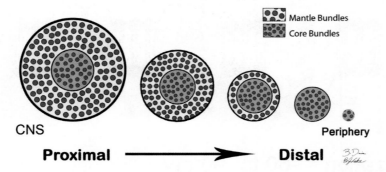

■ **FIGURE 3–15** Distribution of Core and Mantle Bundles. Mantle bundle fibers in a particular location tend to innervate structures in close proximity. Core bundle fibers in that same location tend to innervate structures peripheral to the location. In the example of the inferior alveolar nerve, posterior teeth are innervated by mantle fibers. This results in the molars being anesthetized earlier and more easily than anteriors.

While the absence of signs and symptoms of anesthesia is a good indication that profound anesthesia has not been achieved, the presence of these signs and symptoms is not necessarily a guarantee of profound anesthesia. The lack of profound anesthesia may be due to incomplete penetration of the local anesthetic drug to the deepest core bundles (pulpal fibers tend to be more centrally located) and to accessory innervation (see Chapter 16, "Troubleshooting Inadequate Anesthesia").

INTRODUCTION TO LOCAL ANESTHESIA

Local anesthesia may be defined as a temporary loss of sensation in a specific, usually small area of the body (Malamed, 2004). A primary distinction between local and general anesthesia is that when local anesthesia alone is in effect, patients remain conscious (Daniel et al., 2008).

This distinction is important when procedures are to be performed while a patient is under the influence of sedation or general anesthesia, because in the absence of specific procedures to anesthetize local tissues no local anesthesia exists. For example, a third molar extraction under general anesthesia is typically performed after the administration of local anesthesia. It is important to add that, in the majority of dental procedures, sedation and general anesthesia are seldom necessary in order to achieve good pain control outcomes.

Local anesthesia can be induced by various methods. The applications of pressure, cold, electrical stimulation, and trauma have the potential to cause temporary losses of sensation. While not commonly thought of as local anesthetics, some of these alternatives to injectable drugs are frequently utilized in medicine. In dentistry, combinations of commercial preparations of topical and injectable local anesthetic drugs are more commonly used when discomfort is anticipated. This is accomplished by anesthetizing specific teeth and tissues without anesthetizing all of the teeth and all of the tissues. It is important to note that even when all of the teeth and their surrounding tissues are anesthetized, the anesthesia is still described as local.

Local Anesthetic Drugs and How They Work

Local anesthetic drugs all work similarly. Local anesthetic molecules have a greater affinity for protein receptor sites within the nerve membrane compared to Ca^{+2} ions and subsequently displace them. Different local anesthetic drugs have varying affinities for these receptor sites, which account for clinically significant differences in drug action. One drug, for example, bupivacaine, aggressively bonds to the receptor sites resulting in the longest duration of action of all local anesthetic drugs in current use in dentistry today (Danielsson et al., 1986; Fawcett, Kennedy, Kimar, & Ledger, 2002; Moore & Dunsky, 1983).

Local anesthetic drugs are effective on both sensory and **motor nerves.** They typically anesthetize smaller nerves before larger nerves and sensory nerves before motor nerves (Jastak et al., 1995). While the desired effects of these drugs are localized, their inevitable systemic absorption exposes other tissues to their potentially toxic actions, including the central nervous system (CNS), the cardiovascular system (CVS), and skeletal muscle (Basson & Carlson, 1980; Dudkiewicz, Schwartz, & Laliberte, 1987). All of the currently available injectable dental local anesthetics interrupt the transmission of nerve impulses. The five local anesthetic drugs packaged for injection in dentistry today include articaine, bupivacaine, lidocaine, mepivacaine, and prilocaine.

CHAPTER QUESTIONS

1. Which of the following statements most accurately describe(s) the major differences between sensory and motor neurons?
   1. Sensory neurons are afferent and conduct impulses toward the CNS.
   2. Motor neurons are efferent and conduct impulses to effector tissues and organs.
   3. Sensory neuronal cell bodies do not participate in impulse conduction and they are located away from the axon.
   4. Motor neuronal cell bodies participate in impulse conduction and are located along the length of the neuron at their terminal arborizations.
      a. 3 only
      b. 1 and 2
      c. 1, 3, and 4
      d. All of the above

2. Which of the following sequences best describes the events in a successful impulse generation?
   a. Stimulation, slow depolarization, firing threshold, rapid depolarization, recovery
   b. Stimulation, firing threshold, rapid depolarization, slow repolarization, resting state
   c. Resting state, stimulation, slow depolarization, rapid depolarization, firing threshold
   d. Resting state, stimulation, slow depolarization, rapid depolarization, slow depolarization

3. How are Schwann cells and nodes of Ranvier related?
   a. Schwann cells are nodes of Ranvier.
   b. At the nodes of Ranvier, Schwann cells are one layer thick.
   c. Gaps between Schwann cells are called nodes of Ranvier.
   d. They are not related.

4. Which fiber types are responsible for providing sensory information from dental and periodontal tissues?
   a. C and B fibers
   b. B and A delta fibers
   c. Gamma and C fibers
   d. A delta and C fibers

5. Which of the fibers in question #4 are myelinated?
   a. Both A delta and C fibers
   b. Both B fibers and C fibers
   c. A fibers
   d. None of the above

6. What are three divisions of the dental plexus?
   a. Interdental, interradicular, and periodontal
   b. Inner dental, interradicular, and dental
   c. Interdental, interradicular, and dental
   d. Inner dental, interradicular, and periodontal

REFERENCES

Basson, M. D., & Carlson, B. M. (1980). Myotoxicity of single and repeated injections of mepivacaine in the rat. *Anesthesia & Analgesia, 59,* 275–282.

Beers, M. H., & Berkow, R. (1999). [The] *Merck Manual of Diagnosis and Therapy* (17th ed., pp. 1474–1477). Hoboken, NJ: John Wiley & Sons.

Bennett, C. R. (1978). *Monheim's local anesthesia and pain control in dental practice* (6th ed.). St. Louis: Mosby.

Blanton, P. L., & Jeske, A. H. (2003, June). The key to profound local anesthesia, neuroanatomy. *Journal of the American Dental Association [JADA],* 753–760.

Daniel, S. J., Harfst, S. A., & Wilder, R. S. (2008). *Mosby's dental hygiene: Concepts, cases, and competencies* (2nd ed.). St. Louis: Mosby.

Danielsson, K., Evers, H., Holmlund, A., Kjellman, O., Nordenram, A., & Persson, N. E. (1986). Long-acting local anaesthetics in oral surgery. *International Journal of Oral and Maxillofacial Surgery, 15,* 119–126.

Disalvo, E. A., Simon, S. A. (1995). Permeability and stability of lipid bilayers. Boca Raton, FL: CRC Press.

Dudkiewicz, A., Schwartz, S., & Laliberte, R. (1987). Effectiveness of mandibular infiltration in children using the local anesthetic Ultracaine (articaine hydrochloride). *Journal of the Canadian Dental Association, 53,* 29–31.

Fawcett, J. P., Kennedy, J. M., Kumar, A., & Ledger, R. (2002). Comparative efficacy and pharmaco-kinetics of racemic bupivacaine and s-bupivacaine in third molar surgery. *Journal of Pharmacy and Pharmaceutical Sciences, 5*(2), 199–204.

Guidotti, G. (1972). The composition of biological membranes, *Archives of Internal Medicine, 129,* 194–201.

Hodgkin, A. L., & Huxley, A. F. (1954). A quantitative description of membrane current and its application to conduction and excitation in nerve, *Journal of Physiology* (London), *117,* 500–544.

Jastak, J. T., Yagiela, J. A., & Donaldson, D. (1995). *Local anesthesia of the oral cavity.* Philadelphia: Saunders.

Malamed, S. F. (2004). *Handbook of local anesthesia* (5th ed., pp. 3–26). St. Louis: Elsevier Mosby.

Moore, P. A., & Dunsky, J. L. (1983). Bupivacaine anesthesia— A clinical trial for endodontic therapy. *Oral Surgery,* 1983, 55: 176–179.

Narhi, M., Yamamoto, H., Ngassapa, D., & Hirvonen, T. (1994). The neurophysiological basis and the role of inflammatory reactions in dentine hypersensitivity. *Archives of Oral Biology, 39*(Supplement), 23S.

Noback, C. R., & Demarest, R. J. (1981). *The human nervous system: Basic principles of Neurobiology* (3rd ed.). New York: McGraw-Hill.

Pashley, D. H. (1990). Mechanisms of dentin sensitivity, *Dental Clinics of North America, 34,* 449.

Pogrel, M. A., Schmidt, B. L., Sambajon, V., & Jordan, R. C. K. (2003). Lingual nerve damage due to inferior alveolar nerve blocks. A possible explanation. *JADA, 134*(2), 195–199.

Seeley, R. R., Tate, P., & Stephens, T. D. (2008). *Anatomy & physiology* (8th ed). Boston: McGraw Hill.

Tetzlaff, J. E. (2000). *Pharmacology of local anesthetics* (pp. 3–8). Woburn, MA: Butterworth-Heinemann.

Vree, T. B., & Gielen, M. J. (2005). Clinical pharmacology and the use of articaine for local and regional anaesthesia. *Best Practice and Research Clinical Anaesthesiology,* 19293–19308.

Events in a Successful Nerve Impulse Generation

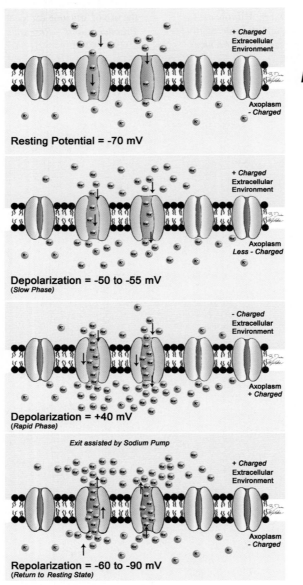

Pharmacology of Local Anesthetic Pain Control

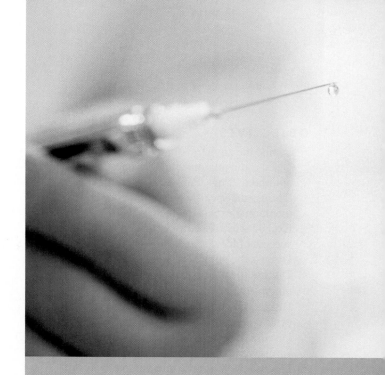

Chapter **4**

Pharmacology Basics

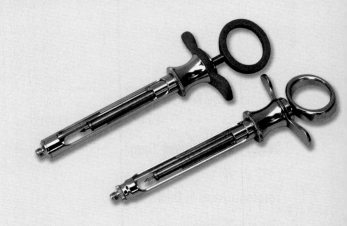

OBJECTIVES

- Define the key terms in this chapter.
- Discuss the pharmacologic properties of local anesthetic drugs and vasoconstrictors.
- Discuss the specific receptor theory and membrane expansion theory.
- Explain why tissue inflammation affects the success of local anesthesia.
- Discuss the clinical relevance of pH and pKa.
- Discuss the pharmacodynamics and pharmacokinetics of local anesthetic drugs.
- Discuss the effects of local anesthetics on the central nervous system (CNS).
- Discuss the effects of local anesthetics on the cardiovascular system (CVS).
- Discuss the biotransformation pathways of amides and esters and the concept of elimination half-life.

INTRODUCTION

The pharmacology of local anesthetic solutions in dentistry includes the pharmacology of local anesthetic drugs and the vasoconstrictors used in combination with them. Understanding the mechanisms of action, **biotransformation** (metabolic pathways), and toxic effects of each drug on local and systemic tissues is necessary for safe and effective administration.

It is also important to understand that pharmacology is far from a static discipline. Clinicians are encouraged to follow developments in this area as new drugs, new drug combinations, and new delivery technologies are introduced to clinical practice. Upon mastering the principles in this chapter, clinicians should be well-prepared to integrate future developments into clinical practice.

LOCAL ANESTHESIA

The primary benefit of local anesthesia is that pain sensations can be suppressed without significant central nervous system (CNS) depression (Daniel, Harfst, & Wilder, 2008; Hardman et al., 1996). As mentioned in Chapter 3, this allows the majority of dental procedures to be performed under local anesthesia without exposing patients to the risks of general anesthesia.

Regardless of the particular type of healthcare procedure, loss of sensation in local anesthesia is produced by preventing the generation and conduction of impulses. The purpose of these impulses is to alert the CNS to localized stimulation or tissue injury. While there are many local anesthesia techniques, the majority of which are used in medicine and some of which do not utilize drugs, this discussion will be confined to local anesthetic drugs used specifically for dentistry.

A sound knowledge of local anesthetic drugs and techniques is the foundation for safe and successful administration. An understanding of the impact of compromised physiologic function, susceptibility to adverse reactions, and awareness of all drugs the patient may be using whether prescribed or not, is equally important. Legal and ethical principles mandate that those licensed to inject drugs into the human body are responsible for these considerations and, ultimately, their consequences.

The drugs used for dental local anesthesia today are remarkably safe (Malamed, 2004a). Few pharmaceuticals, in fact, have such extensive safety records. This does not mean that clinicians can ignore manufacturers'

recommendations, nor does it mean that information provided by experts in the field may be ignored. For example, disregard for maximum recommended doses, especially when considering age, body weight, and physiologic compromise has lead to serious and even fatal consequences in the past (Moore, 1999). Failure to take appropriate steps to avoid depositing solution into blood vessels has met with equally regrettable consequences (Aldrete & Narang, 1975). The use of **vasoconstrictors** (drugs that constrict peripheral vasculature) greatly increases the overall safety of local anesthetic drugs; however, their use must be carefully considered to avoid adverse events (Okada, Suzuki, & Ishiyama, 1989).

Five local anesthetic drugs are packaged for injection in dentistry today. While this number may seem small, it has proven to be adequate in most applications. In addition to these drugs, others that are not packaged for dental use will be discussed due to rare occasions where patients may be allergic to all five. In addition to the injectable drugs, topical anesthetics provide an important adjunct in pain management.

ROUTES OF DELIVERY

There are two primary routes of delivery of dental local anesthetic drugs, topical and submucosal injection. Topical application of local anesthetic drugs is more effective on mucosa than on skin due to the ease of penetration through mucosal barriers. Subcutaneous (SC) and submucosal (SM) injections are more effective than topical routes of administration because they allow direct placement of drugs in close proximity to nerves.

DESIRABLE PROPERTIES OF LOCAL ANESTHETIC DRUGS

An ideal local anesthetic drug would have the following specific properties: a high level of biocompatibility with no systemic effects; a rapid onset; no toxicity to tissue, including nerve tissue; and a therapeutic duration and potency without inducing hypersensitivity or unconsciousness (Malamed, 2004a). Further, it would be sterilizable, readily biotransformed, and provide excellent topical effects at low concentrations (Malamed, 2004a) (see Box 4–1).

All five available local anesthetic agents in dentistry have reasonably low systemic toxicities with adequate onsets and durations. All are readily biotransformed and

Box 4–1   **Desirable Properties of Local Anesthetic Drugs**

Biocompatibility:

1. Nonirritable
2. Nontoxic to neural structures
3. Nonallergenic
4. Biotransformable and easily eliminated
5. Completely reversible effects

Safety and Efficacy (at therapeutic doses):

1. Effective in tissues and mucous membranes
2. Short onsets and no residual effects
3. Reasonable durations
4. Adequate potency
5. Sterilizable
6. Patients remain conscious

Source: Malamed, 2004.

relatively nonallergenic. Only two are acceptable as both topical and injectable agents in dentistry and all are minimally irritating and have the potential to damage nerve tissues (Pogrel & Thamby, 2000). Table 4–1 ■ and Table 4–2 ■ list the drugs, suppliers, and basic formulations.

PHARMACOLOGY OF LOCAL ANESTHETIC AGENTS

Injectable local anesthetic drugs in dentistry are classified as either **amides** or **esters.** Each has two separate and very different chemical components linked by what are known as **intermediate chains.** The distinction of these drugs as either amide or ester is based on the chemical nature of their intermediate chains. A relatively easy way to distinguish between the two formulas is that the amide chain contains a nitrogen atom while the ester chain does not. The chemical formulas of these drugs and their components are demonstrated

Table 4–1	Injectable Dental Local Anesthetic Drugs (2009)	
Generic Drug	*Drug's Trade Name (All trade names are the property of their respective parent companies)*	*Sources Retailed in U.S. Market (2009)*
Articaine	Zorcaine	Cook-Waite (Kodak)
	Septocaine	Septodont
Bupivacaine	Marcaine	Cook-Waite (Kodak)
	Vivacaine	Septodont
	Bupivacaine	Hospira Worldwide
Lidocaine	Lidocaine	Cook-Waite (Kodak)
	Xylocaine	Denstsply
	Lidocaine	Henry Schein
	Octocaine	Novocol
	Lignospan	Septodont
Mepivacaine	Carbocaine	Cook-Waite (Kodak)
	Polocaine	Denstsply
	Mepivacaine	Henry Schein
	Isocaine	Novocol
	Scandonest	Septodont
Prilocaine	Citanest	Denstsply
	Citanest Forte	Denstsply
Procaine	Not available in dental cartridges	

Table 4–2	Available Dental Local Anesthetic Drug Formulations	
Drug	*Concentration*	*Vasoconstrictor*
Articaine	4%	1:100,000 epinephrine
	4%	1:200,000 epinephrine
Bupivacaine	0.5%	1:200,000 epinephrine
Lidocaine	2%	None
	2%	1:50,000 epinephrine
	2%	1:100,000 epinephrine
Mepivacaine	3%	None
	2%	1:20,000 levonordefrin
Prilocaine	4%	None
	4%	1:200,000 epinephrine

For additional information on specific drugs, consult the manufacturers' product inserts.

in Figure 4–1 ■ highlighting the major distinctions between them.

The amide and ester linkages between the separated chemical components serve two important functions (see Figure 4–1). The first is to provide proper spacing between the chemical components, an aromatic (lipophilic) end and a secondary or tertiary amine (hydrophilic) end, which allows the anesthetic to be effective in the tissues (Jastak, Yagiela, & Donaldson, 1995a). The second is to provide for major pathways of biotransformation.

PHARMACODYNAMICS AND PHARMACOKINETICS

The two activities of a drug are referred to as its **pharmacodynamics** and **pharmacokinetics.** Pharmacodynamics refers to the actions of a drug on the body (local anesthesia) which will be discussed in this chapter and to a lesser extent in Chapter 17, "Local Anesthesia Complications and Management." Pharmacokinetics refers to the manner in which the body manages a drug, specifically the mechanisms of **absorption, distribution, metabolism** (biotransformation), and **elimination,** which will be discussed primarily in this chapter.

A major difference between local anesthetics and the majority of drugs is that systemic effects are not desired with local anesthetics (Malamed, 2004a). The primary emphasis in this chapter therefore is the localized tissue effects of the anesthetic drugs.

While the intermediate linkages in local anesthetic drugs provide an easy way to categorize them, it is the dissociation of anesthetic molecules in solution that determines the effects of these drugs. Those commonly used in dentistry are prepared as acid salts. Once dissolved in sterile water, the drugs dissociate into two forms, a positively charged molecule (**cation** also referred to as the ionic molecule) and an uncharged or neutral molecule (**neutral base).** In solution, the cation is more stable.

Local anesthetic drug actions are dependent upon the actions of both the base and cation. Despite the greater stability of cations in solution, it is the behavior of both the base and cation within a nerve membrane that determines the potency, duration, and overall efficacy of local anesthetic drugs. The solutions in dental cartridges are designed to provide an optimal initial balance of cation and neutral base molecules for stable and effective local anesthetics.

Pharmacodynamics of Local Anesthetic Drugs

The pharmacodynamics of local anesthetic drugs include their actions on peripheral nerves, the CNS, CVS, and other tissues. These actions interrupt the normal generation and conduction of nerve impulses and will be explained in the following section.

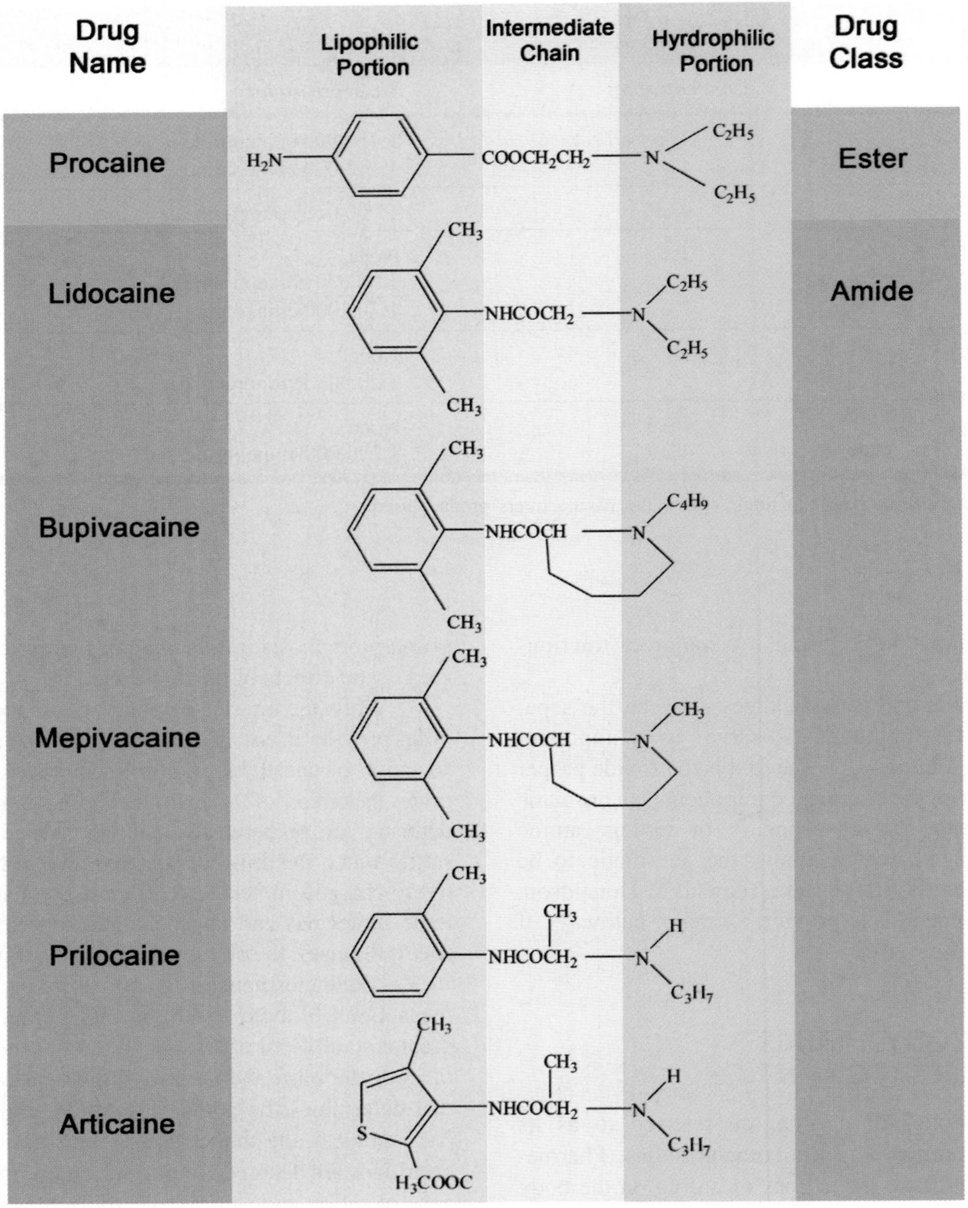

FIGURE 4-1 Chemical Formulas of Amide and Ester Local Anesthetic Drugs.

The Specific Protein Receptor Theory

The mechanism for the effect of local anesthetic drugs on nerve membranes is best explained by the **specific protein receptor theory.** Calcium ions, bound to receptor sites in ion channels during normal nerve function, are displaced when a membrane is stimulated. This allows sodium ion influx, impulse conduction, and stimulation of the CNS.

As discussed in Chapter 3, sodium ion influx appears to occur through selective channels with higher densities of these channels found in the nodes of Ranvier (Tetzlaff, 2000). The opening (and closing) of sodium ion channels is referred to as gating and is controlled by changes in the structural proteins of the nerve membrane adjacent to the ion channels (Haydon & Kimura, 1981).

The action of local anesthetics on nerve membranes is largely explained by the binding of local anesthetic molecules to these structural proteins known as specific protein receptor sites in the ion channels, which temporarily transform nerve membranes to nonexcitable states. Sodium ions cannot pass through channels that are blocked by anesthetic molecules. These channels close, preventing the influx of sodium. It is estimated that approximately 90 percent of the actions of local anesthetic drugs are due to the binding of specific protein receptor sites by local anesthetic cations (Malamed, 2004a).

The Membrane Expansion Theory

A second theory, the **membrane expansion theory,** describes a modification of the membrane structure in the presence of local anesthetic drugs that is not explained by the specific receptor theory (Lee, 1976; Malamed, 2004a). Membrane alterations have been demonstrated along affected nerve membranes, which may be caused by diffusion of local anesthetic molecules to lipophilic regions of the membranes, in the process narrowing the diameters of ion channels and further limiting their permeability to sodium ions (Seeman, 1972). While neither the specific receptor nor the membrane expansion theory is able to explain the actions of local anesthetic drugs entirely, both emphasize the actions of local anesthetic molecules on nerve membranes (Jastak et al., 1995). The dissociation of anesthetic molecules to cations explains the majority of the actions of local anesthetic drugs in the specific receptor theory (~90%). The actions of neutral base molecules in the membrane expansion theory explain approximately 10 percent of the anesthetic effect (Malamed, 2004a).

The Ionic Basis of Local Anesthesia

The process by which anesthesia is induced according to the specific protein receptor theory may be explained as follows. The base molecule is lipophilic and passes through the membrane. Once beyond the influence of the extracellular environment, base molecules combine with hydrogen ions to form cations, which are hydrophilic. Only cations are able to bind to receptor sites in the sodium ion channels of nerve membranes to block nerve impulse generation and transmission. Uncharged

base molecules are necessary to provide adequate concentrations of cations in the channels. In order for anesthesia to develop, cations displace calcium ions, which ordinarily bind receptor sites in the ion channels.

In the formula $RN + H^+ \rightleftarrows RNH^+$, RN represents the neutral base anesthetic molecule, RNH^+ represents the cationic anesthetic molecule, and H^+ is the hydrogen ion. This equation describes the equilibrium between base molecules and cations in local anesthetic drug solutions (ADA/PDR, 2006; Bennett, 1974; Jastak et al., 1995).

As previously mentioned, cations (RNH^+) represent the predominant form in local anesthetic drug solutions because neutral base molecules (RN) are far less stable.

As the drug is injected into the tissues, it is predominantly in the cationic (RNH^+) form; however, more base molecules typically develop in response to normal tissue pH of about 7.4. Once at the nerve membrane, cations (RNH^+) must convert to bases (RN) in order to pass through. In the environment of normal tissue pH, the equilibrium in the previous equation shifts to the left to favor an increase in neutral base molecule production outside the membrane:

$$\mathbf{RN} + H^+ \rightleftarrows RNH^+$$

This provides more base molecules for membrane penetration. As base molecules (RN) penetrate the membrane, fewer exist in the extracellular fluid. This temporary extracellular depletion of base molecules fuels the equilibrium shift to favor base molecule production.

In order to provide cations (RNH^+) to bind to receptor sites, base molecules pass through the nerve membrane. Once exposed to the axoplasmic environment, the equilibrium shifts to the right, resulting in the formation of cations (RNH^+):

$$RN + H^+ \rightleftarrows \mathbf{RNH^+}$$

Hydrogen ions (H^+) are available for this association in the axoplasm (pH ~ 7.4).

To summarize, base molecules (RN) must first penetrate nerve membranes before they can convert to cations (RNH^+). Cations, and *only* cations, are able to bind to receptor sites in sodium ion channels. If adequate numbers of base molecules do not penetrate the membrane and convert to cations, profound local anesthesia will not develop.

Inflammation and Local Anesthesia

When tissues are inflamed at the site of deposition of local anesthetic drugs, the lower pH inhibits the production of base molecules. This inhibition may result in insufficient numbers of base molecules (RN) penetrating nerve membranes. Profound anesthesia may become difficult to achieve or, if initially achieved, to sustain. In addition to the increase in hydrogen ions, localized edema and increased circulation may also contribute to failure of profound anesthesia by removing drugs from the delivery site.

The Relevance of pKa and pH to Local Anesthetics

Manufacturers manipulate the percentages of cations and bases in local anesthetic solutions by adjusting the pH of the solution for optimal therapeutic benefit. The inclusion of more cations than base molecules in solution has other specific benefits, including greater stability, increased solubility of the initially powdered local anesthetic drugs in water, and ease of sterilization (Jastak et al., 1995). Increasing the pH in solution will increase base molecule concentrations while lowering the pH will favor cation concentrations. These adjustments are calibrated for injection into normal tissue pH.

The equilibrium concentrations of cationic and base molecules in solution are described by the **pKa,** also known as the **dissociation constant.** When pKa = pH, there is an equal distribution of cations (RN^+) and uncharged base molecules (RN) in solution.

The **Henderson-Hasselbach equation** is an expression of pH as a function of the concentrations of weak acids and bases in solution. It may also be thought of as a formulaic definition of the dissociation constant, pKa. The Henderson-Hasselbach provides manufacturers a means of determining the percentage of cations and base molecules in solution at a specific pH. It is written:

$$\text{Log (Base/Acid)} = \text{pH} - \text{pKa}$$

Alternatively, it may be expressed in this manner:

$$\text{pKa} = \text{pH} - \text{Log (Base/Acid)}$$

Clinical Application of pKa

In local anesthesia, narrow pKa ranges of around 7.7 to 8.1 are common and include all five of the injectable amides available in dentistry. These values provide clinically useful onsets of anesthesia. As a general rule, the higher the pKa, the longer the onset of anesthesia. pKa values for the five amide dental local anesthetic drugs and the ester, procaine, are listed in Table 4–3 ■. Procaine (pKa 9.1) has both a longer onset (6 to 10 minutes)

Table 4–3	pKa of Local Anesthetic Drugs in Dentistry		
Injectable Drugs		**Topical Drugs**	
Mepivacaine		**Benzocaine**	
pKa = 7.7	Onset 2–4 min.	pKa = 3.5	Onset 1–2 min.
Lidocaine		**Tetracaine**	
pKa = 7.7	Onset 2–4 min.	pKa = 8.6	Onset 10–15 min.
Prilocaine			
pKa = 7.7	Onset 2 min.		
Articaine			
pKa = 7.8	Onset 1–6 min.		
Bupivacaine			
pKa = 8.1	Onset 2–10 min.		
Procaine			
pKa = 9.1	Onset 6–10 min.		

Source: See individual manufacturer product monographs and for procaine, Malamed, S. F.: *Handbook of Local Anesthesia*, 5th ed., St. Louis, Elsevier Mosby, 2004.

and shorter duration compared to the amides, which limits its clinical usefulness in dentistry. Despite falling outside of this range (7.7 to 8.1), some agents used only as topical anesthetics in dentistry are clinically quite effective, such as benzocaine (pKa 3.5) and tetracaine (pKa 8.4).

Vasoactivity of Local Anesthetic Drugs

An important property of the amide dental local anesthetic drugs and the ester, procaine, is their vasoactivity. All are peripheral vasodilators. This means that vessels in the area of deposition will dilate when these drugs are injected. Each drug expresses a different degree of vasodilation. Articaine, bupivacaine, lidocaine, and procaine are potent vasodilators and systemic uptake will be more rapid compared to mepivacaine and prilocaine, which are weak vasodilators.

Vasodilation is not a desirable characteristic of local anesthetic drugs and limits their duration and efficacy unless vasoconstrictors are added to the solutions. Some amides, such as prilocaine and mepivacaine, are frequently used without vasoconstrictors due to their weak vasodilative properties. Others, such as lidocaine, are not particularly useful in dentistry without the addition of vasoconstrictors due to their rapid uptake away from the site into the circulation, limiting their duration.

Not only are the duration and efficacy of local anesthetic drugs affected by their vasoactivity but their toxicity is as well. Drugs that act locally and remain in areas of injection for longer periods are less available to the systemic circulation. Rapid uptake into the systemic circulation can lead to more rapid overdose. Vasoconstrictors oppose rapid uptake.

CNS and CVS Actions of Local Anesthetic Drugs

It has been estimated that 5 to 10 percent of all reported adverse reactions to anesthetic drugs occur due to the administration of *local* anesthetic drugs (Atanassoff & Hartmannsgruber, 2002). The CNS is particularly susceptible to the effects of these drugs. Local anesthetic molecules bound to receptor sites within nerve membranes are temporarily unavailable to the circulation. Unbound molecules are distributed to local tissue or absorbed into the systemic circulation. It is important to note that molecules absorbed into the systemic circulation are quickly distributed to highly sensitive cells of the CNS and CVS. With the exception of bupivacaine, all of the dental local anesthetic drugs affect the CNS well before they impact the CVS and require significantly higher blood concentrations before they affect the CVS (Levsky & Miller, 2005).

Factors that may precipitate toxic overdose from local anesthetic drugs include excessive doses, intravascular administration, rapid delivery or absorption, and/or slower than normal biotransformation or elimination. Other factors that may contribute to overdose include an individual's age, weight, health status, and the route of administration (Malamed, 2004b).

CNS Effects

At therapeutic blood levels, local anesthetic drugs usually exert no clinically significant effects on the CNS (Jastak et al., 1995; Malamed, 2004a). At high blood levels, local anesthetic overdose manifests as CNS depression. The symptoms of CNS depression have been characterized as **biphasic** (occurring in two phases) and are consistent with a progression from early signs of CNS excitation (phase I) to signs of CNS depression (phase II), which can lead to tonic-clonic convulsions, coma, and respiratory arrest (Council on Clinical Affairs, 2005).

An important consideration when identifying CNS effects is that temporary signs of excitation that may be seen in local anesthetic overdose are also unfortunately seen in nonoverdose-related reactions to fear and anxiety in dental settings. To distinguish between a fear reaction and a true overdose, a clinician must be alert to the development of signs of CNS depression. If the excitation represents an early phase of overdose and the excitation is replaced by signs and symptoms of CNS depression, it is due to an overdose (see Box 4–2). This means that the excitatory pathways of the CNS are being depressed by the drug, leaving only signs and symptoms of CNS depression (Malamed, 2004a). The initial phase of excitation may be explained as an early loss of the normal inhibitory pathways of the CNS. These pathways are lost due to earlier depressive effects on those pathways. This early loss of inhibition may be absent in some cases (see Box 4–3). For further discussion on the impact of fear and anxiety see Chapter 18, "Insights for the Fearful Patient."

CVS Effects

Similar to local anesthetic drug effects on the CNS, at therapeutic blood levels there are usually no clinically significant CVS effects (Jastak et al., 1995). The CVS effects of local anesthetic drugs at higher blood levels can be harmful and therapeutically beneficial. For

---

Box 4-2 **Signs and Symptoms of CNS Overdose Toxicity**

(in alphabetical order)

Apprehension, excitedness, talkativeness

Bilateral numbness of tongue

Disorientation

Drowsiness *more common with lidocaine*

Elevated BP, pulse, breathing

Headache

Lightheadedness

Loss of consciousness

Muscle twitching/tremors in muscles of face, extremities

Perioral numbness

Shivering, chilled feeling of skin

Slurred speech

Visual/Auditory disturbances

Warm flushed feeling of skin

Box 4-3 **Special Considerations for Overdose Toxicity of the CNS**

The presentation of symptoms of lidocaine and procaine overdose is the notable exception to the biphasic progression of local anesthetic overdose of the CNS. Often patients do not present with signs and symptoms of excitability; instead they present with initial signs and symptoms of depression only.

Although bupivacaine has specific benefits for longer periods of anesthesia, it is the most toxic of the five local anesthetics. Both CNS and CVS toxicity thresholds are lower and unlike other local anesthetic drugs, CNS and CVS susceptibility is nearly equal. This characteristic, along with bupivacaine's prolonged duration of action, limits its choice as a primary drug for routine use in dentistry.

Source: Levsky & Miller, 2005; Malamed, 2004a.

---

example, toxic overdose of both lidocaine and procaine can ultimately cause cardiovascular collapse, while at the same time both have proven quite useful in treating cardiac arrhythmias (see Box 4–4) (Council on Clinical Affairs, 2005; Malamed, 2004a).

Similar to the CNS effects of local anesthetic drugs, typical CVS events are biphasic. Initially, heart rate and blood pressure may increase. As dosing continues, vasodilation occurs, leading to depression of the myocardium, which may result in a fall in blood pressure. The contractility of the myocardium may be so impaired that cardiac output is reduced. When combined with CNS seizure activity, cardiac and respiratory arrest may result.

With the exception of bupivacaine, this is the usual course of local anesthetic overdose (Prilocaine Product Insert). Bupivacaine is nearly equally toxic to both the CNS and the CVS (see Box 4–3). It is more likely to induce an overdose and once that overdose occurs, it is typically more difficult to reverse compared to other agents. For example, when comparing bupivacaine to lidocaine, it has been demonstrated in animal studies that bupivacaine is up to sixteen times more cardiotoxic than lidocaine (Levsky & Miller, 2005).

Fortunately, most overdoses are self-limiting. The drugs are continuously biotransformed. Their effects on the CNS and CVS, similar to those on the skin, mucosa, periodontium, pulp, and other tissues are transient, disappear rapidly once their concentrations fall below depressant levels. This is why many mild overdoses may go unnoticed.

Box 4-4 **Effects of Local Anesthetics on the CVS**

Effects on myocardium result in depression of:
    Electrical excitability
    Conduction rate
    Force of contraction

Effects on smooth muscle result in vasodilation* of:
    Peripheral vasculature

Effects on blood pressure result in:
    Hypotension with increasing doses (more frequent with procaine and lidocaine)

---

*Except with cocaine, when used as a local anesthetic, which produces vasoconstriction.
Source: Malamed, 2004a.

Pharmacokinetics of Local Anesthetic Drugs

Before discussing the pharmacology of each specific drug, pharmacokinetic properties common to all of the available injectable dental local anesthetic drugs will be discussed in order to better understand the similarities and differences among them.

Absorption and Distribution

Once absorbed into the systemic circulation, drugs are distributed throughout the body (see Figure 4–2 ■). Organs that are highly perfused with blood such as the lungs, brain, heart, and kidneys will receive more of systemically-distributed drugs than those with less perfusion (Malamed, 2004a). Similarly, injection into highly vascular regions will result in faster absorption

and distribution away from sites of deposition. In contrast, deposition into less vascular regions with slower vascular uptake prolongs the local actions of drugs.

Biotransformation and Elimination

Biotransformation, or metabolism of local anesthetic drugs, reduces or eliminates their toxicity. This is accomplished by biologically breaking the drug down into components called metabolites. This process occurs primarily through one of two pathways, either in the liver or in the blood. The pathway of biotransformation in the liver is known as the hepatic **p450 isoenzyme system.** This is a slower process compared to metabolism in the blood by **pseudocholinesterase** (also referred to as cholinesterase and plasma cholinesterase), which is the enzyme responsible for breaking down esters. Manufactured primarily but not

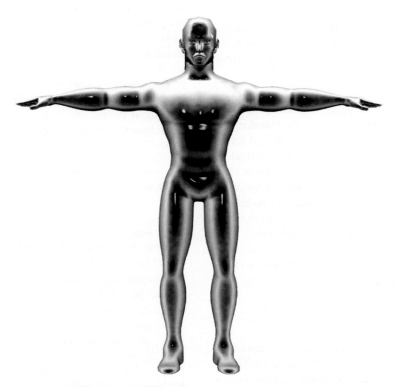

■ **FIGURE 4–2** Systemic Circulation, Absorption, and Distribution of Local Anesthetic Drugs. Local anesthetic drugs are absorbed into the systemic circulation, and distributed throughout the body. Highly perfused organs such as the lungs, brain, heart, and kidneys will receive more systemically distributed drugs than less perfused tissues. Muscle by mass receives the highest percentage of drug.

exclusively in the liver, pseudocholinesterase is widely distributed. When referring to this enzyme in the liver, it is known simply as cholinesterase.

Once metabolites reach the kidneys, they are eliminated along with any unmetabolized fractions of drug.

Biotransformation of Amides

Bupivacaine, lidocaine, and mepivacaine are primarily biotransformed in the liver by hepatic enzymes. This pathway is complex and involves a number of steps. Mepivacaine is less easily biotransformed compared to lidocaine, and bupivacaine is more slowly biotransformed compared to either mepivacaine or lidocaine.

In addition to the liver, prilocaine is biotransformed in the kidneys and the lungs with very little excreted unchanged (Jastak et al., 1995; Prilocaine Product Insert).

Articaine is an exception in its biotransformation pathways. Product monographs state that only 5 to 10 percent of articaine is metabolized via the liver's isoenzyme system. It is a true amide, yet in intraoral administration the majority of its metabolism is non-hepatic, primarily via cholinesterase similar to esters (Jastak et al., 1995).

Biotransformation of Esters

Benzocaine, procaine, and tetracaine are biotransformed in the blood via cholinesterase. Benzocaine and tetracaine are used in dentistry as topical anesthetics. Injectable esters, such as procaine, may be administered submucosally when there is documented allergy to amides. While ester local anesthetic drugs are no longer packaged in dental cartridges they are still occasionally used in dentistry and frequently used in medicine.

Procaine undergoes very rapid metabolism by cholinesterase. Tetracaine's metabolic pathway is similar, but slower, compared to other esters including procaine and benzocaine.

Elimination Half-Life (t½)

The **elimination half-life** of a drug may be defined as the rate at which it is removed from the systemic circulation. It has also been expressed as the time necessary to metabolize and excrete 50 percent of a drug (Malamed, 2004a; Pickett & Terezhalmy, 2006) (see Box 4–5). Lidocaine, for example, has a half-life of 1.6 hours. This means that it will take more than six half-lives to clear this drug or more than nine hours before only a trace remains. In dentistry, a variety of drugs with

---

Box 4–5   Elimination Half-Life

	Drug	Reduction
	100%	
1st ½ life	↓	
2nd ½ life	50	50%
3rd ½ life	25	50%
4th ½ life	12.5	50%
5th ½ life	6.25	50%
6th ½ life	3.12	50%
	↓	

---

different half-lives are currently used. Understanding these differences can impact drug selection and treatment planning (see Box 4–6). Based on pharmacological principles, elimination half-life values may become important when calculating additional dosing after maximum recommended doses (MRD) have been administered (see Box 4–7). Shorter half-life drugs may be readministered sooner with less risk of overdose.

A list of the elimination half-life for each of the five local dental anesthetic drugs available in dental cartridges may be found in Table 4–4 ■.

Box 4–6   Half-Life Consideration for Treatment Planning

Consider the situation of a nursing mother. Selecting a drug that will quickly clear her system reduces the likelihood of the drug being passed to the child while nursing. If articaine is administered for treatment, its half-life is the shortest of all amides at approximately 45 minutes after *maximum* dosing. It was demonstrated in one study that articaine's half-life, after *oral* administration, was approximately 16–20 minutes when no more than 120 milligrams (approximately ¾–1½ cartridges) were administered (Oertel, Ulrike, Rahn, & Kirch, 1999).

It should be noted that, despite distribution into breast milk, there is no documentation of trouble with lidocaine in lactating females. This is likely true of the other local anesthetics as well.

Source: ADA/PDR, 2006; Oertel et al., 1999.

Box 4–7 **Maximum Recommended Dose**

Maximum recommended dose (MRD) represents the maximum quantity of drug that can be *safely* administered in most situations. These values are provided by manufacturers in drug monographs (product inserts) for each drug and have been independently reviewed by the ADA Council on Dental Therapeutics and the United States Pharmacopeial Convention. Conservative recommendations suggested by Malamed are based on the preceding recommendations and use the lowest values from all of the sources when considering MRD values for the drugs (Malamed, 2004a). MRD values will be further discussed and applied in Chapter 7, "Dose Calculations for Local Anesthetic Solutions," and Malamad's published MRD values will be used for this text.

Table 4–4 **Elimination Half-Life Value**

Drug	Half-Life (hrs)
Articaine*	0.75*
Prilocaine	1.6
Lidocaine	1.6
Mepivicaine	1.9
Bupivacaine	2.7–3.5

*Septocaine® Product monograph
Source: Malamed, 2004; Oertel et al., 1999.

CHAPTER QUESTIONS

1. Elimination half-life refers to which *one* of the following?
   a. The time it takes for a drug to be half-metabolized
   b. The time it takes for half of a drug to be out of the system
   c. The time it takes for half of a drug to be out of the circulation
   d. The time it takes for a drug to be out of half of the circulation

2. Ester local anesthetics are metabolized in which *one* of the following pathways?
   a. In the liver
   b. In the blood
   c. In the kidneys
   d. In the brain

3. CNS toxicity occurs due to:
   a. The expected response of neurons in the CNS to the drug dose.
   b. Frank neural tissue damage due to the excessive dose.
   c. Compromised vascular supply in the CNS due to vasoconstrictor doses.
   d. None of the above.

4. CVS toxicity occurs due to:
   a. Compromised vascular supply.
   b. Frank tissue damage.
   c. Decreased myocardial contractility, vasodilation and hypotension.
   d. Decreased myocardial contractility, vasoconstriction, and hypertension.

5. Which portion of the anesthetic molecule is responsible for binding to the receptor site inside the nerve membrane, thereby preventing depolarization?
   a. Calcium ion
   b. Anesthetic free base
   c. Anesthetic anion
   d. Anesthetic cation

6. Which part of a local anesthetic molecule determines the classification of the drug as an ester or amide?
   a. Lipophilic portion
   b. Hydrophilic portion
   c. Intermediate chain
   d. Caine linkage

7. Which of the following is *not* a systemic reaction to an overdose of a local anesthetic agent?
   a. CNS stimulation
   b. Depression of myocardium
   c. Vasodilation of peripheral blood vessels
   d. Respiratory arrest

REFERENCES

ADA/PDR Guide to Dental Therapeutics (4th ed). Montvale, NJ: Thompson PDR Corporation, 2006.

Aldrete, J. A., & Narang, R. (1975). Deaths due to local anesthesia in dentistry. *Anaesthesia, 30*, 685–686.

Atanassoff, P. G., & Hartmannsgruber, M. W. B. (2002). Central nervous system side effects are less important after IV regional anesthesia with ropivacaine 0.2% compared to lidocaine 0.5% in volunteers, *Canadian Journal of Anesthesia, 49*, 169–172.

Bennett, C. R. (1974). *Monheim's local anesthesia and pain control in dental practice* (5th ed). St. Louis: Mosby.

Council on Clinical Affairs: Guideline on appropriate use of local anesthesia for pediatric dental patients, *American Academy of Pediatric Dentistry, 2005.*

Covino, B. G., & Vasallo, H. G. (1976). *Local anesthetics: mechanisms of action and clinical use.* New York: Grune & Stratton.

Daniel, S. J., Harfst, S. A., & Wilder, R. S. (2008). *Mosby's dental hygiene: Concepts, Cases, and Competencies* (2nd ed). St. Louis: Mosby.

Haas, D. A., & Lennon, D. (1995). A 21-year retrospective study of reports of paresthesia following local anesthetic administration. *Journal of the Canadian Dental Association 61*(4), 319–320, 323–326, 329–330.

Hardman, J. G., Limbird, L. E., Molinoff, P. B., Ruddon, A. G., & Goodman, A. G. (1996). *Goodman and Gilman's the pharmacological basis of Therapeutics* (9th ed). New York: McGraw-Hill.

Harn, S. D., & Durham, T. M. (1990). Incidence of lingual nerve trauma and postinjection complications in conventional mandibular block anesthesia, *Journal of the American Dental Association, 121,* 523.

Haydon, D. A., & Kimura, J. E. (1981). Some effects of n-pentane on the sodium and potassium currents of the squid giant axon, *Journal of Physiology, 312, 57–70.*

Horrobin, D. F., Durand, I. G., & Manku, M. S. (1977). Prostaglandin E1 modifies nerve conduction and interferes with local anesthesic action. *Prostaglandins, 14,* 103–108.

Jastak, J. T., Yagiela, J. A., & Donaldson, D. (1995). *Local anesthesia of the oral cavity.* Philadelphia: Saunders.

Keetley, A., & Moles, D. R. (2001). Eastman Dental Institute for Oral Health Care Science, London. *Primary Dental Care, 8*(4), 139–142.

Kitagawa, N., Oda, M., & Totoke, T. (2004). Possible mechanism of irreversible nerve injury caused by local anesthetics: Detergent propertied of local anesthetics and membrane disruption. *Anesthesiology, 100*(4), 962–967.

Lee, A. G. (1976). Model for action of local anesthetics, *Nature, 262,* 545–548.

Levsky, M. E., & Miller, M. A. (2005). Cardiovascular collapse from low dose bupivacaine. *Canadian Journal of Clinical Pharmacology, 12*(3), e(240)–e(245).

Malamed, S. F. (2004a). *Handbook of local anesthesia* (5th ed., pp. 3–26). St. Louis: Elsevier Mosby.

Moore, P. A. (1999, April). Adverse drug interactions in dental practice: interactions associated with local anesthetics, sedatives and anxiolytics series. *Journal of the American Dental Association,* 541–554.

Oertel, R., Rahn, R., & Kirch, W. (1997). Clinical pharmacokinetics of articaine. *Clinical Pharmacokinetics, 33,* 417–425.

Oertel, R., Ulrike, E., Rahn, R., & Kirch, W. (1999). The effect of age on phamacokinetics of the local anesthetic drug articaine. *Regional Anesthesia and Pain Medicine, 24*(6), 524–528.

Okada, Y., Suzuki, H., & Ishiyama, I. (1989). Fatal subarachnoid hemorrhage associated with dental local anesthesia. *Australian Dental Journal, 34,* 323–325.

Pickett, F. A., & Terezhalmy, G. T. (2006). *Dental drug reference with clinical applications.* Baltimore, MD: Lippincott Williams & Wilkins.

Pogrel, M. A., & Thamby, S. (2003). Permanent nerve involvement resulting from inferior alveolar nerve blocks. *Journal of the American Dental Association, 134*(2), 901–907.

Prescribing information: Ravocaine and Novocain with Levophed (1993). New York: Cook-Waite, Sterling Winthrop.

Prilocaine Product Insert, Dentsply Pharmaceutical. York, PA.

Quinn, C. L. (1995). Injection techniques to anesthetize the difficult tooth, *Journal of the California Dental Association.*

Seeman, P. (1972). The membrane actions of anesthetics and tranquilizers. *Pharmacol Rev, 24,* 583–655.

Tetzlaff, J. E. (2000). Clinical pharmacology of local anesthetics. Woburn, MA: Butterworth-Heinemann.

Wilson, W., Taubert, K. A., Gewitz, M., Lockhart, P. B., Baddour, L. M., & Levison, M., et al. (2007). Prevention of ineffective endocarditis: Guidelines from the American Heart Association, by the Committee on Rheumatic Fever, Endocarditis, and Kawasaki Disease. *Circulation,* April 19, 2007, 10.1161 AHA.106.183095. Council on Cardiovascular Disease in the Young, and the Council on Clinical Cardiology, Council on Cardiovascular Surgery and Anesthesia, and the Quality of Care and Outcomes Research Interdisciplinary Working Group.

Wong, J. K. (2001). Success rate of the conventional inferior alveolar nerve block. *Journal of the Canadian Dental Association, 67,* 391–397.

Chapter 5

Dental Local Anesthetic Drugs

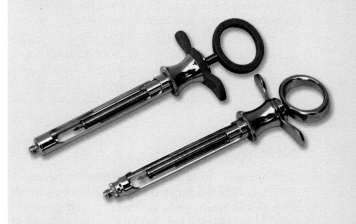

OBJECTIVES

- Define and discuss the key terms in this chapter.
- Discuss similarities and differences between dental local anesthetic drugs.
- Apply this knowledge to clinical situations in which the choice of local anesthetic and/or vasoconstrictor may directly affect safety and success.
- Discuss and determine some situations in which specific drugs are indicated or contraindicated.
- Discuss which local anesthetic solutions work reasonably well without vasoconstrictors and why they are more effective in those clinical situations.
- Discuss when and why solutions with epinephrine and levonordefrin are indicated or contraindicated.

KEY TERMS

articaine **67**
bupivacaine **71**
epinephrine **52**
levonordefrin **62**
lidocaine **52**
maximum
  recommended dose
  (MRD) **54**

mepivacaine **61**
methemoglobinemia
  56
paresthesia **68**
prilocaine **65**
procaine **74**
vasoconstrictors **53**

CASE STUDY: Elena Gagarin

Elena Gagarin, a 30-year-old mother of a nursing infant is in need of dental treatment to relieve pain in two of her teeth. Her main concerns are to be rid of the nagging pain she has experienced for the last several weeks and to make sure she doesn't pass on any of the local anesthetic drugs to her infant.

She is currently nursing every 3 to 4 hours and has made no provisions for reserves for the baby, who is not able to consume formula.

Which of the dental local anesthetic drugs is able to provide adequate pain relief and will not be passed on to the baby in significant quantities 2 to 3 hours after her appointment?

INTRODUCTION

The injectable local anesthetic drugs introduced in Chapter 4, "Pharmacology Basics," share common characteristics in their chemical structures and properties. These characteristics help to explain similarities in the manner in which they may be used.

Local anesthetic drugs are selected by balancing patient factors with the requirements of treatment. In order to administer the most appropriate agent, it is important to recognize the differences among the drugs. For example, a drug may provide safe and reliable anesthesia in the majority of individuals yet may wear off so quickly that it proves to be of limited usefulness for others. In these situations the use of a longer-acting drug may be beneficial.

This chapter will highlight similarities and differences in injectable local anesthetic drugs for dentistry in an effort to promote clinically safe and successful local anesthesia. For a quick-reference table of the properties of each drug discussed, consult Appendix 5–1.

LIDOCAINE

Background

Lidocaine was the first amide local anesthetic drug, developed by Lofgren in 1943. Despite the introduction of other amides since that time, lidocaine remains the standard against which local anesthetic drugs are compared. It has a long and impressive record of reliability, with a rapid onset, rare reports of hypersensitivity, typical pulpal durations of 60 minutes or more, and soft tissue durations of up to 5 hours. Lidocaine has been described as a *versatile* drug due to its nearly universal applicability in all areas of health care delivery (Jastak, Yagiela, & Donaldson, 1995b). Despite its universal appeal, it is particularly well suited for dentistry. Combined with various dilutions of vasoconstrictors, lidocaine has made profound and durable pain control a routine expectation in dentistry (Malamed, 2004a; Xylocaine hydrochloride).

Allergic reactions to lidocaine have not been documented and the drug shows no cross-allergenicity with other currently available amides.

Lidocaine has been noted to have anticonvulsant properties and in large doses has been used to terminate seizures or decrease their durations. Similar to other local anesthetics with anticonvulsant properties, lidocaine acts to prevent or terminate seizures by depressing the excitability of cortical neurons thus raising seizure thresholds (Malamed, 2004a).

Formulations for Use in Dentistry

Lidocaine is provided in the following formulations:

2% lidocaine plain (without vasoconstrictor) (see Figure 5–1A ■)

2% lidocaine with 1:100,000 epinephrine (see Figure 5–1B ■)

2% lidocaine with 1:50,000 epinephrine (see Figure 5–1C ■)

Drugs with vasoconstrictors are written in two common conventions; for example, lidocaine with **epinephrine** may be written as either 2% lidocaine with 1:100,000 epinephrine, or as 2% lidocaine, 1:100,000 epinephrine (epinephrine is a vasoconstrictor added to increase the safety and duration of local anesthetic drugs). These conventions are used interchangeably throughout this text.

Duration of Action

2% lidocaine plain (without vasoconstrictor)
Very short duration = 5–10 minutes pulpal; 60–120 minutes soft tissue

2% lidocaine with 1:100,000 epinephrine
Intermediate duration = 60 minutes pulpal; 180–300 minutes soft tissue

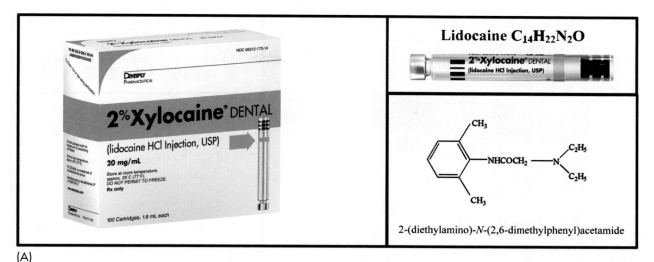

(A)

(B)

(continued)

■ **FIGURE 5–1**   A—2% Lidocaine Plain. B—2% Lidocaine, 1:100,000 Epinephrine.
Source: Modified courtesy of DENTSPLY Pharmaceutical.

2% lidocaine with 1:50,000 epinephrine
> *Intermediate* duration = 60 minutes pulpal;
> 180–300 minutes soft tissue

Local anesthetic drugs are commonly classified as *short, intermediate,* or *long* acting based on the duration of pulpal and hard tissue anesthesia (ADA/PDR, 2006) (see Table 5–1 ■). A *short* pulpal duration in dentistry typically lasts from approximately 20 to 40 minutes. Intermediate durations last up to 70 minutes and long durations up to 8 hours depending on the injection technique. Soft tissue durations are usually much greater,

even when no **vasoconstrictors** are used (ADA/PDR, 2006; Malamed, 2004a).

The receptor binding strength of a local anesthetic and its vasoactivity are key considerations in its duration of action. Lidocaine without a vasoconstrictor has a moderately strong binding strength to affected protein receptors; however, it is a vigorous vasodilator. Due to its strong vasodilating effects, it provides only a very short duration of action when used without a vasoconstrictor. When injected with a vasoconstrictor, lidocaine provides profound and durable anesthesia, enough, in

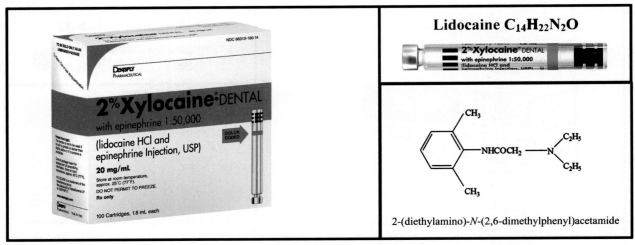

(C)

■ **FIGURE 5–1** C—2% Lidocaine, 1:50,000 Epinephrine.
Source: Modified courtesy of DENTSPLY Pharmaceutical.

Table 5–1	Comparison of Local Anesthetic Durations	
Drug	**Classification (Duration of Action)**	
Articaine	Intermediate	
Bupivacaine	Long	
Lidocaine	Short* Intermediate	
Mepivacaine	Short* Intermediate	
Prilocaine	Short* Intermediate	
Procaine	Short	

*Represents drugs without the addition of vasoconstrictors.

fact, for most dental procedures (see Appendix 5–1). Vasoconstrictors, which prolong local anesthetic durations by constricting local vasculature, are discussed in Chapter 6, "Vasoconstrictors in Dentistry."

Similarity to Other Local Anesthetics

Lidocaine's formula has less similarity to the other amide drugs discussed than to etidocaine, a long-acting amide no longer packaged for dentistry and formerly marketed as Duranest. Etidocaine is still available for use in other healthcare settings.

MRD (Maximum Recommended Dose)

2.0 mg/lb (4.4 mg/kg)

The **maximum recommended dose (MRD)** of a local anesthetic drug represents the maximum quantity of drug that can be *safely* administered during an appointment in most situations. The absolute MRD for lidocaine is 300 mg per appointment (Tetzlaff, 2000).

Lidocaine-induced overdose reactions may differ from other amides in that the initial excitatory phase may be short-lived or nonexistent (DeToledo, 2000). For more detailed information on MRD values see Chapter 7, "Dose Calculations for Local Anesthetic Solutions."

Relative Potency

Lidocaine is twice as potent as its predecessor, procaine, equal in potency to mepivacaine and prilocaine, approximately two-thirds as potent as articaine, and approximately one-fourth as potent as bupivacaine (see Figure 5–2 ■ and Figure 5–3 ■).

Many dental procedures require extended durations of profound anesthesia that are often significantly longer than many medical administrations. These extended durations may be unpleasant and may increase the risk of self-injury. As is the case with all the local anesthetic drugs, lidocaine is not ideal in this respect; however, it has a therapeutic potency that balances the need for profound and durable dental anesthesia without excessive duration.

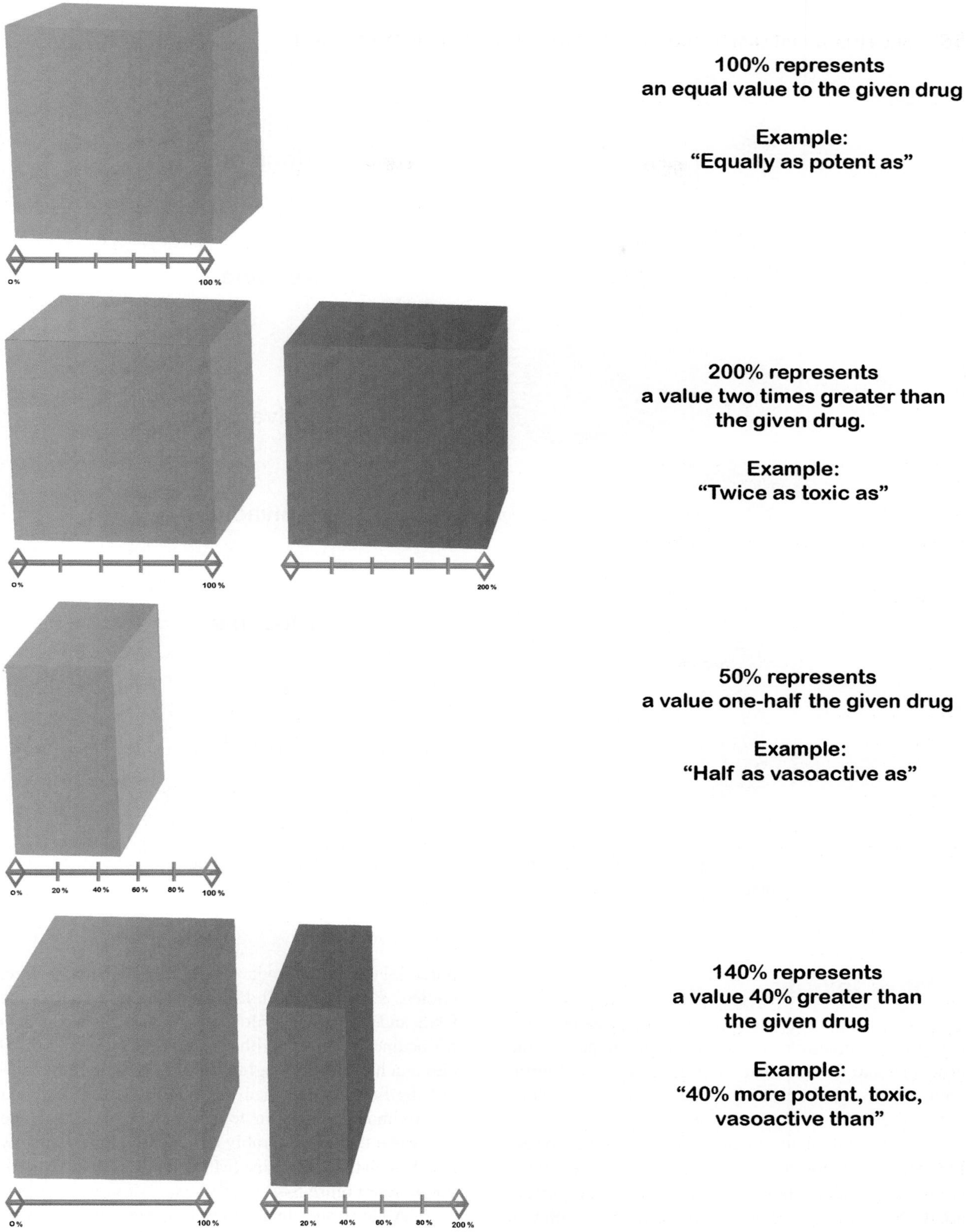
0%
100%
100% represents
an equal value to the given drug
Example:
"Equally as potent as"
0%
100%
200%
200% represents
a value two times greater than
the given drug.
Example:
"Twice as toxic as"
0%
20%
40%
60%
80%
100%
50% represents
a value one-half the given drug
Example:
"Half as vasoactive as"
0%
100%
20%
40%
60%
80%
200%
140% represents
a value 40% greater than
the given drug
Example:
"40% more potent, toxic,
vasoactive than"

■ **FIGURE 5–2** Comparison Values. This scale will be applied for the purpose of discussion and comparison of potency, toxicity, and vasoactivity.

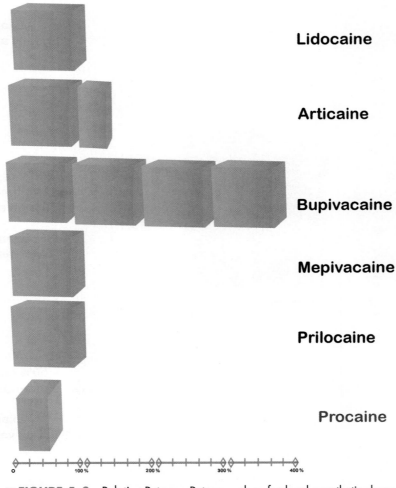

Lidocaine

Articaine

Bupivacaine

Mepivacaine

Prilocaine

Procaine

0   100%   200%   300%   400%

■ **FIGURE 5–3**   Relative Potency. Potency values for local anesthetic drugs compared with lidocaine.

Relative Toxicity

Lidocaine is approximately twice as toxic as procaine and prilocaine, similar in toxicity to mepivacaine and articaine, and *far less toxic* (approximately one-fourth) compared with bupivacaine (Jastak et al., 1995a; Tetzlaff, 2000) (see Figure 5–4 ■).

These statements are accurate but, similar to toxicity statements for other local anesthetic drugs, do not completely address lidocaine's relative toxicity in all areas. For example, while reported to be similar to articaine in toxic potential, lidocaine has been demonstrated in studies to have greater overdose-inducing potential (Oertel, Berndt, & Kirch, 1996; Simon, Vree, Gielen, & Booij, 1997). Lidocaine is more toxic to the CNS and CVS than prilocaine but far less toxic than prilocaine in patients with blood oxygenation deficiencies, such as **methemoglobinemia.** These deficiencies will be further discussed in Chapter 10. Lidocaine *is* approximately equal in toxicity to mepivacaine and bupivacaine is considerably more toxic (approximately four times) than lidocaine (Marcaine; Levsky & Miller, 2005) (see Figure 5–4).

All local anesthetic drugs, if administered intravascularly, may be potentially life threatening, particularly if they are administered rapidly. The relative toxicity values

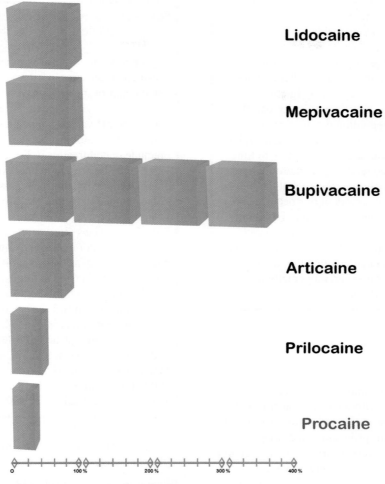

■ **FIGURE 5–4**   Relative Toxicity. Toxicity values for local anesthetic drugs as compared with lidocaine.

of the drugs discussed in this chapter assume that drugs have not been administered intravascularly. Comparisons take into account the normal mechanisms of metabolism. For example, the drug procaine, which will be discussed later in this chapter, is the least toxic of all drugs mentioned. If administered intravascularly, however, it may be as toxic as the other drugs discussed.

Metabolism

Lidocaine is metabolized by hepatic enzymes also known as oxidases and amidases (Tetzlaff, 2000). This process is complex and involves multiple steps. Hydrolysis accounts for about one-third of lidocaine elimination

(Jastak et al., 1995; Tetzlaff, 2000). Several of lidocaine's byproducts (metabolites) are pharmacologically active. For example, monoethylglycinexylidide (MEGX) retains most of the pharmacological activity of lidocaine. One of lidocaine's biotransformation products, 2, 6-xylidine, has raised concerns in the past and has been investigated as a carcinogen in rats (Jastak et al., 1995a) (see Box 5–1).

Excretion

Less than 10% of lidocaine is excreted unchanged by the kidneys.

Higher excretion rates may be more common when the pH of urine is low (Tetzlaff, 2000) (see Box 5–2).

> **Box 5–1   Concerns Regarding Lidocaine and Carcinogenicity**
>
> Patients may sometimes ask about or refer to sources of information that tend to indict certain pharmaceuticals. These sources may ignore, misstate, exaggerate, or modify scientifically-based evidence, especially regarding the dose-related nature of drug toxicity. Lidocaine, for example, has been mentioned as a carcinogen from time to time due to its demonstrated tendency to cause malignant tumors in rats. It is important to note that the induction of malignant nasal tumors in rats occurred *only* after *very large doses* were administered. Not only would comparable dosing in humans far exceed manufacturers' recommended maximum doses, but concerned patients can be reassured that there is no evidence to support similar carcinogenicity in humans (Jastak et al., 1995a).

> **Box 5–2   Factors Impacting Urine pH Related to Excretion**
>
> Higher concentrations of nonmetabolized local anesthetic molecules in urine confirm that higher percentages of the drugs have avoided metabolic breakdown, rendering them potentially more toxic. Low urine pH values can be present in a surprising number of conditions, many of which do not preclude dental treatment. For example, low uric pH values may be present in anorexia and starvation, emphysema, gout, diarrhea, persistent fever, frequent kidney stone formation, infections, and hyperkalemia (increased levels of potassium in the blood). Some vegetarians along with other dental patients with suspected or confirmed nutritional deficiencies may be affected, as well as individuals taking drugs such as chlorothiazide diuretics, methenamine mandelate, ammonium chloride, and aldosterone. In addition, uncontrolled diabetics and those with metabolic syndrome, in general, can have low uric pH values (Kamel, Cheema-Dhadli, & Halperin, 2002; Luthra, Davids, Shafiee, & Halperin, 2004; Maalouf, Cameron, Moe, Adams-Huet, & Sakhaee, 2007; Takahashi, Inokuchi, Kobayashi, Ka, Tsutsumi, Moriwaki, et al., 2007; Tetzlaff, 2000).

Vasoactivity

Lidocaine is a potent vasodilator with a very short duration when administered without a vasoconstrictor. It is a less potent vasodilator compared with procaine but greater compared with prilocaine and mepivacaine, which limits its use to very short procedures if used without a vasoconstrictor (see Figure 5–5 ■).

pKa

The pKa of lidocaine is 7.7.

Values for pKa in dentistry range from 3.5 for benzocaine to 9.3 for procaine. pKa is a valuable measurement of the relative numbers of base molecules initially available in local anesthetic solutions as affected by their pH. The most useful pKa range for injectable anesthetics falls between 7.6 and 8.1. Drugs with pKa values in this range provide more rapid onsets of anesthesia. Lidocaine, mepivacaine, and prilocaine all have pKa values of 7.7, while articaine's is 7.8 and bupivacaine's is 8.1 (Xylocaine hydrochloride; Malamed, 2004a) (see Table 5–2 ■).

pH

The pH of lidocaine plain solutions is 6.5.

The pH of lidocaine solutions with vasoconstrictors ranges from 3.3 to 5.5.

When a vasoconstrictor is added, the pH of local anesthetic drugs is decreased.

Solutions containing vasoconstrictors are more acidic in order to preserve the vasoconstrictors, which would otherwise oxidize, shortening shelf life considerably. Cartridges with vasoconstrictors that are approaching their shelf-life expirations typically experience an additional decrease in pH value that reflects the ongoing and selective oxidation of bisulfite preservatives over the vasoconstrictors (see Table 5–2). This decrease in pH can cause increased burning sensations upon administration.

Onset of Action

The onset of action of lidocaine is approximately 2 to 3 minutes.

The onsets of most injectable amides available in dentistry are considered to be rapid. There is little

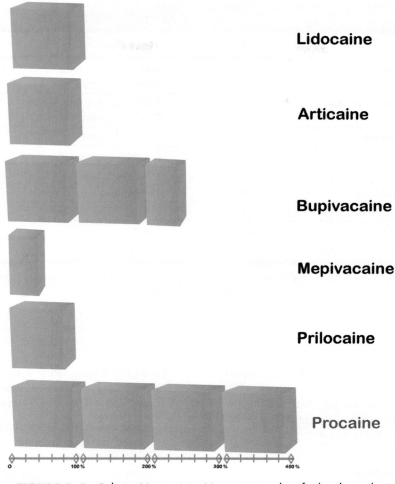

Lidocaine

Articaine

Bupivacaine

Mepivacaine

Prilocaine

Procaine

| 0 | 100% | 200% | 300% | 400% |

■ **FIGURE 5–5**   Relative Vasoactivity. Vasoactivity values for local anesthetic drugs as compared with lidocaine.

clinically noticeable difference in onset between the amides, with the exception of bupivacaine, which has a much slower onset.

Vasoconstrictor

Lidocaine is available with epinephrine in dilutions of 1:50,000 and 1:100,000.

A general pharmacological principle holds that whenever a drug maintains its therapeutic value in lower concentrations its use should be considered. Lidocaine with a 1:50,000 dilution of epinephrine contains twice the quantity of vasoconstrictor drug as a 1:100,000 dilution.

While there may be therapeutic benefit to higher concentrations at times, such as when more vigorous hemostasis is desired in order to control bleeding, there is questionable rationale for the *routine* use of dilutions of 1:50,000 epinephrine (Jastak et al., 1995b).

Half-Life (t½)

The elimination half-life of lidocaine is 1.6 hours (96 minutes).

The elimination half-lives of all dental local anesthetic drugs are considered to be relatively short. Some bisphosphonates prescribed for osteoporosis and

Table 5–2 Comparative pKa and pH Values			
Drug	*pKa*	*Onset Time*	*pH*
Articaine[6] w/ epinephrine 1:100,000	7.8	Infiltration: 1–2 mins Block: 2–2½ mins	4.4–5.2
Articaine[6] w/ epinephrine 1:200,000	7.8	Infiltration: 1–2 mins Block: 2–3 mins	4.6–5.4
Bupivacaine[5] w/ epinephrine	8.1	Up to 6–10 mins	3.0–4.5
Lidocaine[1] w/ epinephrine	7.7	2–3 mins.	3.3–5.5
Mepivacaine[4] plain	7.6	2–4 min.	4.5–6.8
Mepivacaine w/ levonordefrin	7.6	1½–2 mins.	3.0–3.5
Prilocaine[3] plain	7.7	2–4 min.	6.0–7.0
Prilocaine[2] w/ epinephrine	7.9	2–4 min.	3.0–4.0
Procaine[7] w/ vasoconstrictor	9.1	6–10 mins.	3.5–5.5

Sources: Product inserts for [1]Xylocaine®, [2]Citanest®, [3]Citanest Forte®, [4]Carbocaine®, [5]Marcaine® and [6]Septocaine® and for procaine, Malamed, S. F.: *Handbook of Local Anesthesia*, 5th ed., St. Louis, Elsevier Mosby, 2004; Drugs.com (http://www.drugs.com/mmx/ultracaine-d-s-forte.html).

malignancies, for example, have half-lives approximating 10 years.

The half-life of lidocaine falls between the much shorter half-life of articaine and the much longer half-life of bupivacaine (see Table 5–3 ■).

Topical Preparations

Lidocaine is effective as a topical anesthetic. It is available for use in concentrations ranging from 2% to 10% in various ointments, viscous solutions, and mixtures. When used topically, the onset of anesthesia occurs within 1 to 2 minutes, with peak effects available from 2 to 5 minutes (Jastak et al., 1995c). For further discussion on topical preparations see Chapter 8, "Topical Anesthetics."

Pregnancy Category

Lidocaine is in FDA Category B drug.

Lidocaine, in all formulations, is safe to use in pregnancy once the patient's physician has confirmed that there are no exceptional risks. The FDA Pregnancy Category B rating does *not* suggest that there are no risks to the use of a category B drug; rather it suggests that the risks are acceptable *in most circumstances* (ADA/PDR, 2006; Meadows, 2001). Category B status means either that:

1. studies have concluded that there were no demonstrated risks in animals and no human studies available, or
2. there are demonstrated risks in animals but well-controlled studies fail to demonstrate those same risks in the human fetus.

A summary of local anesthetic drugs used in dentistry with their FDA Pregnancy Category ratings may be found in Table 5–4 ■. FDA Pregnancy Categories are discussed in further detail at the end of this chapter and in Table 5–5 ■.

Safety During Lactation

Lidocaine enters breast milk (small amounts); use caution (ADA/PDR, 2006).

Most drugs are available in breast milk once introduced. Product information generally states that caution must be exercised when nursing after lidocaine administration.

Table 5–3   Elimination Half-Life Values

Drug	Half-Life (hrs)	Comparisons
Lidocaine	1.6	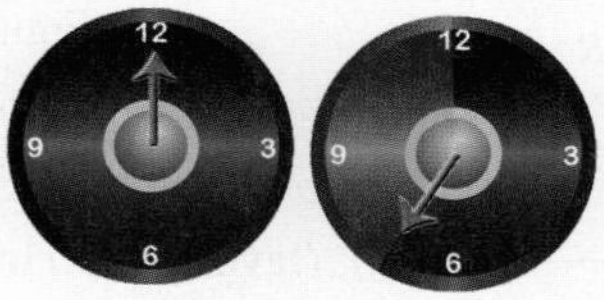
Articaine*	0.75*	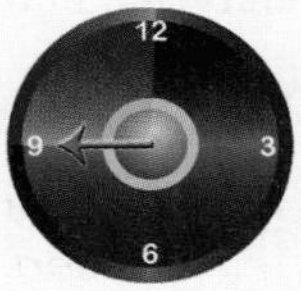
Bupivacaine	2.7–3.5	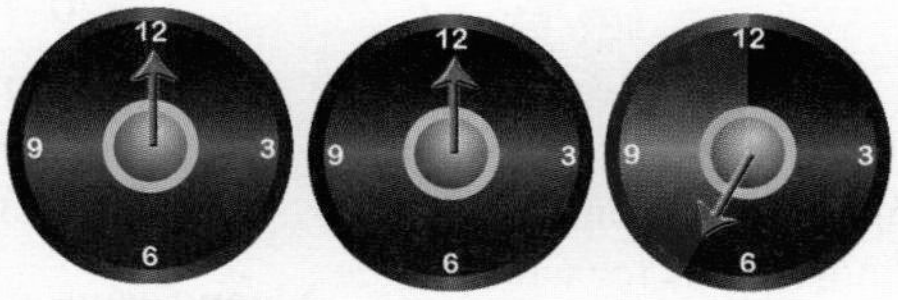
Mepivacaine	1.9	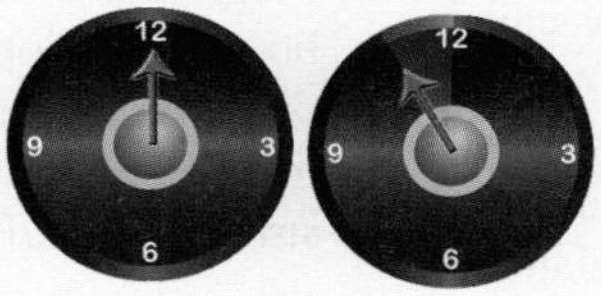
Prilocaine	1.6	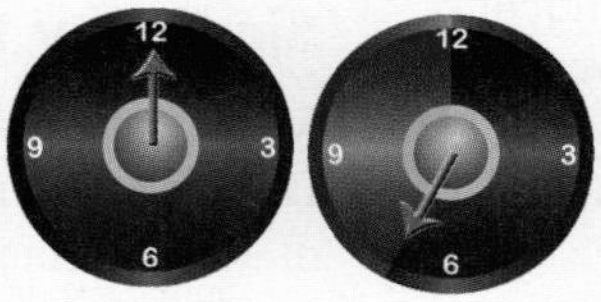
Procaine	0.1	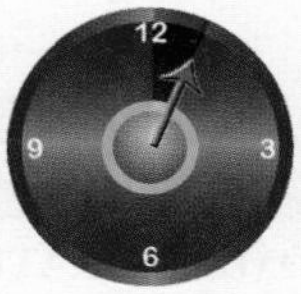

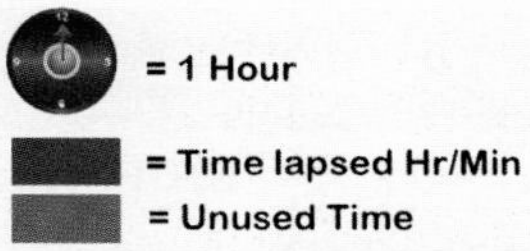

= 1 Hour

= Time lapsed Hr/Min

= Unused Time

*Septocaine product monograph

Source: ADA/PDR, 2006; Tetzlaff, 2000.

MEPIVACAINE

Background

Mepivacaine was introduced in Sweden (1957) as an alternative to lidocaine by A. F. Eckenstam. The pharmacology of mepivacaine is similar to lidocaine's despite its closer chemical resemblance to bupivacaine (Carbocaine, Malamed, 2004a). Its duration, onset of action, potency, and toxicity are all similar to lidocaine's (Tetzlaff, 2000) (see Figure 5–6 ■ and Appendix 5–1).

Unlike lidocaine, mepivacaine is a weak vasodilator and is effective for short durations without a vasoconstrictor. The 3% formulation without vasoconstrictor, for example, is capable of providing approximately 20 to 40 minutes of pulpal anesthesia compared with

Table 5–4	Summary of FDA Pregnancy Ratings for Dental Local Anesthetic Drugs

Dental Local Anesthetic Drug	*FDA Pregnancy Rating*
Articaine	C
Bupivacaine	C
Lidocaine	B
Mepivacaine	C
Prilocaine	B

Source: ADA/PDR, 2006; Meadows, 2001.

plain solutions of 2% lidocaine, which provide only 5 to 10 minutes of pulpal anesthesia. In individuals for whom vasoconstrictors are contraindicated, 3% mepivacaine solutions are particularly useful.

As with lidocaine, mepivacaine has been noted to have anticonvulsant properties and has been used to terminate seizures or decrease their durations (Malamed, 2004a). Similar to other local anesthetics with anticonvulsant properties, mepivacaine acts to prevent or terminate seizures by decreasing the excitability of cortical neurons (raising seizure thresholds) (Malamed, 2004a).

Formulations for Use in Dentistry

Mepivacaine is provided in the following formulations:

> 3% mepivacaine plain (without vasoconstrictor) (see Figure 5–6A)

> 2% mepivacaine with 1:20,000 levonordefrin (see Figure 5–6B)

(**levonordefrin** is a vasoconstrictor used to increase the safety and duration of mepivacaine)

Duration of Action

> 3% mepivacaine plain
>> *Short* duration = 20–40 minutes pulpal; 120–180 soft tissue

> 2% mepivacaine with 1:20,000 levonordefrin
>> *Intermediate* duration = 60 minutes pulpal; 180–300 minutes soft tissue

Mepivacaine provides durable, short-term anesthesia in both infiltrations and nerve blocks without added vasoconstrictors. Mepivacaine prepared with a vasoconstrictor provides durations similar to lidocaine with a vasoconstrictor (ADA/PRA, 2006; Malamed, 2004a).

Similarity to Other Local Anesthetics

Mepivacaine is chemically similar to bupivacaine. Despite this similarity, mepivacaine lacks the duration of action of bupivacaine.

Table 5–5	FDA Drug Categories in Pregnancy

U.S. FOOD AND DRUG ADMINISTRATION	
Category A	Adequate, well-controlled studies in pregnant women have not shown an increased risk of fetal abnormalities.
Category B	Animal studies have revealed no evidence of harm to the fetus; however, there are no adequate and well-controlled studies in pregnant women. **Or** Animal studies have shown an adverse effect, but adequate and well-controlled studies in pregnant women have failed to demonstrate a risk to the fetus.
Category C	Animal studies have shown an adverse effect and there are no adequate and well-controlled studies in pregnant women. **Or** No animal studies have been conducted and there are no adequate and well-controlled studies in pregnant women.
Category D	Studies, adequate well-controlled or observational, in pregnant women have demonstrated a risk to the fetus. However, the benefits of therapy may outweigh the potential risk.
Category X	Studies, adequate well-controlled or observational, in animals or pregnant women have demonstrated positive evidence of fetal abnormalities. The use of the product is contraindicated in women who are or may become pregnant.

Source: ADA/PDR, 2006; Meadows, 2001.

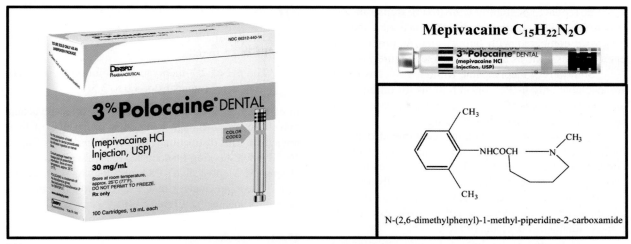

(A)

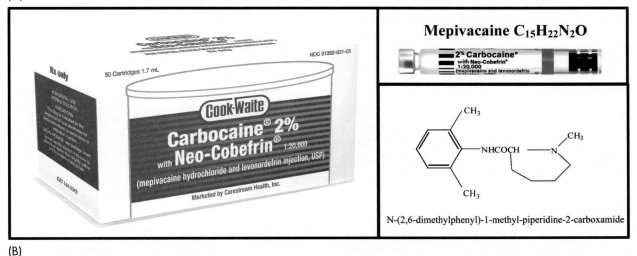

(B)

■ **FIGURE 5–6**   A—3% Mepivacaine Plain. B—2% Mepivacaine, 1:20,000 Levonordefrin.
Source: Courtesy of Carestream Health Inc.; Modified courtesy of DENTSPLY Pharmaceutical.

Mepivacaine is most similar to lidocaine in its pharmacodynamic and pharmacokinetic behaviors. For example, both drugs express anticonvulsant properties (Malamed, 2004a).

MRD

2.0 mg/lb (4.4 mg/kg)

300 mg absolute maximum recommended dose per appointment

Relative Potency

Mepivacaine is twice as potent as procaine, equal in potency to lidocaine and prilocaine, two-thirds as potent as articaine, and approximately one-fourth as potent as bupivacaine (see Figure 5–3).

Relative Toxicity

Mepivacaine is twice as toxic as procaine, approximately twice as toxic as prilocaine, similar in toxicity to articaine (equal to or slightly *more* toxic), similar in toxicity to lidocaine (equal to or slightly *less* toxic), and *far less toxic* compared with bupivacaine (approximately one-fourth as toxic as bupivacaine) (see Figure 5–4).

Solutions of mepivacaine without vasoconstrictor are available only in 3% concentrations for minimal effectiveness. There is 50% more drug in each cartridge of any 3% drug compared with 2% drugs.

Some published maximum recommended doses for mepivacaine reflect a higher toxicity compared with lidocaine (Tetzlaff, 2000b). Mepivacaine tends to produce higher blood levels than lidocaine initially after injection; however, studies suggest that patients tolerate higher levels of mepivacaine before toxic effects become evident (Jastak et al., 1992b).

Studies suggest that both prilocaine and articaine are tolerated better than mepivacaine largely due to their avoidance of liver metabolism (Citanest and Citanest Forte; Jastak et al., 1992b; Oertel, Bernst, & Kirch, 1996; Tetzlaff, 2000).

Metabolism

Mepivacaine is metabolized in the liver but the pathways are different compared with lidocaine. Unlike lidocaine, amidase activity is insignificant. Its elimination half-life of 1.9 hours reflects its less efficient metabolic pathways (Jastak et al., 1995a; Tetzlaff, 2000).

Excretion

Excretion is variable with anywhere from virtually none to up to 16% excreted unchanged. As is true with other local anesthetic drugs, higher excretion rates are more common when urine pH is low.

Vasoactivity

Mepivacaine is a weak vasodilator, characterized as producing only slight vasodilation, which allows it to be used without vasoconstrictors. It is the weakest vasodilator of the five injectable drugs available in dental cartridge form and provides useful short-term durations in both infiltrations and nerve blocks in *plain* (no vasoconstrictor) solutions (see Figure 5–5).

pKa

The pKa of mepivacaine is 7.6 (see Table 5–2).

pH

The pH of 3% mepivacaine plain solutions ranges from 4.5 to 6.8.

The pH of 2% mepivacaine solutions with vasoconstrictor ranges from 3.0 to 3.5.

In certain situations, 3% plain solutions of mepivacaine may have an advantage over other drugs due to their higher pH. This distinction is further discussed in Chapter 16, "Troubleshooting Inadequate Anesthesia," Box 16–2, "Using 3% Mepivacaine's Pharmacology to Your Advantage." These advantages may also extend to plain solutions of prilocaine (see Table 5–2).

Onset of Action

The onset of action for mepivacaine is approximately 1.5 to 2 minutes.

Mepivacaine's onset of action is rapid and similar to most of the other available injectable drugs in dentistry. Some clinicians elect to administer 3% mepivacaine plain as an initiating drug prior to the administration of bupivacaine, which has a much slower onset. This technique allows treatment to begin while bupivacaine is taking effect.

Vasoconstrictor

2% mepivacaine with levonordefrin is available in a dilution of 1:20,000.

With the addition of levonordefrin, the 2% formulation of mepivacaine provides adequate depth and duration of pain control for most dental procedures equivalent to the anesthetic effect of 2% lidocaine with 1:100,000 epinephrine.

Half-Life (t½)

The elimination half-life of mepivacaine is 1.9 hours (114 minutes).

The elimination half-life of mepivacaine is prolonged compared with lidocaine (96 minutes), prilocaine (96 minutes), and articaine (44–45 minutes) (see Table 5–3).

Topical Preparations

There are no topical solutions containing mepivacaine for dental application.

Pregnancy Category

Mepivacaine is in FDA Pregnancy Category C.

Category C suggests that there should be strong rationale for the use of a drug prior to its administration in pregnancy (ADA/PDR 2006; Meadows, 2001).

Safety During Lactation

It is not known whether mepivacaine is excreted in human milk. Caution is recommended.

PRILOCAINE

Background

Prilocaine was first prepared by Lofgren and Tegner in 1953 and approved by the FDA in 1965. Pharmacologically, prilocaine is very similar to mepivacaine (Citanest and Citanest Forte; EMLA Cream and Anesthetic Disc; Malamed, 2004a; Oraqix). See Appendix 5–1.

Prilocaine entered the market with the promise of providing similar clinical effectiveness to lidocaine with significantly decreased toxicity (Tetzlaff, 2000). Unfortunately, prilocaine can reduce the blood's oxygen-carrying capacity, which may lead to a specific anemia known as methemoglobinemia. This will be discussed further under "Relative Toxicity" and in Chapter 16.

Formulations for Use in Dentistry

Prilocaine is provided in the following formulations:

4% prilocaine plain (without vasoconstrictor) (see Figure 5–7A ■)

4% prilocaine with 1:200,000 epinephrine (see Figure 5–7B ■)

Duration of Action

4% prilocaine plain
Short duration (infiltration) = 10–15 minutes pulpal; 90–120 soft tissue
Intermediate duration (block) = 40–60 minutes; 120–240 soft tissue

4% prilocaine with 1:200,000 epinephrine
Intermediate duration = 60–90 minutes pulpal; 180–480 soft tissue

Despite prilocaine's weak vasodilative properties, it is not effective at providing long durations in infiltrations without a vasoconstrictor. This phenomenon, whereby infiltrations are far less effective compared with nerve blocks has also been observed in more potent drugs such as bupivacaine. It is suggested that the 4% formulation with 1:200,000 epinephrine be considered whenever prilocaine is to be used for longer procedures with infiltration anesthesia.

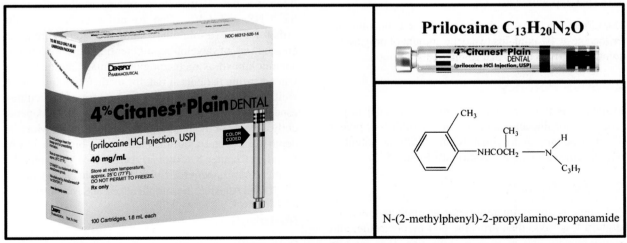

Prilocaine C₁₃H₂₀N₂O

N-(2-methylphenyl)-2-propylamino-propanamide

(A)

(*continued*)

■ **FIGURE 5–7**   A—4% Prilocaine Plain.
Source: Modified courtesy of DENTSPLY Pharmaceutical.

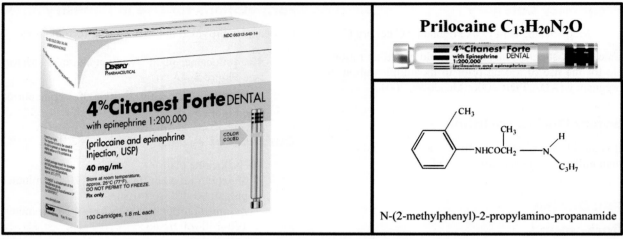

(B)

■ **FIGURE 5–7** B—4% Prilocaine, 1:200,000 Epinephrine.
Source: Modified courtesy of DENTSPLY Pharmaceutical.

Similarity to Other Local Anesthetics

Prilocaine's aromatic ring is linked to a secondary amine, unlike lidocaine, mepivacaine, articaine, and bupivacaine, which all are linked to tertiary amines.

MRD

2.7 mg/lb (6.0 mg/kg)

400 mg absolute maximum recommended dose per appointment

Overdose reactions with prilocaine are uncommon. Prilocaine at 4% contains twice the amount of drug as 2% solutions and 1.5 times that found in 3% solutions.

Relative Potency

Prilocaine is twice as potent as procaine, equal in potency to lidocaine and mepivacaine, two-thirds as potent as articaine, and approximately one-fourth as potent as bupivacaine (Malamed, 2004a) (see Figure 5–3).

Relative Toxicity

Prilocaine is approximately twice as toxic as procaine, slightly less toxic than articaine and mepivacaine, and approximately half as toxic as lidocaine. It is *far less toxic* compared with bupivacaine (approximately one-fifth or less as toxic as bupivacaine) (Jastak et al., 1995a; Tetzlaff, 2000) (see Figure 5–4).

When considering CNS and CVS toxicity, prilocaine is reportedly less toxic compared with lidocaine largely due to the availability of multiple extra-hepatic metabolic pathways (Citanest and Citanest Forte; Tetzlaff, 2000).

Relative Toxicity: Special Considerations With Prilocaine

As previously described in the toxicity discussion of lidocaine, not all toxicity is related to the effects on the CNS and CVS. Due to prilocaine's metabolite orthotoluidine (o-toluidine), some individuals are at increased risk of developing a potentially life-threatening anemia known as methemoglobinemia. Cautions apply when treating patients at risk for methemoglobinemia as well as any patients with oxygenation difficulties, especially those taking medications that are independently capable of inducing methemoglobinemia. More in-depth discussions regarding methemoglobinemia may be found in Chapter 8, "Topical Anesthetics," Chapter 10, "Patient Assessment for Local Anesthesia," and Chapter 17, "Local Anesthesia Complications and Management."

Metabolism

Prilocaine has a simpler hepatic metabolism compared with lidocaine and mepivacaine. Much of the drug, however, is cleared before it is able to reach the liver (Jastak et al., 1995a). The lungs and kidneys are alternate sites of metabolism when the liver is not utilized (Jastak et al., 1995a; Citanest and Citanest Forte).

Excretion

Only small percentages of prilocaine and its metabolites are found in the urine (Jastak et al., 1995a). As with other local anesthetic drugs, higher excretion rates are more common when the pH of urine is low.

Vasoactivity

Prilocaine is a weak vasodilator, making it effective without the addition of vasoconstrictors, although prilocaine is a stronger vasodilator compared with mepivacaine (see Figure 5–5).

pKa

The pKa of prilocaine is 7.9 (see Table 5–2).

pH

The pH of prilocaine plain solutions is 6.0 to 7.0. The pH of prilocaine solutions with 1:200,000 epinephrine is 3.0 to 4.0 (see Table 5–2).

Onset of Action

The onset of action for prilocaine is 2 to 4 minutes.

Prilocaine has a slightly slower onset of action compared with lidocaine, mepivacaine, and articaine as might be predicted from its pKa.

Vasoconstrictor

Prilocaine is available with epinephrine in dilutions of 1:200,000 epinephrine.

Due to prilocaine's weak vasodilative effects, less vasoconstrictor is required. Dilutions of 1:200,000 epinephrine are sufficient to provide profound and durable infiltration and nerve block anesthesia (see Box 5–3).

Half-Life (t½)

The elimination half-life of prilocaine is 1.6 hours (96 minutes).

Although similar to lidocaine and mepivacaine half-lives, the initial amount of drug becomes a factor in this calculation because each cartridge of prilocaine delivers 72 mg of drug, twice as much as 2% lidocaine solutions

---

> **Box 5–3   Clinical Opportunities: LA Drugs with Epinephrine 1:200,000**
>
> Drugs with 1:200,000 epinephrine dilutions compared with those with 1:100,000 formulations can be beneficial when it is necessary to limit vasoconstrictor doses. Some situations in which vasoconstrictors should be limited or avoided altogether include significant cardiovascular compromise, tricyclic antidepressant use, and insulin-resistant diabetes with underlying cardiovascular disease.

and one-fourth more than 3% mepivacaine plain solutions (see Table 5–3).

Topical Preparations

Topical use of prilocaine is found only in combination with other drugs, typically lidocaine. Concentrations of 2.5% lidocaine with 2.5% prilocaine are found in two popular products, Oraqix (Dentsply Pharmaceutical) and EMLA (AstraZeneca). See Chapter 8.

Pregnancy Category

Prilocaine is in FDA Pregnancy Category B.

Both injectable and topical solutions of prilocaine are classified as Pregnancy Category B (ADA/PDR, 2006; Meadows, 2001).

Safety During Lactation

It is unknown whether prilocaine is excreted in human milk. Caution is recommended.

ARTICAINE

Background

Articaine, synthesized in 1969 by H. Rusching, is the most recent FDA-approved injectable local anesthetic drug (2000) (Malamed, 2004a; Septocaine). It is roughly equivalent to lidocaine in both safety and efficacy (Malamed, Gagnon, & Leblanc, 2001). See Appendix 5–1.

Although classified as an amide, articaine has a distinctly different aromatic ring structure with an ester component attached. This unique configuration provides several beneficial pharmacologic behaviors. Unlike other amides, the addition of the ester component promotes rapid biotransformation. The presence of a sulfur atom within the ring structure makes it highly lipophilic, easing articaine's passage through neural membranes.

Offsetting these pharmacologic advantages is articaine's controversial association with a higher than typical incidence of post-operative nerve damage **(paresthesia),** particularly during inferior alveolar nerve blocks and some palatal injections. This concern will be discussed in Chapter 17.

Effective Concentrations in Dentistry

Articaine is provided in the following formulations:

4% articaine with 1:100,000 epinephrine (see Figure 5–8A ■)

4% articaine with 1:200,000 epinephrine (see Figure 5–8B ■)

New local anesthetic drugs are required to be as safe and as effective as 2% lidocaine. While articaine

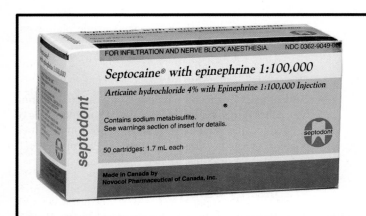

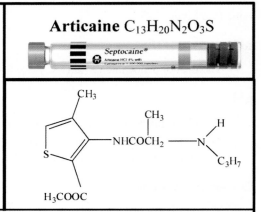

methyl 4-methyl-3-(2-propylaminopropanoylamino)thiophene-2-carboxylate hydrochloride

(A)

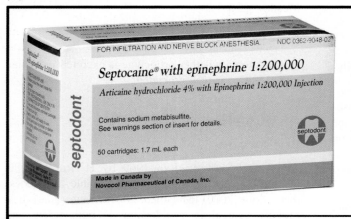

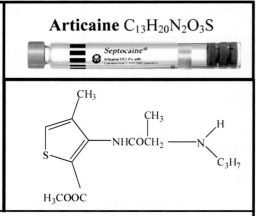

methyl 4-methyl-3-(2-propylaminopropanoylamino)thiophene-2-carboxylate hydrochloride

(B)

■ **FIGURE 5–8** A—4% Articaine, 1:100,000 Epinephrine. B—4% Articaine, 1:200,000 Epinephrine.
Source: Courtesy of Septodont.; Modified courtesy of DENTSPLY Pharmaceutical.

concentrations of less than 4% would certainly be desirable from a safety standpoint, they are not as reliably effective as 2% lidocaine.

Duration of Action

> 4% articaine with 1:100,000 epinephrine
> *Intermediate* duration = 60–75 minutes pulpal;
> 180–360 soft tissue

> 4% articaine with 1:200,000 epinephrine
> *Intermediate* duration = 45–60 minutes pulpal;
> 120–300 soft tissue

Although the product monograph indicates a slightly decreased duration with 1:200,000 epinephrine solutions, they are roughly clinically equivalent to durations with 1:100,000 solutions.

Similarity to Other Local Anesthetics

Articaine is most similar to prilocaine. It has few similarities to the other dental local anesthetic drugs, however, including prilocaine.

MRD

> 3.2 mg/lb (7 mg/kg)
> 500 mg absolute maximum recommended dose per appointment

It is interesting to note that the MRD for articaine 4%, in healthy individuals weighing 150 lbs or greater, is almost 7 cartridges (500 mg maximum) compared with lidocaine 2% (8.3 cartridges, or 300 mg maximum) despite its higher concentration. This means that more than 1.6 times as many milligrams (500 mg/300 mg) of articaine can be safely administered compared with lidocaine in most individuals.

Relative Potency

Articaine is more than twice as potent as procaine, approximately one-third more potent than lidocaine, mepivacaine, and prilocaine, and approximately one-third as potent as bupivacaine (Malamed, 2004a) (see Figure 5–3).

Even though articaine is more potent than lidocaine, its potency does not necessarily translate into increased clinical efficacy. As with all drugs, variability in response among individuals can offset any predicted benefits based upon pharmacological activities.

Relative Toxicity

Articaine is more toxic to the CNS and CVS than procaine, slightly more toxic than prilocaine, slightly less toxic than mepivacaine and lidocaine, and *far less* toxic compared with bupivacaine (Jastak et al., 1995a; Oertel, Berndt, & Kirch, 1996) (see Figure 5–4).

While articaine is considered nearly equal in toxicity to lidocaine, it has been characterized as being less toxic than lidocaine in intraoral administration and as causing less severe reactions when overdoses have been induced (Jastak et al., 1995a; Oertel, Berndt, & Kirch, 1996).

Relative Toxicity: Special Considerations with Articaine

In addition to potential CNS and CVS toxicity, articaine *may* induce methemoglobinemia when used in *higher* than therapeutic doses (Haas & Lennon, 1995; Septocaine; Septocaine hydrochloride). Articaine has also been associated with a higher-than-typical incidence of nerve damage (paresthesia) but the actual tendency is unknown. Some experts have suggested relatively low rates for all paresthesias, including those that are transient, possibly as low as 3 per million for articaine, which is the highest rate when considering all injectable dental local anesthetic drugs (Haas & Lennon, 1995; Harn & Durham, 1990a; Xylocaine hydrochloride). Pogrel and Thamby have suggested that the incidence of *permanent* nerve damage may be much greater than previously thought, at between one in 26,762 and one in160,571 in inferior alveolar blocks, for *all* drugs, including articaine (Pogrel & Thamby, 2000). The true neurotoxic potential of all the local anesthetics, including articaine, is unknown at this time.

Paresthesia

Paresthesia is nerve injury that may be defined as a prolonged temporary or permanent, partial or complete loss or alteration of sensation. Fortunately, the vast majority of paresthesias are transient.

Many clinicians are concerned that paresthesia will develop after the use of articaine. Risks may be *lessened* by reducing volumes administered, adhering to slow injection rates, and avoiding inferior alveolar nerve blocks (Haas & Lennon, 1995; Malamed, 2004c).

Avoiding blocks is recommended by some authorities, not due to any proven increased incidence of paresthesia with articaine (see Box 5–4 and Chapter 17) but

---

Box 5–4   Research Notes: Articaine
and Paresthesia

Despite the extensive scope of one retrospective
survey, it is important to note that not all studies have
demonstrated statistical increases in the incidence of
paresthesia due to articaine (Haas & Lennon, 1995).
Some have demonstrated even greater risks (Pogrel &
Thamby, 2000). Others, such as a 2001 randomized,
double-blind investigation of the safety of articaine in
1,325 subjects did not demonstrate any exceptional
risks. Two-thirds of the subjects received articaine and
one-third received lidocaine for inferior alveolar nerve
blocks. The investigators reported that "the total
number of subjects who reported these symptoms
[of paresthesia] four to eight days after the procedure
was eight (*1 percent*) for the articaine group and five
(*1 percent*) for the lidocaine group" (Malamed,
Gagnon, & Leblanc, 2000).

For a more detailed discussion of paresthesia
and articaine, see Chapter 17.

---

due to the opinion that articaine may cause paresthesia
more frequently than other drugs (Haas & Lennon, 1995;
Dower, 2007). Since it is known that an inferior alveolar
block is the primary associated technique that results in
paresthesia, avoiding blocks with articaine is similar to
administering an area-appropriate antibiotic when the
source of an infection is unknown. Both can meet with
reasonable success even when many questions remain.

Metabolism

Compared with other amide drugs, articaine has a rapid
half-life. Not only is additional dosing safer but should adverse toxic reactions occur, they generally resolve quickly
(Jastak et al., 1995a; Oertel, Ulrike, Rahn, & Kirch, 1999;
Septocaine; Vree, Baars, Van Oss, Booij, 1988).

Articaine's metabolism is unique. Five to ten
percent is metabolized via hepatic p450 enzymes. The
majority of articaine's removal is accomplished by
rapid plasma cholinesterase metabolism to articainic
acid, its inactive primary metabolite, prior to reaching
the liver. Articaine is further metabolized to articainic
acid glucoronide, a minor metabolite, also considered
to be pharmacologically inert (van Oss, Vree, Baars,
Termond, & Booij, 1988; van Oss, Vree, Baars,
Termond, & Booij, 1989).

Excretion

Very little articaine, about 2%, is excreted unchanged
(Septocaine hydrochloride). Metabolites excreted in
urine include articainic acid and small amounts of articainic acid glucoronide (Septocaine hydrochloride). As
with other local anesthetic drugs, higher excretion rates
are more common when the pH of urine is low.

Vasoactivity

Articaine is approximately equal in vasodilating activity
compared with lidocaine, greater compared with mepivacaine and prilocaine, and much weaker compared
with procaine and bupivacaine (see Figure 5–5).

Due to this activity, articaine is not useful without
the addition of a vasoconstrictor. Even though articaine
is a powerful vasodilator, it is nearly as effective with
both 1:100,000 and 1:200,000 dilutions of epinephrine.

pKa

The pKa of articaine is 7.8.

Articaine's pKa is slightly higher than lidocaine's (7.7),
which translates to somewhat fewer base molecules
available initially. Articaine is more lipophilic, however,
and its base molecules have higher affinities for nerve
membranes, which may contribute to a reported slightly
faster onset of anesthesia than lidocaine (see Table 5–2).

pH

The pH of articaine with 1:100,000 epinephrine
ranges from 4.0 to 5.2.

The pH of articaine with 1:200,000 epinephrine
ranges from 4.6 to 5.4 (see Table 5–2).

Onset of Action

The onset of action for articaine in *infiltration*
anesthesia is 1 to 2 minutes.

The onset of action for articaine in *nerve block*
anesthesia is 2 to 3 minutes.

Articaine's onset of action is variable depending upon
the technique, although in all techniques, articaine provides a rapid onset (Malamed, 2004a). In infiltrations,
articaine provides the most rapid onset of all five injectable drugs in dentistry, 1 to 2 minutes. In nerve
blocks, articaine's onset is comparable to lidocaine but
slightly slower than mepivacaine's, 1.5 to 2 minutes.

Vasoconstrictor

Articaine is available with epinephrine in dilutions of 1:100,000 and 1:200,000.

Both of these formulas provide clinically useful vasoconstriction (see Box 5–4).

Half-Life (t½)

At 476 mg (~6.5 cartridges) with 1:100,000 epinephrine articaine t½ = 43.8 minutes.

At 476 mg (~6.5 cartridges) with 1:200,000 epinephrine articaine t½ = 44.4 minutes.

A recent study suggests that the elimination half-life of articaine may be age and dose dependent (Oertel, Ulrike et al., 1999). When administering 60–120 mg or approximately 0.8–1.5 cartridges using *common dental local anesthetic techniques,* the observed half-life of articaine was reported to range from about 16 to 20 minutes, depending on the age of the recipient (Oertel, Rahn, et al, 1997; Oertel, Ulrike, et al., 1999). While not as specific, product monographs agree that articaine's half-life may be age and/or dose-dependent (Septocaine hydrochloride; Zorcaine). Until recently, a primary worldwide supplier of articaine listed the half-life of articaine as 1.8 hours. The revised half-life value in recent monographs (2006 to present) represents a major adjustment in this value, which can impact clinical dose decision making (Septocaine hydrochloride; Zorcaine). See Appendix 5–1 and Table 5–3.

Topical Preparations

Articaine is not available as a topical anesthetic.

Pregnancy Category

Articaine is in FDA Pregnancy Category C.

Category C suggests that there should be strong rationale for the use of a drug prior to administering in pregnancy (ADA/PDR, 2006; Meadows, 2001).

Safety During Lactation

Caution is recommended. Safe use in lactation has not been established (Malamed, Gagnon, & Leblanc, 2001).

BUPIVACAINE
Background

Bupivacaine was prepared by A. F. Ekenstam in 1957 and approved by the FDA in 1972. It is related structurally to lidocaine and mepivacaine (Malamed, 2004; Marcaine). See Appendix 5–1. Due to its long durations, bupivacaine may not be appropriate in many clinical situations, but it does have several important clinical indications:

1. When extended postoperative pain control is needed (bupivacaine can provide up to 12 hours of relief).
2. In situations where profound and durable anesthesia have proven to be difficult if not impossible to achieve with all the other available drugs.
3. For extended procedures requiring longer than 60-to-90-minute durations.

Self-injury is an important consideration when using bupivacaine, particularly if the individuals are at higher risk of self-inflicted postoperative trauma such as young children (see Box 5–5).

Formulations for Use in Dentistry

Bupivacaine is provided in the following formulation:

0.5% bupivacaine with 1:200,000 epinephrine (see Figure 5–9 ■)

The strength of bupivacaine's receptor site binding allows for lower concentrations of epinephrine to be used.

Duration of Action

0.5% bupivacaine with 1:200,000 epinephrine
Long duration = up to 12 hours; pulpal and soft tissue

Despite bupivacaine's intense vasodilating characteristics, it is capable of producing prolonged anesthesia due to its strong protein receptor binding in sodium channels. When used for lengthy dental procedures, pulpal and soft tissue anesthesia may last up to 12 hours. Bupivacaine may provide sufficient anesthesia to relieve pain overnight and is often used for that purpose when post-operative pain is anticipated. In patients who metabolize other drugs quickly and in

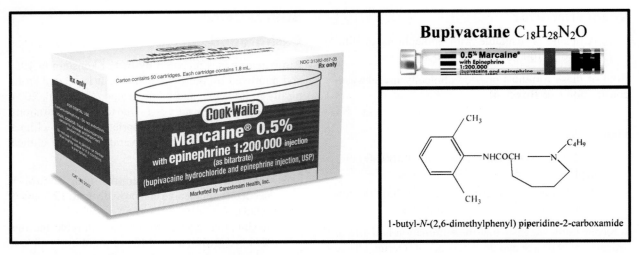

■ **FIGURE 5–9**   0.5% Bupivacaine, 1:200,000 Epinephrine.
Source: Courtesy of Carestream Health Inc.; Modified courtesy of DENTSPLY Pharmaceutical.

Box 5–5   Special Postoperative
Considerations for Bupivacaine

Postoperative Pain Management: Bupivacaine is frequently administered for pain management when significant postoperative pain is anticipated. In these situations, it is administered after treatment has been completed. The value of this strategy is that the patient can benefit from an extended period of pain relief, up to 12 hours. This can allow time for oral pain medications to take effect.

Postoperative Self-Injury: An important factor when considering the use of bupivacaine is that it is not appropriate for individuals in which there is significant risk of self-injury due to prolonged anesthesia.

---

those requiring extended management of postoperative pain, or for unusually long treatment times, bupivacaine has proven quite effective (see Box 5–5).

Similarity to Other Local Anesthetics

Bupivacaine is chemically similar to mepivacaine.

MRD

0.6 mg/lb (1.3 mg/kg)

Absolute maximum recommended dose per appointment is 90 mg.

Bupivacaine will not be metabolized or cleared as quickly in the presence of a compromised cardiovascular system. Overdoses tend to be more severe and less easily reversed due to bupivacaine's greater cardiotoxicity (circulation is more likely to be compromised and cannot reduce blood levels as quickly, prolonging the overdose).

Relative Potency

Bupivacaine is eight times more potent than procaine, four times more potent than lidocaine, mepivacaine, and prilocaine, and nearly three times more potent than articaine. This accounts for the dilute concentration available in dentistry, 0.5% (see Figure 5–3).

Relative Toxicity

Bupivacaine is nearly eight times more toxic than procaine, five to six times more toxic than prilocaine, and nearly four times more toxic than lidocaine, mepivacaine, and articaine.

Bupivacaine toxicity is nearly equal to both the CNS and CVS (Levsky & Miller, 2005). In overdoses, two main factors contribute to the increased risk versus other drugs, bupivacaine's lengthy half-life and early CVS involvement (see Figure 5–4).

Reports of overdose have been characterized as *uncommon* but when they do occur, these events tend to be more difficult to reverse due to the early CVS involvement, which slows the removal of drugs from circulation (Levsky & Miller, 2005).

In dentistry, adverse events have been rare with bupivacaine for two important reasons: easier tracking of total doses with cartridges and lower maximum recommended doses compared with medicine, where MRDs may run as much as 2.5 times greater (Jastak et al, 1995; Levsky & Miller; Younessi & Punnia-Moorthy, 1999). While precautions based on toxicity are recommended when considering bupivacaine, there should be no hesitation to use it when circumstances clearly indicate an advantage over the other drugs, such as inadequate duration or the need for longer periods of pain relief (Younessi & Punnia-Moorthy, 1999).

Metabolism

Bupivacaine's metabolism is complex. The liver provides the major amidase metabolic pathway (Malamed, 2004a). Biotransformation of bupivacaine is much slower compared with the other local anesthetic drugs (Tetzlaff, 2000).

Excretion

Very little, to up to 16%, is excreted in the urine unchanged (Tetzlaff, 2000). As with other local anesthetic drugs higher excretion rates are more common when the pH of urine is low.

Vasoactivity

Bupivacaine is a very potent vasodilator; nevertheless it has long durations due to its strong protein receptor binding strength (see Figure 5–5).

In contrast to lidocaine, mepivacaine, articaine, and prilocaine, bupivacaine is a more aggressive vasodilator. It is distinguished not only as being the second most potent vasodilator of those discussed in this chapter (procaine is the most potent) but as the most durable of all drugs in dentistry, as well.

pKa

The pKa of bupivacaine is 8.1.

Bupivacaine's higher pKa translates into slower onset times. When bupivacaine is to be used, other rapid onset drugs such as mepivacaine and lidocaine may be administered first in order to allow treatment to begin sooner (see Table 5–2).

pH

The pH of bupivacaine solutions with 1:200,000 epinephrine = 3.0–4.5.

See Table 5–2.

Onset of Action

The onset of action for bupivacaine is 6 to 10 minutes.

Bupivacaine has the slowest onset of all the injectable drugs in dentistry and is up to five to ten times slower than mepivacaine and articaine in some situations.

Vasoconstrictor

Bupivacaine is available with epinephrine in dilutions of 1:200,000.

Bupivacaine in dentistry is prepared with epinephrine due to its vigorous vasodilative activity.

Despite inducing vigorous vasodilation in tissues, bupivacaine requires minimal epinephrine concentrations due to its potency.

Half-Life (t½)

The elimination half-life of bupivacaine is reported from 2.7–3.5 hours.

Bupivacaine has the longest half-life of all dental injectable local anesthetics (see Table 5–3).

Topical Applications

There are no topical applications of bupivacaine available in dentistry.

Pregnancy Category

Bupivacaine is in FDA Pregnancy Category C.

As previously stated, bupivacaine is not appropriate for routine use in dentistry, including in pregnancy (ADA/PDR, 2006; Meadows, 2001). Careful consideration and compelling rationale are necessary prior to using any Category C drug.

Safety in Lactation

It is unknown whether or not bupivacaine is excreted in human milk. Caution is advised (see Table 5–4).

PROCAINE

Background

Procaine was introduced by Alfred Einhorn in the early 1900s as an alternative to cocaine due to the desire to eliminate addictive tendencies when using local anesthetic drugs as well as the systemic toxicity and local tissue injury that too often accompanied cocaine's use (Tetzlaff, 2000). See Appendix 5–1.

Procaine is no longer available in dental cartridges; however, it is included in this discussion to represent the ester class of local anesthetics, none of which is currently packaged for dental administration. Procaine's proprietary name, Novocaine, has been synonymous with dental anesthesia for many years (Malamed, 2004a).

In the rare event a patient is allergic to all of the amide dental local anesthetic drugs, procaine or other selected esters may be substituted. Although not packaged for dentistry, procaine and other esters may be obtained in medical vials for use with hypodermic needles (see Figure 5–10 ■).

Formulations for Use in Dentistry

Although not currently available in dental cartridges, procaine can be obtained in medical vials in the following formulations (Malamed, 2004a):

   2% procaine plain (without vasoconstrictor)

   4% procaine plain (without vasoconstrictor)

   2% procaine with 1:100,000 epinephrine

   4% procaine with 1:100,000 epinephrine

Duration of Action

   2% procaine plain (without vasoconstrictor)

   4% procaine plain (without vasoconstrictor)
      Very short duration = no pulpal, 15–30 minutes soft tissue

   2% procaine with 1:100,000 epinephrine

   4% procaine with 1:100,000 epinephrine
      Intermediate duration = 60 minutes pulpal

Procaine is a vigorous vasodilator and is rapidly metabolized by plasma cholinesterase. Despite the 60 minute duration that may be available when combined with a vasoconstrictor, results have been variable with a greater number of individuals experiencing incomplete pain control during dental appointments compared with lidocaine. When considered along with procaine's *relatively* high incidence of inducing allergic reactions, procaine's disappearance from the dental market is understandable.

Similarity to Other Local Anesthetics

Procaine is similar to tetracaine. Both are esters. As is true of many of local anesthetics, procaine is an anticonvulsant (Tetzlaff, 2000).

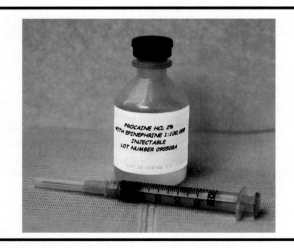

Procaine $C_{13}H_{20}N_2O_2$

H_2N —⟨ ⟩— $COOCH_2CH_2$ — N ⟨ C_2H_5 / C_2H_5 ⟩

2-(diethylamino)ethyl 4-aminobenzoate

■ **FIGURE 5–10**   2% Procaine, Epinephrine 1:100,000.

MRD

Consult product information monograph.

The potential for overdose is *very* low as long as solution is not deposited in vessels and doses do not exceed the MRD (Tetzlaff, 2000).

Relative Potency

Procaine is *significantly* less potent compared with all of the injectable amides in dentistry (Malamed, 2004a). This property, along with procaine's relatively high incidence of inducing allergic reactions (see Relative Toxicity discussion below), accounts for the decision by manufacturers to cease preparing procaine in dental cartridges by 1989.

It is half as potent as lidocaine, mepivacaine, and prilocaine, and approximately one-third as potent as articaine. It has only about 12% as potent as Bupivacaine. Except for situations in which no amides may be used, procaine is not desirable in dentistry (see Figure 5–3).

Relative Toxicity

Procaine is significantly less toxic compared with all of the amides in dentistry. Its rapid metabolism and complete avoidance of liver metabolism make it the safest drug of the six. When high plasma levels are reached quickly, as may happen in successive intravascular administrations, procaine has the ability to inhibit plasma cholinesterase activity, which may actually increase its potential for toxicity (Tetzlaff, 2000) (see Figure 5–4).

Procaine is a derivative of para-aminobenzoic acid (PABA), which is also its primary metabolite. PABA is thought to be responsible for procaine's relatively high rate of allergenicity (Jastak et al., 1995a). The recorded incidence of allergy to procaine is significant more for its rate of occurrence compared with the amides, than for its high overall rate of occurrence (Wilson, Deacock, Downie, & Zaki, 2000).

Metabolism

Procaine is rapidly metabolized via plasma cholinesterase. There are no hepatic pathways for its biotransformation (Malamed, 2004a; Tetzlaff, 2000).

Excretion

More than 2% is excreted unchanged by the kidneys (Malamed, 2004a). Higher excretion rates are more common when the pH of urine is low.

Vasoactivity

Procaine is a potent vasodilator (see Figure 5–5).

pKa

The pKa of procaine is 9.1.

As might be expected from procaine's high pKa value, onset of anesthesia is slow. Few base molecules are available initially. In addition to the availability of fewer base molecules, procaine has poor lipid solubility (Tetzlaff, 2000) (see Table 5–2).

pH

The pH of procaine plain is 5.0 to 6.5.

The pH of procaine with a vasoconstrictor is 3.5 to 5.5.

Procaine is virtually worthless as a plain preparation in dentistry; therefore its higher pH in plain form is not significant. When vasoconstrictors are added, pH levels drop to those approximating pH levels in other similar solutions (see Table 5–2).

Onset of Action

The onset of action for procaine is 6–10 minutes.

The onset of action of procaine is similar to bupivacaine. Procaine's pKa is high at 9.1.

Vasoconstrictor

Procaine can be obtained with epinephrine in dilutions of 1:100,000.

Half-Life (t½)

The elimination half-life of procaine is 6 minutes.

Due to its rather rapid hydrolysis via plasma cholinesterase, procaine is one of the safest drugs available (Tetzlaff, 2000). The elimination half-life is shortest of all dental local anesthetic injectable drugs (see Table 5–3).

Topical Applications

There are no topical applications for procaine in dentistry (Tetzlaff, 2000).

Pregnancy Category

Procaine is in FDA Pregnancy Category B.

Procaine is equal in safety during pregnancy to lidocaine and prilocaine. (ADA/PDR, 2006; Meadows, 2001).

Safety During Lactation

It is unknown whether or not procaine is excreted in human milk. Use with caution (ADA/PDR, 2006).

FDA PREGNANCY CATEGORIES

In determining the safe use of a drug in pregnancy, FDA guidelines and prescribing information should be consulted. The FDA provides guidance in the form of *drug categories in pregnancy* (ADA/PDR, 2006; Meadows, 2001). This information can be readily accessed online at http://www.fda.gov.

The following interpretations describe the categories for local anesthetic drugs included in this chapter:

Category A—No demonstrated increased risk of fetal abnormalities

Category B—No demonstrated increased risk in animal studies but no studies available in humans or animal studies have shown an increased risk, but well-controlled studies in humans failed to demonstrate any risk

Category C—Not enough information to determine at this time

A complete list of FDA Pregnancy Categories and their rationale is included in Table 5–5.

Dental local anesthetic drugs, including topical anesthetics, generally fall within Categories B and C. Injectable and topical lidocaine, prilocaine, and epinephrine in smaller doses (found in 2% lidocaine with 1:100,000 epinephrine, for example) fall within Category B. Articaine, benzocaine, bupivacaine, levonordefrin, and mepivacaine fall within Category C, as does epinephrine in larger doses.

What does this mean? In pregnancy, lidocaine, prilocaine, and smaller doses of epinephrine have demonstrated no increased risk of inducing or contributing to fetal abnormalities and, while not proven absolutely safe, are considered safe to use. Articaine, bupivacaine, levonordefrin, mepivacaine, and larger doses of epinephrine, while not necessarily unsafe, cannot refer to studies in pregnant women demonstrating fetal safety and they may actually have caused harm in animal studies. Careful consideration must be given before using any Category C drug.

CASE MANAGEMENT: Elena Gagarin

While most drugs may be found in breast milk, this is not seen as a particular problem. Amides are first pass drugs, which means they pass through the liver first and only lesser quantities would be available in breast milk. Even though the administration of local anesthetic drugs to nursing mothers is not thought to be significant, mothers who are concerned can be reassured if articaine is used because articaine possesses the anesthetic efficacy of the other amides yet it is much more quickly biotransformed by pseudocholinesterase.

Case Discussion: The half-life of articaine, even when maximum safe doses have been administered, is approximately 45 minutes. When less than maximum safe doses have been administered intraorally, the half-life has been demonstrated to be even less. In three hours, regardless, levels drop to a fraction of what they were initially (only about 1/8 to 1/16 the initial dose). This compares with lidocaine where there is nearly half the initial dose present at 3 hours. The percentage of any drug that actually enters breast milk is unknown and probably variable. If nursing mothers time their dental appointments carefully and articaine is used, only insignificant traces would be present once nursing commences. If blocks of the mandible are needed, Gow-Gates or Vazirani-Akinosi techniques are recommended due to the possible increased risk of paresthesia in inferior alveolar blocks.

CHAPTER QUESTIONS

1. The definition of the maximum recommended dose (MRD) of a drug best fits which *one* of the following definitions?
   a. A safe dose to administer in all situations
   b. A dose that a 150 pound individual can have
   c. A dose that cannot be exceeded under any circumstance
   d. A safe guideline when administering local anesthetic drugs

2. Which *one* of the following best describes articaine's metabolism?
   a. Articaine is metabolized approximately 25% in the liver.
   b. Articaine is metabolized primarily via plasma cholinesterase.
   c. Much of articaine is excreted unchanged.
   d. Articaine's metabolism is similar to prilocaine's.

3. You are treating a patient with significant cardiovascular compromise who suffers from significant liver damage. Which one of the following drugs would be most appropriate for this patient when you are anesthetizing the maxillary right quadrant?
   a. 2% lidocaine, 1:100,000 epinephrine
   b. 3% mepivacaine plain
   c. 4% articaine, 1:200,000 epinephrine
   d. 0.5% bupivacaine, 1:200,000 epinephrine

4. A periodontist requires hemostasis on palatal tissues in the maxillary left quadrant prior to elevating a surgical flap. Which one of the following drugs would furnish the most vigorous hemostasis?
   a. 2% mepivacaine, 1:20,000 levonordefrin
   b. 4% prilocaine, 1:200,000 epinephrine
   c. 2% lidocaine, 1:50,000 epinephrine
   d. 4% articaine, 1:100,000 epinephrine

5. Which characteristic of a local anesthetic drug determines how well it works without a vasoconstrictor?
   a. Potency
   b. Vasoactivity
   c. pKa
   d. Lipophilic ability

6. If a patient is taking a tricyclic antidepressant and a beta-blocker, which *one* of the following drugs would be most appropriate to administer?
   a. 2% lidocaine, 1:100,000 epinephrine
   b. 2% mepivacaine, 1:20,000 levonordefrin
   c. 3% mepivacaine plain
   d. 4% articaine, 1:200,000 epinephrine

7. Methemoglobinemia is a life-threatening condition that may be precipitated by which *one* of the following drugs?
   a. lidocaine
   b. mepivacaine
   c. prilocaine
   d. bupivacaine

8. Arrange the injectable local anesthetic drugs in descending order of *overall* CNS and CVS toxicity.
   a. Bupivacaine, mepivacaine, lidocaine, prilocaine, articaine
   b. Bupivacaine, mepivacaine, lidocaine, articaine, prilocaine
   c. Bupivacaine, mepivacaine, articaine, lidocaine, prilocaine
   d. Bupivacaine, lidocaine, mepivacaine, articaine, prilocaine

REFERENCES

ADA/PDR Guide to Dental Therapeutics (4th ed.). Montvale, NJ: Thompson PDR Corporation, 2006.

Atanasov, N., Popivanova, N., & Yochev, S. (1981). Liver carboxylesterase in the serum of viral hepatitis patients. *Folia Med (plovdiv), 23*(3–4), 61–63.

Carbocaine: Prescribing information available from Carestream Health, Atlanta, GA; www.kodakdental.com.

Chan, Lingtak-Neander, PharmD, BCNSP, Associate Professor, Department of Pharmacy and Graduate Program in Nutritional Sciences, University of Washington, Seattle, WA. Personal correspondence.

Citanest and Citanest Forte: Prescribing information available from AstraZeneca, Wilmington, DE; www.astra.com.

Daniel, S. J., Harfst, S. A. (2007). *Dental hygiene concepts, cases, and competencies* (2nd ed.). St. Louis: Mosby.

Dasgupta, D. D., Tendulkar, B. A., Paul, T. T., Satoskar, R. S. (1984) Comparative study of centbucridine and lignocaine for subarachnoid block. *Journal of Postgraduate Medicine, 30,* 207–209.

De Toledo, J. C. (2000). Lidocaine and seizures, *Therapeutic Drug Monitoring, 22,* 320–322.

Dower, J. S. (2007). Letter to the American Dental Association: Anesthetic study questioned. *Journal of the American Dental Association, 138*(6), 708–709.

Dower, J. S. (2003, February). A review of paresthesia in association with administration of local anesthesia. *Dentistry Today,* 8–13.

EMLA Cream and Anesthetic Disc: Prescribing information available from Astra Pharmaceuticals, Wayne, PA; www.astra.com. 1999.

Haas, D. A., & Lennon, D. (1995). A 21-year retrospective study of reports of paresthesia following local anesthetic administration. *Journal of the Canadian Dental Association, 61*(4), 319–320, 323–326, 329–330.

Harn, S. D., & Durham, T. M. (1990a). Incidence of lingual trauma and postinjection complications in conventional mandibular block anesthesia. *Journal of the American Dental Association, 121*(4), 519–523.

Harn, S. D., & Durham, T. M. (1990b). Incidence of lingual nerve trauma and postinjection complications in conventional mandibular block anesthesia. *Journal of the American Dental Association, 121*(4), 523.

Hawkins, M. (2006, October 16). *Local anesthesia: Technique and pharmacology, problems and solutions.* ADA Annual Session. Las Vegas, NV.

Hjelle, J. J., & Grauer, G. F. (1986). Acetaminophen-induced toxicosis in dogs and cats, *Journal of American Veterinary Medical Association, 188*(7), 742–749.

Jastak, J. T., Yagiela, J. A., & Donaldson, D. (1995a, pp. 87–126). *Local anesthesia of the oral cavity.* Philadelphia: Saunders.

Jastak, J. T., Yagiela, J. A., & Donaldson, D. (1995b, pp. 96–98). *Local anesthesia of the oral cavity.* Philadelphia: Saunders.

Jastak, J. T., Yagiela, J. A., & Donaldson, D. (1995c, p. 115). *Local anesthesia of the oral cavity.* Philadelphia: Saunders.

Jastak, J. T., Yagiela, J. A., & Donaldson, D. (1995d, p. 100–102). *Local anesthesia of the oral cavity.* Philadelphia: Saunders.

Jastak, J. T., Yagiela, J. A., & Donaldson, D. (1995e, p. 104–107). *Local anesthesia of the oral cavity.* Philadelphia: Saunders.

Kamel, K. S., Cheema-Dhadli, S., & Halperin, M. L. (2002). Studies on the pathophysiology of the low urine pH in patients with uric acid stones. *Kidney International, 61,* 988–994.

Kitagawa, N., Oda, M., Totoke, T. (2004). Possible mechanism of irreversible nerve injury caused by local anesthetics: Detergent properties of local anesthetics and membrane disruption. *Anesthesiology, 100*(4), 962–967.

Levsky, M. E., & Miller, M. A. (2005, October 24). Cardiovascular collapse from low dose bupivacaine. *Canadian Journal of Clinical Pharmacology, 12*(3), e240–245.

Luthra, M., Davids, M. R., Shafiee, M. A., & Halperin, M. L. (2004). Anorexia nervosa and chronic renal insufficiency: A prescription for disaster. *Quarterly Journal of Medicine, 97,* 167–178.

Maalouf, N. M., Cameron, M. A., Moe, O. W., Adams-Huet, B., & Sakhaee, K. (2007). Low urine pH: A novel feature of the metabolic syndrome. *Clinical Journal of the American Society of Nephrology, 2,* 883–888.

Malamed, S. F. (2004a) *Handbook of local anesthesia* (5th ed., pp. 27–81). St. Louis: Elsevier Mosby.

Malamed, S. F. (2004b) *Handbook of local anesthesia* (5th ed., pp. 60–61). St. Louis: Elsevier Mosby.

Malamed, S. F. (2004c) *Handbook of local anesthesia* (5th ed., pp. 213–217). St. Louis: Elsevier Mosby.

Malamed, S. F. (2004d) *Handbook of local anesthesia* (5th ed., pp. 349–360). St. Louis: Elsevier Mosby.

Malamed, S. F., Gagnon, S., & Leblanc, D. (2001). Articaine hydrochloride: A study of the safety of a new amide local anesthetic. *Journal of the American Dental Association, 132,* 177–185.

Malamed, S. F., Gagnon, S., & Leblanc, D. (2000). Efficacy of articaine: A new amide local anesthetic. *Journal of the American Dental Association, 131,* 635–642.

Marcaine 0.5%: Prescribing information available from Eastman Kodak, Rochester, NY; www.kodakdental.com.

Meadows, M. (2001, May–June). Pregnancy and the drug dilemma. *FDA Consumer Magazine.*

Moore, P. A. (1999, April) Adverse drug interactions in dental practice: Interactions associated with local anesthetics, sedatives and anxiolytics. *Journal of the American Dental Association,* 541–554.

Oertel, R., Berndt, A., & Kirch, W. (1996). Saturable in vitro metabolism of articaine by serum esterases: Does it contribute to the persistence of the local anesthetic effect? *Regional Anesthesia and Pain Medicine, 21,* 576–581.

Oertel, R., Rahn, R., Kirch, W.: Clinical pharmacokinetics of articaine. *Clinical Pharmacokinetics, 33,* 417–425, 1997.

Oertel, R., Ulrike, E., Rahn, R., & Kirch, W. (1999). The effect of age on phamacokinetics of the local anesthetic drug articaine. *Regional Anesthesia and Pain Medicine, 24*(6), 524–528.

Oraqix: Prescribing information available from Dentsply Pharmaceuticals, York, PA, www.dentsplypharma.com.

Park, C. J., Park, S. A., Yoon, T. G., Lee, S. J., Yum, K. W., & Kim, H. J. (2005, September). Bupivacaine induces apoptosis via ROS in the Schwann cell line. *Journal of Dental Research, 84*(9), 852–857.

Pogrel, M. A., Schmidt, B. L., Sambajon, V., & Jordan, R. C. K. (2003). Lingual nerve damage due to inferior alveolar nerve blocks: A possible explanation. *Journal of the American Dental Association, 134*(2), 195–199.

Pogrel, M. A., &, Thamby, S. (2000). Permanent nerve involvement resulting from inferior alveolar nerve blocks. *Journal of the American Dental Association, 131*(7), 901–907.

Prescott, L. F. (1996). *Paracetamol (acetaminophen): A critical bibliographic review.* Philadelphia: Taylor & Francis.

Septocaine hydrochloride: Prescribing information available from Septodont, Inc., New Castle, DE; www.septodontinc.com.

Simon, M. A., Vree, T. B., Gielen, M. J., & Booij, L. H. (1997, April). Comparison of the disposition kinetics of lidocaine and (+/−) prilocaine in 20 patients undergoing intravenous regional anaesthesia during day case surgery. *Journal of Clinical Pharmacology and Therapeutics, 22,* 141–146.

Takahashi, S., Inokuchi, T., Kobayashi, T., Ka, T., Tsutsumi, Z., Moriwaki, Y. et al. (2007). Relationship between insulin resistance and low urinary pH in patients with gout, and effects of PPAR alpha agonists on urine pH. *Hormone and Metabolic Research, 39*(7), 511–514.

Tetzlaff, J. E. (2000). Clinical pharmacology of local anesthetics (1st ed.). Woburn, MA: Butterworth-Heinemann.

Vacharajani, G. N., Parikh, N., Paul, T., & Satoskar, R. S. (1983). A comparative study of centbucridine and lidocaine in dental extraction. *International Journal of Clinical Pharmacology Research, 3*(4), 251–255.

van Oss, G. E. C. J. M., Vree, T. B., Baars, A. M., Termond, E. F. S., & Booij, L. H. D. J. (1988). Clinical effects and pharmacokinetics of articainic acid in one volunteer after intravenous administration. *Pharmaceutisch Weekblad (Scientific edition) 10,* 284–286.

van Oss, G. E. C. J. M., Vree, T. B., Baars, A. M., Termond, E. F. S., & Booij, L. H. D. (1989). Pharmacokinetics, metabolism, and renal excretion of articaine and its metabolite articainic acid in patients after epidural administration. *European Journal of Anaesthesiology, 6,* 49–56.

Vree, T. B., Baars, A. M., van Oss, G. E. C. J. M., & Booij, L. H. D. J. (1988). High-performance liquid chromatography and preliminary pharmacokinetics of articaine and its 2-carbomethoxy metabolite in human serum and urine. *Journal of Chromatography, 424,* 440–444.

Wahl, M. J., Schmitt, M. M., Overton, D. A., & Gordon, M. K. (2002). Injection pain of bupivacaine with epinephrine vs. prilocaine plain. *Journal of the American Dental Association, 133*(12), 1652–1656.

Wilson, A. W., Deacock, S., Downie, I. P., & Zaki, G. (2000). Allergy to local anesthetic: the importance of thorough investigation, *British Dental Journal, 188,* 320–322.

Younessi, B. S., Punnia-Moorthy, A. (1999). Cardiovascular effects of bupivacaine and the role of this agent in preemptive dental analgesia. *Journal of the American Dental Society of Anesthesia, 46*(2), 56–62.

Xylocaine dental ointment 5%: Prescription information available from Astra Pharmaceutical Products, Westborough, MA; www.astra.com.

Xylocaine hydrochloride: Prescription information available from Astra Pharmaceutical Products, Westborough, MA; www.astra.com.

Zorcaine (Articaine hydrochloride 4%), local anesthetic with epinephrine 1:100,000: Prescription information available from Kodak Dental Systems, Carestream Health, Rochester, NY; www.kodakdental.com.

Dental Local Anesthetic Drugs*

Local Anesthetic Drugs Color Coded Box	MRD (mg/lb)	MRD (mg/kg)	MRD Absolute	pH	Half-Life t½	Pulpal Anesthesia (in minutes)
4% Articaine (w/ vaso)	3.2	7.0	500	4.4–5.2	45**	75
4% Articaine (w/ vaso)	3.2	7.0	500	4.4–5.2	45**	45
0.5% Bupivacaine (w/ vaso)	0.6	1.3	90	3.0–4.5	260	90–180
2% Lidocaine (plain)	2.0	4.4	300	6.5	96	5–10
2% Lidocaine (w/ vaso)	2.0	4.4	300	3.3–5.5	96	60
2% Lidocaine (w/ vaso)	2.0	4.4	300	3.3–5.5	96	60
3% Mepivacaine (plain)	2.0	4.4	300	4.5–6.8	114	20–40
2% Mepivacaine (w/ vaso)	2.0	4.4	300	3.0–3.5	114	60
4% Prilocaine (plain)	2.7	6.0	400	4.5–6.8	96	10–15 infiltration(I) 40–60 block (B)
4% Prilocaine (w/ vaso)	2.7	6.0	400	3.0–4.0	96	60–90

*Drug inserts for each drug should be consulted prior to use. Recommended doses in this table may be equal to or lower than those recommended by manufacturers.

**Values after maximum recommended dosing per Septocaine product monographs (SEPTODONT, Inc., New Castle, DE).

Soft Tissue Anesthesia (in minutes)	Vasoconstrictor	Relative Potency	Relative Toxicity	Duration Category
		(Reference value = lidocaine @100%)		
180–300	Epinephrine 1:100,000	150%	100%	Intermediate
120–300	Epinephrine 1:200,000	150%	100%	Intermediate
240–540	Epinephrine 1:200,000	400%	Less than 400%	Long
60–120	None	100%	100%	Very short
180–300	Epinephrine 1:50,000	100%	100%	Intermediate
180–300	Epinephrine 1:100,000	100%	100%	Intermediate
120–180	None	100%	75%–100%	Short
180–300	Levonordefrin 1:20,000	100%	75%–100%	Intermediate
90–120 (I) 120–240 (B)	None	100%	60%	Short (I) Intermediate (B)
180–480	Epinephrine 1:200,000	100%	60%	Intermediate

Chapter 6

Vasoconstrictors in Dentistry

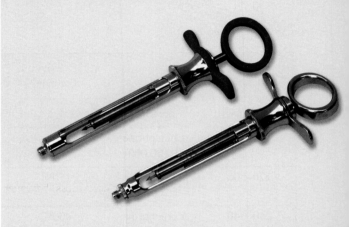

OBJECTIVES

- Define and discuss the key terms in this chapter.
- Discuss the overall similarities and differences among vasoconstrictors.
- Discuss clinical situations in which the choice of vasoconstrictor may directly affect anesthetic success.
- Discuss and determine situations in which specific vasoconstrictors may be indicated or contraindicated.
- Discuss the difference in potency between epinephrine and levonordefrin.

KEY TERMS

adrenergic **83**
adverse events **85**
epinephrine **83**
catecholamine **83**
felypressin **90**

levonordefrin **83**
norepinephrine **83**
phenylephrine **90**
sympathomimetic **83**
vasopressors **83**

CASE STUDY: Elena Gagarin

Elena Gagarin is free of dental pain or any other dental problems. Her doctor prescribed a tricyclic antidepressant for her and shortly after she started taking it, a cusp fractured on #14, which already had a very large restoration.

INTRODUCTION

Vasoconstrictors enhance local anesthetic drugs in a number of important ways (Agency for Healthcare Research and Quality [AHRQ], 2002; Jastak, Yagiela, Donaldson, 1995; Yagiela, 1999). They constrict local vessels, increasing safety by slowing systemic absorption. This constriction also prolongs the local actions of the drugs, increases their profoundness, and provides hemostasis (Jastak et al., 1995).

Vasoconstrictors are particularly useful in dental settings where long durations and more profound anesthesia are routinely required. Their usefulness, however, comes at the expense of physiologic and pharmacologic considerations. A 1999 report prepared for the American Dental Association, for example, states that vasoconstrictors have been associated with more drug interactions than any other drugs in dentistry (Yagiela, 1999). An interesting and frequently overlooked fact is that the systemic uptake of vasoconstrictors is increased by the vasodilating properties of the local anesthetic drugs with which they are combined (Yagiela, 1999). In other words, while vasoconstrictors decrease the systemic toxicity of local anesthetic drugs, local anesthetic drugs increase the toxicity of vasoconstrictors (Yagiela, 1999).

When clinicians are knowledgeable about the physiologic and pharmacologic effects of vasoconstrictors and administer them appropriately, the benefits usually outweigh the risks and they remain an essential part of the practice of pain control in dentistry.

This chapter will discuss the pharmacology of vasoconstrictors used in dentistry with an emphasis on epinephrine and levonordefrin.

VASOCONSTRICTORS IN DENTISTRY

There are two vasoconstrictors, also known as **vasopressors,** which are routinely found in dental local anesthetic drugs in North America, epinephrine and levonordefrin. Epinephrine represents the benchmark for vasoconstrictors in dental local anesthesia. Levonordefrin is a useful substitute.

Adrenergic Actions of Vasoconstrictors

Epinephrine is a naturally occurring **catecholamine** or neurotransmitter, along with **norepinephrine** and dopamine. Unlike epinephrine, **levonordefrin** is a *synthetic* catecholamine. Both epinephrine and levonordefrin stimulate **adrenergic** receptors, the targets of the catecholamines within the tissues. They belong to a larger group of drugs that include both catecholamine and noncatecholamine adrenergic stimlators known as sympathomimetic amines (see Table 6–1 ■) (Malamed, 2004).

Epinephrine (Adrenalin) is also referred to as a **sympathomimetic** drug, which means it mimics sympathetic nervous system mediators such as endogenous epinephrine and norepinephrine. The sympathetic nervous system may be described as quickly responsive ("fight or flight") while the parasympathetic system may be described as functioning more slowly ("rest and digest"). Other sympathomimetic drugs used in local anesthetic solutions include levonordefrin (Neo-Cobefrin) and phenylephrine.

Sympathomimetic drugs can be classified as direct-acting, indirect-acting, and mixed-acting. These classifications refer to the manner in which the drugs exert their influence on adrenergic receptors. An example of adrenergic receptor activity is found in their effects on the smooth muscle walls of peripheral blood vessels. An initial adrenergic (sympathomimetic) receptor effect on these structures results in vasoconstriction, slowing the uptake of anesthetic drugs into vessels (see Table 6–2 ■).

Table 6–1	Common Sympathomimetic Amines	
Catecholamines	*Noncatecholamines***
Epinephrine*	Amphetamine
Norepinephrine*	Methamphetamine
Levonordefrin	Ephedrine
Dopamine*	Phenylephrine

*Naturally-occurring chemicals
**All are examples of chemicals found in street drugs, diet pills and cold medications
Source: Malamed, 2004.

Table 6–2 Sympathomimetic Drug Influence on Adrenergic Receptors		
Direct Acting	*Indirect Acting*	*Mixed Acting*
Epinephrine	Tyramine	Metaraminol
Norepinephrine	Amphetamine	Ephedrine
Levonordefrin	Methamphetamine	
Isoproterenol	Hydroxyamphetamine	
Dopamine		
Methoxamine		
Phenylephrine		

Source: Malamed, 2004.

Direct-acting drugs are similar to endogenous epinephrine and norepinephrine, providing direct stimulation of adrenergic receptors on susceptible cells and tissues. Examples of direct-acting sympathomimetic drugs include synthetic or exogenous epinephrine and norepinephrine, levonordefrin (Neo-Cobefrin), dopamine, isoproterenol, methoxamine, and phenylephrine.

Indirect-acting drugs block the removal or recycling of epinephrine and norepinephrine, resulting in a buildup of both, which in turn causes overstimulation of adrenergic receptors. Indirect-acting drugs include amphetamine, methamphetamine, and hydroxyamphetamine. Cocaine, an ester-type local anesthetic drug, also has significant indirect adrenergic stimulating effects.

Mixed-acting drugs have both direct and indirect effects on adrenergic receptors. Mixed-acting drugs include metaraminol and ephedrine.

Vasoconstriction is provided by the temporary actions of these drugs on smooth muscle walls of blood vessels. The slowing of vascular uptake in the areas in which local anesthetic drugs with vasoconstrictors are deposited allows more time for the drugs to enter nerve membranes and block receptor sites. In addition to enabling more efficient activity of local anesthetic drugs on nerve membranes, there is at least some direct action of epinephrine that results in decreased sensation (Tetzlaff, 2000).

Two types of adrenergic receptors were identified by Ahlquist in 1948, alpha (α) and beta (β) (Ahlquist, 1948). Since that time, subcategories have been identified, which explain specific actions of vasoconstrictors. Alpha (α) receptors are responsible for smooth muscle contraction in peripheral arterioles and veins throughout the body (peripheral vasoconstriction) (ADA/PDR,

2006). Beta 1 (β_1) receptors are responsible for cardiac stimulation and Beta 2 (β_2) receptors are responsible for smooth muscle relaxation such as bronchodilation and vasodilation (ADA/PDR, 2006). Both α and β receptors contribute to the potential for cardiac dysrhythmias (ADA/PDR, 2006). A summary of selected effects and affected organs and can be found in Table 6–3 ■.

Use or Avoidance of Vasoconstrictors

The use or avoidance of vasoconstrictors in some situations remains a controversial topic (AHRQ, 2002). Avoiding vasoconstrictors based on their impact on blood pressure alone, for example, may be misguided. Plain drugs, such as 3% mepivacaine, may not always provide profound anesthesia. A lack of profound anesthesia can result in unmanageable pain, which in turn can lead to unpredictable spikes in blood pressure due to the endogenous release of epinephrine. The endogenous release can exceed administered doses of epinephrine.

When discussing vasoconstrictors, it is helpful to remember that dental appointments can be stressful and that endogenous epinephrine released from the adrenal glands may increase prior to and during appointments. Endogenous release can increase the adverse adrenergic effects of exogenous (injected) epinephrine. It has been suggested that exogenous epinephrine may actually stimulate endogenous release by its direct action on adrenergic receptors of the adrenal glands (Takahashi, Nakano, Sano, & Kanri, 2005). This type of release might occur, for example, if a patient who is particularly fearful of dental appointments is given modest amounts of epinephrine yet displays signs and symptoms of an epinephrine overdose where none technically exists.

Table 6–3   Selected α and β Adrenergic Effects on CVS and Respiratory Systems*

CARDIOVASCULAR SYSTEM		
	Receptors Affected	*Action(s)*
Heart rate	β_1, β_2	Increased (may be blocked or reversed by vagal reflex activity)
Contractile force	β_1, β_2	Increased
Coronary arterioles	$\alpha_1, \alpha_2, \beta_2$	Constriction/Dilation (subject to local control)
Peripheral resistance	$\alpha_1 \ \alpha_2, \beta_2$	Increased/Decreased
RESPIRATORY SYSTEM		
Bronchiole smooth muscle	β_1	Relaxation
Pulmonary arterioles	α_1, β_2	Constriction/Dilation (subject to local control)

*Data from Table 3–3: Systemic Effects of Adrenergic Amines, in J. T. Jastak, J. A. Yagiela, & D. Donaldson D, *Local Anesthesia of the Oral Cavity*, Philadelphia, 1995, WB Saunders, p. 7.

The endogenous release might be responsible for the excessive amounts of epinephrine in the circulation. While current protocol recognizes that exogenous epinephrine from dental cartridges causes more significant stimulation than endogenous release, the impact of the potential endogenous release is far less predictable due to the difficulty in anticipating quantities that might be released (Cryer, 1980; Yagiela, 1991).

Adrenergic vasoconstrictors used in dental procedures typically do not produce noticeable effects but are capable of causing undesired local and systemic reactions (Yagiela, 1999). Local effects may include ischemia and necrosis while systemic effects may include changes in arterial blood pressure, palpitations, dysrhythmias, and even permanent injury or death due to ventricular fibrillation, heart attack, or stroke (Yagiela, 1999). Overdose, intravascular administration, drug interactions, and intolerance increase the risks of these adverse events (Yagiela, 1999).

Fortunately, most **adverse events** associated with the use of vasoconstrictors are short-lived. This is due to their efficient reuptake in synapses and the rapid removal and biotransformation of any residual portions that enter the bloodstream (Jastak et al., 1995). The term *adverse events* refers to the undesired effects which occur in response to the pharmacologic actions of a drug, including the events surrounding its administration.

While highly unlikely, clinicians must nevertheless be aware of the possibility of more serious consequences when using these drugs. Malamed refers to the American Dental and American Heart Association joint statement on vasoconstrictors in local anesthetics when addressing this topic: "Vasoconstrictor agents should be used only when it is clear that the procedure will be shortened or the analgesia rendered more profound. When a vasoconstrictor is indicated, extreme care should be taken to avoid intravascular injection. The minimum possible amount of vasoconstrictor should be used" (Malamed, 2004).

EPINEPHRINE

As previously mentioned, epinephrine is a naturally occurring catecholamine. Epinephrine is used in dentistry as a potent vasoconstrictor that both enhances profound anesthesia and increases the safe use of local anesthetic drugs.

In both medicine and dentistry, epinephrine has other important uses including the reversal of generalized anaphylaxis and bronchospasm. In ophthalmology and optometry, epinephrine-induced mydriasis (dilation of the pupils) is used to augment diagnosis and treatment.

Epinephrine provides nearly equal α and β effects, however not at the same time. Initial α vasoconstriction of peripheral vasculature allows time for anesthetic drugs to bind to receptor sites. Later, β_2 vasodilation predominates. This has been observed before and after surgery where epinephrine has been administered. Initially, α effects enhance profound, durable anesthesia and reduce hemorrhaging at surgical sites. Postoperatively, the dominant β_2 effects can result in increased bleeding approximately 6 hours after surgery (Malamed, 2004; Sveen, 1979).

Due to its nearly equal effects on both α and β adrenergic receptors, epinephrine is the drug of choice in responding to generalized anaphylaxis. Simply stated, anaphylaxis presents as peripheral vasodilation and bronchial constriction. Epinephrine's α adrenergic stimulation provides peripheral vasoconstriction (reversing the vigorous vasodilation) and its β adrenergic stimulation provides bronchodilation (relieving breathing difficulties).

Vasoconstrictor concentration is expressed as a dilution ratio of milligrams of drug to milliliters of solution (mg/ml) into which it is dissolved. A dilution ratio of 1:1000 epinephrine is equivalent to one gram in one liter, expressed as 1000 mg/1000 ml = 1mg/ml. A dilution ratio of 1:100,000 is equivalent to one gram in 100 liters, expressed as 1000 mg/100,000 ml = 1mg/100 ml or 0.01 mg/ml.

Epinephrine is added to local anesthetic solutions in North America in concentrations of 1:50,000, 1:100,000, and 1:200,000 (see Figure 6–1 ■). Dilutions of 1:50,000 contain four times the quantity of vasoconstrictor as 1:200,000. While there may be therapeutic benefit at times, such as the more vigorous hemostasis provided by this higher concentration to control bleeding during surgical procedures, there is questionable rationale for the use of dilutions of 1:50,000 epinephrine in a majority of clinical situations (Malamed, 2004). Its use may be more common in dental specialties. All

dilutions contribute to profound and durable anesthesia in combination with local anesthetic drugs.

The maximum dose of epinephrine for use in dentistry in healthy individuals has been determined to be 0.2 mg per appointment. In significant cardiovascular compromise (ASA categories III & IV), the maximum dose is reduced to 0.04 mg, which is 20% of the standard maximum dose of epinephrine (Special Committee of the New York Heart Association, 1955; see Chapter 7, "Dose Calculations for Local Anesthetic Solutions"; see Chapter 10, "Patient Assessment for Local Anesthesia").

Other dose reductions may apply in selected situations, including elderly populations and in the presence of a number of specific drug interactions (Lindquist & Ettinger, 2003; Special Committee of the New York Heart Association, 1955; Yagiela, 1999).

Summary of Actions on Specific Systems and Tissues

Myocardium: Increased cardiac output and heart rate

Pacemaker cells: Increased incidence of dysrhythmias

Coronary arteries: Increased coronary artery blood flow

Blood Pressure: Increased systole; decreased diastole (except increased in higher doses)

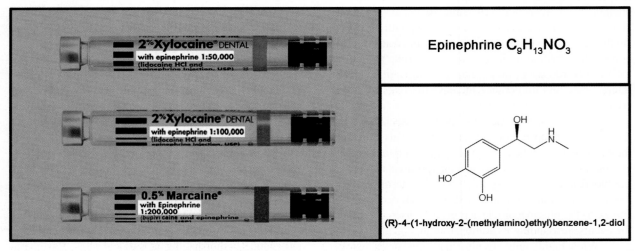

Epinephrine $C_9H_{13}NO_3$

(R)-4-(1-hydroxy-2-(methylamino)ethyl)benzene-1,2-diol

■ **FIGURE 6–1** Epinephrine Dilutions. Epinephrine is added to local anesthetic solutions in dilutions of 1:50,000, 1:100,000, and 1:200,000.

Source: Modified courtesy of DENTSPLY Pharmaceutical.

CVS: Decreased cardiac efficiency

Vasculature: α vasoconstriction in skin and mucous membranes; β$_2$ vasodilation in skeletal muscle vasculature (lower doses); α vasoconstriction (higher doses)

Hemostasis: α vasoconstriction initially (higher doses), then β$_2$ vasodilation after six hours

Respiratory: β$_2$ vasodilation of bronchiole smooth muscle

CNS: In therapeutic doses, not a potent stimulant

Other Noncardiac Effects: Increased oxygen consumption in all tissues may occur.

In addition, epinephrine can decrease the hypoglycemic effects of insulin resulting in elevated blood sugar levels (see Box 6–1).

Termination of Action: Reuptake by adrenergic nerves and once absorbed, catechol-0-methyltransferase (COMT) and monamine oxidase (MAO) inactivation

Effect on Endogenous Epinephrine Release: The exact mechanism is unknown although it has been suggested by some that adrenomedullary stimulation by exogenous epinephrine on presynaptic β-receptors may be responsible for endogenous releases (Takahashi et al., 2005).

Sources: Jastak et al., 1995; Malamed, 2004; Sveen, 1979; Takahashi et al., 2005.

LEVONORDEFRIN

Levonordefrin is the only synthetic catecholamine available in dental cartridges in North America. It is considered to have about one-sixth the potency of epinephrine and therefore requires more concentrated dilutions in dental cartridges to exert effects similar to epinephrine (Malamed, 2004). It also differs from epinephrine in its actions on adrenergic receptors. Unlike epinephrine's 50% α and 50% β effects, levonordefrin's action is primarily α, 75% versus 25% β (Jastak et al., 1995). As a weak stimulator of beta adrenergic receptors, it is similar to norepinephrine, which is approximately 90% α (Jastak et al. 1995). Despite levonordefrin's major effect on α receptors, epinephrine is a more powerful vasoconstrictor of peripheral vasculature, thus providing much better hemostasis (control of bleeding).

Box 6–1   Others Considerations Prior to Using Vasoconstrictors

Other important considerations before the use of vasoconstrictors include evaluation for situations where specific tissues of the body are at greater risk of injury due to vasoconstriction. For example, this may be the case when there is a history of stroke, radiation therapy, or *brittle* diabetes with underlying cardiovascular disease, as described below.

A history of a cerebrovascular accident (CVA or stroke) increases the risk of experiencing a subsequent CVA due to increases in blood pressure in response to vasoconstrictors.

Radiation therapy increases the risk of osteonecrosis (known as osteoradionecrosis after irradiation of the bone in question) due to a resultant compromise of the vascular bed. Vasoconstrictors can further compromise the vascular bed depriving the bony tissues of oxygen, nutrients, and bone-forming cells needed to maintain vitality.

Epinephrine can decrease the hypoglycemic effects of insulin. This may be a particular problem in diabetics who are taking large doses of insulin, frequently referred to as *brittle* diabetics, especially those with underlying cardiovascular disease. The insulin they take is often ineffective at maintaining consistent blood sugar levels, instead alternating between severe hypo- and hyper-glycemic episodes. A consultation with the patient's physician can help determine their status. Epinephrine can generally be given to well-controlled diabetics without special precautions.

Source: Budenz, 2000; Little, Falace, Miller, & Rhodus, 2008; Malamed, 2004.

Levonordefrin is less potent compared with epinephrine and is formulated in dilutions of 1:20,000, which are five times more concentrated (less diluted) than 1:100,000 epinephrine solutions (see Figure 6–2 ■). Two percent mepivacaine with 1:20,000 levonordefrin provides an excellent alternative to 2% lidocaine with 1:100,000 epinephrine in most clinical situations, and in specific situations in which epinephrine may be contraindicated, such as when other specific drugs are being taken.

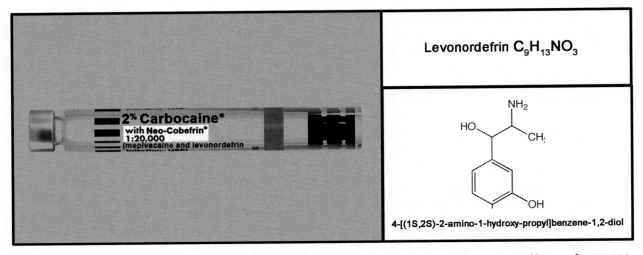

FIGURE 6–2 Levonordefrin Dilutions. Levonordefrin is added to local anesthetic solutions in a dilution of 1:20,000. Levonordefrin is much weaker than epinephrine and is formulated in a dilution that is five times more concentrated (less diluted) to provide similar efficacy of the local anesthetic drug.
Source: Modified courtesy of DENTSPLY Pharmaceutical.

Summary of Actions on Specific Systems and Tissues

In general, levonordefrin has less effect on the adrenergic receptors of the cardiovascular and cardiopulmonary systems compared to epinephrine (Jastak et al., 1995; Malamed, 2004). The lack of significant β stimulation tends to negate the advantages of levonordefrin's widespread decreases in adrenergic stimulation. Epinephrine's ability to dilate the smooth muscles of the bronchioles gives it a significant advantage over levonordefrin. Epinephrine also provides much better hemostasis, as previously mentioned.

In the concentrations found in the single dental formulation (2% mepivacaine with 1:20,000), levonordefrin provides an equivalent duration of local anesthetic activity compared to 1:100,000 epinephrine. When comparing their relative abilities to provide durable anesthesia in *appropriate* concentrations, levonordefrin and epinephrine are essentially equivalent.

Myocardium: Increased cardiac output and heart rate, but less than epinephrine

Pacemaker cells: Increased incidence of dysrhythmias, but less than epinephrine

Coronary arteries: Increased coronary artery blood flow, but less than epinephrine

Blood Pressure: Increased systole, but less than epinephrine. Decreased diastole, except increased in higher doses

CVS: Decreased cardiac efficiency

Vasculature: α vasoconstriction in skin and mucous membranes but less than epinephrine; β₂ vasodilation in skeletal muscle vasculature (lower doses); α vasoconstriction (higher doses) but less than epinephrine

Hemostasis: Much less effective than epinephrine

Respiratory: Vasodilation of bronchiole smooth muscle but much less than epinephrine

CNS: In therapeutic doses, a less potent stimulant compared to epinephrine

Metabolism: Elevated blood sugar but less than epinephrine. Increased oxygen consumption in all tissues but less than epinephrine

Termination of Action: Reuptake by adrenergic nerves and COMT inactivation

Effect on Endogenous Epinephrine Release: Unknown mechanism but less than epinephrine

DOSAGE DISCUSSION

Determining the dose of vasoconstrictor drug in a given volume of solution requires an understanding of dilution ratios, standard cartridge volumes, the defined maximum recommended dose for each drug, and relevant patient factors such as general health status and weight.

A thorough discussion of methods for calculation of vasoconstrictor doses can be found in Chapter 7, "Dose Calculations for Local Anesthetic Solutions."

TOXICITY & BIOTRANSFORMATION OF VASOCONSTRICTORS

Vasoconstrictor toxicity results from excessive stimulation of adrenergic receptors. High plasma levels of epinephrine have been described as inevitable soon after administration and typically result in increased heart rate and systolic blood pressure (Clutter, Bier, Shah, & Cryer, 1991; Tetzlaff, 2000; Tolas, Pflug, & Halter, 1982). Peak plasma concentrations, for example, have been shown to occur within the first few minutes (Jastak et al., 1995). Outward signs and symptoms of transient high plasma levels are only *occasionally* noted clinically but tend to be quite frightening when they occur (Jastak et al., 1995). These signs and symptoms include nausea, restlessness, a racing heart, severe headaches, palpitations, tremors, and shakiness. Fortunately, these unpleasant effects are usually short-lived due to the efficiency of vasoconstrictor metabolism (Jastak et al., 1995). Levonordefrin is similar to epinephrine in this respect although to a lesser extent (Jastak et al., 1995). Table 6–4 ■ demonstrates typical signs and symptoms of vasoconstrictor overdose and adverse events. Note that many of the signs and symptoms of overdose mimic those observed in anxiety and fear as discussed in Chapter 2,

"Fundamentals of Pain Management" and Chapter 18, "Insights for the Fearful Patient."

The absorption of vasoconstrictors from areas of deposition is slowed by their own actions and may take several hours (Jastak et al., 1995). Once absorbed, however, biotransformation of adrenergic vasoconstrictors is rapid with expected plasma half-lives of only about 1 to 2 minutes (ADA/PDR, 2006).

Epinephrine is recycled in the synaptic junctions. The enzyme, catecholamine-O-methyltransferase (COMT) is responsible for the biotransformation of any epinephrine that is not recycled. Further breakdown may occur via monamine oxidase (MAO) (Jastak et al., 1995, Malamed, 2004). Levonordefrin is also biotransformed by COMT; however, it is not subject to significant MAO metabolism due to its chemical structure (Jastak et al., 1995). Its systemic effects and the termination of its actions are similar to epinephrine's (Jastak et al., 1995). Responses to suspected overdoses or other reactions to vasoconstrictors and local anesthetic drugs are discussed in Chapter 17, "Local Anesthesia Complications and Management."

Despite the administration of only very small doses of vasoconstrictors, signs and symptoms of overdose or other adverse events may occur in some individuals either during or shortly after administration. These effects pass rather quickly. Individuals affected in this way may state or record on health histories that they are "allergic" to the "adrenalin" in the anesthetic. Although it is possible this was the result of intravascular deposition, it may actually reflect a hyper-response to absorbed doses, particularly if it occurred on repeated occasions (see Box 6–2). It is important to note that this type of sensitivity is not allergenic since it lacks humoral, cell-mediated, and/or antigen-antibody reactions (see Table 6–5 ■). Instead, it relates to a rapid, direct, and vigorous stimulation of adrenergic receptors. These events can be dramatic and frightening and provide convincing rationale for limiting or avoiding epinephrine-containing local anesthetics in these individuals. They do not, however, reflect a true epinephrine allergy, which is not possible because epinephrine in local anesthetics is identical to endogenous epinephrine (Pickett & Terezhalmy, 2006.)

Table 6–4	Adverse Events in Vasoconstrictor Overdose

Comparison of Signs and Symptoms Vasoconstrictor Overdose versus Anxiety and Fear

Vasoconstrictor Overdose	*Anxiety/Fear Responses*
Nausea	Nausea
Restlessness	Restlessness
Heart racing	Heart racing
Intense anxiety	Intense anxiety
Weakness	Weakness
Tremor	Tremor
Severe headache	Headache
Hyperventilation	Hyperventilation
Palpitation	Palpitation
Shakiness	Shakiness
	Fainting

OTHER VASOCONSTRICTORS USED IN DENTISTRY

Norepinephrine, phenylephrine, and felypressin are not currently available in dental local anesthetic

Some confusion exists among patients regarding their experiences with epinephrine and what constitutes an allergy in general. Since it is physiologically impossible to have an allergy to epinephrine, they most likely experienced what has been termed a hyper-response to the drug. The term *hyper-response* refers to overdose manifestations to doses that typically would not result in noticeable effects. These doses are always less than maximum recommended doses.

In these individuals, this is the normal response and, although below maximum recommended levels, they are dose-related.

Hypersensitivity refers to an allergic process that involves humoral, cell-mediated, and/or antigen-antibody reactions. True allergic responses are *not* dose related.

Source: Jones & Mason, 1990; *Mosby's Medical, Nursing, and Allied Health Dictionary*, 1994.

Table 6–5   **Contrasting Overdose vs Allergic Responses**

Comparison of Signs and Symptoms Vasoconstrictor Overdose versus Allergy

Vasoconstrictor Overdose	Allergic Response*
Nausea	Hives
Restlessness	Rash
Heart racing	Bronchospasms
Intense anxiety	Vasodilatation
Weakness	
Tremor	
Severe headache	
Hyperventilation	
Palpitation	
Shaky	

*Allergic response to epinephrine is impossible, signs and symptoms of allergy may be in response to other contents of the cartridge.

preparations in North America; however, all three vasoconstrictors have been in use in other regions of the world for many years.

Norepinephrine

Norepinephrine is a naturally-occurring catecholamine whose activity on adrenergic receptors is approximately 90% α (Malamed, 2004). It is similar to levonordefrin in its actions on these receptors and much different compared to epinephrine in that norepinephrine's vasoconstrictive actions lack significant β_2 activity thus they are virtually unopposed (Jastak et al., 1995; Malamed, 2004). The vigorous and sustained vasoconstriction (hemostasis) induced by norepinephrine has a higher tendency to induce necrosis, especially on the palate (Malamed, 2004).

Phenylephrine

Phenylephrine is a synthetic non-catecholamine with weak vasoconstrictive effects, approximately 95% α activity (Malamed, 2004). It is formulated in much higher concentrations (1:2500) compared to epinephrine and levonordefrin in order to overcome its weaker vasoconstrictive effects (Malamed, 2004). It has been described as an excellent drug with few significant side effects; however, plasma levels of lidocaine were found to be elevated when phenylephrine was administered for epidural block compared to similar solutions with epinephrine (Malamed, 2004; Stanton-Hicks, Berges, & Bonica, 1973). This directly relates to its weak vasoconstrictive action. Phenylephrine was previously available in North America in a 4% procaine, 1:2500 dilution. With the demise of procaine as a primary local anesthetic, this formulation is no longer available.

Felypressin

Felypressin is a synthetic hormone that has vasoconstrictive properties with more smooth muscle effects on the venous rather than the arteriolar microcirculation. It has a wide margin of safety, with little to no effect on the myocardium and no adrenergic nerve influence. It is therefore safe to use for patients with dysrhythmias or hyperthyroidism, and for patients using tricyclic antidepressant medication (Inagawa, Ichinohe, & Kaneka, 2005; Jastak et al., 1995; Malamed, 2004).

For additional information on norepinephrine, phenylephrine, and felypressin, the clinician is urged to consult the references for this text.

CASE MANAGEMENT: Elena Gagarin

Due to precautions surrounding tricyclic antidepressant use, it is decided that a drug without a vasoconstrictor or with limited vasoconstrictor doses will be used. The first choice, 4% prilocaine plain, failed to provide adequate anesthesia or duration for a crown which was the treatment agreed upon. The second choice, 3% mepivacaine provided profound anesthesia of #14 but it lasted only 5 minutes. Four percent articaine with 1:200,000 epinephrine was selected because it provides adequate profoundness and duration, it has a very short half-life, and it has the least amount of epinephrine per millimeter available.

Case Discussion: A severe spike in blood pressure and reflexive bradycardia are more likely to occur in the presence of tricyclic antidepressants if vasoconstrictors are used. Epinephrine may be administered but the total quantities of drug should be limited. A 1:200,000 dilution is safer than a 1:100,000 dilution because it contains half the amount of epinephrine. Three drugs are packaged in this dilution: 4% prilocaine, 0.5% bupivacaine, and 4% articaine with 1:200,000 epinephrine. Any of the three might work in this situation, however, if Elena is still nursing the half-life of prilocaine (1.6 hours) and bupivacaine (2.7 hours) are significantly greater than the half-life of articaine (less than 45 minutes) may then be the better choice.

Levonordefrin increases the potential for hypertensive episodes and reflexive bradycardia to such an extent that it should be avoided altogether.

CHAPTER QUESTIONS

1. Which *one* of the following vasoconstrictors is most useful in providing hemostasis?
   a. Phenyephrine
   b. Epinephrine
   c. Levonordefrin
   d. Felypressin

2. A patient has significant cardiovascular disease and requires a restorative procedure on tooth #5. Retraction cord and hemostasis are needed in order to keep the restorative site dry. Which *one* of the following drugs would be most indicated in this situation?
   a. 4% articaine, 1:200,000 epinephrine
   b. 2% mepivacaine, 1:20,000 levonordefrin
   c. 2% lidocaine, 1:50,000 epinephrine
   d. 4% prilocaine plain

3. Which *one* of the following statements is true?
   a. Levonordefrin is more potent compared to epinephrine.
   b. Cardiac stimulation from levonordefrin is greater compared to epinephrine.
   c. Cardiac stimulation from levonordefrin is less compared to epinephrine.
   d. Levonordefrin is equal in potency compared to epinephrine.

4. Epinephrine's metabolism is relatively rapid after local anesthesia administration.
   a. True
   b. False

5. Metabolic enzymes for epinephrine include which of the following?
   a. COMT and MAO
   b. Hepatic isoenzymes
   c. Renal isoenzymes
   d. COMT only

6. A diabetic patient requires periodontal therapy on the upper and lower right quadrants. She is well-controlled and otherwise healthy. Which *one* of the following represents the safest and most effective local anesthesia regime?
   a. 4 cartridges of 2% lidocaine, 1:100,000 epinephrine
   b. 2 cartridges of 2% lidocaine, 1:100,000 epinephrine and 2 cartridges of 3% mepivacaine plain
   c. 2 cartridges of 2% lidocaine, 1:100,000 epinephrine and 2 cartridges of 4% articaine, 1:200,000 epinephrine
   d. 2 cartridges of 2% lidocaine 1:100,000 epinephrine and 2 cartridges of 2% mepivacaine, 1:20,000 levonordefrin

REFERENCES

ADA/PDR Guide to Dental Therapeutics (4th ed.). (2006). Montvale, NJ: Thompson PDR.

Ahlquist, R. P. (1948). A study of the adrenotropic receptors. *American Journal of Physiology, 153,* 586–600.

Agency for Healthcare Research and Quality. (2002, March). *Cardiovascular effects of epinephrine in hypertensive dental patients.* Summary, Evidence Report/Technology Assessment Number 48, AHRQ Publication Number 02-E005.

Budenz, A. W. (2000, August). Local anesthetics and medically complex patients. *Journal of the California Dental Association, 28*(8), 611–619.

Clutter, W. E., Bier, D. M., Shah, S. D., & Cryer, P. E. (1991). Epinephrine plasma metabolic clearance in healthy volunteers and in patients having third molar surgery. *British Dental Journal, 170,* 373–376.

Cryer, P. E. (1980). Physiology and pathophysiology of the human sympathoadrenal neuroendocrine system. *New England Journal of Medicine, 303,* 436–444.

Inagawa, M., Ichinohe, T., & Kaneka, Y. (2005). *Felypressin contained in dental local anesthetics aggravates myocardial oxygen balance.* Tokyo Dental College, Chiba-shi Chiba, Japan 2005. Accessed July 26, 2007, at http://iadr.confex.com/iadr/2005Balt/techprogram/abstract_63639.htm.

Jastak, J. T., Yagiela, J. A., & Donaldson, D. (1995). *Local anesthesia of the oral cavity.* Philadelphia: Saunders.

Jones, J. H., & Mason, D. K. (1990). *Oral manifestations of systemic disease* (2nd ed.). Philadelphia: Saunders.

Lipp, M., Dick, W., Daublander, M., Fuder, H., & Stanton-Hicks, M. (1993). Exogenous and endogenous plasma levels of epinephrine during dental treatment under local anesthesia. *Regional Anesthesia and Pain Medicine, 18,* 6–12.

Lindquist, T. J., & Ettinger, R. L. (2003). The complexities involved with managing the care of an elderly patient. *Journal of the American Dental Association, 134,* 593–600.

Little, J. W., Falace, D. A., Miller, C. S., & Rhodus, N. L. (2008). *Dental management of the medically compromised patient* (7th ed.). St. Louis: Mosby Elsevier.

Malamed, S. F. (2004). *Handbook of local anesthesia* (5th ed.). St. Louis, Elsevier Mosby.

Mosby's Medical, Nursing, and Allied Health Dictionary (4th ed.). St. Louis, Mosby-Year Book, Inc.

Pickett, F. A., & Terezhalmy, G. T. (2006). *Dental drug reference with clinical implications.* Lippincott Williams & Wilkins.

Special Committee of the New York Heart Association. (1955). Use of epinephrine with procaine in dental procedures. *Journal of the American Dental Association, 50,* 108.

Stanton-Hicks, M., Berges, P. U., & Bonica, J. J. (1973). Circulatory effects of peridural block. IV. Comparison of the effects of phenylephrine and epinephrine. *Anesthesiology, 39,* 308–314.

Sveen, K. (1979). Effect of the addition of a vasoconstrictor to local anesthetic solution on operative and postoperative bleeding, analgesia, and wound healing. *International Journal of Oral Surgery, 8,* 301–306.

Takahashi, Y., Nakano, M., Sano, K., & Kanri, T. (2005). The effects of epinephrine in local anesthetics on plasma catecholamine and hemodynamic responses. *Odontology, 93,* 72–79.

Tetzlaff, J. E. (2000). *Clinical pharmacology of local anesthetics* (1st ed.). Woburn, MA: Butterworth-Heinemann.

Tolas, A. G., Pflug, A. E., & Halter, J. B. (1982). Arterial plasma epinephrine concentrations and hemodynamic responses after dental injection of local anesthetic with epinephrine. *Journal of the American Dental Association, 104,* 41–43.

Yagiela, J. A. (1999). Adverse drug interactions in dental practice: Interactions associated with vasoconstrictors, Part V of a series. *Journal of the American Dental Association, 130,* 701–709.

Yagiela, J. A. (1991). Epinephrine and the compromised heart. *Orofacial Pain Management, 1,* 5–8.

Zhang, C., Banting, D. W., Gelb, A. W., & Hamilton, J. T. (1999). Effect of β-adrenoreceptor blockade with nadolol on the duration of local anesthesia. *Journal of the American Dental Association,* 1773–1780.

Chapter 7

Dose Calculations for Local Anesthetic Solutions

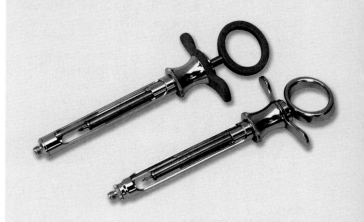

OBJECTIVES

- Define and discuss the key terms in this chapter.
- Define and discuss the significance of the maximum recommended dose of a drug.
- List maximum recommended doses for each local anesthetic drug and vasoconstrictor.
- Identify and discuss the relevant information and mathematical operations required to calculate drug doses.
- Demonstrate accurate calculations of recommended doses for local anesthetic drugs and vasoconstrictors in clinical situations.
- Demonstrate accurate calculations of recommended doses when multiple drugs with differing concentrations are administered.
- Define dose modification for vasoconstrictors in patients with significant cardiovascular compromise.
- Demonstrate accurate calculations of recommended doses for local anesthetic drugs and vasoconstrictors for patients with significant cardiovascular compromise.
- Demonstrate accurate calculation of recommended doses for children using Clark's Rule and Young's Rule.

KEY TERMS

cardiac dose **101**
cartridge volume **96**
Clark's Rule **102**
dilution ratio **98**
drug concentration **94**
drug percentage **94**
drug ratio **101**
limiting drug **100**
maximum recommended dose (MRD) **94**
Young's rule **103**

CASE STUDY: Elena Gagarin

After administering one cartridge of 4% articaine with 1:200,000 epinephrine for a crown on #14, which limits the total amount of epinephrine administered to Elena Gagarin, it was later decided that additional anesthetic would be necessary because #14 was becoming sensitive during the placement of a temporary crown.

Three percent mepivacaine plain was selected for two reasons. The first is that it has no vasoconstrictor and the second is that temporary fabrication would require only brief additional anesthesia.

Elena Gagarin weighs 120 lbs and is otherwise healthy. Calculate the total volume of 3% mepivacaine that she can receive at her appointment. How many milligrams of drug does this represent? What is the total dose of epinephrine that she received?

INTRODUCTION

Treatment planning and accurate documentation of local anesthetic agents require careful calculation and recording of drug doses. Local anesthetic solutions used in dentistry contain one or more drugs (a local anesthetic drug with or without a vasoconstrictor). The maximum recommended dose for each solution is dependent on the drug that limits the total volumes that may be delivered. In most cases, when solutions with an anesthetic and vasoconstrictor drug are used, the limiting drug will be the local anesthetic agent. In some situations, the vasoconstrictor will limit the volumes administered. These differences will be discussed in this chapter.

CALCULATING LOCAL ANESTHETIC DRUG DOSES

Necessary information for calculating recommended doses and/or determining the dose of local anesthetic drugs administered requires an understanding of the following:

1. *Concentration* for the selected anesthetic drug
2. *Dilution percentages* for vasoconstrictors
3. *Standard cartridge volumes*
4. Defined *maximum recommended dose* for each drug
5. Relevant *patient factors* such as weight and general health status, including medications

Definition of Maximum Recommended Doses for Local Anesthetic Drugs

As introduced in Chapter 4, "Pharmacology Basics," **maximum recommended dose (MRD)** represents the maximum quantity of drug that can be *safely* administered during an appointment in most situations. Dose recommendations are provided by manufacturers in product inserts for each drug. These values have been independently reviewed by the United States Pharmacopeial Convention and previously by the ADA Council on Dental Therapeutics (Malamed, 2004). Conservative recommendations suggested by Malamed are based on the preceding recommendations and are the lowest values for any drug. These values also simplify monitoring drug dosing by using a common value for all forms of a drug (Malamed, 2004).

The acronym MRD is also used to indicate the manufacturer's recommended dose, which may lead to some confusion. For the purposes of this text, MRD will refer to maximum recommended dose, which conforms to Malamed's more conservative recommendations. Table 7–1 ■ provides MRD values for all five injectable dental local anesthetic drugs.

Factors Required for Drug Dose Calculations

Clinicians commonly express and document doses of local anesthetic drugs as the number of cartridges, milliliters of solution, and/or milligrams of drug administered. Regardless of the manner in which they are expressed, these doses are all calculated based upon milligrams.

The **drug concentration** of a local anesthetic in a cartridge is expressed as a percentage, for example 2%, 3%, 4%. The **drug percentage** is an expression of the relative amount of drug in a cartridge. A 4% drug contains twice as much drug as a 2% drug.

In order to understand the percentages on which the contents of local anesthetic drug solutions are based, it may be helpful to consider that a 100% solution, by definition,

Table 7–1	Maximum Recommended Doses of Local Anesthetic Drugs		
	Maximum Recommended Dose per Appointment Based on Local Anesthetic Drug ONLY*		
Drug	**mg/lb**	**mg/kg**	**mg per appt.***
Articaine	3.2	7.0	500 mg
Bupivacaine	0.6	1.3	90 mg
Lidocaine	2.0	4.4	300 mg
Mepivacaine	2.0	4.4	300 mg
Prilocaine	2.7	6.0	400 mg

Note: "per appt." values represent dosages for a healthy, 150–160 pound adult. Values must be adjusted for children, adults of low weight and medically compromised.
Source: ADA/PDR, 2006; Malamed, 2004.

Box 7–1   Drug Percentage Conversions

100% solution = one gram (1000 mg) of drug per milliliter of solution = 1000 mg/ml

10% solution = one-tenth the milligrams (100 mg) of drug per milliliter of solution = 100 mg/ml

1% solution = one-hundredth the milligrams (10 mg) of drug per milliliter of solution = 10 mg/ml

---

contains 1 gram or 1000 mg of drug per milliliter of solution. This may be expressed as 1000 mg/ml. A 10% solution therefore would contain one-tenth the milligrams per milliliter, expressed as 100 mg/ml, and a 1% solution (only available for use in medicine) would contain one-hundredth the milligrams per milliliter or 10 mg/ml (see Box 7–1). Considering that a standard North American cartridge contains 1.8 ml of solution, not 1.0 ml (see Box 7–2), at a concentration of 1%, 1 cartridge would contain 18 mg of drug (10 mg/ml × 1.8 ml/cartridge = 18 mg/cartridge). Box 7–3 and Appendix 7–1, "Local Anesthetic Solutions—Dose Calculation Facts" provide a comprehensive summary of key factors for determining drug dosages.

Injectable local anesthetic drugs for use in dentistry are provided in concentrations of 0.5%, 2%, 3%, and 4%. Compared to a 1% solution with 10 mg/ml of drug, a 0.5% solution, for example, contains half this quantity, or 5 mg/ml of drug. A 2% solution contains twice this quantity, or 20 mg/ml; a 3% solution contains three times this quantity, or 30 mg/ml of drug; and a 4% solution contains 40 mg/ml of drug. To determine the dose of drug per cartridge, multiply the mg/ml times 1.8 (see Box 7–3).

Calculating Local Anesthetic Drug Doses

Methods used to determine the number of milligrams of local anesthetic drug delivered vary among clinicians. A common method will be demonstrated for the following situation. Assume that 2 cartridges of 2% lidocaine plain have been administered to a 100 lb patient. The first step in calculating the dose is to identify the key factors. For this situation these factors are:

1. In a 2% solution, there are 36 mg of drug per cartridge
2. 2 cartridges have been delivered
3. The MRD for lidocaine is 2 mg/lb or 300 mg maximum
4. The patient's weight is 100 lbs

Milligrams Delivered

To calculate the milligrams of drug delivered, first multiply the total number of cartridges by the total mg of drug in each cartridge for a 2% drug:

2 (cartridges) × 36 mg = 72 mg

This patient received 72 mg of lidocaine.

Box 7–2   Cartridge Volume Variations

There is no international standard regarding **cartridge volume**. Cartridges distributed in North America are designed to contain 1.8 ml of solution. In some cases, the manufacturer's insert, in compliance with FDA regulations, will state that the cartridge liquid capacity guarantee is 1.7 ml. This represents a manufacturing variation of $+/-$ 0.1 ml and assures that *no less than* 1.7 ml is present in each cartridge. This will not alter the basic formulas for calculation and allows for volumes up to 1.8 ml of solution (which may be present in any standard cartridge, even if it is not *guaranteed* to be there). The standard for calculating dosages is considered 1.8 ml. Applying this standard provides a margin of safety when near-maximum doses are delivered.

When considering 2 cartridges, this reflects a variance of 0.2 ml. With eight, this would reflect 0.8 ml. In any case, for cartridges that truly contain 1.7 ml, the patient would receive less than the dose calculated at 1.8 ml and the MRD would not be compromised.

Cartridges in the United Kingdom and Australia typically contain 2.2 ml of solution. Some have been noted in Japan to be 1.0 ml. Dental clinicians must be aware of the cartridge capacities in the countries in which they practice and calculate drug doses accordingly.

Dose Related to MRD

To determine the maximum dose *for this patient,* multiply the MRD for this drug by the patient's weight:

$$2 \text{ mg/lb} \times 100 \text{ lbs} = 200 \text{ mg}$$

The MRD for lidocaine for this patient is 200 mg.

Although the absolute MRD for lidocaine is 300 mg, when adjusted for weight, this patient may only receive 200 mg of drug. With some exceptions, MRDs are based on a healthy 150 lb adult ($2 \text{ mg/lb} \times 150 \text{ lbs} = 300 \text{ mg}$). If a patient weighs more than 150 lbs, the MRD would remain 300 mg.

Appendix 7–2, "Local Anesthesia and Vasoconstrictor Reference," provides a comprehensive look-up table for determining total cartridges of drug by body weight. A conversion formula for kilograms to pounds is also included in Appendix 7–2.

Calculating Additional Doses of the Same Drugs

This patient has received 72 mg of 2% lidocaine. She can safely receive a maximum of 200 mg. Subtract the total dose already delivered from the MRD for this patient to determine the additional allowed dose:

$$200 \text{ mg} - 72 \text{ mg} = 128 \text{ mg}$$

An additional 128 mg of lidocaine may be delivered.

Box 7–3   Local Anesthetic Drugs—Dose of Drug per Cartridge

Drug dose and "per cartridge" facts:

1 ml = 1 cc

1 cartridge = 1.8 ml solution (1.8 cc)

1% solution = 10 mg/ml

1 cartridge of a 1% local anesthetic = 10 mg/ml $\times$ 1.8 ml/cartridge = 18 mg/cart

Common Dental Concentrations:

0.5% solution ml/cartridge =   5 mg/ml

2% solution ml/cartridge = 20 mg/ml

3% solution ml/cartridge = 30 mg/ml

4% solution ml/cartridge = 40 mg/ml

Cartridge Conversions:

0.5 mg/ml $\times$ 1.8 =   9 mg/cartridge

20 mg/ml $\times$ 1.8 = 36 mg/cartridge

30 mg/ml $\times$ 1.8 = 54 mg/cartridge

40 mg/ml $\times$ 1.8 = 72 mg/cartridge

Converting Milligrams to Cartridges

To convert this number (128 mg) into clinically useful terms, determine the number of cartridges this would represent. To do this, divide the additional mg allowed by the mg per cartridge:

$$128 \text{ mg} \div 36 \text{ mg/cartridge} = 3.5 \text{ cartridges}$$

This patient may receive 3.5 additional cartridges of 2% lidocaine.

Calculating Additional Doses of Different Drugs

The following discussion assumes that the toxic effects of local anesthetic drugs in combination may be synergistic. When considering additional administrations of different drugs, this means that the toxic risks would be greater than the sum of the individual risks of the drugs. In addition to administering 3% mepivacaine plain after administering 0.5% bupivacaine, for example, there would be a greater risk associated with their use than the sum of the individual risks.

It may be safest to assume, therefore, that local anesthetic drug combinations are synergistic rather than additive, which would have the effect of increasing the combined toxic potential beyond that which would ordinarily be expected when using more than one drug at a single appointment (Pickett & Terezhalmy, 2006). While the extent of this synergy (if it exists) is not known at this time, clinicians are advised to use caution and to follow closely the recommendation of using the absolute maximum dose of the most toxic drug when calculating maximum doses of combinations (Pickett, 2006). In other words, this assumes that all drugs delivered are as toxic as the most toxic drug, which may well be the safest calculation under the circumstances. It is important to remember that manufacturers are not obligated to supply information on the risks of additional administrations of *different* local anesthetic drugs.

Assume therefore that 4% articaine plain will be added to the 2 cartridges of 2% lidocaine plain that were administered in the previous example. Before adding another drug, additional key factors are:

1. The patient initially received 72 mg of lidocaine.
2. The MRD for lidocaine for this patient is 200 mg.

3. In a 4% solution, there are 72 mg of drug per cartridge.
4. The MRD for articaine is 3.2 mg/lb or 500 mg maximum.

When multiple drugs are administered with different MRDs, the lowest MRD (most toxic drug) is applied when calculating total drug doses. To determine the MRD of articaine for this patient, multiply the MRD for this drug by the patient's weight:

$$3.2 \text{ mg/lb} \times 100 \text{ lbs} = 320 \text{ mg}$$

The MRD for articaine for this patient is 320 mg.

Although the MRD for articaine is 500 mg, when adjusted for weight, this patient may receive only 320 mg of drug. In this example, the MRD for lidocaine (the most toxic drug = 200 mg) is lower than the MRD for articaine (320 mg) and will be used for calculating dose limits.

This patient has received 72 mg of lidocaine. Since the MRD for lidocaine will limit this example, she can safely receive a maximum of 200 mg of drug. Subtract the total dose already delivered from the MRD for this patient to determine the allowed additional dose:

$$200 \text{ mg} - 72 \text{ mg} = 128 \text{ mg}$$

For this patient, 128 mg of 4% articaine can be delivered.

To convert this number (128 mg) into clinically useful terms, determine the number of cartridges this would represent. Divide the additional mg allowed by the mg per cartridge:

$$128 \text{ mg} \div 72 \text{ mg/cartridge} = 1.7 \text{ cartridges}$$

This patient may receive 1.7 cartridges of 4% articaine in addition to the two cartridges of 2% lidocaine.

Alternate Method for Calculating Doses Delivered

Another approach to calculating doses of local anesthetic drugs administered applies only the mg/ml values previously discussed for 0.5%, 2%, 3%, and 4% drugs. After determining the total volume in milliliters of solution administered, multiply that times the mg/ml for the concentration of drug used. For example, for the previously presented situation:

1. A 2% solution contains 20 mg of drug per milliliter
2. A 4% solution contains 40 mg of drug per milliliter

3. 2 cartridges of lidocaine (3.6 ml) and 1.7 cartridges of articaine (~3 ml) are allowed
4. Total of 2% idocaine = 20 mg × 3.6 ml = 72 mg
5. Total of 4% articaine = 40 mg × 3 ml = 120 mg

In this example, 72 mg of lidocaine and 28 mg of articaine were delivered.

Milligrams Delivered

To calculate the milligrams of drug delivered, first multiply the total number of cartridges by the total ml per cartridge:

$$2 \times 1.8 \text{ ml} = 3.6 \text{ ml}$$

Now, multiply this times the mg/ml based on the drug percentage (2% drug = 20 mg)

$$3.6 \text{ ml} \times 20 \text{ mg} = 72 \text{ mg}$$

This patient received 72 mg of a 2% drug.

For one-half cartridge, the calculation would be:

$$0.9 \text{ ml} \times 20 \text{ mg} = 18 \text{ mg}$$

For two-thirds cartridge, the calculation would be:

$$1.2 \text{ ml} \times 20 \text{ mg} = 2.4 \text{ mg}$$

Table 7–2 ■ provides a summary of the milligrams of drug based on drug concentrations and cartridges delivered.

CALCULATING VASOCONSTRICTOR DOSES

Determining the dose of vasoconstrictor in a given volume of solution requires an understanding of dilution percentages, standard cartridge volumes, the defined maximum recommended doses for epinephrine and levonordefrin, and relevant patient factors such as general health status.

Calculations of vasoconstrictor doses are different compared with those used to determine local anesthetic drug doses. The main differences are that vasoconstrictors are expressed as **dilution ratios** rather than concentration percentages and maximum doses of vasoconstrictors are not weight dependent.

Definition of Maximum Recommended Doses for Vasoconstrictor Drugs

The limits on vasoconstrictor doses (MRDs) are based on recommendations of the 1954 Special Committee of the New York Heart Association, and more recently the American Heart Association, for patients with ischemic heart disease (Malamed, 2004; Special Committee of the New York Heart Association, 1955).

For the purposes of this text, MRDs for vasoconstrictors also conform to the 2006 ADA/PDR Guide to Dental Therapeutics (ADA/PDR, 2006). Table 7–3 ■ provides values for epinephrine and levonordefrin.

Vasoconstrictor Dilutions

To understand vasoconstrictor dilutions, ratios are expressed as milligrams to milliliters. A dilution ratio of 1:1000 epinephrine is equivalent to one gram in one liter, expressed as 1000 mg/1000 ml = 1mg/ml. A dilution ratio of 1:100,000 is equivalent to one gram in 100 liters, expressed as 1000 mg/100,000 ml = 1 mg/100 ml, or 0.01 mg/ml (see Box 7–4).

Since each cartridge contains 1.8 ml of solution, 1 cartridge with 1:100,000 epinephrine contains 0.018 mg of epinephrine (0.01 mg/ml × 1.8 ml = 0.018 mg). Vasoconstrictor dilutions used in dentistry are provided in ratios of 1:20,000, 1:50,000, 1:100,000, and 1:200,000. Compared with a 1:100,000 solution with 0.018 mg of drug, a 1:20,000 solution contains five times the quantity or 0.09 mg of drug; a 1:50,000 solution contains twice the quantity or 0.036 mg of drug, and, a 1:200,000 solution contains half the quantity or 0.009 mg of drug (see Box 7–4).

Table 7–2 Examples of Local Anesthetic Doses in Total mg per Cartridge(s)				
	% Local Anesthetic Drug			
Cartridge = Volume	**0.5%** (× 5 mg)	**2%** (× 20 mg)	**3%** (× 30 mg)	**4%** (× 40 mg)
1 = 1.8 ml	9 mg	36 mg	54 mg	72 mg
2 = 3.6 ml	18 mg	72 mg	108 mg	144 mg
3 = 5.4 ml	27 mg	108 mg	162 mg	216 mg
4 = 7.2 ml	36 mg	144 mg	216 mg	288 mg

Table 7–3	Maximum Safe Doses for Epinephrine and Levonordefrin				

	Maximum Safe Dose per Appointment Based on Vasoconstrictor ONLY				
Drug Ratio	*Healthy Patient**	*Maximum Cartridges*	*Ischemic Heart Disease*	*Maximum Cartridges*
EPINEPHRINE				
1:50,000	**0.2 mg**	5.5	0.04 mg	1.1
1:100,000	**0.2 mg**	11	0.04 mg	2.2
1:200,000	**0.2 mg**	22	0.04 mg	4.4
LEVONORDEFRIN				
1:20,000	**1 mg**	11	0.2 mg	2.2

Source: Medical Office Pharmacology Review, 2008; Special Committee of the New York Heart Association, 1955.
*Note that for healthy patients, with the exception of 1:50,000 dilutions, the MRD (maximum cartridges) for the local anesthetic drugs will be reached well before the MRD for epinephrine.

Box 7–4   Vasoconstrictor Drugs—Volume of Drug per Cartridge

Drug dose and "per cartridge" facts:

The relative amounts of vasoconstrictors in cartridges are commonly referred to as dilution ratios.

1:1000 = 1 g or 1000 mg of vasoconstrictor per 1000 ml solution = 1 mg/ml

1:10,000 = 1 ml of 1:1000 vasoconstrictor + 9 ml water = 0.1 mg/ml

1:100,000 = 1 ml of 1:10,000 vasoconstrictor + 9 ml water = 0.01 mg/cartridge

1.8 ml cartridge of 1:100,000 = 0.01 mg/ml $\times$ 1.8 ml = 0.018 mg/cartridge

Common Dental Concentrations

1:20,000 = 0.05 mg/ml or 0.05 $\times$ 1.8 ml = 0.09 mg/cart

1:50,000 = 0.02 mg/ml or 0.02 $\times$ 1.8 ml = 0.036 mg/cart

1:100,000 = 0.01 mg/ml or 0.01 $\times$ 1.8 ml = 0.018 mg/cart

1:200,000 = 0.005 mg/ml or 0.005 $\times$ 1.8 ml = 0.009 mg/cart

---

Calculating Vasoconstrictor Drug Doses

In order to calculate the total milligrams of vasoconstrictors in local anesthetic solutions that are administered, start by identifying the key factors. Assume that 2 cartridges of 2% lidocaine with 1:100,000 epinephrine have been administered to a 100 lb female. For this situation these factors are:

1. For a 1:100,000 dilution there are 0.018 mg of vasoconstrictor drug per cartridge
2. 2 cartridges have been delivered
3. The maximum recommended dose for epinephrine in a healthy patient is 0.2 mg
4. The MRD for 2% lidocaine is 2 mg/lb or 300 mg maximum.

Milligrams Delivered

From the previous local anesthetic drug calculation, it was determined that this patient received 72 mg of lidocaine. To calculate the milligrams of vasoconstrictor delivered, multiply the total number of cartridges by the total mg of drug in each cartridge for a 1:100,000 solution:

$$2 \times 0.018 \text{ mg} = 0.036 \text{ mg}$$

This patient received 0.036 mg of epinephrine.

Determining the Limiting Drug

As stated earlier in this chapter, the maximum recommended dose for each anesthetic solution is dependent on which individual drug limit will determine the total amount of solution that may be delivered. In most cases, the **limiting drug** will be the local anesthetic agent while occasionally it will be the vasoconstrictor. For example, this patient may receive a total of 5.5 cartridges of 2% lidocaine based on local anesthetic drug limitations, whereas *based on epinephrine only* she could receive a total of 11 cartridges.

Since 5.5 cartridges is the smaller number of the two, the limiting drug for this patient is the local anesthetic drug.

With the exception of epinephrine at 1:50,000, the local anesthetic drug will be the limiting drug for healthy patients (see Table 7–4 and Appendix 7–2).

Maximum cartridge values for local anesthetic and vasoconstrictor drugs prepared for use in dentistry illustrate this point and may be found in Table 7–4 ■. Consult Table 7–1 for MRDs in milligrams for local anesthetic drugs and Table 7–3 for maximum safe doses for epinephrine and levonordefrin.

MRD Related to Both Local Anesthetic and Vasoconstrictor

Previously it was determined that the MRD for lidocaine for this patient is 200 mg. Assuming this is a

Table 7–4 Maximum Local Anesthetic Doses for *Healthy Patients*		
Local Anesthetic Drugs	*Maximum Cartridges* Based on LA Only*	*Maximum Cartridges Based on Vaso Only*
0.5% Bupivacaine w/ 1:200,000 epi	10	22
2% Lidocaine Plain	8	–
2% Lidocaine w/ 1:50,000 epi*	8	5.5
2% Lidocaine w/ 1:100,000 epi	8	11
2% Lidocaine w/ 1:200,000 epi	8	22
2% Mepivacaine w/ 1:20,000 levo	8	11
3% Mepivacaine Plain	5.5	–
4% Articaine w/ 1:100,000 epi	6	11
4% Articaine w/ 1:200,000 epi	6	22
4% Prilocaine Plain	5	–
4% Prilocaine w/ 1:200,000 epi	5	22

*Note: For *healthy patients*, the local anesthetic drug is the controlling agent for all drugs *except* 2% lidocaine with 1:50,000 epinephrine.
Source: ADA/PDR, 2006; Malamed, 2004; Special Committee of the New York Heart Association, 1955.

healthy patient, the established recommended dose for epinephrine is 0.2 mg per appointment.

It has been calculated that the patient received 0.036 mg of epinephrine, which is well under the established recommended dose for epinephrine of 0.2 mg.

Calculating Additional Doses of Same Drugs

From the previous local anesthetic drug calculation, it was determined that an additional 128 mg of 2% lidocaine or 3.5 cartridges could be delivered. This patient received 0.036 mg of epinephrine. She can safely receive a maximum 0.2 mg. Subtract the total dose already delivered from the recommended dose for this patient to determine the allowed additional dose:

$$0.2 \text{ mg} - 0.036 \text{ mg} = 0.164 \text{ mg}$$

This patient may receive an additional 0.164 milligrams of epinephrine.

Converting Milligrams to Cartridges

In previous calculations, it was determined that this patient may receive an additional 128 mg of 2% lidocaine, or 3.5 cartridges and 0.164 milligrams of epinephrine. To convert the dose of epinephrine (0.164 milligrams) into clinically useful terms, determine the number of cartridges this would represent. Divide the additional mg allowed by the mg per cartridge:

$$0.164 \text{ mg} \div 0.018 \text{ mg/cartridge} = 9 \text{ cartridges}$$

This patient may receive an additional 9 cartridges based on epinephrine ONLY but the limiting drug is lidocaine (3.5 cartridges).

Cardiac Considerations for Vasoconstrictors

When applying limits to doses for patients with ischemic heart disease, restrictions on vasoconstrictors are based on recommendations of the Special Committee of the New York Heart Association and more recently the American Heart Association, as previously noted (ADA/PDR, 2006). As listed in Table 7–5 ■, this reduced value, also referred to as the **cardiac dose,** is 0.04 mg per appointment for epinephrine and 0.2 mg levonordefrin. Table 7–5 states the maximum number of cartridges this represents for each **drug ratio.**

CALCULATING PEDIATRIC DOSES

Calculating drug doses for children applies the same principles as determining adult doses; however, there may be some exceptions with obese children (see Box 7–5). The key to correct dosing for children is to determine their actual weight rather than rely on "guessing." Clinicians can deliver overdoses to children both by failing to make appropriate adjustments based on weight and by making erroneous estimates of weight. An available scale can eliminate any problems due to overestimating a child's weight (Medical Office Pharmacology Review, 2008).

Table 7–5   Cardiac Doses of Vasoconstrictors by Drug Ratio

Cardiac Doses of Vasoconstrictors by Drug Ratio
Total Milligrams Available
Cardiac Dose = 0.04 mg epinephrine & 0.2 mg levonordefrin
Shaded boxes indicate excessive doses of the drug by total cartridges

Number of Cartridges	Epinephrine 1:50,000	Epinephrine 1:100,000	Epinephrine 1:200,000	Levonordefrin 1:20,000
1	0.036 mg	0.018 mg	0.009 mg	0.09 mg
2	0.072 mg	0.036 mg	0.018 mg	0.18 mg
3	0.108 mg	0.054 mg	0.027 mg	0.27 mg
4	0.144 mg	0.072 mg	0.036 mg	0.36 mg

Source: ADA/PDR, 2006; David & Vogel, 1996; Malamed, 2004; Medical Office Pharmacology Review, 2008.

Box 7–5 Impact of Obesity on Child Local Anesthetic Doses

Childhood obesity may pose a unique concern when calculating safe drug doses. Relying solely on a child's weight when establishing safe doses in obese children can be problematic. Assumptions that these children can receive doses that correspond to their weight do not take into account the immaturity of their organ development. An obese 7-year-old, for example, cannot metabolize drugs as efficiently as a 20-year-old of the same weight (Ball & Bindler, 2008). In this situation, it may be useful to consult standard pediatric age specific height-weight charts (see Table 7–6 ■). For further discussion see Chapter 19, "Insights from Pedodontics," Box: 19–1, "Special Consideration in Child Obesity,"and Table 19–2, "Impact of Body Weight on Drug Dosage—Example: 2% Lidocaine."

There are two approaches frequently used for determining pediatric drug doses in addition to the calculation methods already discussed. These are *Clark's Rule* and *Young's Rule;* Clark's rule is applied in this text.

Clark's Rule

Clark's Rule is based upon a child's weight and states that the child's weight (in pounds) is divided by 150 to get the approximate fraction of the adult dose to give to the child. For example, to calculate the maximum safe dose for a 6-year-old, 50 lb child, using 2% lidocaine:

1. $50 \div 150 = 0.33$ (1/3)
2. $300 \text{ mg} \times 0.33 = 99 \text{ mg}$ (child's dose)

The dose would be approximately 1/3 of the adult MRD of 300 mg (8 cartridges) and the child's dose would be ~100 mg, or about 2.5 cartridges (100 mg/36 mg per cartridge = 2.77, which rounds down to 2.5). It is

---

Table 7–6 Child and Adolescent Height Weight Average*

Male			Female		
Age (years)	Height (inches)	Weight (pounds)	Age (years)	Height (inches)	Weight (pounds)
1 year old	28–29	22	1 year old	28–29	~22
2 years old	31	~28	2 years old	30	~28
3 years old	33	33	3 years old	33	~31
4 years old	37	35–37	4 years old	37	~35
5 years old	40	~42	5 years old	40	~40
6 years old	42	~46	6 years old	41	~46
7 years old	44	~51	7 years old	43	~51
8 years old	45	~57	8 years old	45	~57
9 years old	49	~62	9 years old	47	~64
10 years old	51	~70	10 years old	51	~70
11 years old	52	77	11 years old	52	~80
12–13 years old	58–62	85–100	12–13 years old	60–63	95–105
14–15 years old	63–66	105–125	14–15 years old	63–64	105–115
16–17 years old	67–70	130–150	16–17 years old	64	115–120
18–20 years old	68–70	150–160	18–20 years old	66	125–130

*This data is based on averages from CDC tables for child and adolescent height weight averages (2000 CDC Growth Charts for the United States, http://www.cdc.gov/growthcharts) and is provided only as a conservative average for making clinical judgments of appropriate dosages of local anesthetic drugs for children.

important to remember that this is a *maximum* dose not a routine or recommended dose regime.

This method is most similar to the methods discussed previously. Knowing the child's weight and the MRD in milligrams per pound allows for easy calculations. For example, for 2% lidocaine the MRD is 2 mg/lb, for a 50 pound child this is:

$$2 \text{ mg/lb} \times 50 \text{ lbs} = 100 \text{ mg}$$

The MRD for 2% lidocaine for this patient is 100 mg.

Young's Rule

Young's Rule is based on a child's age regardless of weight. This "rule of thumb" states that the child dosage is equal to the adult dosage multiplied by the child's age in years, divided by the sum of 12 plus the child's age. For example, to calculate the dose for a 6-year-old, 50 lb child, the adult MRD for 2% lidocaine would be 300 mg. The calculation would be:

1. $300 \text{ mg} \times 6 = 1800$
2. $1800 \div (12 + 6) = 100$

The child's dose would be 100 mg.

CASE MANAGEMENT: Elena Gagarin

Elena weighs 120 lbs. She received one cartridge of 4% articaine with 1:200,000 epinephrine which has an absolute maximum dose of 500 milligrams during any one appointment for all individuals 150 or greater and a maximum dose of 3.2 mg per lb. Based on this limit, *Elena can receive up to 384 mg of articaine (120 lbs × 3.2 mg/lb MRD).*

Elena received 72 mg of articaine (the volume contained in one cartridge).

Switching to 3% mepivacaine means that absolute maximums must be identified for both drugs and the lowest is selected when drugs are combined. The absolute maximum for mepivacaine is 300 mg and the absolute maximum for articaine is 500 mg. The lower maximum of 300 mg will be used for all calculations after the initial dose of articaine.

A total of 300 mg is allowed for individuals weighing 150 lbs or more when using mepivacaine. This figure is reduced for anyone weighing less than 150 lbs.

Elena weighs 120 lbs, therefore she can have 240 mg of mepivacaine (120 lbs × 2 mg/lb MRD).

Each cartridge of 4% articaine contains 72 mg of drug. 240 mg (mepivacaine MRD) – 72 mg (initial articaine dose) = 168 mg (additional dose allowed). This is the additional number of milligrams of mepivacaine Elena can have following the dose of articaine.

To be clinically useful, this information can be converted to cartridges by the following calculation: 168 mg (available) ÷ 54 mg (dose in a 1.8 ml cartridge) = 3.0 additional cartridges of 3% mepivacaine (rounded down from 3.1)

CHAPTER QUESTIONS

1. All of the following are correct when considering MRDs, *except:*
   a. Articaine = 500 mg (3.2 mg/lb, 7 mg/kg)
   b. Bupivicaine = 90 mg (0.6 mg/lb, 1.3 mg/kg)
   c. Lidocaine = 200 mg (2 mg/lb, 4.4 mg/kg)
   d. Mepivicaine = 300 mg (2 mg/lb, 4.4 mg/kg)

2. Relevant information and mathematical operations required to calculate drug doses for local anesthetics and vasoconstrictors include all but which *one* of the following?
   a. Dilution percentages
   b. Standard cartridge volumes
   c. Defined MRD for each drug
   d. Height and weight

3. Which *one* of the following is *not* related to the MRD for 2% lidocaine, 1:100,000 epinephrine?
   a. 8 cartridges
   b. 11 cartridges
   c. 2 mg/lb for a 150 lb individual
   d. 300 mg for a 150 lb individual

4. What is the MRD for vasoconstrictors when administering 2% lidocaine, 1:100,000 epinephrine to a healthy individual?
   a. 0.02 mg
   b. 0.1 mg
   c. 0.2 mg
   d. 1.0 mg

5. An individual has received 4 cartridges of 2% lidocaine, 1:100,000 epinephrine and is not profoundly anesthetized. How many cartridges of 4% articaine, 1:200,000 epinephrine may be administered if the individual weighs 160 lbs?
   a. 1
   b. 2
   c. 3
   d. 4

6. How many cartridges of 4% articaine, 1:200,000 epinephrine may be administered for an individual with significant cardiovascular compromise?
   a. 1
   b. 2
   c. 3
   d. 4

7. Which *one* of the following accurately describes available formulations?
   a. 2% lidocaine, 1:100,000 epinephrine; 3% lidocaine, 1:200,000 epinephrine
   b. 2% lidocaine, 1:100,000 epinephrine; 4% lidocaine, 1:200,000 epinephrine
   c. 2% lidocaine, 1:100,000 epinephrine; 2% lidocaine, 1:50,000 epinephrine
   d. 2% lidocaine, 1:200,000 epinephrine; 2% lidocaine, 1:20,000 levonordefrin

8. The maximum dose per weight of 4% articaine, 1:100,000 epinephrine for children is:
   a. 2 mg/lb
   b. 3 mg/lb
   c. 2.2 mg/lb
   d. 3.2 mg/lb

9. 0.5% bupivacaine, 1:200,000 epinephrine contains how many milligrams of anesthetic drug per cartridge?
   a. 9
   b. 18
   c. 36
   d. 54

REFERENCES

ADA/PDR Guide to Dental Therapeutics (4th ed.). (2006). Montvale, NJ: Thompson PDR.

Ball, J. W., & Bindler, R. C. (2008). *Pediatric nursing, caring for children* (4th ed.). Upper Saddle River, NJ: Pearson Prentice Hall.

2000 CDC Growth Charts for the United States, http://www.cdc.gov/growthcharts/, Accessed September 29, 2008.

Council on Dental Therapeutics of the American Dental Association. (1984). *Accepted dental therapeutics* (40th ed.). Chicago: American Dental Association.

Davis, M. J., & Vogel, L. D. (1996). Local anesthetic safety in pediatric patients. *New York State Dental Journal, 62*(2), 32–35.

Finder, R. L., & Moore, P. A. (2002). Adverse drug reactions to local anesthesia. *Dental Clinics of North America, 46* (4), 747–757.

Malamed, S. F. (2004). *Handbook of local anesthesia* (5th ed.). St Louis: Elsevier Mosby.

Medical Office Pharmacology Review; http://www.mapharm.com, Accessed March 29, 2008.

Pickett, F. A., & Terezhalmy, G. T. (2006). *Dental drug reference with clinical applications.* Baltimore: Lippincott Williams & Wilkins.

Special Committee of the New York Heart Association. (1955). Use of epinephrine with procaine in dental procedures. *Journal of the American Dental Association, 50*, 108.

Local Anesthetic Solutions— Dose Calculation Facts

Local Anesthetic Drugs—Volume of drug per Cartridge

Local Anesthetic Drugs used in dentistry are diluted and commonly referred to as a *concentration*

Drug dose and "per cartridge" facts:
$$1 \text{ ml} = 1 \text{ cc}$$
$$1 \text{ cartridge} = 1.8 \text{ ml solution (1.8 cc)}$$
$$1\% \text{ solution} = 10 \text{ mg/ml}$$
$$1\% = 10 \text{ mg/ml} \times 1.8 \text{ ml/cartridge} = 18 \text{ mg/cart}$$

Common Dental Concentrations—1.8 ml Cartridge Conversions:

Concentration		*Drug per ml*		*Drug per cartridge*
0.5% solution ml/cartridge	$\rightarrow$	5 mg/ml	$\rightarrow$	0.5 mg/ml $\times$ 1.8 = **9 mg**/cartridge
2% solution ml/cartridge	$\rightarrow$	20 mg/ml	$\rightarrow$	20 mg/ml $\times$ 1.8 = **36 mg**/cartridge
3% solution ml/cartridge	$\rightarrow$	30 mg/ml	$\rightarrow$	30 mg/ml $\times$ 1.8 = **54 mg**/cartridge
4% solution ml/cartridge	$\rightarrow$	40 mg/ml	$\rightarrow$	40 mg/ml $\times$ 1.8 = **72 mg**/cartridge

---

Vasoconstrictor Drugs—Volume of drug per Cartridge

Vasoconstrictors used in dentistry are diluted and commonly referred to as a *ratio*

Drug dose and "per cartridge" facts:

$1{:}1000 = 1$ g or 1000 mg of vasoconstrictor per 1000 ml solution (1 mg/ml)

$1{:}10,000 = 1$ ml of 1:1000 vasoconstrictor $+$ 9 ml water $= 0.1$ mg/ml

$1{:}100,000 = 1$ ml of 1:10,000 vasoconstrictor $+$ 9 ml water $= 0.018$ mg/cartridge

$1{:}100,000 = 0.01$ mg/ml $\times$ 1.8 ml $= 0.018$ mg/cartridge

Common Dental Ratios—1.8 ml Cartridge Conversions:

Ratio		*Drug per ml*		*Drug per cartridge*
1:20,000	$\rightarrow$	0.05 mg/ml	$\rightarrow$	0.05 $\times$ 1.8 ml = **0.09** mg/cart
1:50,000	$\rightarrow$	0.02 mg/ml	$\rightarrow$	0.02 $\times$ 1.8 ml = **0.036** mg/cart
1:100,000	$\rightarrow$	0.01 mg/ml	$\rightarrow$	0.01 $\times$ 1.8 ml = **0.018** mg/cart
1:200,000	$\rightarrow$	0.005 mg/ml	$\rightarrow$	0.005 $\times$ 1.8 ml = **0.009** mg/cart

---

(continued)

Maximum doses for vasoconstrictors
Doses *based SOLELY on vasoconstrictor*

Epinephrine
Healthy patient—0.2 mg/appointment
= 10 ml of 1:50,000 (5 cartridges)
= 20 ml of 1:100,000 (11 cartridges)
= 40 ml of 1:200,000 (22 cartridges)

"Cardiac Dose"—0.04 mg/appointment
= 2 ml of 1:50,000 (1 cartridge)
= 4 ml of 1:100,000 (2 cartridges)
= 8 ml of 1:200,000 (4 cartridges)

Levonordefrin
Healthy patient—1 mg/appointment
= 20 ml of a 1:20,000 (11 cartridges)

"Cardiac Dose"—0.2 mg/appointment
= 4 ml of a 1:20,000 (2 cartridges)

"Cardiac Dose" = 20% (1/5) of healthy pt. dose
"Reduce" for Compromised/Geriatric patients

Local Anesthesia and Vasoconstrictor Maximum Dose Reference

bupivacaine	lidocaine	mepivacaine	
0.5% = 9 mg drug per cartridge Maximum dose 90 mg 0.6 mg/lb = 1.3 mg/kg **MRD* 10 cartridges**	2% = 36 mg drug per cartridge Maximum dose 300 mg 2 mg/lb = 4.4 mg/kg **MRD* 8 cartridges**	2% = 36 mg drug per cartridge 3% = 54 mg drug per cartridge Maximum dose 300 mg 2 mg/lb = 4.4 mg/kg **MRD* 5.5 cartridges**	**MRD* 8 cartridges**

0.5%	2%			3%	2%
w/ epi 1:200,000	w/o epi	1:50,000	1:100,000	w/o vaso	w/ levonordefrin 1:20,000

Max cartridges by body weight	Max cartridges by body weight			Max cartridges by body weight	

bupivacaine — Max cartridges by body weight

10 max	≥150 lbs+
9.5–10	143–149
9–9.5	135–142
8.5–9	128–134
8–8.5	120–127
7.5–8	113–119
7–7.5	105–112
6.5–7	98–104
6–6.5	90–97
5.5–6	83–89
5–5.5	76–82
4.5–5	68–75
4–4.5	60–67
3.5–4	53–59
3–3.5	
2.5–3	
2	

lidocaine — Max cartridges by body weight

	8 max	≥150 lbs+
	7.5–8	135–149
	7–7.5	126–134
	6.5–7	117–125
	6–6.5	108–116
	5.5–6	99–107
	5–5.5	90–98
1:50,000	4.5–5	81–89
	4–4.5	72–80
	3.5–4	63–71
	3–3.5	54–62
	2.5–3	45–53
1:100,000	2–2.4	
	1.5–2	
1:50,000	1.6 (1 @ 1:50,000)	

Lidocaine w/ 1:50,000 epi
limiting factor for **healthy** patient
epinephrine **NOT** lidocaine
Maximum Dose = 5 cartridges

mepivacaine — Max cartridges by body weight

5.5 max	≥150 lbs+	8 max	≥150 lbs+
5–5.5	135–149	7.5–8	135–149
4.5–5	122–134	7–7.5	126–134
4–4.5	108–121	6.5–7	117–125
3.5–4	95–107	6–6.5	108–116
3–3.5	81–94	5.5–6	99–107
2.5–3	68–80	5–5.5	90–98
2–2.4	54–67	4.5–5	81–89
1.5–2	41–53	4–4.5	72–80
1.1		3.5–4	63–71
		3–3.5	54–62
		2.5–3	45–53
		2–2.4	
		1.5–2	
		1.6	

Converting Pounds to Kilograms

(lbs→kg = lbs/2.2) (kg→lbs = kg × 2.2)

(continued)

articaine		prilocaine		Medically Compromised Individual
4% = 72 mg drug per cartridge Maximum dose 500 mg 3.2 mg/lb = 7 mg/kg **MRD* 6 cartridges**		4% = 72 mg drug per cartridge Maximum dose 400 mg 2.7 mg/lb = 6 mg/kg **MRD* 5 cartridges**		Restrict to *smallest effective* dose **Shaded Box represents ~ 20% of LA**

4%		**4%**		*"Cardiac Dose"* **epinephrine = 0.04 mg** (20% of **normal 0.2** mg dose) *"Cardiac Dose"* **levonordefrin = 0.2 mg** (20% of **normal 1.0 mg** dose)
w/epi 1:100,000	w/ epi 1:200,000	w/o vaso	w/ epi 1:200,000	

Max cartridges by body weight			**Max cartridges by body weight**			**Based *only* on *Vasoconstrictor* Maximum Cartridges**
	6 max	**≥150 lbs+**		**5 max**	**≥150 lbs+**	levonordefrin **1:20,000 = 2 cartridges**
	5.5–6	124–149		4.5–5	120–149	epinephrine **1:50,000 = 1 cartridge**
	5–5.5	113–123		4–4.5	107–119	epinephrine **1:100,000 = 2 cartridges**
	4.5–5	102–112		3.5–4	93–106	epinephrine **1:200,000 = 4 cartridges**
	4–4.5	91–101		3–3.5	80–92	
1:200,000	3.5–4	79–90		2.5–3	67–79	*All volumes on this list are rounded down*
	3–3.5	68–78		2–2.4	53–66	*to nearest 1/2 cartridge.*
	2.5–3	57–67		1.5–2	40–52	
	2–2.4	45–56		1–1.5		
1:100,000	1.5–2			1		
	1.2					

*MRD = Maximum Recommended Dose (based on Malamad 5th edition)

108

Chapter 8

Topical Anesthetics

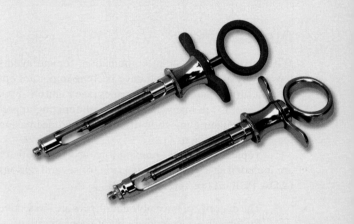

OBJECTIVES

- Define and discuss the key terms in this chapter.
- Discuss the clinical applications of topical anesthetic drugs.
- Discuss the most common methods of application.
- Understand indications and contraindications of topical anesthetic drugs.
- Discuss maximum recommended doses when provided by manufacturers and safe application habits when they are not provided.
- Describe and recognize the signs and symptoms of adverse topical anesthetic drug reactions, both local and systemic.
- Define and discuss eutectic mixtures including factors that determine their effectiveness.
- Discuss what is meant by compounded drugs and proper guidelines for their use.

CASE STUDY: Elena Gagarin

Elena Gagarin believes that she has a high tolerance for pain. Despite this belief, when palatal injections were necessary for the placement of a rubber dam clamp on the right posterior palatal tissues, she cried during the injection. She said that she was fine at the time but requested an alternative to the palatal injections at subsequent visits, if possible.

INTRODUCTION

Whether used alone or in combination, topical agents have many applications and have become important options in current pain control strategies (see Figure 8–1 ■). Their benefits are many and include minimizing apprehension, managing injection discomfort, and decreasing the need for injections.

Topical anesthetic preparations used in dentistry are included as a separate discussion for several reasons (ADA/PDR, 2006; Tetzlaff, 2000):

1. The majority of injectable anesthetics are ineffective for topical use in dentistry in safe concentrations.
2. Ester local anesthetic drugs are both useful and popular as topicals.

3. Some agents, such as dyclonine hydrochloride, which have no injectable counterparts or are too toxic for injection, can nevertheless provide capable and safe topical anesthesia.
4. Paraben preservatives such as methylparaben, banned in injectable preparations, are beneficial and can be found in some multiuse topical preparations.

Topical anesthetic agents have many uses in dentistry. The most common is for penetration site anesthesia prior to needle insertion. Topicals are also useful for discomfort related to radiographic film placement, periodontal evaluation and treatment, procedures confined to superficial mucosa, the placement of retraction cord and rubber dams (when anesthesia has not been established prior to placement), and controlling gag reflexes.

Topical agents are widely accepted based on an extensive history of safe and effective use. Despite this history, there have been rare deaths associated with the *excessive* use of topical preparations. Although adverse reactions are primarily seen in medicine, a recent incident illustrates the inherent dangers of *excessive* applications (see Box 8–1).

Generally formulated in concentrations exceeding those approved for use in injectable local anesthetic drugs, topical preparations are potentially more toxic. This is complicated by the wide variety of application

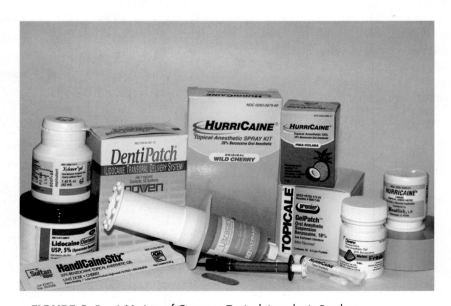

■ **FIGURE 8–1** A Variety of Common Topical Anesthetic Products.

Box 8–1 Rare Death Related to Lidocaine Topical

(01/18/05—RALEIGH)–A young woman's family says she was on her way to have laser hair-removal treatment in Raleigh when something went terribly wrong. Doctors say the young woman suffered brain damage and heart failure due to high levels of lidocaine in her blood.

. . . December 28th, [the young woman] had an appointment for laser hair removal, but she never made it to the treatment.

She had been given tubes of lidocaine cream to apply in preparation for that treatment . . . [It is known] that she applied some of the cream on the morning of December 28th.

About 45 minutes before the scheduled treatment, a member of the DOT's Motorist Assistance Patrol found [the young woman] in her car, on the side of Interstate 40 having a seizure.

[The] death certificate indicates a cause of death was elevated blood lidocaine levels.

. . . a . . . drug information specialist, says lidocaine is commonly used as a local anesthetic, but it comes with a warning.

Excerpt from: "Commonly Used Drug Leads to Mysterious Death . . . Eyewitness News Exclusive" - Angela Hampton http://abclocal.go.com/wtvd/story?section=News&id=2633185. Accessed July 27, 2007.

cartridges containing specific concentrations of drugs, tracking topical dosages can be problematic. Patches and metered sprays offer more precise calculations as do some single dose application systems. Liquids and gels in multiuse containers, and nonmetered sprays present problems even when maximum doses are known because there is no easy way to determine how much was dispensed or how much was absorbed before being washed away in saliva.

Another factor in topical anesthetic application is that there is no rationale for exceeding peak uptake intervals (the period during which the majority of absorption occurs) because the risk of tissue damage increases the longer they contact mucosa. When there is no therapeutic benefit, excessive durations of topical application should be avoided.

In addition to standard commercial topical preparations, **compounded drugs** formulated by compounding pharmacies (see Figure 8–2 ■) should be accompanied by a set of instructions specific for their intraoral use and are intended for use only on what the FDA describes as *identified* patients (see Box 8–2). Strict adherence to all instructions accompanying these preparations is recommended.

Factors that may affect topical anesthetic toxicity include concentration, the relative ability to penetrate tissue, the speed of systemic absorption, and the total area of coverage. Any situation that slows the metabolism of topical anesthetics increases their toxic potential.

methods and the frequent lack of any clear way to determine the dose applied.

This chapter will discuss the most common topical anesthetic drugs in dentistry. Special attention will be given to describing common signs and symptoms of adverse events, the benefits of topical drug combinations, and guidelines for the use of compounded formulations.

GENERAL CONSIDERATIONS

Unlike their injectable counterparts, maximum dose recommendations for many topical products do not exist (Yagiela, 2005). Even when manufacturers provide MRD information, clinicians often have difficulty determining how much was dispensed or absorbed. Compared to injectable administrations with calibrated

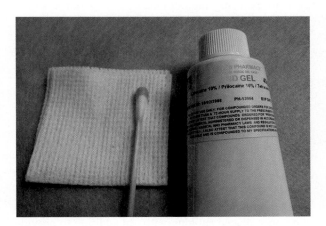

■ **FIGURE 8–2** Example: Compounded Topical Anesthetic Product.

Box 8–2 Compounding Rules

When choosing to use topical agents from compounding pharmacies, it is important to be familiar with the FDA Modernization Act of 1997. This legislation states: "The compounded product must be individually prescribed for an identified patient" (FDA, 1977). This language may be interpreted to mean that it is contrary to the act to acquire a multi-dose package intended for use on patients yet to be identified. An example of one interpretation of this rule would be that a product shared with a different office could not be used in that office because those patients were not identified when the prescription was filled. Copies of the act may be obtained at the FDA website, http://www.fda.gov.

COMMON APPLICATION METHODS

Available in a variety of commercial forms, topical anesthetics may be dispensed as liquids, gels, creams, ointments, metered and unmetered sprays, and subgingival dual-phase systems.

Application methods include the use of cotton swabs, sprays, patches, air injection systems, and subgingival delivery systems with blunt-tipped devices (see Figure 8–3 ■, Figure 8–4 ■ and Figure 8–5 ■).

Topical anesthetics in liquid form have been used for many years. Liquid rinses can provide widespread topical effects, for example, controlling gag reflexes prior to exposing radiographs or taking impressions. This form has proven less useful prior to needle penetration because it is difficult to maintain site-specific, durable coverage of tissue. Gels, on the other hand, are less useful for widespread pain control or controlling the gag reflex but are more useful in smaller areas such as prior to needle penetration. Creams may contain single drugs or mixtures of drugs. Ointments provide excellent topical anesthesia and have been used for years. Metered sprays have significant benefit over unmetered sprays when considering toxicity. One of the newest applications, a subgingival liquid-to-gel system is easily applied due to its liquid state at room temperature and its rapid transformation to a gel-like state once placed subgingivally. In addition to providing excellent tissue anesthesia and occasional pulpal anesthesia, this system has wide margins of safety, a

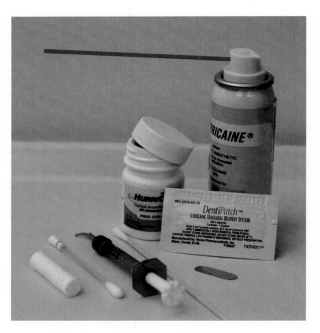

■ **FIGURE 8–3** Various Topical Anesthetic Application Methods. Topical anesthetic agents are applied by a variety of methods mostly dependent on the viscosity of the product and desired application sites.

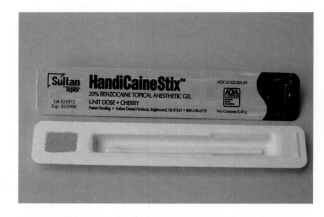

■ **FIGURE 8–4** Single-Dose Commercial Applicators.

known maximum safe dose, and easily quantified volumes dispensed due to its packaging in cartridge form (Oraqix, Dentsply Pharmaceuticals).

Typical application methods for gels include cotton swabs and single-dose commercial applicators (see Figure 8–4). Sprays include disposable intraoral tips and are either metered (the dose is related to the length of time

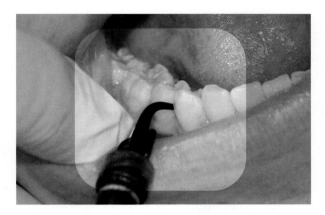

■ **FIGURE 8–5**   Secondary Syringe Delivery.

the nozzle is depressed) or unmetered (unknown quantities are administered) (see Figure 8–6 ■). Interestingly, some sprays call for depressing the nozzle only one-half second per application. This rather limited spray interval is difficult to accomplish clinically, and applications may routinely exceed the half-second interval.

Patches contain specific doses of anesthetic drug per area of surface contact. For example, applying half a patch administers exactly half the dose that is included in the entire patch. One popular patch, DentiPatch

(Noven Pharmaceuticals, Miami, Florida) delivers 46.1 mg of lidocaine per patch (see Figure 8–7 ■). While not necessarily recommending the practice (follow all manufacturer's instructions), cutting a patch in half and applying this reduced surface area to the mucosa, for example, would administer exactly 23.05 mg of lidocaine. In a 2001 study, peak uptake was reported to occur at 15 minutes and the topical anesthetic benefit lasted up to 45 minutes (Carr & Horton, 2001). In order to avoid tissue damage, it is suggested that the patch be left on tissue no more than 15 minutes.

When calculating systemic doses delivered by patches, consult manufacturers' product inserts. In the case of the DentiPatch, the systemic dose resulting from the recommended administration of one patch is equal to one-tenth the number of milligrams administered. If an entire patch is applied to mucosa the delivered dose would be 46.1 mg of lidocaine but the systemic dose would be only 4.61 mg.

Patches are particularly useful in the palate where injection anesthesia has a reputation for discomfort. When injections in several areas of the mouth are anticipated, some clinicians find it useful to place the patch first, allowing it to remain in contact with the tissues for the recommended time, while proceeding with other

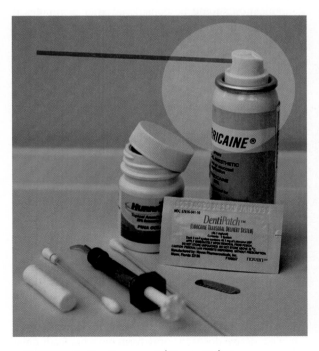

■ **FIGURE 8–6**   Commercial Spray Delivery.

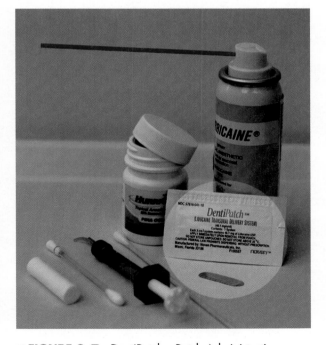

■ **FIGURE 8–7**   DentiPatch—Patch Administration.

injections. In order for good adhesion to the tissues, the patch should be held firmly in place for a full 40 seconds (the patient can be instructed to do this), and longer if it is not well-adhered at 40 seconds, to avoid detachment and possible swallowing. The patch is firmly adhered if it remains in place despite gentle tugging with cotton forceps.

COMMON TOPICAL AGENTS

A number of drugs can be used alone and in combinations to provide effective topical anesthesia for common dental procedures. These preparations include the following drugs, which will be discussed individually and in combination according to their approved formulations: benzocaine, dyclonine hydrochloride, lidocaine, tetracaine hydrochloride, butamben, and prilocaine.

Benzocaine

Benzocaine, an ester, is one of the most widely used topical anesthetic agents (Jastak, Yagiela, & Donaldson, 1995; Hurricaine). Existing nearly 100% in the base form it is poorly absorbed into the systemic circulation, which gives it a very low potential for systemic toxicity. It may be acquired in gel, transdermal patch, liquid, and spray forms in concentrations ranging from 6% to 20% (see Figure 8–8 ■). The most commonly used concentration is 20%, which provides adequate topical effect in 30 seconds with a peak effect occurring at 2 minutes. Durations range from 5 to 15 minutes.

Similar to prilocaine, benzocaine can induce methemoglobinemia and should be avoided in individuals who are at risk. It is best to avoid both drugs in this situation (see Table 8–1 ■).

Similarity to other topical anesthetics
Benzocaine is an ester.

It has been characterized as nonionic and remains nearly 100% nonionic (in its neutral base form) even if swallowed (Tetzlaff, 2000). Other ester topical anesthetics include tetracaine and butamben.

Effective concentrations in dentistry
Benzociane is formulated in 6% to 20% preparations.

Onset of action
The onset of anesthesia for benzocaine is 0.5 minutes, with peak effect at 2 minutes.

While the onset of action with benzocaine is rapid, a more reliable time elapse in terms of comfort before injection is 1 to 2 minutes.

Duration of action
The average duration of anesthesia for benzocaine is 5 to 15 minutes.

Fifteen minutes is seldom needed before injection but once the initial 5 minutes have elapsed, there is no guarantee that an acceptable topical effect is still present. Reapplication should be considered after 5 minutes if the injection has not occurred during that time.

MRD (maximum recommended dose)
There is no established MRD for benzocaine.

It is recommended that clinicians follow manufacturer's recommendations whenever available. With spray preparations of benzocaine, never exceed a 2 second administration period (ADA/PDR, 2006).

Toxicity
Toxic reactions to benzocaine in dentistry are rare.

Precautions increase when tissues are highly abraded, when used in children and adults of very low weight, and when applied to large areas of tissue (see Box 8–3).

Although uncommon, this potential nevertheless exists, especially if sprays are used in larger volumes, such as might occur from excessive numbing of the oral cavity prior to exposing radiographs or taking impressions.

While unlikely, methemoglobinemia has occurred when excessive doses in spray form have been administered (FDA, 2006). The risk of methemoglobinemia is

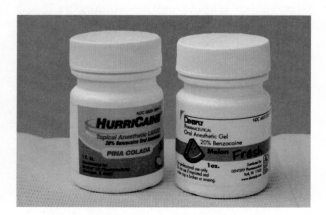

■ **FIGURE 8–8** Benzocaine Topical.

Table 8–1 **Dental Single Drug Topical Anesthetic Preparations**

Drug	Class	Effective Concentrations	Onset of Action (minutes)	Duration of Action (minutes)	MRD (mg)	FDA Pregnancy Category*
benzocaine	ester	6–20%	0.5–2	5–15	unknown	C
dyclonine	ketone	1%	up to 10	30	200	C
lidocaine	amide	2–5%	1–2	15	200–300	B
tetracaine	esther	0.25–0.5	up to 20 (slow)	20–60	20	C

*During lactation all of these drugs should be used with caution.

Box 8–3 **Special Considerations When Using Topical Anesthetics**

Broken skin and inflamed or damaged mucosa, such as the linings of diseased periodontal pockets, are more easily penetrated because the drugs bypass the protective epithelial barrier, moving directly to exposed blood vessels in the connective tissue and from there into the systemic circulation. Topical anesthetics applied in this manner must be considered more carefully when monitoring safe doses.

---

increased in small children, probably due to their low body weight (Tetzlaff, 2000). Although by no means typical, it is important to point out that benzocaine gel for teething pain has resulted in symptomatic methemoglobinemia in the past (Tetzlaff, 2000).

Benzocaine has also been reported to be an antagonist to the actions of the sulfonamide antibacterials (Alston, 1992).

As an ester, benzocaine metabolizes to PABA, which is an FDA-identified antigen. Allergies are more frequent to ester agents. In the case of topical anesthetics, allergic reactions, while not restricted to local areas of tissue, tend to involve delayed responses and are usually limited to areas of contact only. Benzocaine allergies are almost always restricted to these areas. Lidocaine topical is an appropriate substitute should this occur.

Metabolism
Benzocaine is metabolized by ester hydrolysis (via cholinesterase).

Principal metabolites include PABA and ethanol, which may further metabolize to carbon dioxide and water.

Excretion
Benzocaine is excreted as PABA, ethanol, carbon dioxide, and water in variable ratios.

Pregnancy category
Benzocaine FDA Pregnancy Category C.

Lactation
Caution is recommended in nursing.

Most drugs are available in breast milk once introduced. Product information generally states that caution must be exercised when nursing after benzocaine administration.

Proprietary names by application category
(variable concentrations)
Some prescription and over-the-counter products containing benzocaine are listed in Table 8–2 ■.

Sources: FDA, 2006; Tetzlaff, 2000.

Dyclonine Hydrochloride

Dyclonine hydrochloride, formerly available as Dyclone (0.5% solution), is a nonester, nonamide, ketone topical anesthetic (the aromatic and amino ends are joined by a ketone linkage) (Jastak et al., 1995). Dyclonine provides a relatively safe and very durable topical effect. With a slow onset of between 2 and 10 minutes and duration of about 30 minutes, it is particularly useful when amides and esters may not be used. Dyclonine is occasionally available as a spray (a 1% solution) and is currently available through compounding pharmacies (see Figure 8–9 ■). It can also be found in over-the-counter (OTC) products such as Sucrets Children's, Regular Strength, and Maximum Strength lozenges and Cepacol Sore Throat Lozenges and Sprays (see Figure 8–10 ■) (Malamed, 2004).

Table 8–2 Some Topical Anesthetic Products Containing Benzocaine

Aerosols
- Americaine 20%
- Hurricaine 20%
- Topex 20%

Creams
- Benzocaine 5%
- Orajel PM Maximum Strength 20%

Gels
- HDA Toothache 6.5%
- Baby Anbesol 7.5%
- Baby Oral Pain Reliever 7.5%
- Dentane 7.5%
- Orajel Baby Happy Smiles Kit 7.5%
- Orajel Teething Medication 7.5%
- Orajel 10%
- Orajel Nightime
  Teething Baby Medicine 10%
- Zilactin Baby Extra Strength 10%
- Zilactin B 10%
- Orajel Denture Plus 15%
- Orajel Ultra Mouth Sore 15%
- Americaine Anesthetic Lubricant 20%
- Anbesol Maximum Strength 20%
- Comfortcaine 20%

- Darby Super-Dent
  Benzocaine Topical Anesthetic Gel 20%
- Dentsply Benzocaine Oral Anesthetic Gel 20%
- Dentapaine 20%
- Gingicaine 20%
- Hurricaine 20%
- Kank-A Soft Brush Lubricant 20%
- Oral Anesthetic 20%
- Orabase-B 20%
- Orajel Maximum Strength 20%
- Orajel Mouth Aid 20%
- Patterson 20%
- Topex 20%
- Topicale 20%

Gel Patch
- Topicale GelPatch 36 mg/patch

Gum
- Dent's Extra Strength Toothache 20%

Ointments
- Anacaine 10%
- Benzodent 10%
- CoraCaine 20%
- Red Cross Canker 20%
- Topicale 20%

Liquid Solutions
- Orasept 1.53%
- Gumsol 2%
- Babee Teething Lotion 2.5%
- Rid-A-Pain 6.5%
- Miradyne-3 9%
- Tanac Liquid 10%
- Anbesol Maximum Strength 20%
- Dent's Maximum Strength Toothache Drops 20%
- Gingicaine 20%
- Hurricaine 20%
- Kank-A 20%
- Topex 20%

Lozenges
- Chloroseptic Sore Throat 6 mg
- Cepacol Extra Strength 10 mg
- Spec-T 10 mg
- BiZets 15 mg

Swabs
- Orajel Baby Teething Swabs 7.5%
- Dentemps Oral Pain Relief 10%
- Gingicaine One SwabStick 20%
- Hurricaine 20%
- Orajel Medicated Mouthsore Swab 20%
- Orajel Medicated Toothache Swab 20%
- Topex 20%
- Zilactin Toothache Maximum Strength 20%

*Product examples in this chapter current as of October 2008.

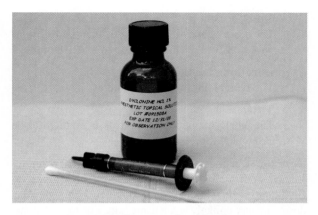

■ **FIGURE 8-9** Dyclonine Hydrochloride.

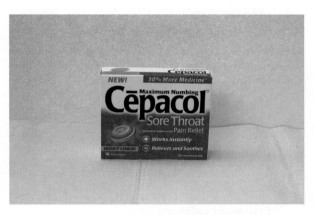

■ **FIGURE 8-10** OTC Source of Dyclonine Hydrochloride. OTC oral anesthetic lozenges containing dyclonine hydrochloride.

Similarity to other topical anesthetics
Dyclonine is a ketone.

It is chemically unique compared to other local anesthetics used in dentistry and medicine.

Effective concentrations in dentistry
Dyclonine is commonly formulated in 1% preparations.

Onset of action
The onset of anesthesia for dyclonine is up to 10 minutes.

Duration of action
The average duration of anesthesia for dyclonine is about 30 minutes (effects may last as long as 1 hour).

MRD
The MRD for dyclonine is 200 mg, or 20 ml of a 1% solution.

Doses are reduced for children and medically compromised adults as well as for situations in which tissues are heavily abraded prior to application. Safe doses have not been determined for children under 12. Allergic reactions are uncommon.

Toxicity
Although toxicity is unlikely and the toxic potential of dyclonine is very low due to poor water solubility, in excessively large doses it may affect sensitive neural tissues similar to other local anesthetic agents resulting in progressive signs and symptoms of CNS and CVS depression.

Metabolism
No information is available on dyclonine metabolism.

Excretion
No information is available on dyclonine excretion.

Pregnancy category
Dyclonine hydrochloride FDA Pregnancy Category C.

Lactation
Caution is recommended in nursing.

Most drugs are available in breast milk once introduced. Product information generally states that caution must be exercised when nursing.

Proprietary names and available preparations
Some prescription and over-the counter products containing dyclonine hydrochloride are listed in Table 8–3 ■.

Sources: ADA/PDR, 2006; Jastak et al., 1995; Malamed, 2004; Tetzlaff, 2000.

Lidocaine

Lidocaine is an effective topical anesthetic drug and an excellent alternative to esters when esters are contraindicated (Jastak et al., 1995). The most common preparation of lidocaine topical is as an ointment in multiuse jars (see Figure 8–11 ■). It is also available in 2–5% concentrations primarily in liquid and gel forms. Toxic reactions, although uncommon, have occurred with lidocaine topical, particularly in the spray form (see Box 8–1). Dental preparations of lidocaine in spray form appear to be

Table 8–3	Examples of Topical Anesthetic Products Containing Dyclonine

Solution
- Dyclone 1% (available from compounding pharmacies and some medical suppliers)

Lozenges
- Sucrets lozenges:
    Children's 1.2 mg
    Regular Strength 2 mg
    Maximum Strength 3 mg

Spray
- Cepacol Sore Throat, Maximum Strength 0.1%

Source: Tetzlaff, 2000.

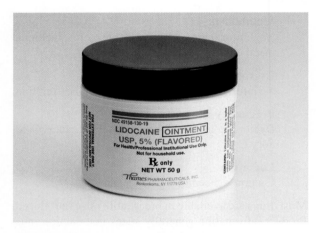

■ **FIGURE 8–11** Lidocaine Topical.
Source: Courtesy of Septodont USA.

unavailable in North America at this time (2009). Onset times vary between 2 and 10 minutes with an expected duration of 15 minutes. Lidocaine is available as a predominantly acid salt preparation (lidocaine hydrochloride) or as a neutral base formulation (lidocaine base). Base preparations have lower systemic absorptions in comparison to acid salt formulations and therefore less toxicity (Mehra, Caiazzo, & Maloney, 1998).

Similarity to other topical anesthetics
Lidocaine is most similar to prilocaine compared to other topicals in dentistry.

Effective concentrations in dentistry
Lidocaine topical is commonly formulated in 2% to 5% preparations.

Onset of action
The onset of anesthesia for lidocaine is 1 to 2 minutes, peak effects may take up to 5 to 10 minutes.

Duration of action
The typical duration is 15 minutes.

MRD
The MRD for lidocaine topicals is reported to be 200 to 300 mg.

Overdose reactions are similar to overdoses from injectable forms of lidocaine with typical progression to CNS depression without initial excitation, although overdoses are very unlikely when using lidocaine topical alone.

Toxicity
Lidocaine topical is a CNS depressant, however, toxic reactions are rare.

Precautions increase when tissues are highly abraded, when used in children and adults of very low weight, and when applied to large areas of tissues.

Metabolism
Lidocaine is metabolized in the liver by hepatic oxidases and amidases.

Excretion
Less than 10% of lidocaine is excreted unchanged by the kidneys.

Pregnancy category
Lidocaine is FDA Pregnancy Category B.

Lactation
Caution is recommended in nursing.

Most drugs are available in breast milk once introduced. Product information generally states that caution must be exercised when nursing.

Proprietary names by application category
Some prescription and over-the-counter products containing lidocaine are listed in Table 8–4 ■.

Sources: ADA/PDR, 2006; Jastak et al., 1995; Malamed, 2004.

Tetracaine Hydrochloride

Tetracaine is a potent ester topical anesthetic. In dentistry, tetracaine is used only in combination with other topical anesthetics.

Historically, it replaced cocaine as an equally effective yet less irritating substitute when applied to the

Table 8–4 Examples of Topical Anesthetic Products Containing Lidocaine	

Patch (base formulation)
• DentiPatch – 46.1 mg
  4.61 mg systemic dose for entire patch
  (proportionately less when fractions
  of the patch are used)
	Gel (hydrochloride salt formulation)
	• Xylocaine Jelly 2%

Ointment (base formulation) • Octocaine 5% (50 mg/ml) • Xylocaine 5% (50 mg/ml)	**Oral Topical Solution** • Xylocaine Viscous 2%
Solution (base formulation) • Zilactin – 2.5%	**Solution** (hydrochloride salt formulation) • Xylocaine 4%

Source: ADA/PDR, 2006; Jastak et al., 1995.

eyes. Repeated or long-term eye contact is now discouraged. Excessive dosing and too-frequent application may result in serious adverse reactions, including those requiring resuscitation.

Similarity to other local anesthetics
Tetracaine is an ester similar to benzocaine and butamben.

Effective concentrations in dentistry
Tetracaine is commonly formulated in 0.25% to 0.5% preparations.

Onset of action
The onset of anesthesia for tetracaine is slow and variable, with peak effects taking up to 20 minutes.

Duration of action
The average duration of anesthesia for tetracaine is 20 to 60 minutes.

MRD
The MRD for tetracaine is 20 mg (1 ml of a 2% solution).

Tetracaine is rapidly absorbed through mucous membranes with a very slow metabolism. Precautions increase when tissues are highly abraded and when used in smaller children.

Toxicity
Tetracaine is the most potent of the dental topical anesthetics. Serious adverse reactions have occurred in conjunction with tetracaine topical anesthesia, particularly in medicine. Excessive doses and too-frequent administrations should be avoided. Extreme caution has been urged with the use of tetracaine due to its potential for systemic toxicity.

Metabolism
Tetracaine undergoes hydrolysis via plasma cholinesterase.

Primary metabolites of tetracaine include PABA and diethylaminoethanol, both of which have an unspecified activity.

Excretion
Tetracaine is excreted by the kidneys.

Pregnancy category
Tetracaine is FDA Pregnancy Category C.

Lactation
Caution is recommended in nursing.

Most drugs are available in breast milk once introduced. Product information generally states that caution must be exercised when nursing.

Proprietary names by application category
Some prescription products containing tetracaine are listed in Table 8–5 ■.

Sources: ADA/PDR, 2006; Jastak et al., 1995; Malamed, 2004; Patel, Chopra, & Berman, 1989; Synera Patch.

TOPICAL DRUG COMBINATIONS

Some topical anesthetics are formulated in combinations to provide enhanced onsets and durations beyond the properties of each drug individually. These combinations are formulated to provide more useful clinical ranges of onset and duration for optimal therapeutic effect.

Table 8–5	Examples of Topical Anesthetic Products Containing Tetracaine

Solution
- Pontocaine 0.25% and 0.5% topical solutions

Nebulized Spray
- Pontocaine 0.5%

Tetracaine in combination will be discussed later as "Benzocaine, Butamben, and Tetracaine combination."

Source: ADA/PDR, 2006; Jastak et al., 1995.

Some are designed for enhanced effectiveness in specific applications. For example, prilocaine is found in combination with lidocaine for topical use in dentistry. This combination of anesthetic drugs is known as a **eutectic mixture** (Jastak et al., 1995, Tetzlaff, 2000). Prilocaine and lidocaine mixtures are described later in this chapter in the discussion of Eutectic Mixtures.

Benzocaine, Butamben, and Tetracaine (combination)

When formulated in combination, these three ester drugs provide a much more useful range of topical anesthesia compared to any of the individual drugs acting alone:

2% tetracaine (long-acting, slow-onset)

14% benzocaine (short-acting, fast-onset), and

2% **butamben** (intermediate-acting, intermediate-onset).

This particular example, Cetacaine (Cetylite Industries Inc., Pennsauken, NJ) enables a rapid onset and a very long duration of topical anesthesia (see Figure 8–12 ■).

Similarity to other topical anesthetics
All three drugs are esters.

Effective concentrations in dentistry
Tetracaine, butamben, and benzocaine are commonly formulated with 2% tetracaine, 2% butamben and 14% benzocaine.

Onset of action
The onset of action of tetracaine, butamben, benzocaine combinations is about 30 seconds.

Duration of action
The duration of the combination may be as much as 45 minutes.

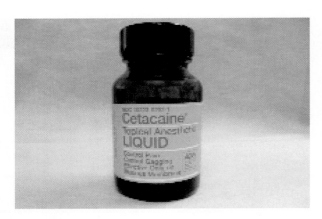

■ **FIGURE 8–12** Cetacaine—Benzocaine, Butamben, and Tetracaine (combination).

MRD
See product inserts for specific MRDs for this combination.

Toxicity
Overdose reactions are similar to overdoses from injectable esters with signs and symptoms of CNS depression followed by CVS toxicity. Precautions increase when tissues are highly abraded, when used in children and adults of very low weight, and when applied to large areas of tissue.

Metabolism
Esters are metabolized via cholinesterase.

Excretion
Excretion occurs primarily through the kidneys.

Pregnancy category
Benzocaine, Butamben, and Tetracaine are all FDA Pregnancy Category C.

Lactation
Caution is recommended in nursing women.

Most drugs are available in breast milk once introduced. Product information generally states that caution must be exercised when nursing.

Proprietary names by application category
Some prescription and over-the counter products containing benzocaine, butamben, and tetracaine combined are listed in Table 8–6 ■.

Sources: ADA/PDR, 2006; Jastak et al., 1995; Malamed, 2004.

Table 8–6	Examples of Topical Anesthetic Products Containing Benzocaine, Butamben, and Tetracaine

Aerosol
* Cetacaine (14%, 2%, 2%)

Solution
* Cetacaine (14%, 2%, 2%)

Gel
* Cetacaine Hospital (14%, 2%, 2%)

Source: ADA/PDR, 2006; Jastak et al., 1995.
*Product examples current as of September 2008.

EUTECTIC MIXTURES

Eutectic mixtures of local anesthetics provide a more rapid onset on skin and a greater depth of topical penetration on both skin and mucosa compared to any of the ingredients acting alone. This is the result of very specific properties of the mixture.

In preparing eutectic mixtures, powdered drugs are suspended in water and oil to form a cream (Tetzlaff, 2000). Concentrations of the drugs are typically higher than those used in injectable forms and are present in the cream largely as base molecules (Tetzlaff, 2000).

Enhanced properties of eutectic mixtures result from higher concentrations of base molecules, the homogeneous nature of the cream, and the lower melting point of the mixture compared with any of the melting points of the individual components. These properties assure increasing depths of anesthesia, an even distribution, and a faster onset on skin compared with other topicals, but not on mucosa, where most individual topicals have similar onsets. The longer the mixtures are left in contact with skin or mucous membranes, however, the deeper their penetration. Contact on skin for 2 hours will typically yield a greater penetration of anesthesia compared to 1 hour.

Compared to mucosa, skin is a more significant barrier to diffusion of topical drugs and requires longer application times, typically 60 minutes or longer. As previously stated, onsets of eutectic mixtures on mucous membranes are considered rapid compared with skin but still require similar time compared to other commonly available topical agents. A eutectic's advantage on mucosa over any faster-acting topicals is the *depth* of topical anesthesia it is able to provide. The difference is considerable enough, in fact, that eutectic mixtures have been used at times as the sole method of anesthesia, especially in

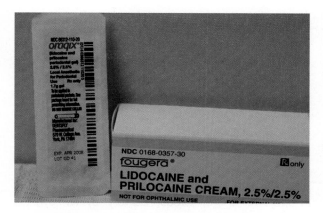

■ **FIGURE 8–13** Oraqix and Lidocaine and Prilocaine Periodontal Eutectic Mixture.

pediatric dentistry where their enhanced depth may be sufficient to provide pulpal anesthesia in the youngest patients (Malamed, 2004). Pulpal effects were found to be less reliable for adults and older children (Malamed, 2004).

Two common eutectic mixtures of local anesthetic drugs commercially available are EMLA and Oraqix (see Figure 8–13 ■). EMLA is formulated for skin but has been used successfully on mucous membranes in both medicine and dentistry. It is approved only for medical use, however, and instructions for use in dentistry do not exist. It is a combination of lidocaine and prilocaine. Oraqix, also a mixture of lidocaine and prilocaine, is formulated for subgingival application although it has a uniquely different method of application. Due to the inclusion of prilocaine, the risk of methemoglobinemia exists in both preparations.

Lidocaine and Prilocaine Periodontal Eutectic Mixture

Oraqix (Dentsply Pharmaceuticals, York, Pennsylvania) is a eutectic mixture designed for "intrapocket" use in dentistry (ADA/PDR, 2006; Oraqix). It is a liquid at room temperature that thickens to a gel-like consistency (dual-phase) when placed subgingivally. The Oraqix delivery system includes a syringe-type carrier (see Figure 8–14 ■) that holds a specialized cartridge and a blunt-tipped applicator (see Figure 8–15 ■). The drugs are *applied,* rather than *injected,* into the sulcus via the blunt-tipped applicator (see Figure 8–16 ■). The product insert suggests a wait of 20 to 30 seconds after initial application in the gingival sulcus before deeper application into periodontal pockets. Deeper application is discontinued once the gel

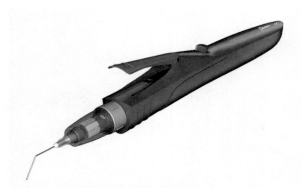

■ **FIGURE 8-14** Oraqix Delivery System Syringe. Modified courtesy of Dentsply Pharmaceutical.

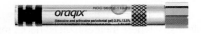

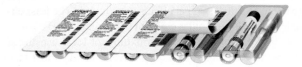

■ **FIGURE 8-15** Oraqix Delivery System Cartridge and Needle. Modified courtesy of Dentsply Pharmaceutical.

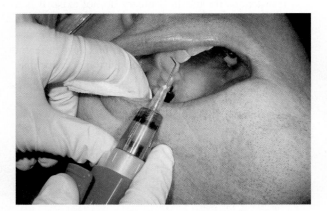

■ **FIGURE 8-16** Oraqix Subgingival Delivery.

becomes visible at the gingival margin. Features enhancing the safety of Oraqix include:

1. Low systemic toxicity with only 20 to 40% of the dispensed drug available systemically.
2. Ease of dose tracking compared with multidose packaging common with other topicals. (Standard calculation methods can be used with the 1.7 ml cartridges.)

3. A specialized *safety collar* (see Figure 8–17 ■) prevents accidental placement of the cartridge into standard aspirating syringes, avoiding accidental submucosal injection of the drugs.

Oraqix can substitute for injectable local anesthetics in some situations, although pulpal anesthesia is not expected but may be provided to some extent (Oraqix).

Similarity to other topical anesthetics
Lidocaine and prilocaine are amides.

Lidocaine is similar to etidocaine and prilocaine is similar to articaine. There is no equivalent combination to Oraqix due to its unique liquid-to-gel transformation at physiologic temperatures.

Effective concentrations in dentistry
Lidocaine and prilocaine in eutectic mixtures for topical use are commonly formulated with 2.5% lidocaine and 2.5% prilocaine.

Onset of action
The onset of anesthesia for topical lidocaine and prilocaine combinations is about 1 minute.

Duration of action
The overall duration of action of Oraqix is 20 minutes (ranging between 14 and 31 minutes).

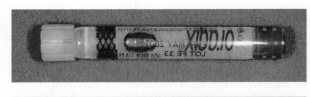

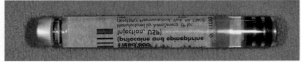

■ **FIGURE 8-17** Oraqix Delivery System Cartridge Safety Feature. There are two key safety features of Oraqix cartridges (top) when compared to standard local anesthetic cartridges (bottom) that prevent insertion into standard syringes and inadvertent submucosal injection. An Oraqix cartridge has a white plastic *safety collar* over the end cap and needle penetration end. The size prohibits insertion into a standard syringe. The second feature is the unique "crosshatched" colored band near the *safety collar*. On a standard dental cartridge a bar code is present while a drug identification color band is near the stopper.

Duration is variable and depends upon the time of application and the type of tissue on which Oraqix is applied.

MRD
The MRD for topical lidocaine and prilocaine in a eutectic mixture is 5 cartridges per appointment maximum (Oraqix).

Toxicity
Only about 20 to 40% is absorbed systemically.

Overdose reactions are similar to overdoses from injectable amides with signs and symptoms of CNS depression followed by CVS toxicity. Prilocaine increases the possibility of the development of methemoglobinemia in individuals with congenital and idiosyncratic tendencies.

Metabolism
Lidocaine is metabolized by hepatic oxidases and amidases.

Prilocaine is metabolized in the liver by amidases, and in the lungs and kidneys.

Excretion
Excretion occurs primarily through the kidneys.

Pregnancy category
Both lidocaine and prilocaine are FDA Pregnancy Category B.

Lactation
Caution is recommended in nursing women.

Most drugs are available in breast milk once introduced. Product information generally states that caution must be exercised when nursing.
Source: Oraqix.

Lidocaine and Prilocaine Eutectic Mixtures

Another eutectic mixture of lidocaine and prilocaine is available as EMLA (Eutectic Mixture of Local Anesthetics, AstraZeneca, Wilmington, Delaware). The same concentration of drugs found in Oraqix is available in EMLA, 2.5% lidocaine and 2.5% prilocaine; however, EMLA is not a dual-phase system (see EMLA reference). EMLA is also available in generic preparations (see Figure 8–18 ■).

In pediatric dentistry, EMLA can be particularly useful by providing complete pulpal anesthesia for some procedures due to its significant depth of penetration (Munshi, Hegde, & Latha, 2001). As with Oraqix, EMLA has gained popularity by providing deep topical

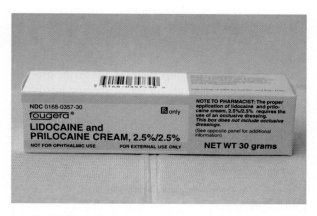

■ **FIGURE 8-18** Lidocaine and Prilocaine Eutectic Mixture (Generic EMLA).

effects that may provide specific benefits (Malamed, 2004). While not originally recommended for dental use, clinical trials have demonstrated that it can be effective in dentistry (Bernardi, Secco, & Benech, 1999; Munshi et al., 2001). Product information accompanying EMLA does not provide specific information regarding its use on oral mucous membranes.

Similarity to other topical anesthetics
Lidocaine and prilocaine are amides.

Lidocaine is similar to etidocaine and prilocaine is similar to articaine.

Effective concentrations
No information is available for intra-oral applications.

Effective concentrations and application have been established for medical use only (see Box 8–4).

MRD
0–3 months or less than 5 kg (body weight) = 1 gram

3–12 months or greater than 5 kg = 2 gram

1–6 years or greater than 10 kg = 10 grams

7–12 and greater than 20 kg = 20 grams

Typically, up to 5 to 10 grams must be applied on genital mucosa for effective topical anesthesia.

Overdose reactions are similar to overdoses from injectable amides with signs and symptoms of CNS depression followed by CVS toxicity. Prilocaine increases the possibility of the development of methemoglobinemia in individuals with congenital and idiosyncratic tendencies.

Box 8–4 *Dose Considerations for the Medical Use of EMLA*

EMLA is not approved by the FDA for dental use. For this reason, there are no dental-specific instructions included with the product. On the other hand, the FDA has not banned it from use in dentistry. So-called off-label use implies knowledge on the part of clinicians in the appropriate and reasonable use of such products.

The directions for **medical** *use include the following:*

Apply 1 to 2 grams in each 10 cm^2

Supplied in 5- and 30-gram tubes and as an adhesive anesthetic disc

---

Toxicity

Approximately 1/20 the amount of the lidocaine applied on skin is absorbed systemically while approximately 1/36 the amount of the prilocaine applied on skin is absorbed systemically.

When 10 grams were applied to genital mucosa, the absorbed doses of lidocaine and prilocaine, respectively, were 148–641 ng/ml and 40–346 ng/ml, which is well below the concentrations anticipated to give rise to systemic toxicity (5000 ng/ml for both lidocaine and prilocaine).

Onset of action

5 to 10 minutes are required on genital mucosa for sufficient anesthesia. No information is available on oral mucosal uses.

The longer EMLA is held against the tissues, the greater the depth of anesthesia it provides. Applications on skin are usually adequate in 1 hour.

Duration of action

No information is available for intra-oral applications.

MRD

No information is available for intra-oral applications.

Toxicity

No information is available for intra-oral applications.

Metabolism

Lidocaine is metabolized by hepatic oxidases and amidases.

Prilocaine is metabolized in the liver by amidases, and in the lungs and kidneys.

Excretion

Excretion occurs primarily through the kidneys.

Pregnancy category

Lidocaine and prilocaine eutectic mixtures are FDA Pregnancy Category B.

Lactation

Caution is recommended in nursing women (see EMLA reference).

Most drugs are available in breast milk once introduced. Product information generally states that caution must be exercised when nursing.

Source: EMLA.

CONSIDERATIONS IN THE ADMINISTRATION OF TOPICALS

Although toxic reactions are rare, the higher concentrations of many topical anesthetics compared with injectable agents give them a potentially greater risk of toxicity. As these agents become more popular and gain acceptance as alternatives to traditional injectable anesthesia, it is important to consider the increased risks when using them. Careful monitoring of administered volumes and of the time between successive applications, as well as minimizing areas of coverage, are all important considerations.

Local Adverse Reactions

Local reactions with topical agents include tissue sloughing, edema, delayed hypersensitivity, redness, pain, and burning at the sites of application. Increased likelihood of adverse events follows application on abraded or broken tissue, including that caused by trauma during application, prolonged contact with skin or mucosa, and undiagnosed hypersensitivities to any of the ingredients. These reactions generally respond well to palliative strategies and discontinuation of the agent. Localized edema following an allergic reaction is shown in Figure 8–19 ■.

Systemic Reactions

Topicals are readily absorbed through oral and bronchial mucosa but only weakly absorbed through GI mucosa.

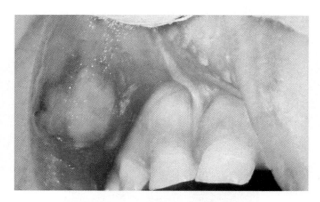

■ **FIGURE 8–19** Local Adverse Reaction. Local edema following application of benzocaine topical.

Swallowing does not promote significant systemic uptake (Malamed, 2004).

Allergic reactions to ester topical agents are rare but not impossible, while allergies to amide topicals have been described as virtually unknown (Yagiela, 2005). Some multiuse amide topicals, however, may contain methylparaben. These preparations benefit from methylparaben's antioxidant, bacteriostatic, and fungistatic properties, particularly in a container that is repeatedly opened and closed, compared with sealed sterile cartridges, which are designed to be used once and then discarded (Malamed, 2004). The United States Food and Drug Administration ordered the removal of methylparabens from dental cartridges in 1984, in response to increasing reports of allergenicity and the absence of a continued need for their inclusion. The order did not affect topicals (Malamed, 2004). It is recommended that product information be consulted for the possible inclusion of methylparaben.

Despite the very low risk of systemic allergic reaction, systemic reactions are possible and have occurred. These have typically been overdose reactions and have ranged from sub-clinical to life-threatening. Overdoses may manifest as mild CNS depression (restlessness, agitation, and increased heart rate) or more severe CNS and CVS depression (unconsciousness, convulsions, decreased force of myocardial contraction, respiratory collapse, and cardiovascular collapse).

When systemic signs and symptoms occur due to methemoglobinemia, they may manifest as lethargy, cyanosis, and respiratory difficulty (Malamed, 2004). Adverse methemoglobinemic events have occurred due to difficulties in determining applied doses, particularly in spray forms. Benzocaine, for example, one of the most widely used and certainly one of the safest topicals, has been linked, in excessive volumes in spray form, to serious methemoglobinemia (Abu-Laban, Zed, Purssell, & Evans, 2001). The following excerpt appeared in the FDA Patient Safety News: Advisory on Benzocaine Sprays and Methemoglobinemia Show #50, April 2006: "The FDA recently issued a public health advisory to remind health care professionals that the overuse of benzocaine anesthetic sprays can cause methemoglobinemia, a potentially life-threatening condition that can result in cyanosis, confusion, hemodynamic instability and coma. . . . Patients with methemoglobinemia can suffer effects ranging from headache to cyanosis (turning blue due to lack of oxygen) that can be life-threatening in the most severe cases." The link to methemoglobinemia also applies to prilocaine in both topical and injectable forms (MMWR, 1994). It is important to point out that recent FDA warnings were prompted by the results of excessive application related to the removal of leg hair and prior to intubation (FDA, 1997). Nevertheless, the potential exists for life-threatening adverse reactions following the inappropriate and excessive use of spray topicals prior to exposing radiographs, for controlling gag reflexes, and for widespread topical anesthesia in dental hygiene procedures.

In some circumstances, particular caution is advisable. Underlying conditions that may predispose to methemoglobinemia according to the April 2006 FDA Advisory include: ". . . patients with breathing problems, such as asthma or emphysema, patients with heart disease, and those who smoke. . . ."

A number of other medications, such as acetaminophen and sulfonamides, and some additives and dyes are also linked to methemoglobinemia. Methemoglobinemia is discussed in depth in Chapter 5, "Dental Local Anesthetic Drugs," Chapter 10, "Patient Assessment for Local Anesthesia," and Chapter 17, "Local Anesthesia Complications and Management."

Jet Injection Devices

Jet injection devices, which propel solution into tissues using air, may be particularly useful in needle-phobic individuals and children. Technically, they *inject* anesthetics, effecting complete local anesthesia for some procedures (Malamed, 2004). They may also be used to provide deeper topical anesthesia prior to needle penetration (see Figure 8–20 ■). Their greatest advantage appears to arise from the ability to propel solutions into

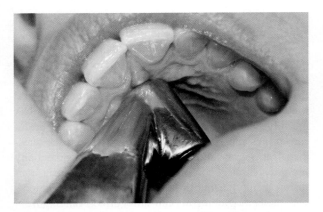

■ **FIGURE 8–20**   Palatal Pre-anesthesia "Jet" Injection.

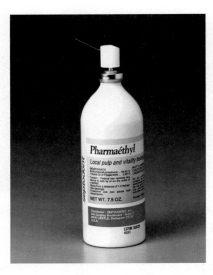

■ **FIGURE 8–21**   Future Developments in Topical Anesthetics. Refrigerants, similar to the cryo-anesthetic ("cold spray") sprays used for pulp testing, may have future applications as topical anesthetics.
Source: Courtesy of Septodont USA.

tissues at significant depth without the use of needles, deep enough at times to provide pulpal anesthesia. According to a 2001 evaluation of 100 children, the degree of pulpal anesthesia provided was deemed "completely successful" and there was a statistically significant bias in favor of the use of a needleless jet syringe over conventional syringes in children (Munshi, Hegde, & Bashir, 2001). Other authors have referred to these devices as inadequate substitutes for traditional needles and syringes and as providing primarily topical anesthesia (Malamed, 2004).

The impact of jet-propelled solutions, themselves, is objected to by some and well tolerated by others (Malamed, 2004). There is often some local tissue damage at the site of injection in the form of transient bruising, especially in the palate.

Despite the costs of these devices, some will find them invaluable in the treatment of children and in other patients with greater dental anxieties, including needle phobias.

Currently available devices include the Syrijet Mark II Needleless Injector (Mizzy Division, Keystone Industries, Cherry Hill, New Jersey) and the MadaJet XL (MADA Medical Products Inc., Carlstadt, New Jersey). These devices are further discussed in Chapter 9, "Local Anesthetic Delivery Devices."

Future Developments in Topical Local Anesthesia

Current research may result in the medical use of a refrigerant, similar to those used for pulp testing (see Figure 8–21 ■), to provide topical anesthesia.

A study comparing the use of a refrigerant as a topical anesthetic versus more time-consuming gel topicals found that pain was significantly reduced when the refrigerant was used (Kosaraju & Vendewalle, 2009). The refrigerant used was 1,1,1,3,3-pentafluoropropane/1,1,1,2-tetrafluoroethane (Gebauer's Pain Ease, 2009). In arriving at that favorable comparison, only a 5- to 10-second application of the refrigerant was necessary.

Medical uses of refrigerants as topicals on skin have demonstrated similar results in immunizations compared to patch preparations. Adverse inflammatory reactions on skin, which can apparently alter pigmentation patterns under exposed areas, were described as not having been identified specifically for mucosa. The manufacturer indicates that the product should not be used on diabetics or those with poor circulation or on any skin with a sensitivity deficit. In addition, cautions include the possible development of postoperative discomfort, irritation, and frostbite. Further study was recommended.

CASE MANAGEMENT: Elena Gagarin

Adequate topical anesthesia can desensitize the maxillary palatal tissues in areas being treated. Slow injection and expressing a few drops of anesthetic solution ahead of the needle often works well, but Elena requested no needles in the palate. Topical patches, which provide greater depths of penetration compared with other topicals, also work well and do not usually require injections afterward in order to place comfortable rubber dam clamps.

Case Discussion: Some patients are adamant regarding not wanting to receive palatal injections. This attitude often arises from painful injections in the palate during previous dental visits. Placement of topical ahead of injection with enough time to diffuse through the surface layer, the application of pressure in the area to further "prenumb" the tissues, and *very* slow deposition rates will help to prevent fear of pain from palatal injections. When these guidelines have not been observed in the past, it is sometimes necessary to rely on patch topicals or interpapillary injections originating from the buccal aspects of teeth in order to desensitize palatal tissues.

CHAPTER QUESTIONS

1. Eutectic mixtures have which of the following characteristics?
   a. They work more rapidly than most other topicals.
   b. They penetrate more deeply on skin than mucosa.
   c. Their melting points exceed that of their ingredients acting alone.
   d. Their formulations facilitate deeper and more efficient penetrations of tissues compared to their ingredients acting alone.

2. Which of the following lists is most accurate when describing topical anesthetic uses?
   a. Prior to exposing radiographs, prior to injections, prior to placing retraction cord
   b. Prior to dental hygiene therapy and in subgingival tissues
   c. In procedures confined to mucosa and prior to taking impressions
   d. All of the above

3. Which *one* of the following statements is *incorrect* regarding maximum recommended doses of topical anesthetics?
   a. They are sometimes difficult to track.
   b. MRDs are not always provided.
   c. Spray forms have easy-to-track dosing.
   d. DentiPatch has easy-to-track dosing.

4. Generous quantities of topical and injected anesthesia have been administered, when the patient begins to shake and appears agitated and anxious. Is there reason for concern?
   a. Yes, because these may be early signs of CNS depression.
   b. No, because this is a very nervous patient and she hates dental appointments.
   c. No, because the doses of injectable anesthetic were within safe guidelines.
   d. Yes, because the patient is a dental phobic.

5. Topical anesthetic mixtures may be of benefit in all but which *one* of the following ways?
   a. Combinations may increase therapeutic ranges.
   b. Combinations may increase penetration depths.
   c. Mixtures may allow drugs to be used as topicals that are not suitable when used alone.
   d. Mixtures decrease the potential for adverse reaction.

6. All of the following statements are true regarding compounded drugs, *except*:
   a. Compounded drugs are formulated for individuals for whom they are prescribed.
   b. Compounded drugs may be used on other individuals as long as the use is the same as the original use.
   c. Compounded drugs may contain much larger quantities of drug compared to multiuse commercial preparations.
   d. Compounded topicals are dispensed by prescription.

7. The predominantly base form of lidocaine topical anesthetic is safer than the predominantly hydrochloride salt.
   a. True
   b. False

8. Dyclonine hydrochloride is an excellent and very durable topical anesthetic and belongs to which *one* of the following classes of anesthetic?
   a. Amide
   b. Ketone
   c. Ester
   d. None of the above

REFERENCES

Abu-Laban, R. B., Zed, P. J., Purssell, R. A., & Evans, K. G. (2001, January). Severe methemoglobinemia from topical anesthetic spray: Case report, discussion and qualitative systematic review. *Canadian Journal of Emergency Medicine, 3*(1), 51–56.

ADA/PDR Guide to Dental Therapeutics (4th ed.). (2006). Montvale, NJ: Thompson PDR.

Alston, T. A. (1992). Antagonism of sulfonamides by benzocaine and chloroprocaine. *Anesthesiology, 76*, 375–476.

Bernardi, M., Secco, F., & Benech, A. (1999). Anesthetic efficacy of a eutectic mixture of lidocaine and prilocaine (EMLA) on the oral mucosa: Prospective double-blind study with a placebo. *Minerva Stomatol, 48*, 9–43.

Carr, M. P., & Horton, J. E. (2001). Evaluation of a transoral delivery system for topical anesthesia. *Journal of the American Dental Association, 132*(12), 1714–1719.

EMLA: Product information available from AstraZeneca, Wilmington, DE; www.astra.com.

FDA Modernization Act of 1997. Available at: http://www.fda .gov/fdac/features/2000/400_compound.html. Accessed July 17, 2006.

FDA Patient Safety News. (2006, April). Advisory on Benzocaine Sprays and Methemoglobinemia: Show #50. Available at: http://www.accessdata.fda.gov/scripts/cdrh/cfdocs/ psn/printer.cfm?id=418. Accessed July 17, 2006.

Gebauer's Pain Ease, topical aerosol skin refrigerant. Technical data document available at www.gebauerco.com/ Contentpages/ResourceCenter/PDFs/TechSheets/ PETS_ENGPdf. Accessed January 13, 2009.

Hurricaine topical anesthetic: Product information available from Beutlich LP, Pharmaceuticals, Waukegan, IL; www.beutlich.com.

Jastak, J. T., Yagiela, J. A., & Donaldson, D. (1995). *Local anesthesia of the oral cavity*. Philadelphia: Saunders.

Kosaraju, A., & Vandewalle, K. S. (2009). A comparison of a refrigerant and a topical anesthetic gel as preinjection anesthetics. *Journal of the American Dental Association, 140*, 68–72.

Malamed, S. F. (2004). *Handbook of local anesthesia* (5th ed.). St. Louis: Elsevier Mosby.

Mehra, P., Caiazzo, A., & Maloney, P. (1998). Lidocaine toxicity. *Journal of the American Dental Society of Anesthesia, 45*(1), 38–41.

MMWR (Morbidity and Mortality Weekly Report). (1994, September 9). CDC Centers for Disease Control and Prevention. Prilocaine-induced methemoglobinemia— Wisconsin, 1993, *43*(35), 655–657.

Munshi, A. K., Hegde, A., & Bashir, N. (2001). Clinical evaluation of the efficacy of anesthesia and patient preference using the needle-less jet syringe in pediatric dental practice. *Journal of Clinical Pediatric Dentistry, 25*, 131–136.

Munshi, A. K., Hegde, A. M., & Latha, R. (2001). Use of EMLA: Is it an injection free alternative, *Journal of Clinical Pediatric Dentistry, 25*, 215–219.

Oraqix: Product information available from Dentsply Pharmaceuticals, York, PA; www.dentsplydental.com.

Patel, D., Chopra, S., & Berman, M. D. (1989). Serious systemic toxicity resulting from use of tetracaine in upper endoscopic procedures. *Digestive Diseases and Sciences, 34*(6), 882–884, 1989.

Synera Patch (lidocaine and tetracaine): Product information available from Endo Pharmaceuticals, Inc., Chadds Ford, Pennsylvania; www.endo.com.

Tetzlaff, J. E. (2000). *Clinical pharmacology of local anesthetics* (1st ed.). Woburn, MA: Butterworth Heinemann.

Yagiela, J. A. (2005, May). Safely easing the pain for your patients. *Dimensions, 3*(5), 20–22.

Injection Fundamentals

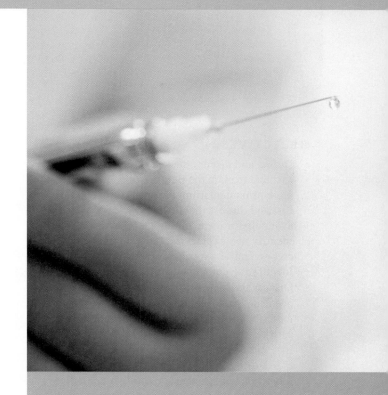

Chapter 9

Local Anesthetic Delivery Devices

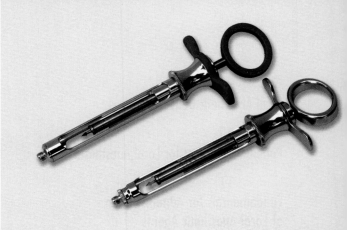

OBJECTIVES

- Define and discuss the key terms in this chapter.
- List and explain the purpose of each item in the basic armamentarium for anesthetic injections.
- List and discuss the different types of syringes available for local anesthetic injections.
- Identify and explain the function of each component of a local anesthetic syringe.
- Identify the components of a needle.
- Discuss the factors to consider when selecting needles.
- Describe the components of a local anesthetic cartridge.
- List and describe the purpose of the contents in a cartridge.
- Identify local anesthesia cartridges according to the ADA labeling system.
- Discuss and demonstrate safe needle recapping and disposal procedures.

KEY TERMS

armamentarium **131**
bevel **137**
breech-loading **134**
cartridge **142**
carpule **142**
computer-controlled local anesthetic delivery (CCLAD) **150**
devices **131**
diaphragm **142**
end cap **142**
Engineering Controls (EC) **140**
finger grip **134**
gauge **136**
harpoon **136**
hub **138**
jet injection **154**

lumen **137**
medical devices **131**
needles **136**
needle adaptor **136**
needle caps **140**
penetrating end **137**
piston **136**
scoop technique **141**
shaft **137**
shank **137**
stopper **142**
syringe **131**
syringe adaptor **137**
syringe barrel **134**
thumb ring **135**
window **134**
Work Practice Controls (WPC) **140**

CASE STUDY: Elena Gagarin

When the clinician approached the operator's chair, the patient had already been seated and a cotton-tipped applicator with topical anesthetic was protruding from her mouth. The assistant had preloaded the syringe with 2% lidocaine, 1:100,000 epinephrine before leaving. She had also displayed the results of the most recent health history on the monitor to show that there were no contraindications to lidocaine or epinephrine and that the patient had received both drugs previously with no adverse reactions.

After removing the cotton-tipped applicator and rinsing the patient's mouth, the clinician pressed lightly on the tissues under the applicator to test for sensitivity. The patient responded that she didn't feel a thing. The needle was positioned over the penetration site and was advanced beneath the mucosa without pain, continuing the penetration until the target area was reached. The clinician pulled back slightly on the thumb ring to create negative pressure in the cartridge in order to aspirate. No signs of blood appeared in the cartridge and the clinician depressed the thumb ring to deposit solution but noticed that the plunger did not move, no matter how hard it was pushed. The syringe was withdrawn from the mouth.

INTRODUCTION

This chapter discusses devices required for the delivery of local anesthetic agents. A thorough knowledge of these devices is necessary for appropriate selection and use. Practices for safe handling and disposal of the devices will also be discussed.

ARMAMENTARIUM FOR DENTAL LOCAL ANESTHESIA

After determining which procedures will be performed, the injection techniques and devices that will best meet the anesthetic requirements of the procedures can be selected. The term **devices** specifically refers to **medical devices** in accordance with the Federal Food Drug & Cosmetic (FD&C) Act, section 201(h). See Box 9–1. These include syringes, cartridges, needles, and recapping and disposal

> ### Box 9–1   FDA Definition of Medical Device
>
> The Federal Food Drug & Cosmetic (FD&C) Act defines a device as ". . . an instrument, apparatus, implement, machine, contrivance, implant, in vitro reagent, or other similar or related article, including any component, part or accessory, which is intended for use in the diagnosis of disease or other conditions, or in the cure, mitigation, treatment, or prevention of disease, in man or other animals, or intended to affect the structure of any function of the body and which does not achieve its primary intended purpose through chemical action and which is not dependent upon being metabolized for the achievement of its primary intended purposes."

Source: Section 201(h) of the Federal Food Drug & Cosmetic Act at http://www.fda.gov.

items (National Institute for Occupational Safety and Health, 2002). The term **armamentarium** refers to *all* equipment, materials, devices, and methods used during the delivery of local anesthetic agents.

Basic armamentarium appropriate for dental local anesthetic injections includes (see Figure 9–1):

1. mouth mirror (may also include a cheek retractor)
2. devices for safe needle recapping and disposal
3. syringe devices
4. cotton pliers or hemostat
5. gauze squares for drying tissues and enhancing retraction
6. cotton swabs for application of topical anesthetic agents and predetermination of penetration sites and angles
7. needles of appropriate gauge and length
8. cartridges of drugs
9. topical anesthetic agents

Syringes, cartridges, needles, and recapping and disposal devices and their variations will be discussed in the following sections.

Dental Local Anesthetic Syringes

A local anesthetic **syringe** is a device for injecting anesthetic agents submucosally or subcutaneously. Syringes are metallic or plastic piston pump devices into which

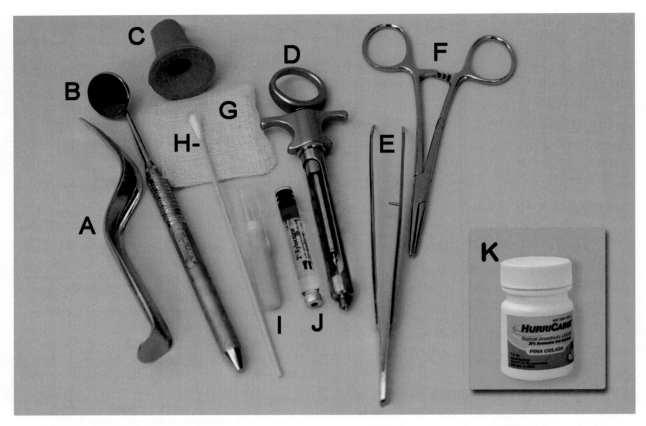

■ **FIGURE 9–1**   Injection Armamentarium. A—cheek retractor or B—mouth mirror, C—safe needle recapping device, D—syringe, E—cotton pliers or F—hemostat, G—gauze squares, H—cotton swabs, I—needle, J—anesthetic cartridge, K—topical anesthetic.

disposable glass cylinders (cartridges) of anesthetic solution are inserted. After attaching a needle to the syringe and activating gentle pressure on a plunger, the device is used to administer local anesthetics.

Several different types of syringes are available in dentistry, including those that are: sterilizable stainless steel or plastic; disposable plastic; manual and self-aspirating; ratcheted for delivering small doses under pressure; needleless; and, computer-controlled. Figure 9–2 ■ provides examples. Most types have one or more designs available. Preference and availability will usually determine which type is selected.

The most common design in dentistry is the sterilizable, breech-loading, cartridge-type, aspirating syringe since inadvertent intravascular injection is a primary

hazard of local anesthetic injections. This syringe has easy-to-master aspirating capabilities to allow testing and visual inspection before drugs are administered.

Anatomy of a Dental Syringe

Syringes for dental local anesthesia consist of a syringe barrel, finger grip portion (with spring and bearing guide), sliding piston with thumb ring and harpoon, and needle adaptor. Figure 9–3 ■ shows a disassembled syringe and its individual components. The function of each component is discussed next.

Syringes have traditionally come in two standard designs and sizes (see Figure 9–4 ■). Those with winged thumb rests are somewhat longer than wingless "petite" designs. Several variations in size are now available to

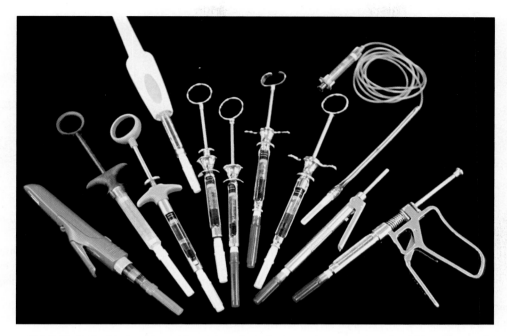

■ **FIGURE 9–2**   Various Dental Local Anesthetic Syringes. Syringes are selected based on technique and clinician preference. They include a number of manual and computer controlled devices.

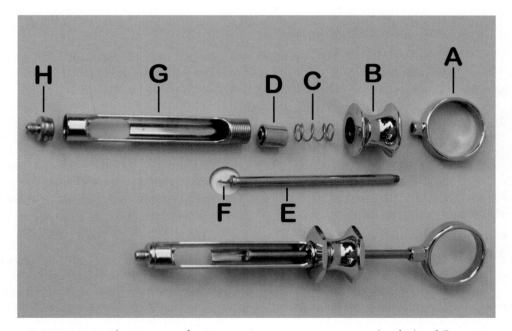

■ **FIGURE 9–3**   The Anatomy of a Syringe. Syringe components are identified as follows: A—thumb ring, B—finger grip, C—spring, D—guide bearing, E—piston with attached F—harpoon, G—syringe barrel, and H—needle adaptor.

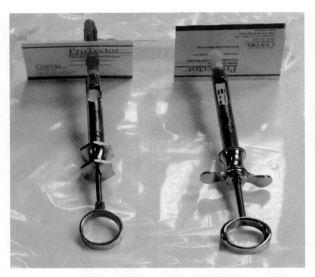

■ **FIGURE 9–4** Commonly Used Syringes. These examples are breech-loading, manual aspiration, cartridge-type devices. The syringe on the left is a "wingless" design and the one on the right is "winged."

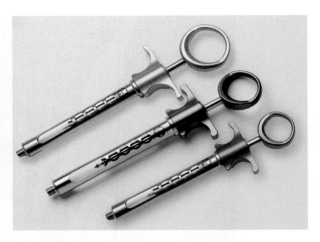

■ **FIGURE 9–6** Small, Medium, and Large Syringes. Septodont USA has redesigned their syringes to accommodate small, medium, and large hands. Note the graduated sizes of the thumb ring.
Source: Courtesy of Septodont USA.

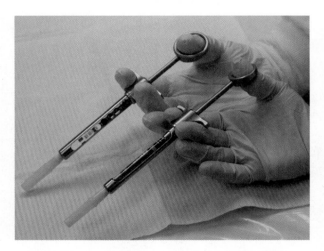

■ **FIGURE 9–5** Syringe Size and Design. Syringes vary in size and design; clinician preference may be based on hand size.

accommodate small to large hand sizes (Figures 9–5 ■ and 9–6 ■). Syringes distributed in North America accommodate standard 1.8 ml cartridges.

Although manual aspiration syringes are more common, some clinicians prefer self-aspirating hybrids, which differ from manual syringes in that they do not have harpoons and they do not require thumb movements in a direction away from deposition sites in order to aspirate (see Figure 9–7 A ■). When using self-aspirating syringes, all accompanying instructions must be followed for proper aspiration testing (see Box 9–2). An extra step is frequently required in order to initiate aspiration prior to injection.

The **syringe barrel** (Figure 9–3 G) is designed to hold glass cartridges of local anesthetic solutions. The most common style has a large side opening allowing for **breech-loading** of cartridges into syringe barrels. This large side opening (**window**) also provides for direct visibility of cartridges throughout injections. Although less common, some syringes load from the end of the barrel. The finger rest portion articulates open to provide entry into the end of the barrel. Figure 9–8 ■ shows examples of breech-loading and articulating devices.

The **finger grip** (Figure 9–3 B) component encircles the diameter of the syringe barrel and the piston passes through the middle of the finger grip. During use, clinicians hold the syringe with the index and middle fingers on the finger grip to balance and control movements of the syringe. There are two basic styles of finger rests, winged and wingless. See Figure 9–4 for examples of winged and wingless finger rests. The spring (Figure 9–3 C) and bearing guide (Figure 9–3 D)

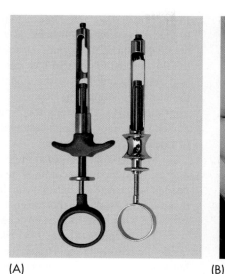
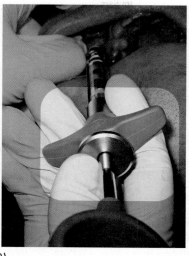

(A)   (B)

■ **FIGURE 9–7**   Self Aspirating Syringes. A—Self-aspirating syringes do not have harpoons to seat into stoppers. B—Some designs require an additional step. The thumb disks must be pressed in order to activate aspiration prior to injection.

Box 9–2   **Design and Technique Modifications for Self-Aspirating Syringes**

Syringes designed to self-aspirate do not have harpoons on their pistons because negative pressure is not dependent on manual "pull-back" motions on stoppers. These syringes have a "thumb disk" on the piston above the finger grip. Prior to initial injection, clinicians press against the thumb disk to activate the aspiration test (Figure 9–7 B). Negative pressure is created by the elastic recoil of the cartridge diaphragm when the cartridge is pushed against the hub in the base of the syringe. During the injection, aspiration is accomplished by gently applying brief pressure on the piston and releasing. In this situation, aspiration occurs when the clinician releases the pressure on the stopper (Aspiject; Astra Self-Aspirating Syringe).

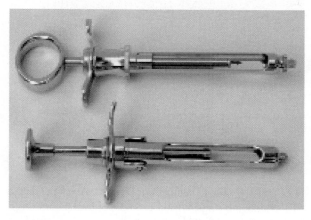

■ **FIGURE 9–8**   Breech-loading Syringe. Top—An example of a breech-loading device (most commonly used today); Bottom—An example of an articulating device. Note the hinge joint just below the finger grip.

slide into the finger grip when the syringe is loaded, which provides tension on the cartridge. At least one syringe is now available with a silicone-coated finger grip and thumb ring, which may improve grip and stability during aspiration (see Figure 9–9 ■).

A **thumb ring** (Figure 9–3 A) is attached to the external end of the piston. Clinicians place their thumbs in the ring to advance or retract pistons. Traditionally, thumb ring components have been available in one standard size and shape, which has been problematic for clinicians with small hands. Current syringes are available in a variety of thumb ring designs in order to

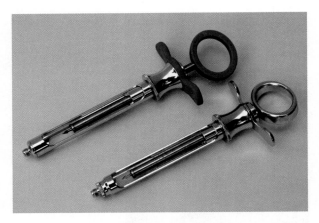

■ **FIGURE 9–9** Silicone-Coated Finger Grip and Thumb Ring Designs. Silicone coatings (top view) may reduce "slipping" during aspiration procedures and are available on both standard and petite syringes.

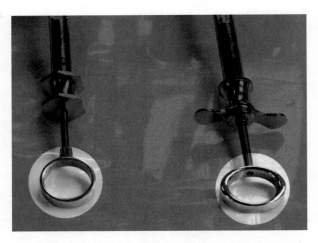

■ **FIGURE 9–10** Thumb Rings Designs. A—An example of round thumb rings; B—An example of oval thumb rings. Note the distance from the piston to the upper inside surface of the ring.

provide for ease of aspiration for all hand sizes. Oval designs require shorter distances to engage the inside of the thumb ring for aspiration. For a comparison of round and oval thumb rings see Figure 9–10 ■. Other syringes have smaller thumb rings. As noted previously, some newer designs have a silicone coating to enhance grip (see Figure 9–9). Figures 9–4 through 9–10 display a number of syringe options.

The **piston** (Figure 9–3 E) passes through the finger grip complex and is attached on one end to the finger ring and on the other end to the harpoon tip. Prior to loading syringes, pull-back movements of the piston create tension on the spring, retracting the bearing guide to allow insertion of cartridges into syringes.

Advancing the piston engages the harpoon in the cartridge stopper to deposit solution and facilitate aspiration tests. The steps for aspiration tests are discussed in Chapter 11, "Fundamentals for Administration of Local Anesthetic Agents."

With smaller (petite) syringes designs, the pistons may be shortened to accommodate the shorter distances needed to activate aspiration tests. It is important to note that it is impossible to expel the entire contents of a 1.8 ml cartridge when pistons are shortened.

The **harpoon** (Figure 9–3 F) is the part of the piston inside the barrel that penetrates the stopper. Embedding harpoons into cartridge stoppers allows for retraction of stoppers to create a slight negative pressure inside the cartridge during aspiration tests. Harpoons are very sharp and can cause injury if syringes are mishandled.

Self-aspirating syringes do not have harpoons, therefore other methods are implemented to create negative pressures required for aspiration tests. Box 9–2 explains how self-aspirating syringes create this pressure. Figure 9–8 shows syringes with and without harpoons.

The **needle adaptor** (Figure 9–3 H) is the threaded surface at the end of the barrel onto which needles are screwed. This component is sometimes referred to as the hub or tip of the syringe. The needle adaptor may be permanently attached or replaceable. For adaptors that can be unscrewed, care should be taken to avoid inadvertent removal and disposal of the needle adaptor when the needle is removed from the syringe.

Syringes should be inspected regularly to assure proper function of each component of the device.

Dental Local Anesthetic Needles

Needles used for dental local anesthesia are slender, hollow, sterile stainless steel devices with sharp points intended to be attached to a syringe to inject local anesthetic solutions. All needles are disposable, single-patient devices. Needles are identified by their lengths and by their diameters, also referred to as their **gauge,** and are selected based on the injection techniques to be used. Removable plastic needle caps protect the needle from contamination prior to and after use. Needle caps are color-coded for ease of identification of lengths and gauges, although there is no standard for this (see

Figure 9–11 ■). While the needle cap has an important role in protection from needlestick injuries, it should not be considered the primary safety device for needlestick protection. If needles are mishandled or bent, their caps can easily be pierced as demonstrated in Figure 9–12 ■. Careful attention to needle handling and recapping is

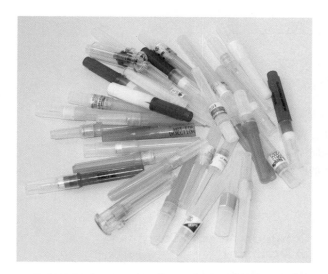

■ **FIGURE 9–11** Dental Local Anesthetic Needles. Needles from various manufacturers have colored caps that designate needle length. There is no uniform color-coding system for needles.

required. Whenever needles are unsheathed, needlestick prevention protocols should remain in effect.

Anatomy of a Local Anesthetic Needle

Needles for dental local anesthesia consist of a shaft (with beveled tip and cartridge penetrating end), a syringe adaptor, and a "hub."

Each needle has a flexible, hollow, stainless steel **shaft.** This one-piece shaft, also referred to as a **shank,** extends from the tip of the needle through the syringe adaptor and hub, to what is known as the cartridge penetrating end (Figure 9–13 A ■). The hollow portion of the needle is referred to as its **lumen,** which runs through the entire length of the shaft. The diameter of the lumen determines the gauge of the needle. Smaller gauges are identified by larger numbers and larger gauges by smaller numbers. Needle gauges will be discussed in more detail later. Some needles are coated with silicone to aid insertion through tissues.

The **bevel** is the diagonal cut that makes the point of a needle (Figure 9–13 B). It is designed to facilitate atraumatic penetration through mucosal and cutaneous tissues.

The cartridge **penetrating end** of the needle shaft opposite the bevel end pierces through the center of the diaphragm of the local anesthetic cartridge (Figure 9–13 C).

The **syringe adaptor** of the needle is the plastic or aluminum hub though which the needle shaft passes (Figure 9–13 D and Figure 9–14 ■). Hubs are either

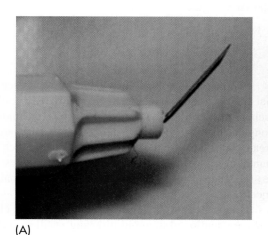

(A)

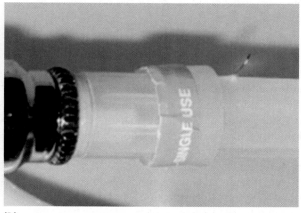

(B)

■ **FIGURE 9–12** Needle Puncture Risks. Needle caps alone cannot prevent needlestick injuries. Close attention to needle use guidelines and Work-Practice Controls must be observed. In this example, a bent needle was not adequately resheathed and the needle tip penetrated the cap.

Courtesy of Albert "Ace" Goerig DDS, MS.

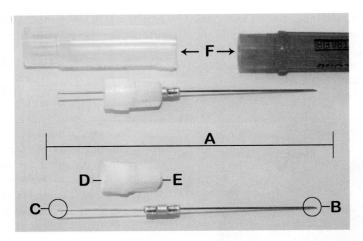

■ **FIGURE 9–13** Anatomy of a Needle. Needle components are identified as follows: A—needle shaft with beveled tip B and cartridge penetrating end C, D—syringe adaptor, and E—"hub," F—needle cap.

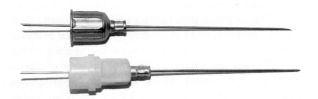

■ **FIGURE 9–14** Needle Hub Variations. Needle hubs are either metal or plastic, and either prethreaded or self-threading.

self-threading or prethreaded (see Figure 9–14) and attach the needle to the syringe. Self-threading adaptors must be pushed and turned onto syringes to seat the needle. Once seated, these plastic adaptors can be adjusted slightly to reorient bevel directions when desired. Most prethreaded adaptors anchor in one position only, locking bevels in one orientation.

Some syringe adaptors have an indicator mark that allows for easy identification of the orientation of the needle bevel. Examples of bevel indicators are shown in Figures 9–15A ■ and 9–15B ■.

The **hub** of a needle is the point at which the shaft joins and secures the needle to the syringe adaptor (Figure 9–13 E). Clinicians commonly refer to the entire syringe adaptor/hub complex as "the hub."

Common Needle Lengths in Dentistry

The length of needle is selected based on the depth of penetration necessary to achieve successful anesthesia. Local anesthetic needles in dentistry are usually identified as long, short, and extra-short. Although needle lengths vary slightly among manufacturers, typical lengths (shown in Figure 9–16 ■) are:

1. long needles average ~32 mm (1½ inches)
2. short needles average ~25 mm (1 inch)
3. extra-short needles average ~12 mm (½ inch)

Short needles are frequently used for injections that do not require significant depths of penetration, such as infiltrations and maxillary block techniques. Long needles are used when deposition sites are at greater distances from penetration sites, such as mandibular block techniques. Extra-short needles can be used when penetrations are shallow such as in palatal injections.

Regardless of the injection technique used, clinicians are cautioned to avoid inserting needles to their hubs. Needle breakage, although rare, is more likely to occur at the hub when excessive lateral pressure is exerted against hub/shaft interfaces (Brunton, Lazo, & Parker, 2006). For this reason, changing the direction of a needle when deeply embedded within tissue is

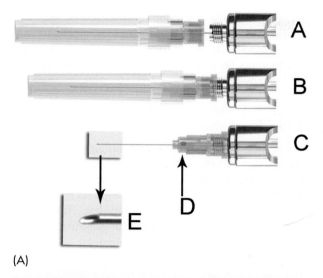

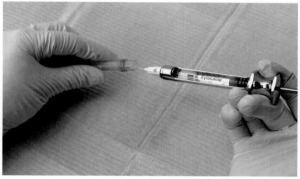

(A)

(B)

■ **FIGURE 9–15** A—Needle Attachment and Bevel Indicators. To attach the needle: A—the cartridge penetrating end is inserted through the cartridge diaphragm; B—the needle is screwed onto the syringe with firm pressure; C—once seated, check the bevel orientation. Some needles have dots, arrows, or other markings on their hubs D that correspond to the locations of the bevel lumens or openings E. B—Bevel Indicators. When checking bevel orientations, keep needle tips shielded by caps to prevent needle stick injury.

Source: (A) Modified courtesy of Dentsplay Pharmaceutical.

not recommended. The best practice when a needle must be redirected, is to withdraw at least half the inserted length before establishing a new pathway (Malamed, 2004). Needle breakage is further discussed in Chapter 17, "Local Anesthesia Complications and Management."

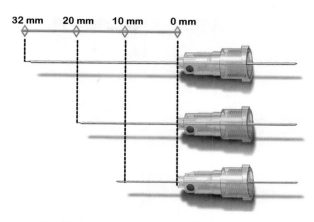

■ **FIGURE 9–16** Needle Lengths. Common needle lengths used in dentistry are: long (average ~32 mm/ 1½ inches), short (average ~25 mm/1 inch), and extra-short (average ~12 mm/½ inch).

Source: Modified courtesy of Dentsply Pharmaceutical.

Common Needle Gauges in Dentistry

Needles in dentistry are available in 25, 27, and 30 gauge sizes (see Figure 9–17 ■). Selection of the gauge to be used is based on the depth of penetration necessary to reach deposition sites, on the relative risks of what is known as positive aspiration, and on clinician preference. Factors impacting this choice are related to needle deflection, ease and accuracy of aspiration, and perceived patient comfort.

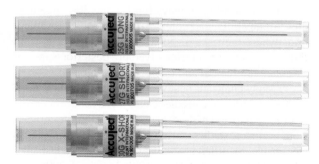

■ **FIGURE 9–17** Needle Gauge Indicators. A common system for indicating gauge size is: Red caps = 25 gauge needles, Yellow caps = 27 gauge needles, and Blue caps = 30 gauge needles.

Source: Courtesy of Dentsply Pharmaceutical.

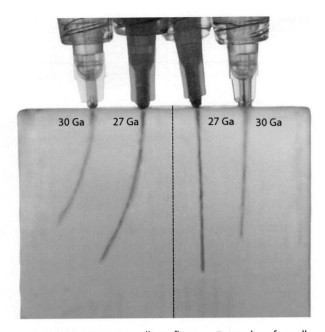

■ FIGURE 9–18 Needle Deflection. Examples of needle deflection with: Left—traditional "straight" insertion technique, and Right—bidirectional rotation technique during needle penetration using Wand® handpieces and needles. Note the greater deflection with the straight insertion pathway and with 30-gauge needles.

In injections such as inferior alveolar blocks, which require deep penetrations through dense tissue, smaller gauge needles deflect less. Higher gauge needles (30 gauge) are the most flexible and have demonstrated the greatest deflection. Figure 9–18 ■ shows an example of needle pathways for 27- and 30-gauge needles. Some clinicians prefer 25-gauge needles for injections where the risks of positive aspiration are greater. Examples include inferior alveolar, posterior superior alveolar, and mental and incisive nerve blocks.

Many clinicians believe that injections administered with 27- or 30-gauge needles cause less discomfort during insertion compared with 25-gauge needles despite comparisons in clinical studies that have demonstrated that patients are unable to differentiate between larger and smaller gauge needles (Evers & Hans, 1993; Malamed, 2004).

Needle Caps

Needle caps and hubs are individually color coded by manufacturers to identify needle gauges and lengths. Although there is no standardized system, many manufacturers use a similar set of criteria to identify needle gauge. See Figure 9–17 for an example.

Each needle cap is fixed to a needle in a manner that requires breaking a seal before using the needle. This step assures sterility.

Needle Safety for Patients and Clinicians

Needlestick injuries present a significant risk for the transmission of infectious diseases to dental healthcare personnel (HCP). Inadvertent needlesticks during intra-oral injections put HCP at risk for contracting hepatitis and acquired immune deficiency syndrome (HIV-AIDS). Attention must be focused on careful handling of dental needles during each step of an injection.

Both the Centers for Disease Control and Prevention and OSHA have published specific guidelines and standards for recommended techniques (**Work Practice Controls—WPC**) and/or devices (**Engineering Controls—EC**) to be implemented for the prevention of needlestick injuries. According to OSHA, "*recapping or needle removal must be accomplished through the use of a mechanical device or a one-handed technique*"; therefore, clinicians are prohibited from managing needles with two-handed manual recapping techniques. Information on accessing these guidelines and standards is provided in Box 9–3.

Box 9–3   Needle Safety Guidelines and Standards

Specific guidelines and standards for the management of needles in the dental workplace can be accessed at:

CDC Guidelines for Infection Control in Dental Health-Care Settings—2003
MMWR, December 19, 2003/52(RR17);1–61

http://www.cdc.gov/mmwr/preview/mmwrhtml/rr5217a1.htm

OSHA Bloodborne Pathogens and Needlestick Prevention
Regulations (Standards—29 CFR), Bloodborne pathogens.—1910.1030

http://www.osha.gov/SLTC/bloodbornepathogens/index.html

There are a number of methods for safely managing needles. The **scoop technique** is a recommended Work Practice Control (WPC) maneuver (CDC, 2003). This technique requires that clinicians slide uncapped needles into needle caps (sheaths) while the needles are lying on instrument trays or tables (see Figure 9–19 ■). A needle cap must not be handled until the point of the needle is protected by the sheath. Care must be taken to avoid contaminating the needle during this process, especially if it may be used again. It is perhaps more convenient to hold the cap with a forceps or hemostat while inserting the needle in order to avoid dragging it over the tray cover. See Figure 9–20 ■.

Engineering Controls (EC) are designed to provide added protection when handling and recapping needles. A variety of devices is available, as demonstrated in Figure 9–21 ■ and Appendix 9–4, "Suggested Needle

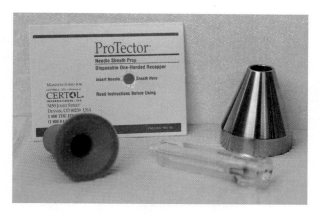

■ **FIGURE 9–21** Needle Recapping Devices. Many different safe recapping devices are available, including single-use and sterilizable devices.

Recapping Techniques—'Best Practices'," The EC should provide a barrier between the tip of the needle and the fingers of the HCP throughout the recapping procedure. These devices prevent accidental needlesticks when properly used as demonstrated in Figure 9–22 ■. Clinicians should never recap needles with their opposite hand or in the hand of an assistant. All clinicians must assure that recapping controls are in place and functioning properly.

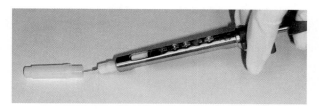

■ **FIGURE 9–19** CDC Suggested Needle Recapping Work Practice Controls. The "scoop-method" is a simple one-handed method of recapping a contaminated needle. Care must be taken to avoid contact with the tray while passing the needle into the needle cap.

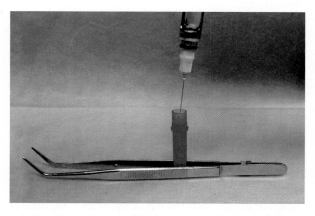

■ **FIGURE 9–20** Modified "Scoop-Method." Stabilizing the needle cap can improve access for ease of insertion in a modified "scoop-method."

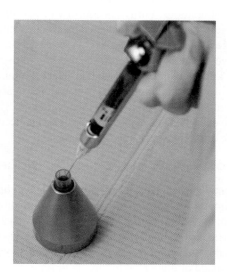

■ **FIGURE 9–22** Engineering Controls (EC) for Recapping Needles. The EC provides a barrier between the tip of the needle and the fingers throughout the recapping procedure and recapping can be one-handed.

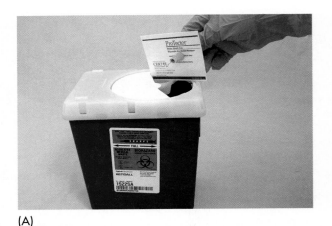
(A)

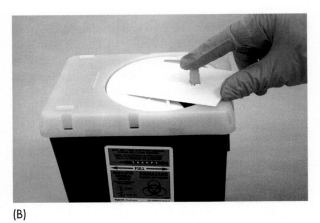
(B)

■ **FIGURE 9–23** Needle Disposal. Needles must be disposed of in appropriate sharps containers, using a one-handed method.
Source: Courtesy of Certol International LLC.

Once needles are removed from syringes they must be placed in appropriate sharps containers for containment and disposal as demonstrated in Figure 9–23 ■.

Local Anesthetic Drug Cartridges

The dental **cartridge** is a glass cylinder that holds local anesthetic drugs and other contents in solution for injection into oral tissues. It is commonly referred to as a **carpule,** which is actually a trademark term of Cook-Waite Laboratories. Purity and sterility of anesthetic solutions are more easily managed in single-unit, glass cartridges. The clear glass also provides easy monitoring of delivered doses and unobstructed views of aspiration tests. Cartridges used in the United States contain up to 1.8 ml of solution. Volumes in other counties vary from 1.5 ml in Japan to 2.2 ml in the United Kingdom. Syringes in these countries are specifically designed to accommodate the differences in cartridge volume and size.

Anatomy of Dental Drug Cartridges

The dental cartridge has four components: a cylindrical glass tube; a rubber (or silicone) stopper; an aluminum end cap; and a rubber diaphragm (see Figure 9–24 ■).

The cylindrical tube contains local anesthetic drugs and other ingredients in solution. It is most commonly made of glass (see Figure 9–24 A).

The **stopper** (or bung) is made of silicone-treated, nonlatex rubber to improve ease of movement through the cylinder (see Figure 9–24 B). The syringe harpoon is engaged into the stopper and pushed by the piston to de-

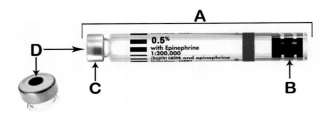

■ **FIGURE 9–24** Standard Local Anesthetic Cartridge for Dentistry. Cartridge components are identified as follows: A—cylindrical glass tube, B—stopper, C—aluminum cap, D—diaphragm.

posit solution. The stopper also creates an airtight seal in the cartridge.

The aluminum **end cap** on the other end of the cylinder fits tightly around the neck of the cartridge (see Figure 9–24 C) and holds the **diaphragm** (or septum) in place (see Figure 9–24 D). The diaphragm is a semipermeable barrier that is centered in the cap. The penetrating end of the needle pierces the center of the diaphragm. As long as the needle does not puncture at an angle, the diaphragm acts as a seal to prevent anesthetic from leaking around the needle.

Until recently, stoppers and diaphragms for dental cartridges were made of latex products. Since latex allergies have become more common, many manufacturers have voluntarily replaced the stoppers and diaphragms with nonlatex materials. For further discussion on latex allergies and local anesthetic devices see Box 9–4 (Shojae & Haas, 2002).

Contents of Anesthetic Cartridges

Each cartridge contains a local anesthetic drug in solution, and most also contain a vasoconstrictor drug. To create an injectable aqueous solution, powdered local anesthetic drug is mixed with hydrochloric acid to create an acidic salt for better water solubility. The hydrochloride salt of the drug is then added to distilled water (the diluent), which makes up the majority of the solution.

When vasoconstrictors are included, sodium bisulfite (a food and drug preservative) is added to the solution to prolong the shelf life and efficacy of the vasoconstrictor drug. Sodium bisulfites increase the acidity of the solution which can result in a burning sensation when administered. Additionally, sodium chloride is included to improve tissue compatibility (isotonicity). These contents are summarized in Box 9–5.

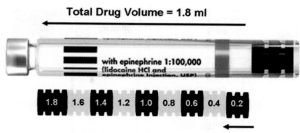

Total Drug Volume = 1.8 ml

with epinephrine 1:100,000 (lidocaine HCl and epinephrine Injection, USP)

1.8   1.6   1.4   1.2   1.0   0.8   0.6   0.4   0.2

Drug Volume Expelled by 1 stopper = 0.2 ml

■ **FIGURE 9–25**   Dosage Calculation Tips. Each stopper displaces approximately 0.2 ml of solution from a 1.8 ml cartridge. Monitoring stopper movement can be used to determine drug doses delivered.

As noted previously, dental cartridges distributed for use in North America are designed to hold 1.8 ml of solution. While all cartridges are capable of holding 1.8 ml, some package inserts state that the cartridge holds at least 1.7 ml. In stating that a cartridge is guaranteed to hold 1.7 ml, a manufacturer is protected against occasions in which a cartridge might contain slightly less than 1.8 ml.

When calculating drug dosages, the standard volume of 1.8 ml is used in all calculations regardless of manufacturers' minimum guarantees of 1.7 ml. This is mandatory because any particular cartridge that is guaranteed to contain *at least* 1.7 ml may contain up to 1.8 ml.

The volume of drug expelled by one cartridge stopper length is a standardized unit for easy calculation of volumes of solution delivered. Each stopper displaces approximately 0.2 ml of solution. Monitoring the distance the stopper moves can be used to determine the portion of solution expelled from a 1.8 ml cartridge. For example, when the stopper is advanced 3 times its length, 0.6 ml of solution have been expelled. Figure 9–25 ■ demonstrates the use of stopper lengths for quick dosage calculations.

Cartridge Labeling and Color Coding

Every cartridge is wrapped in a secure, Mylar label. Each label provides information on the local anesthetic and vasoconstrictor drugs contained in the cartridge. Both trade and generic drug names are provided, along with drug concentrations and dilutions of vasoconstrictor, the manufacturer, an expiration date, a local anesthetic drug color code band, and the lot number and bar code (see Figure 9–26 ■).

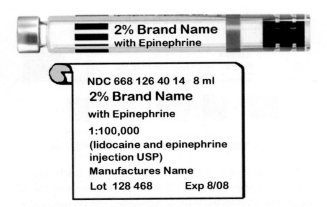

2% Brand Name
with Epinephrine

NDC 668 126 40 14 8 ml
2% Brand Name
with Epinephrine
1:100,000
(lidocaine and epinephrine
injection USP)
Manufactures Name
Lot 128 468   Exp 8/08

■ **FIGURE 9–26** ADA Label Standards and Cartridge Label Information. Cartridge labels provide trade and generic drug names, drug concentrations, dilutions of vasoconstrictor, the name of the manufacturer, and an expiration date. Each drug is identified with color code band and each batch with a lot number.

Each cartridge should be examined prior to injection in order to confirm that the appropriate anesthetic and vasoconstrictor are being administered and that the solution has not expired. It should never be assumed that another individual has loaded a syringe properly. This responsibility rests solely with the individual who administers the drug.

Since June of 2003, manufacturers have been required to apply a uniform cartridge color-coding system for identifying specific local anesthetics and local anesthetic/vasoconstrictor combinations. Box 9–6 describes this color coding system and Figure 9–26 and Figure 9–27 ■ demonstrate the label requirements and color codes for the dental local anesthetic drugs distributed in North America.

Effective April 26, 2006, the FDA published the final *Bar Code Label Requirements for Human Drug Products and Biological Products* regulation. While this rule is intended to improve patient safety in hospital settings by reducing medication errors, it requires pharmaceutical manufacturers to include bar codes on all drug packages. Bar codes can be seen on dental local anesthetic cartridges as demonstrated in Figure 9–26.

Integrity of Cartridges and Contents

Due to high standards for packaging, shipping, and delivery, cartridges generally arrive intact. During normal usage, cartridge integrity is protected by the Mylar label,

---

Box 9–6   ADA Accepted Local Anesthetics Color-Coding System

The ADA criteria for Local Anesthetics Color-Coding states that:

• The color code consists of a band 3.0 ± 0.5 mm wide at a distance of 15 ± 5 mm from the stopper end of the cartridge.
• The end cap of the cartridge may be either color-coded to match the ADA Color-Coding System or given a silver color.
• The stopper will not be color-coded and should not be indicative of the drug or color code.
• Lettering on the cartridge shall be black and font size should follow FDA labeling guidelines (headings at least 8-point type and text at least 6-point type).
• Lettering shall be in durable print that will not be removed by normal office handling.

These criteria are demonstrated in Figures 9–26 and 9–27.

Source: www.dentsplypharma.com/faq_packagefeatbenefits.asp.

which serves as both a protective sleeve and a surface for printing product label information.

Problems with cartridges may include excessive air bubbles, leaking around the cap or stopper, distortion of stoppers, difficulty advancing stoppers, and jamming of cartridges in the barrel.

Air Bubbles in Cartridges

During manufacturing, small air bubbles (1 to 2 mm) are frequently trapped under the diaphragm when the aluminum cap is placed on the cartridge. Clinicians are usually not able to see this bubble because it is very small and concealed by the cap. The bubble is of little consequence because it will never pass through the needle.

Cartridges should be discarded when larger bubbles are noted below the cap when held vertically. Large bubbles can result when solutions have been frozen or contaminated (see Figure 9–28 ■).

Leakage at the Cap

Although it is recommended that cartridges be seated in syringes before attaching needles, many clinicians routinely assemble syringes by screwing the needle on first.

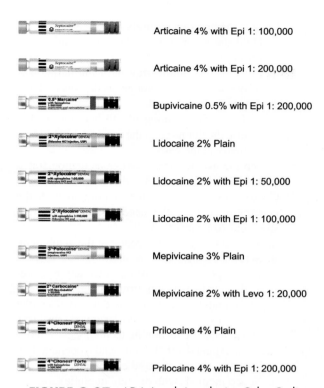

	Articaine 4% with Epi 1: 100,000
	Articaine 4% with Epi 1: 200,000
	Bupivicaine 0.5% with Epi 1: 200,000
	Lidocaine 2% Plain
	Lidocaine 2% with Epi 1: 50,000
	Lidocaine 2% with Epi 1: 100,000
	Mepivicaine 3% Plain
	Mepivicaine 2% with Levo 1: 20,000
	Prilocaine 4% Plain
	Prilocaine 4% with Epi 1: 200,000

■ **FIGURE 9–27**   ADA Local Anesthetics Color-Coding System.

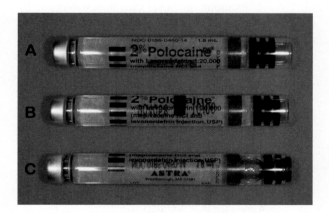

■ **FIGURE 9–28**   Air Bubbles in Cartridges. No air bubbles are visible in cartridge A or B. Cartridge C contains a large air bubble. Note the intruded stopper in cartridge A and the extruded stopper in cartridge C.

This usually does not present a problem; however, when higher gauge needles (such as 30 gauge) are used, there is an increased risk of leakage. Due to the flexibility of higher gauge needles, deflection of the cartridge penetrating end can occur when cartridges are loaded into a syringe. This deflection may cause tearing of the diaphragm and leaking of solution when pressure is applied to the stopper. Inserting cartridges in the syringe when loading, before screwing on needles, can reduce the incidence of this type of damage.

Leakage at the Stopper

When pressure is applied to the syringe piston in a properly assembled syringe, slight expansion of the stopper occurs. This expansion creates even contact between the inner surface of the glass cylinder and the stopper, which in turn prevents leakage from the cartridge. When a syringe piston is damaged or bent, the stopper tips away from the side of the cylinder under the pressure. This allows anesthetic solution to leak.

Displacement of Stoppers

When stoppers are partially extruded from cartridges, it is possible that freezing occurred during shipping or storage or that contamination occurred during storage in disinfectant solution. Disinfectant solutions are able to seep into cartridges and displace stoppers. Affected cartridges should be discarded. Figure 9–28, C shows an extruded stopper caused by freezing.

Cartridge Handling, Storage, and Expiration

Millions of anesthetic cartridges are used worldwide every year. Purity and sterility of drugs are assured through complicated manufacturing processes in carefully controlled environments. Continuous evaluation of samples from each lot (which are set aside for 6 months) helps to maintain a high level of quality control. In addition, every individual cartridge is inspected before shipment.

If solutions have been overheated during shipping and handling, the contents of the cartridge may appear cloudy or sediment may be visible. If there is any question regarding the contents of a cartridge, it should be discarded.

Although damage during shipment rarely occurs, it is important to visually examine each cartridge before administering its contents. Cartridges should be inspected for:

1. integrity
2. clarity of the solution

3. presence of large air bubbles
4. damaged or tarnished caps
5. damaged or leaking stoppers
6. lapsed expiration dates

All local anesthetic solutions should be stored in cool dry areas at temperatures recommended in product inserts. Solutions containing vasoconstrictors should be stored in the dark. Cartridges should never be stored in alcohol or other disinfectant solutions that can leak into them, contaminating the solutions. If cartridges are stored in approved warming devices, it is important to be aware that *long-term* storage at temperatures higher than typical room temperatures may degrade the contents more quickly. Cartridges stored in these devices should be used as soon as possible.

Local anesthetics without vasoconstrictors have a shelf life of approximately 24 months. Those with vasoconstrictors have a shelf life of approximately 18 months.

Steps for Loading Syringes

Preparing and testing syringes for accurate delivery of local anesthetic drugs should be accomplished prior to penetrating mucosa. Comfortable insertion, controlled delivery rates, and effective aspiration testing are all dependent on the proper functioning of the syringe and its components. The following recommended sequence of steps addresses all safety and functional issues. These steps are demonstrated in Appendix 9–3, "Summary of Basic Steps for Loading Syringes."

1. Select the appropriate syringe, needle, and cartridges (see Appendix 9–3).
2. Remove the syringe from the sterile pack.
   a. Confirm that all parts are intact and secure (important with syringes that can be disassembled).
   b. Examine the harpoon and piston for imperfections and debris.
   c. Pull back on the thumb ring to fully retract the piston (this will place tension on the spring and bearing guide) as demonstrated in Appendix 9–3, Step 1.
3. Insert the cartridge into the barrel as demonstrated in Appendix 9–3, Step 2.
   a. The cap should be oriented toward the needle adaptor and the stopper towards the harpoon.
   b. Confirm that the cartridge is firmly seated in the barrel (Appendix 9–3, Step 3).
   c. Release the tension on the piston (cartridge will fit "snugly").

4. Engage the harpoon securely into the stopper.
   a. Hold the syringe in the "ready for injection" position.
   b. Press on the thumb ring until the harpoon is fully seated into the stopper as demonstrated in Appendix 9–3, Step 4.
      i. To confirm seating of the harpoon, gently turn the thumb ring; the cartridge should turn freely in the barrel.
5. Attach the needle to the syringe as demonstrated in Appendix 9–3, Steps 5 and 6.
6. Gently pierce the cartridge diaphragm with the penetrating end of the needle shaft as demonstrated in Appendix 9–3, Step 6.
   a. Take care to pierce the center of the diaphragm.
   b. Screw the needle securely onto the needle adaptor.
      i. For plastic hub needles that are not pre-threaded, maintain firm pressure while attaching the needle to thread it into place (the metal will cut the thread design into the hub).
7. Establish a needle recapping technique as demonstrated in Appendix 9–3, Step 7 and Appendix 9–4, and locate a sharps disposal container.
   a. Scoop method (with or without guide)
      i. Cap on tray, cap stabilized in forceps, stabilization card attached
   b. Recapping Device
      i. Device prepared and/or attached
8. Confirm the needle bevel orientation (when desired) as demonstrated in Appendix 9–3, Step 8.
   a. Gently remove the cap.
      i. Examine the bevel direction, determine by directly viewing bevel direction, or
      ii. Determine orientation by means of the bevel indicator on needle hub.
   b. Using appropriate one-handed recapping technique, reseat the cap as demonstrated in Appendix 9–3, Step 9.
   c. If indicated, redirect the bevel by gently turning the needle at the hub.
   d. Recheck and repeat as necessary.
   e. Recap with one-handed recapping technique.
9. Orient the syringe to display the large window when it is picked up for injection as demonstrated in Appendix 9–3, Step 10.
   a. When there is no assistant present to pass the syringe, it is helpful to set up the syringe for viewing of the large window when first picked up. To do this, place the syringe on the tray with the

window facing down. When ready, pick up the syringe with the palm facing down toward the tray.

10. Retrieve the syringe and proceed with the injection.
    a. Retrieve the syringe.
        i. Once in position for the injection, the large window will be facing the clinician.
    b. Carefully remove the cap (when a recapping guide is used, *always* keep fingers behind the guide).
    c. Set the cap down (with guide or in recapping device).
    d. Proceed with the injection.

These steps are summarized in Box 9–7.

Harpoons may occasionally disengage from stoppers during aspiration testing. The syringe must be withdrawn from the mouth and the needle made safe. Once the needle is removed and safe, reintroduce the harpoon into the stopper by pushing on the thumb ring. A second and less time-consuming method may be used in which the needle is safely capped after withdrawal from the mouth and a quick direct blow is applied to the thumb ring with the palm of the dominant hand while holding the syringe with the other hand, in order to reengage the stopper. The steps for the second method are summarized as follows:

1. Withdraw the syringe from the patient's mouth and recap.
2. Move the syringe clear of the patient and other support individuals (before initiating a "blow" to the thumb ring).
3. Stabilize the syringe in one hand (without wrapping fingers around the barrel and surrounding the cartridge).
4. Apply a *quick,* direct "blow" to the thumb ring. When the blow is administered, it is not necessary to "follow through" with the force. Instead, the hand should be quickly withdrawn in a "forward thrust, rapid backward release" sequence. Glass cartridges are less likely to fracture if the forward thrust is only momentary and is quickly reversed. Ideally, the stopper does not visibly change positions in the cartridge when this maneuver is used, minimizing hydraulic pressures on the glass.
5. Examine the stopper to *confirm* that the harpoon has been reengaged.
6. If a cartridge fractures, replacement is necessary. Safe Work Practices should be observed at all times.

Box 9–7 **Basic Steps for Loading Syringes**

1. Select the appropriate syringe, needle, and cartridge(s).
2. Remove the syringe from the sterile pack and examine.
3. Insert the cartridge into the barrel.
4. Engage the harpoon securely into the stopper.
5. Attach the needle.
6. Establish the needle recapping technique.
7. Confirm the bevel orientation (when desired).
8. Orient the syringe for viewing of the large window.
9. Retrieve the syringe and proceed with the injection.

Steps for Disassembling Syringes and Disposal of Needles and Cartridges

Once an injection has been completed, proper recapping and unloading of syringes is mandatory. The needle is contaminated and primary concerns center around the potential for needlestick injuries and infectious disease transmission. Due to this specific concern, the CDC Guidelines for Infection Control in Dental Health-Care Settings—2003 are explicit in their instructions for handling needles. Appendix 9–1 provides the text of the relevant section of these guidelines.

Prevention of injuries is, of course, the best approach to this health and safety issue. Protocol for the safe handling of needles and for an appropriate response in the event of a needlestick must be in place *before* significant exposure occurs and must be followed at all times (Smith, Cameron, Bagg, & Kennedy, 2001).

The first part of this protocol involves a sequence of steps for disassembling syringes. Recommendations include:

1. Withdraw the syringe from the oral cavity, keeping all patient tissues and all hands in view.
2. Move the syringe to the recapping area with the needle in clear view at all times.
    a. It is safest if the clinician re-sheaths the needle rather than another individual.

3. Using appropriate one-handed Work Practice and Engineering Controls, reinsert the needle into its cap. A variety of methods is demonstrated in Appendix 9–4.
4. Once the needle tip is completely enclosed within the cap, secure the cap to the needle hub.
   a. Ideally this is accomplished by applying gentle pressure with a one-handed technique as demonstrated in Figure 9–29 ■.
5. Remove the needle from the syringe by "rocking" or "twisting" it off the needle adaptor and moving the exposed penetrating end away from the syringe and any hands.
   a. Be sure the needle adaptor remains on the syringe (see Figure 9–30 ■).
      i. If the adaptor is accidentally removed with the needle, it should be removed with a forceps or hemostat. *Never* use unprotected fingers.
   b. For needles with metal hubs, simply unthread the hub.
6. Continue to move the needle to an appropriate sharps container at a predetermined location near chairside.

7. Holding the sheathed end of the needle and cap, insert the needle into the receiving hole of the container according to product instructions (see Figure 9–23).
   a. Some recapping guides will stay in place until this step is completed and aid in placing the needle, sharp end first, into sharps containers.
8. Once the needle is safely disposed of, remove the cartridge.
   a. Pull back on the piston to disengage the harpoon.
   b. Tip the syringe to the side to allow the cartridge to fall free of the barrel.
      i. Occasionally stoppers remain lodged on harpoons. They can be removed safely with a forceps or hemostat after the cartridge has been removed from the syringe. Do not use fingers at any time to dislodge stoppers from harpoons.
      ii. Empty cartridges are contaminated and the glass may be broken. All cartridges must be disposed of in sharps containers.
9. When needles and cartridges have been properly disposed of, syringes may be sterilized along with other contaminated instruments.

These steps are summarized in Box 9–8.

The second part of this protocol is related to the management of needlestick injuries. All healthcare

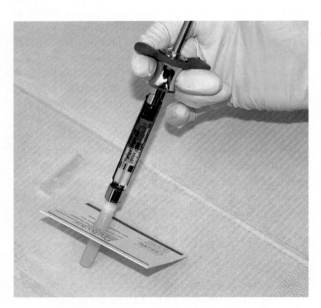

■ **FIGURE 9–29**   Recapping and Making Needles Safe. Using a one-handed technique, completely enclose the needle in the cap and then secure the cap to the needle hub by applying gentle pressure.

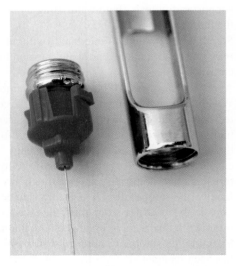

■ **FIGURE 9–30**   Loss of Syringe Parts. When removing needles take care that the needle adaptor does not detach from the syringe and be disposed with the needle.

facilities are required to have procedures in place for the prevention of needlestick injuries and for a standardized response if they occur. In the event of a needlestick injury, clinicians must report the injury to the designated exposure manager as soon as possible and follow established protocol.

Attitudes can play a significant role in the safe handling of needles. Changing long-standing unsafe practices can prove challenging. Observance of standard precautions during all phases of injection administration, however, is both ethically and medically sound.

Response to Needlesticks

If a needlestick (or other puncture injury) occurs, all anesthetic procedures and treatment should be terminated and the injured tissues immediately and thoroughly washed with soap and water. The facility's exposure manager should be notified while appropriate first aid is initiated. According to CDC guidelines, postexposure management should include documentation in both the patient's chart and the exposed individual's health record.

Technique Specific Syringes

In addition to syringes based on the traditional Cook design, a number of specialized devices are routinely used in dentistry. Some syringe devices allow for ease of access and delivery of anesthetic solutions, while reducing physical stress on the hand when drugs are delivered under pressure. Others facilitate controlled rates of delivery to improve patient comfort. Additional features are designed to regulate incremental dosing. Although used in a traditional manner, some syringes are designed as single-use devices with specific safety features intended to reduce the risk of needlesticks.

Five devices will be discussed, including those used for periodontal ligament and intraosseous injections, computer controlled local anesthetic delivery, jet injection, and those whose primary goal is safety (disposable "safety syringes").

Periodontal Ligament Injection Devices

In periodontal ligament (PDL) injections, measured doses of anesthetics are delivered under pressure to confined spaces. Some clinicians find hand pressures associated with PDL injections difficult to sustain when using standard aspirating syringes.

Specialized devices for PDL injections are available in two primary designs, a "pistol grip" and a "pen type" arrangement, both of which reduce hand pressures. Glass cartridges are typically enclosed within syringe barrels with no exposure to the outside or with very small protected windows. Should a cartridge fracture within these syringes, there is no danger of glass falling into the mouth. Pressures compared to hand pressures with traditional syringes are reduced by utilizing mechanical advantages. Devices available for PDL injections include the N-Tralig (Miltex Inc.) and the Paroject (Septodont USA). Some syringes are also able to deliver specific and small volumes of drug and facilitate tracking the volumes of drug delivered.

As discussed in Chapter 15, "Injections for Supplemental Pain Control," achieving the most appropriate angle for needle insertion can be challenging with these and all syringes. For maximum safety, commercially designed syringe adaptors are available that facilitate a 45 degree insertion angle. For example, a 45 degree angle attachment is available for a standard N-Tralig syringe designed for PDL injections. These devices are shown in Figure 9–31 ■ and Figure 9–32 ■. They can eliminate the need for bending needles and their use does not compromise OSHA (or other state) safety standards that prohibit bending of *contaminated* needles in most situations.

Intraosseous Injection Devices

Intraosseous injection techniques require local anesthetic solutions to be deposited within alveolar bone through which they diffuse to nerves. To accomplish this, a small penetration through alveolar bone, known as a perforation, is necessary. A needle is then inserted and the anesthetic delivered. These systems provide

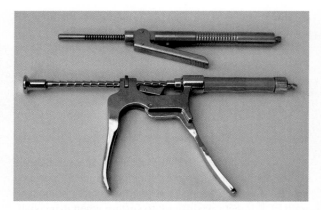

■ **FIGURE 9–31** Common PDL Syringes. Two common PDL syringes are the the Paroject (top) and N-Tralig (bottom).

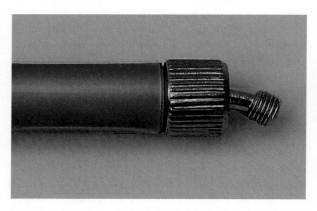

■ **FIGURE 9–32** N-Tralig 45 Degree Angle Adaptor. The 45 degree angle adaptor provides appropriate insertion angles without bending needles.

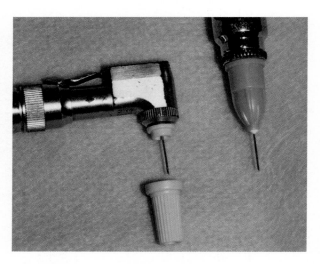

■ **FIGURE 9–33** Stabident Intraosseous Injection Device.

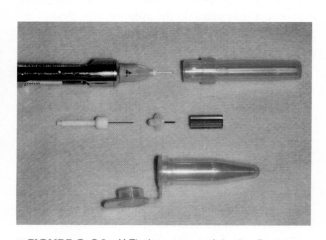

■ **FIGURE 9–34** X-Tip Intraosseous Injection Device.

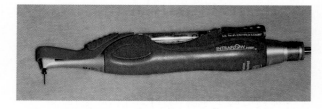

■ **FIGURE 9–35** IntraFlow Intraosseous Injection Device.

both perforator tips and 27 gauge injection needles (8 mm – ultra-short).

Devices available for intraosseous injections include the Stabident system (Faifax Dental Inc.), the X-Tip (Dentsply Maillefer), and the IntraFlow device (Pro-Dex) and are shown in Figure 9–33 ■, Figure 9–34 ■, and Figure 9–35 ■. Instraosseous techniques are discussed in Chapter 15.

Computer Controlled Local Anesthetic Delivery Devices

Computer-controlled local anesthetic delivery (CCLAD) devices are preprogrammed, electronic delivery systems for the administration of anesthetic injections. A key feature of CCLAD devices is the ability

to precisely control the rate of delivery. The initial phase of the injection can start at a very slow rate of delivery for a given period of time. Following this initial deposition, the rate can be increased to a predetermined rate based on the injection technique selected. Clinical research has shown that this approach will produce a more consistent injection than traditional techniques with manual syringes and does not depend on clinicians to assure a slow rate of delivery. Of particular importance when performing injections into dense tissues, such as the palate, attached gingiva, or periodontal ligament, these devices can maintain a specified rate and controlled pressure that can eliminate patient discomfort and adverse tissue reactions occasionally seen when using manual syringes.

Available devices are operated by means of either manual or foot controls that start the flow of anesthetic drugs, signal for aspiration tests, and stop the flow of solution. These devices differ markedly from PDL syringes in that they do not generate high pressures. For this reason, when using one of these devices, one can deposit greater volumes of solution at controlled lower pressures when compared to other PDL devices (and standard syringes).

A second-generation CCLAD device, the STA Single Tooth Anesthesia System™ Instrument (Milestone Scientific Inc., Livingston, New Jersey) designed with an innovative technology called Dynamic Pressure Sensing Technology® Instruments, have also been optimized for single-tooth anesthesia techniques (periodontal ligament injections or PDLs). This is the most recent CCLAD device introduced to the dental market. Unlike its predecessors, this device has real-time pressure feedback providing clinician's feedback information to identify the correct injection sites.

There are three primary devices in use in North America: the Comfort Control Syringe (CCS) (Dentsply/ Professional, York, Pennsylvania); the CompuDent/ Wand Instrument; and the STA Single Tooth Anesthesia System Instrument (Milestone Scientific Inc.). Use of CCLADs for specific injection techniques is discussed in technique chapters 12–15.

Comfort Control Syringe (CCS)

The Comfort Control Syringe (CCS) is distributed by Dentsply/Professional (see Figure 9–36 ■). The design features of the CCS handpiece have some similarities to manual syringes. The CCS utilizes standard cartridges and needles that are attached following basic steps similar to manual syringes. Other features of the CCS include a digital panel that displays the rate, elapsed time, and amount of anesthetic delivered, and a clear plastic cartridge sheath that allows complete visibility of cartridges at all times.

The CCS handpiece is considerably larger than manual syringes and is controlled by buttons on its front surface. It is a two-stage, controlled-rate delivery device.

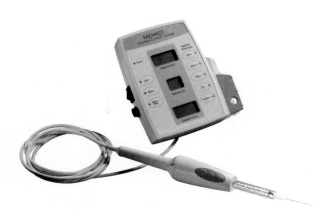

■ **FIGURE 9–36**   Comfort Control CCLAD.
Source: Courtesy of Dentsply Midwest.

The injection begins at a very slow rate for 10 seconds and is programmed to increase to a faster rate of delivery, consistent with the injection technique selected from the control panel. Clinicians with small hands may need to modify their grasps in order to comfortably stabilize, activate, and manage this handpiece. The CCS has 5 preprogrammed delivery rates, listed in Table 9–1 ■.

CompuDent/Wand and STA Single Tooth Anesthesia System Instruments

Milestone Scientific was the first manufacturer to market a CCLAD device (the Wand® Instrument) in 1997, at the same time pioneering the AMSA injection technique (Hochman, Chiarello, Hochman, Lopatkin, & Pergola, 1997; Friedman & Hochman, 1998). The STA Single Tooth Anesthesia System Instrument and the CompuDent Instrument are both manufactured by Milestone Scientific (see Figure 9–37 ■). The CompuDent Instrument was formerly marketed as the Wand Instrument, and the STA Single Tooth Anesthesia System Instrument is newly released.

Table 9–1	Comfort Control Syringe Preset Delivery Rates	
Injection Technique	**Delivery Rate**
Block	0.020 mL/sec
Intraosseous	0.020 mL/sec
Infiltrations	0.017 mL/sec
Palatal	0.008 mL/sec
PDL	0.007 mL/sec

Source: Comfort Control™ Syringe product manual REF 850155.

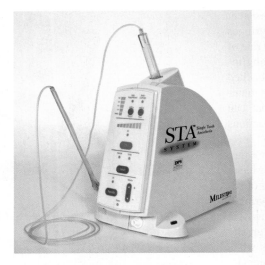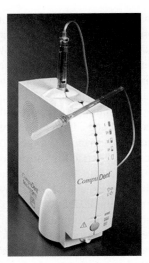

■ **FIGURE 9–37** STA Single Tooth Anesthesia System™ and CompuDent/ Wand® Instruments
Source: Courtesy of Milestone Scientific.

As with other CCLAD systems, the STA Single Tooth Anesthesia System and the CompuDent Instruments operate using a multistage delivery system. To enhance injection comfort, technique steps recommended by Milestone are described as *prepuncture, puncture, penetration,* and *injection.* During the prepuncture and puncture steps a small volume of anesthetic is administered ahead of the needle. This "anesthetic pathway" serves to minimize discomfort from needle penetration and may eliminate the need for topical anesthetics. This may be characterized as a *stealth* technique in which the recipient is unaware of the procedure until it is finished.

Both the STA Single Tooth Anesthesia System and CompuDent Instruments have similar, preprogrammed delivery rates, listed in Table 9–2 ■.

Table 9–2	CompuDent and STA Single Tooth Anesthesia System Preset Delivery Rates		
CompuDent Modes	***Delivery Rate***	***STA Modes***	***Delivery Rate***
slow speed	~ 1.8 mL/50 seconds	***STA*** 1-speed mode *ControlFlo*	~ one drop/2 seconds 0.005 mL/second
fast speed	~ 1.8 mL/25 seconds	***Normal*** 2-speed mode *ControlFlo* *RapidFlo*	~ one drop/second 0.005 mL/second 0.03 mL/second
		Turbo 3-speed mode *ControlFlo* *RapidFlo* *TurboFlo*	 0.005 mL/second 0.03 mL/second 0.06 mL/second

Source: STA Single Tooth Anesthesia System™ and CompuDent® Instruments product manuals, Hochman, MN: Single-tooth anesthesia: pressure-sensing technology provides innovative advancement in the field of dental local anesthesia, *Compendium,* April 2007, *28*(4), 186–193.

The design features of these delivery systems are unique compared with traditional syringes. The components have been described as "slim-line" and are relatively unobtrusive, which may offer a psychological benefit for some patients. See Figure 9–38 ■. Most clinicians, but particularly those with small hands, find it easy to grasp and stabilize the slender ergonomic wand-like handpiece during injection. Clinicians will find that this system can prevent repetitive hand-strain injury because of the overall system design (Murphy, 1998). Additionally, with a simple adaptation of the Wand handpiece (see Figures 9–39 ■ through 9–42 ■), needle approach and insertion may be achieved without stimulating a visual response in the patient as demonstrated in Figure 9–43 ■. Delivery of local anesthetics is initiated and controlled by a foot pedal.

The slim profile of the Wand handpiece enhances the unique insertion technique recommended. During injections with standard syringes, needles deflect away from bevel openings when needles are advanced. With the STA Single Tooth Anesthesia System and CompuDent Instruments, deflection is avoided by rotating the needle during insertion (known as a "pen roll" or "bidirectional" rotation technique), a maneuver that would be difficult if not downright dangerous with standard syringes (Friedman & Hochman, 2000). Figure 9–18 demonstrates this phenomenon with both 27 and 30 gauge needles.

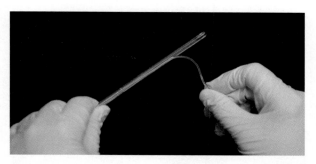

■ **FIGURE 9–39**   Adaptation of the Wand Handpiece—Step 1. Loosen the plastic tubing from the slot in the side of the Wand handpiece.

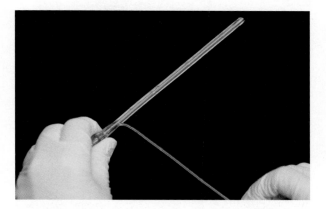

■ **FIGURE 9–40**   Adaptation of the Wand Handpiece—Step 2. Gently "peel" the plastic tubing from the length of the Wand handpiece.

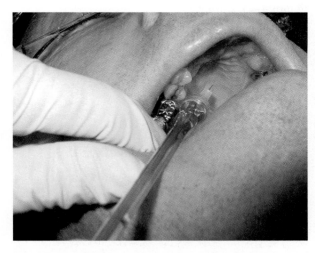

■ **FIGURE 9–38**   Wand Handpiece. The "slim-line" Wand handpiece is designed specifically for use with the STA Single Tooth Anesthesia System and CompuDent Instruments.

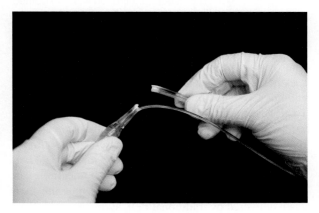

■ **FIGURE 9–41**   Adaptation of the Wand Handpiece—Step 3. With a rocking motion, snap off the slim handle portion of the Wand handpiece, above the needle hub.

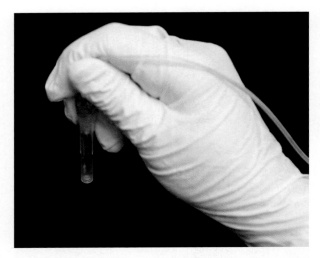

■ **FIGURE 9–42** Modified Wand Handpiece.

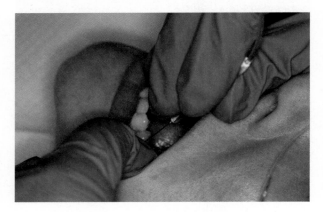

■ **FIGURE 9–43** Mandibular Infiltration with a Modified Wand Handpiece.

A specific design feature of the STA Single Tooth Anesthesia System Instrument facilitates single-tooth anesthesia with the new STA-Intraligamentary injection without associated trauma to the PDL. The STA Single Tooth Anesthesia System Instrument has patented pressure-sensing technology that provides audible and/or visual feedback to the clinician to assure the optimum placement of the needle throughout the injection. When properly placed, intraligamentary (PDL) injections can be accomplished with significantly less pressure than when delivered by traditional PDL syringes.

The Wand® handpiece is also available with a specially designed needle safety device called the Safety Wand® shown in Figure 9–44 ■.

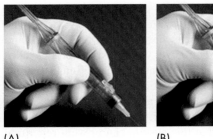

(A)   (B)

■ **FIGURE 9–44** Safety Wand Handpiece. A—needle positioned for injection; B—needle retracted into safety sleeve.

CCLAD systems provide a number of advantages over traditional, manual syringes and have a significant place in future dental anesthesia practices.

Jet Injectors

Jet injection devices use narrow bursts of air, or "jets" to penetrate mucosa without needles. These spring-loaded syringes are used primarily to establish deep prepenetration topical anesthesia but they have also been used in infiltration and shallow block anesthesia with some success. Examples of jet injectors are the Syrijet (Mizzy/ Keystone Products, Cherry Hill, New Jersey) and the Madajet (MADA Medical Equipment International, Carlstandt, New Jersey) shown in Figure 9–45 ■.

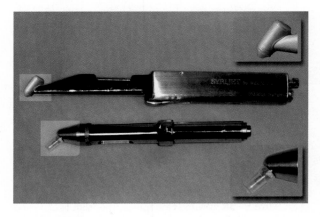

■ **FIGURE 9–45** Jet Injection Devices. Two common jet injection devices are the Syrijet (top) and Madajet (bottom).

Safety Syringes

Safety syringes are plastic single-use, or partially disposable devices designed to reduce the risk of needlestick injuries associated with trapping injection needles. Interest in these devices has become quite limited and many are no longer available. One device that is still available is sold as the Ultra Safety Plus from Septodont USA.

As noted previously, Milestone Scientific also provides a Safety Wand for the CompuDent and STA devices.

CASE MANAGEMENT: Elena Gagarin

Case Discussion: As the clinician discovered when the cartridge was removed from the syringe, it had been loaded backwards and the harpoon had perforated the diaphragm instead of the stopper. The patient would need another injection because the clinician, who was ordinarily very attentive to detail, had failed to check the armamentarium that someone else had set up.

There are at least two important lessons learned from this experience:

1. A seemingly negative aspiration was not even an aspiration.
2. Before inserting needles into tissues, syringes should be checked for easy flow of solution in addition to confirming that the correct drugs were loaded. Had this been done, the clinician would have known that the cartridge was loaded backwards before penetrating any tissues.

CHAPTER QUESTIONS

1. Which *one* of the following statements is correct?
   a. The standard aspirating syringe is designed to provide negative pressure on aspiration, unlike the self-aspirating syringe.
   b. The standard aspirating syringe is designed to provide positive pressure on aspiration, unlike the self-aspirating syringe.
   c. Neither the standard nor the self-aspirating syringes provides negative pressure on aspiration.
   d. The standard aspirating syringe is designed to provide negative pressure on aspiration similar to the self-aspirating syringe.

2. Which *one* of the following is correct when addressing OSHA requirements for medical device safety in dentistry?
   a. Two hands are allowed as long as one hand only secures the needle cap.
   b. Contaminated needles may be bent as long as the bend is accomplished with cotton pliers or a hemostat.
   c. Two hands are never allowed to recap needles even when one hand is holding a hemostat or locking pliers to secure the protective caps.
   d. Uncontaminated needles may be bent.

3. In comparing a 25 gauge needle with a 30 gauge needle, the 25 gauge needle:
   1. Has better aspiration.
   2. Breaks more easily.
   3. Is less comfortable than the 30 gauge.
   4. Has a smaller diameter.
   5. Can be used in highly vascular areas.

   a. 2,4,5
   b. 2,4
   c. 1,3,5
   d. 1,5

4. Long needles are approximately _____ long.
   a. ~12 to 22 mm
   b. ~32 to 36 mm
   c. ~40 to 42 mm

5. When a stopper is extruded, what has likely caused the problem?
   a. The cartridge was overfilled during manufacturing.
   b. Freezing occurred during shipping or handling.
   c. Overheating has caused pressure in the cartridge.
   d. Oxidation of sodium bisulfate has created gas in the cartridge.

6. During an infiltration injection you give the patient three stopper-widths of local anesthetic. How much solution have you injected into the patient?
   a. 0.2 ml
   b. 0.9 ml
   c. 1.8 ml
   d. 0.6 ml

7. What substance is used as the preservative for epinephrine in local anesthetic cartridges?
   a. Sodium bisulfite
   b. Sodium hypochlorite
   c. Methylparaben
   d. Nitrogen

REFERENCES

Aspiject: Product information available from RØNVIG Dental Mfg. A/S, GI, Vejlevej 57-59, DK-8721 Product Insert: Daugaard, Denmark; www.ronvig.com.

Astra Self-Aspirating Syringe, Product Insert: Astra Pharmaceutical Products, Inc., MA 01606.

Brunton, L., Lazo, J., & Parker, K. (2006). *Goodman and Gilman's the pharmacological basis of therapeutics* (11th ed.). New York: McGraw-Hill.

CDC Guidelines for Infection Control in Dental Health-Care Settings—2003 MMWR, December 19, 2003/52(RR17); 1–61 http://www.cdc.gov/mmwr/preview/mmwrhtml/rr5217a1.htm

Centers for Disease Control and Prevention. Sample Screening and Device Evaluation Forms. Available at: http://www.cdc.gov/oralhealth/infectioncontrol/forms.htm. Accessed November 11, 2008.

Comfort Control Syringe REF850155, Product Insert: Dentsply/Professional, 1301 Smile Way, York, PA 17404.

Daniel, S. J., Harfst, S. A., & Wilder, R. S. (2008). *Mosby's dental hygiene: concepts, cases, and competencies* (2nd ed.). St. Louis: Mosby.

Dentsply Pharmaceutical, www.dentsplypharma.com. Accessed November 11, 2008.

Evers, Dds, Hans. (1993). The Dental Cartridge System. Trosa, Sweden: Trosa Tryckeri AB.

Federal Food Drug & Cosmetic (FD&C) Act, section 201(h), 52 FR 30097, Aug. 12, 1987, as amended at 59 FR 63008, Dec. 7, 1994; 66 FR 38799, July 25, 2001.

Friedman, M. J., & Hochman, M. N. (1998). The AMSA injection: A new concept for local anesthesia of maxillary teeth using a computer-controlled injection system. *Quintessence International, 29,* 297–303.

Hochman, M. N., Chiarello, D., Hochman, C. B., Lopatkin, R., & Pergola, S. (1997). Computerized local anesthesia delivery vs. traditional syringe technique. *New York State Dental Journal, 63,* 24–29.

Hochman, M. N., & Friedman, M. J. (2000). In vitro study of needle deflection: A linear insertion technique versus a bi-directional rotation insertion technique. *Quintessence International, 31,* 737–743.

Malamed, S. F. (2004). *Handbook of local anesthesia* (5th ed.). St. Louis: Mosby.

Murphy, D. (1998). *Ergonomics and the dental care worker* (p. 181). ISBN: 0-87553-0233-0. Washington DC: American Public Health Association.

National Institute for Occupational Safety and Health. *Safer medical device implementation in healthcare facilities.* Available at: http://www.cdc.gov/niosh/topics/bbp. Accessed September 17, 2002.

OSHA Bloodborne Pathogens and Needlestick Prevention Regulations (Standards—29 CFR), Bloodborne pathogens—1910.1030 http://www.osha.gov/SLTC/bloodbornepathogens/index.html

Shojaei, A. R., & Haas, D. A. (2002). Local anesthetic cartridges and latex allergy: a literature review. *Journal of the Canadian Dental Association, 68*(10), 622–626.

Smith, A. J., Cameron, S. O., Bagg, J., & Kennedy, D. (2001). Management of needlesticks in general dental practice. *British Dental Journal, 190*(12), 645–650.

Summary of Sharps Management Recommendations

CDC GUIDELINES FOR INFECTION CONTROL IN DENTAL HEALTH-CARE SETTINGS

I Preventing Transmission of Bloodborne Pathogens

  B Preventing Exposures to Blood and OPIM

    1 **General recommendations**

      a **Use standard precautions** (OSHA's bloodborne pathogen standard retains the term universal precautions) for all patient encounters (IA, IC) (*11,13,19,53*).

      b **Consider sharp items** (e.g., needles, scalers, burs, lab knives, and wires) that are **contaminated with patient blood and saliva as potentially infective and establish engineering controls and work practices to prevent injuries** (IB, IC) (*6,13,113*).

      c Implement a written, comprehensive program designed to minimize and manage DHCP exposures to blood and body fluids (IB, IC) (*13,14,19,97*).

    2 **Engineering and work-practice controls**

      a **Identify, evaluate, and select devices with engineered safety features at least annually** and as they become available on the market (e.g., safer anesthetic syringes, blunt suture needle, retractable scalpel, or needleless IV systems) (IC) (*13,97,110–112*).

      b **Place used disposable** syringes and needles, scalpel blades, and other sharp items **in appropriate puncture-resistant containers located as close as feasible to the area in which the items are used** (IA, IC) (*2,7,13,19,113,115*).

      c **Do not recap used needles by using both hands or any other technique that involves directing the point of a needle toward any part of the body. Do not bend, break, or remove needles before disposal** (IA, IC) (*2,7,8,13,97,113*).

      d **Use either a one-handed scoop technique or a mechanical device designed for holding the needle cap when recapping needles** (e.g., between multiple injections and before removing from a nondisposable aspirating syringe) (IA, IC) (*2,7,8,13,14,113*).

Excerpt from: Morbidity and Mortality Weekly Report, *Guidelines for Infection Control in Dental Health-Care Settings—2003*, December 19, 2003 / Vol. 52 / No. RR-17, Page 40, Centers for Disease Control and Prevention.

CDC Sample Device Evaluation Form: Dental Safety Syringes and Needles

Available at www.cdc.gov/OralHealth/infection_control/forms.htm

Sample Device Evaluation Form
Dental Safety Syringes and Needles

This form collects opinions and observations from dental healthcare personnel who have pilot tested a safer dental device. This form can be adapted for use with multiple types of safer devices. Do not use this form to collect injury data because it cannot ensure confidentiality.

Date:_____

Product: Name, brand, company:_____

Number of times used: _____

Your position or title: _____

Your occupation or specialty: _____

1. Did you receive training in how to use this product?
    ❏ Yes **[Go to Next Question]**   ❏ No **[Go to Question 4]**

2. Who provided this instruction? **(Check All that Apply.)**
    ❏ Product representative   ❏ Staff member   ❏ Other

3. Was the training you received adequate?
    ❏ Yes   ❏ No

4. Compared to others of your sex, how would you describe your hand size?
    ❏ Small   ❏ Medium   ❏ Large

5. What is your sex?   ❏ Female   ❏ Male

Please answer all questions that apply to your duties and responsibilities. If a question does not apply to your duties and responsibilities, **please leave it blank**.

During the Pilot Test of this Device . . .	Strongly Disagree	Disagree	Neither Agree nor Disagree	Agree	Strongly Agree
6. The weight of the device was similar to that of a conventional dental syringe.	1	2	3	4	5
7. The device felt stable during assembly, use and disassembly.	1	2	3	4	5
8. The device fit my hand comfortably.	1	2	3	4	5
9. The anesthetic cartridges were easy to change.	1	2	3	4	5
10. Aspiration of blood into the anesthetic cartridge was clearly visible.	1	2	3	4	5
11. I had a clear view of the injection site and needle tip.	1	2	3	4	5
12. The device did not appear to increase patient discomfort.	1	2	3	4	5

May, 14 2002
http://www.cdc.gov/OralHealth/infection_control/forms.htm

During the Pilot Test of this Device . . .	Strongly Disagree	Disagree	Neither Agree nor Disagree	Agree	Strongly Agree
13. The device performed reliably.	1	2	3	4	5
14. I was able to give injections in all mouth sizes and all areas of the mouth.	1	2	3	4	5
15. I used the device for all of the same purposes for which I use the conventional device.	1	2	3	4	5
16. Activating the safety feature was easy.	1	2	3	4	5
17. The safety feature was easy to recognize and use.	1	2	3	4	5
18. The safety feature did not activate inadvertently, causing me to use additional syringes or needles.	1	2	3	4	5
19. The safety feature functioned as intended.	1	2	3	4	5
20. The instructions were easy to follow and complete.	1	2	3	4	5
21. I could have used this product correctly without special training.	1	2	3	4	5
22. The "feel" of the device did not cause me to change my technique.	1	2	3	4	5
23. This device meets my clinical needs.	1	2	3	4	5
24. This device is safe for clinical use.	1	2	3	4	5

Additional comments for any responses of "Strongly Disagree" or "Disagree."

_____

_____

_____

Summary of Basic Steps for Loading Syringes

Select appropriate syringe, needle(s), cartridge(s), and recapping method.

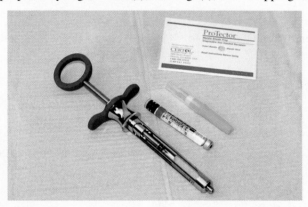

1. Fully retract the piston to allow cartridge to slide into the barrel.

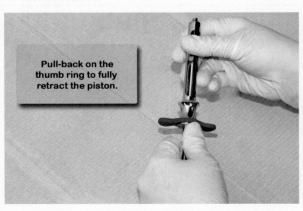

Pull-back on the thumb ring to fully retract the piston.

2. Insert the cartridge with the stopper toward the piston.

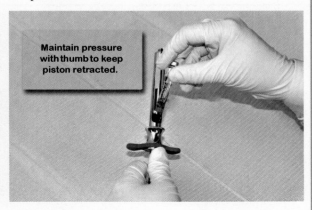

Maintain pressure with thumb to keep piston retracted.

3. Release the tension on the piston and confirm that the cartridge is fully seated.

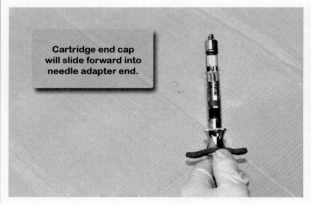

Cartridge end cap will slide forward into needle adapter end.

4. Seat the harpoon securely into the stopper.

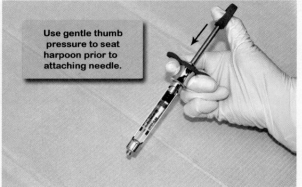

Use gentle thumb pressure to seat harpoon prior to attaching needle.

5. Open the needle by gently turning the cap to break the seal.

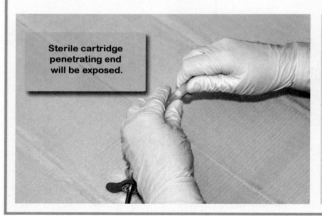

Sterile cartridge penetrating end will be exposed.

6. Screw the needle securely onto the needle adaptor.

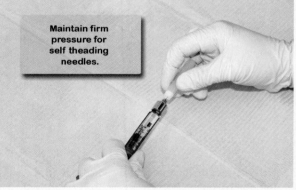

Maintain firm pressure for self theading needles.

7. Prepare needle recapping device (when applicable) if used.

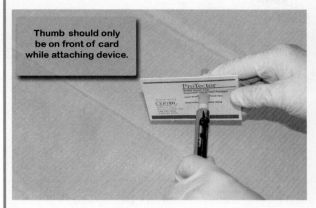

Thumb should only be on front of card while attaching device.

8. Gently loosen and remove the cap to confirm bevel orientation and then orient the syringe for viewing of the large window.

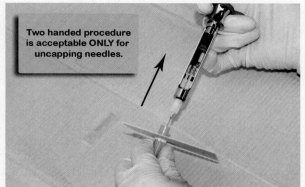

Two handed procedure is acceptable ONLY for uncapping needles.

9. Safely replace the cap with a one-handed technique.

This recapping device serves as a prop for the cap during the "scoop" method.

10. Orient the syringe facing down to achieve ease of retrieval with:
    a. a "palm up" grasp
    b. large window visible

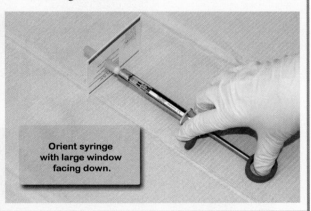

Orient syringe with large window facing down.

Suggested Needle Recapping Techniques—"Best Practices"

Each clinician is obligated to apply safe needle handling and recapping methods based on CDC and OSHA guides for their practice setting. A variety of acceptable techniques apply OSHA Work Practice and Engineering Controls. The *key* to safe needle recapping is sound *one-handed technique*. Examples are provided below.

Basic "scoop" method

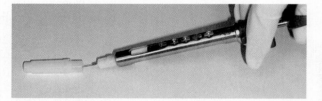

"Scoop" method *assisted* with cotton pliers as cap holder

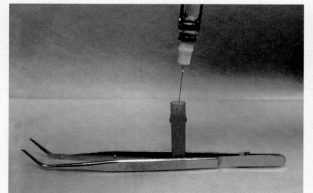

"Scoop" method *assisted* with weighted cap holder

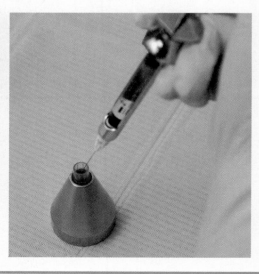

"Scoop" method *assisted* with card prop device cap holder

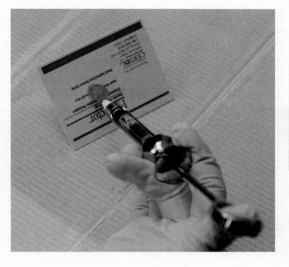

"Scoop" method *assisted* with rubber prop device cap holder

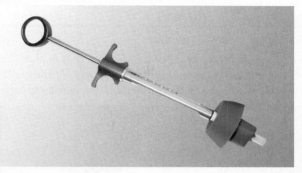

Best Practices allow for (A) removing caps with the assistance of a device, but recapping MUST be done with one hand. With all recapping methods and devices it is important that an unprotected needle is NEVER moved towards clinicians' hands (B).

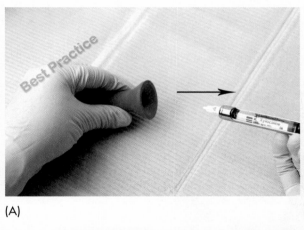

(A)

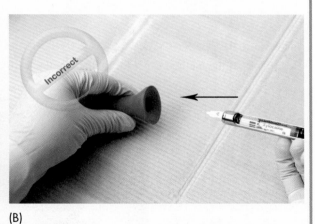

(B)

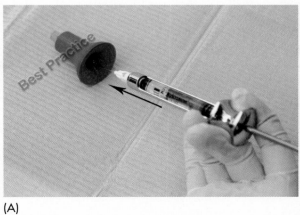

(A)

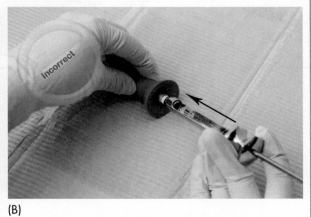

(B)

Note the *unsafe* practice

The thumb is on the front of the device. This device aids recapping by propping up the cap for ease of entry. It is NOT considered a barrier to needle penetration.

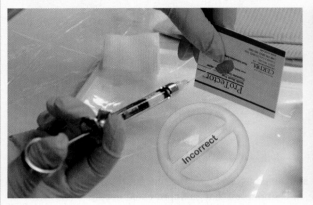

Note the *unsafe* practice

Although the fingers are behind the card, this device is not puncture proof and is not intended for recapping in this manner. This practice can be used to uncap needles.

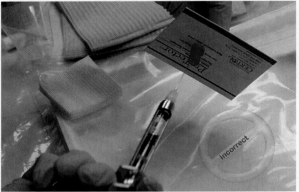

Note the *BEST PRACTICES*

Regardless of the method used, recapping needles with a one-handed method is the **safest** way to render needles safe.

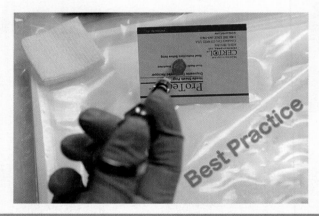

Chapter 10

Patient Assessment for Local Anesthesia

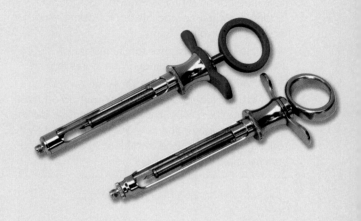

OBJECTIVES

- Define and discuss the key terms in this chapter.
- Identify and discuss the responsibilities associated with the delivery of regional anesthesia.
- Describe the ASA (American Society of Anesthesiologists) Physical Status Classification System categories I–VI (P1–P6).
- Discuss patient assessment tools for the evaluation of physical and psychological tolerance to local anesthesia.
- Discuss the implications of patient evaluation in obtaining informed consent.
- Identify and apply contraindications to the use of local anesthesia.
- Discuss treatment modifications that can be made to increase patient safety and comfort with local anesthesia.
- Discuss situations that require a medical consultation prior to treatment.
- Identify signs and symptoms of undiagnosed medical conditions that can affect local anesthetic administration.
- Discuss the importance of postanesthetic care.

KEY TERMS

CASE STUDY: Carlos Martinez

Carlos Martinez, a 67-year-old male, is a new patient with extensive dental needs. His history includes several positive responses, including to hepatitis C and diabetes. His blood pressure is 142/90 and he is a moderate smoker. On further questioning and after medical consultation, he is found to have sustained significant liver damage, is resistant to insulin therapy, and is on a new medication for hypertension, Corgard (nadalol), which he and his doctor admit is not yet working that well.

He also has a prior family history of methemoglobinemia, although he states that he has never had an episode, personally.

He is ambulatory and otherwise able to visit the dental office without difficulty. Extensive dental and dental hygiene therapy are planned that will require local anesthesia in all four quadrants and numerous restorative appointments.

INTRODUCTION

Local anesthesia can be physically and psychologically demanding (Moore & Brodsgaard, 2001; Meechan, 2005). Comprehensive patient assessment is the foundation for the safe delivery of local anesthetic drugs. In most healthy, uncompromised individuals, local anesthetics can be administered according to standard dose recommendations. In other individuals, the administration of local anesthesia is safe as long as certain precautions are observed. Clinicians must determine when local anesthetic solutions may or may not be used and they must monitor patients before, during, and after the administration of local anesthetic agents. This chapter will discuss specific considerations for local anesthesia and a standardized approach to patient assessment. Treatment modifications will be based on limitations and contraindications for local anesthesia that are identified in this assessment.

ASA Physical Status Classification System

Applying a standardized approach to patient assessment can be useful when determining physical and psychological tolerance to proposed treatment. The assessment process is also valuable in determining appropriate modifications that can reduce the risks of adverse events including medical emergencies associated with treatment.

According to the **American Society of Anesthesiologists (ASA),** patient safety is the most important goal in the delivery of anesthesia (American Society of Anesthesiologists [ASA], 2002). The responsibilities associated with the delivery of local anesthesia are described in the ASA Statement on Regional Anesthesia:

> Anesthesiology in all of its forms, including regional anesthesia, is the practice of medicine. Regional anesthesia involves diagnostic assessment, the consideration of indications and contraindications, the prescription of drugs, and the institution of corrective measures and treatment in response to complications. Therefore, the successful performance of regional anesthesia requires medical as well as technical expertise.

According to the ASA, clinicians who administer regional local anesthesia must conform to a prescribed sequence of care (see Box 10–1). Since regional nerve blocks are routinely administered in dentistry, these guidelines apply equally to all dental professionals who administer them.

Appropriate attention to anesthetic procedures is crucial since it has been reported that the majority of medical emergencies in the dental office are associated with the administration of local anesthesia (Malamed, 2004; Kaufman, Goharian, & Katz, 2000). Following the delivery of local anesthetic agents, patients must be observed and assessed for adverse reactions. Clinicians must

---

Box 10–1 **Elements of the ASA Medical Component of Care**

1. Pre-anesthetic evaluation of the patient
2. Prescription of the anesthetic plan
3. Personal participation in the technical aspects of the regional anesthetic
4. Following the course of the anesthetic
5. Remaining physically available for the immediate diagnosis and treatment of emergencies
6. Providing indicated post-anesthesia care

Source: ASA, 2002.

Box 10–2	ASA Physical Status Classification System
ASA I	A normal healthy patient
ASA II	A patient with mild systemic disease
ASA III	A patient with severe systemic disease
ASA IV	A patient with severe systemic disease that is a constant threat to life
ASA V	A moribund patient who is not expected to survive without the operation
ASA VI	A declared brain-dead patient whose organs are being removed for donor purposes

Source: ASA, 2006.

be prepared to identify and manage all adverse reactions including medical emergencies, should they arise.

Comprehensive patient assessment, including the use of the **ASA Physical Status Classification System,** is a key factor in determining the safety of local anesthesia administration in advance of procedures (see Box 10–2). The ASA system classifies patients into six categories, ASA I–VI (also noted as ASA P1–P6), based on their overall physical health. Examples of medical conditions in each class are provided in Appendix 10–1 (Malamed, 2007; Nield-Gehrig & Willman, 2008).

The majority of healthy patients are classified ASA I or ASA II. Treatment modifications are few, and serious adverse events are uncommon for these patients. Patients who are ASA III with *severe* systemic disease are more likely to experience adverse events. These patients may still be considered for elective dental procedures with local anesthesia; however, treatment modifications to ensure patient safety are frequently necessary. Elective dental care is contraindicated for ASA IV patients.

Since local anesthesia is stressful for many patients, the assessment process should include a determination of psychological tolerance. Anxiety and fear can be measured using **dental fears questionnaires** and dental anxiety scales (DAS) (Corah, 1969; Humphris, Morrison, & Lindsay, 1995). Treatment modification with an appropriate **Stress Reduction Protocol (SRP)** can reduce psychogenically generated medical emergencies (Malamed, 2007; Nield-Gehrig &

Willman, 2008). See Appendix 10–2 for a suggested Stress Reduction Protocol. For further discussion on dental fears related to local anesthesia, see Chapter 18, "Insights for the Fearful Patient."

TOOLS FOR PATIENT ASSESSMENT

Comprehensive Patient Assessment

The following review of patient assessment is presented in order to minimize adverse events related to local anesthesia. Key elements for applying health information to local anesthetic procedures will be highlighted. Dental fears questionnaires and the benefits of consulting with medical professionals will also be discussed.

Medical and Dental History

Information gained from medical and dental histories includes known medical conditions (past and current), prescription medications, and over-the-counter products, including dietary and herbal supplements. Previous experiences with local anesthesia can provide valuable insight; for example, patients may report that they never really get numb, that they are usually fatigued after receiving local anesthetics, that they often pass out during or after receiving anesthesia or from "shots" in any setting, that they usually stay numb for hours, or that they always have to be given a lot of novocaine, among other possible responses.

Prior to the administration of local anesthetics drugs it is necessary to know what other drugs a patient is taking. Box 10–3 outlines a suggested patient drug record. Drugs that are in a patient's system when local anesthetics are administered are referred to as **concomitant.** These drugs may influence the choice of local anesthetic drugs and the quantities administered due to their influence on the efficacy, metabolism, or elimination of anesthetic drugs. The effects of the anesthetic drugs on other drugs are equally important. In other words, some concomitant drugs potentiate the actions or delay the metabolism of local anesthetic drugs while others diminish their actions or hasten their metabolism. In other instances, the drugs are affected in some way by the local anesthetics.

There are many different medical and dental history forms available, including multilingual versions of basic forms (see Box 10–4). Clinicians should select forms that best meet their needs, recognizing that there are regional variations in documentation and that approaches to information gathering are variable.

An additional tool for assessing patient anxiety and fear is a *fears* questionnaire, which can provide helpful

---

Box 10–3 Patient Drug Record

Document the following for *prescription medications:*

1. The drug name
   List both trade and generic if it applies
   (e.g., Coumadin™ [warfarin]).
2. The drug classification
   What is the intended action of this group of drugs (e.g., anticoagulant)?
3. The purpose for taking the drug
   Why is the drug prescribed? This may differ from its classification (e.g., thromboembolytic disorders).
4. The prescribed dose and schedule
   Document deviations from prescribed schedules and the rationale.
5. Side effects and adverse reactions
6. Precautions or contraindications with dental care
7. Drug interactions
8. Treatment modifications indicated

For *nonprescription drugs, vitamins, minerals, and herbals,* document:

1. The product name
   List both trade and generic if they apply
   (e.g., Advil™ [ibuprofen]).
2. The product classification
   What is the intended action of this group of drugs (e.g., analgesic)?
3. The purpose for taking the product
   Why is it being consumed (e.g., mild headache)?
4. The dose and schedule (if applicable)
   Document if the patient exceeds recommended daily doses.
5. Side effects or adverse reactions

Nonprescription drug and herbal references are available for over-the-counter products. Updates should include notations regarding any concerns or changes since the last appointment.

Box 10–4 Multilingual Health History Forms

In a unique project, the University of the Pacific School of Dentistry and MetLife Insurance Company have created a basic health history form available in thirty-six languages, including Arabic, Chinese, Farsi, German, Hmong, Japanese, Portuguese, Russian, Spanish, Thai, Vietnamese, and many others. These forms are available at www.dental.pacific.edu, and at www.metdental.com.

---

information about a patient's level of dental anxiety and fear. According to Newton and Buck, there are fifteen different measures of dental care anxiety (Newton & Buck, 2000). A useful method for measuring anxiety in the dental setting has been developed by Corah (Corah, 1969; Humphris, Morrison, & Lindsay, 1995) (see Box 10–5).

Clinical Examination

Objective information about a patient's physical condition can be obtained from an evaluation of vital signs (blood pressure, pulse, respiration, and weight). Blood

---

Box 10–5 Corah's Dental Anxiety Scale (DAS)

Corah's **Dental Anxiety Scale (DAS)** is a clinical tool for measuring dental anxiety in adults (Corah, 1969; Humphris, Morrison, & Lindsay, 1995). Patients were originally provided with four examples of dental situations, although a fifth question specifically concerning local anesthesia has been added to this scale (Humphris, Morrison, & Lindsay, 1995). Patients are asked to select the response that most closely matches their reaction to one of the hypothetical situations (out of four possible responses of increasing severity). They score between 4 and 20 points on the DAS, with higher values indicating higher anxiety. Scores above 15 indicate phobic levels. These forms are available at www.dentalfearcentral.org/media/dental_anxiety_scale.pdf.

pressure values directly correlate with specific ASA classifications. Acceptable safe ranges for the administration of local anesthesia are listed in Appendix 10–1. Abnormally slow or fast breathing can be an indicator of disease or anxiety or both. Values above 20 or below 12 are considered outside the normal range. Pulse rates may also vary, depending on the general health and fitness of an individual, from 50 to 70 beats per minute. In a disease state, pulses may range from very low to very high. Weight, as previously discussed, is critical when determining appropriate doses of drugs, especially for children and small adults before local anesthesia administration (see Chapter 7, "Dose Calculations for Local Anesthetic Solutions").

General observations of patients may give clues to their overall ability to tolerate local anesthetic procedures. Ideally, they should be well rested and well nourished prior to appointments. It is especially important for patients with diabetes to have had appropriate and adequate nutrition prior to appointments.

Medical Consultation

In order to optimize safety, a consultation with a patient's physician is sometimes necessary prior to local anesthesia. Medical consultations should be considered when patients have not seen a doctor recently, when there are gaps in the information provided, when they are pregnant, or when any other concerns suggest follow-up is necessary. Medical conditions requiring consultation include heart conditions, recent surgeries, uncontrolled high blood pressure, some psychological conditions, compromised liver and kidney function, immune system compromise, and any others that raise concerns regarding local anesthesia and treatment.

Undiagnosed and Undisclosed Medical Conditions

Both medical history and dental fears questionnaires are completed by patients or their representatives and provide both objective and subjective information that is, unfortunately, limited to the information that a patient or his or her representative chooses or is able to disclose. Ideally, patients will be thorough and truthful about their medical and dental histories.

A consult with a patient's physician is also recommended in order to ensure safety during anesthetic procedures. This is especially true if patients are unable to recall or appear to be withholding important details about medical conditions or current medications or when there is no history of recent medical care.

Some patients have undiagnosed medical conditions with no obvious signs or symptoms and for whatever reason do not seek heath care or lack access to it. Many undiagnosed conditions can influence the safety of local anesthetic drugs. In addition to unknown medical conditions, language and cultural barriers, and mental and physical disabilities can limit an individual's ability to relate information on their medical status regardless of whether or not it is known to them. Unusual signs and symptoms detected during patient assessment can serve as clues to undiagnosed medical conditions that may need to be addressed before local anesthesia is administered. For example, uncontrolled high blood pressure is a contraindication to local anesthesia and can sometimes point toward other undiagnosed systemic problems. Frequent thirst and urination may be a sign of undetected and therefore uncontrolled diabetes. In situations such as these, patients should have medical evaluations prior to receiving local anesthesia.

When patients are unable to provide adequate assessment information, it is recommended that a family member, friend, legal guardian, or translator be available, not only for assessment but to assist in obtaining or providing (in the case of a child, or mentally or physically disabled patient) informed consent for proposed treatment. See Chapter 11, "Fundamentals for Administration of Local Anesthetic Agents" for further discussion on informed consent.

SYSTEMS REVIEW

Prior to the administration of local anesthesia, a comprehensive health history, including a thorough review of systems, is indicated. This review includes the cardiovascular, respiratory, nervous, metabolic, and excretory systems.

Cardiovascular System

The systemic effects of local anesthesia include effects on both cardiac and vascular structures. Overall, the experience of stress from a local anesthesia procedure is likely to increase blood pressure, pulse, and possibly respiration. These vital signs serve as baseline comparisons in response to adverse events that may develop after local anesthetics are administered.

According to the most recent American Heart Association guidelines (2007), very few individuals require antibiotic prophylaxis before dental treatment compared with previous recommendations. The exceptions include those who are at exceptional risk of developing infective endocarditis (IE). These include individuals with artificial heart valves or congenital heart disease, and those with a previous history of IE (ADA, 2007). It may be advisable to consult with a patient's cardiologist and to obtain the results of recent echocardiograms before administering anesthesia.

Most local anesthetic injections through tissue are considered to be noninvasive and do not require premedication. The treatment that is to be performed following local anesthesia, on the other hand, may dictate a need for antibiotic prophylaxis (see Box 10–6).

Patients with hemophilia and clotting disorders, and patients on blood thinning medications such as warfarin, may require modifications to the types of injections, types of drugs, and doses of local anesthesia they may receive. Patients who have experienced recent myocardial infarctions or cerebrovascular accidents need to delay elective dental treatment, including local anesthesia, for appropriate periods of time (see Appendix 10–1). Examples of health history questions that focus on the cardiovascular system are presented in Figure 10–1 ∎.

Box 10–6   ADA Recommended Prophylaxis for IE

According to the American Dental Association (ADA):

Endocarditis prophylaxis is reasonable for . . . "All dental procedures that involve manipulation of gingival tissue or the periapical region of teeth or perforation of the oral mucosa.* . . ."

Additionally, according to the ADA: "*The following procedures and events *do not need* prophylaxis: routine anesthetic injections through non-infected tissue, taking dental radiographs, placement of removable prosthodontic or orthodontic appliances, adjustment of orthodontic appliances, placement of orthodontic brackets, shedding of deciduous teeth and bleeding from trauma to the lips or oral mucosa."

Source: ADA, 2007.

Respiratory System

The systemic effects of local anesthesia on the respiratory system are typically minimal. Epinephrine acts on beta adrenergic receptors of the smooth muscles of the bronchial circulation to dilate the vessels.

Do you now have, or have you ever had or taken, any of the following?

1. Artificial heart valves or congenital heart disease — Yes/No
2. Infective endocarditis — Yes/No
3. Rheumatic fever, rheumatic heart disease, or scarlet fever — Yes/No
4. Heart attack, bypass surgery, stents, angina, or other heart problems — Yes/No
5. High blood pressure or low blood pressure — Yes/No
6. Congestive heart failure — Yes/No
7. Stroke (cerebrovascular accident or transient ischemic attack) — Yes/No
8. Heart murmur or mitral valve prolapse — Yes/No
9. Hemophilia or clotting disorders — Yes/No
10. Hematomas following local anesthesia — Yes/No
11. Weight loss medications such as Fen Phen — Yes/No
12. Antibiotic premedications before dental treatment — Yes/No
13. An echocardiogram — Yes/No

∎ **FIGURE 10–1**   Assessment of the Cardiovascular System.

Do you now have, or have you ever had any of the following?

1. Asthma   Yes/No
2. Emphysema   Yes/No
3. Tuberculosis   Yes/No
4. Congestive heart failure   Yes/No
5. Chronic lung disease   Yes/No
6. Sinus or ear problems   Yes/No
7. Persistent or bloody cough   Yes/No
8. Methemoglobinemia, or episodes of "turning blue" after local anesthesia   Yes/No
9. Sensitivity to sulfite preservatives in food or in local anesthetics   Yes/No
10. Episodes of hyperventilation due to anxiety or panic attacks   Yes/No
11. Chronic obstructive pulmonary disease   Yes/No

■ **FIGURE 10–2**   Assessment of the Respiratory System.

Asthma may be induced by allergy, including sulfite sensitivity and physiological and psychological stress related to local anesthesia administration, all of which may decrease a patient's respiratory capacity. Anxiety in susceptible children typically provokes asthmatic episodes. In adults, it more commonly causes hyperventilation.

Congestive heart failure (CHF) impairs lung function, particularly in the pulmonary vessels where blood accumulates (congestion in the lungs). This leads to pulmonary hypertension and compromises both heart and lung function, which may necessitate modifications for local anesthesia. Patients diagnosed with CHF should not be placed in the supine position, which can quickly lead to serious pulmonary edema. Examples of health history questions that focus on the respiratory system are presented in Figure 10–2 ■.

Nervous System

The overall condition of a patient's nervous system has a major influence on the process and outcome of local anesthesia. The patient's ability (or inability) to tolerate the stress of local anesthesia is partially influenced by the health of his or her nervous system. Local anesthetics are central nervous system (CNS) depressants. This depression is additive to any preexisting CNS depression. When CNS depression is suspected, careful evaluation prior to the use of a local anesthetic is indicated. For example, when a patient has taken a large dose of narcotic drugs

prior to anesthesia administration, the local anesthetic can have a more profound effect on the CNS.

If, during the evaluation, signs and symptoms of intraoral paresthesia are evident it should be determined whether or not they are the result of previous local anesthetic procedures. If so, it is important to determine the specific injection(s) performed in order to avoid injections that follow the same pathway. Examples of health history questions that focus on the nervous system are presented in Figure 10–3 ■.

Metabolic Systems

Patients with compromised liver function may not be able to metabolize amide local anesthetic drugs efficiently. Because the liver is the primary source of cholinesterase, ester metabolism may also be compromised. When serious compromise is suspected, a consultation with a physician is indicated. This will help to determine appropriate limitations on the type and dose of local anesthetic used. For example, if the physician reports that there has been extensive liver damage, administering a drug such as articaine, which is only 5 to 10 percent metabolized in the liver can be useful although depending upon the degree of depletion of cholinesterase, articaine may have less advantage (Pickett & Terezhalmy, 2006). Shorter appointments with fewer milligrams of drug administered are recommended, regardless of the anesthetic selected.

The amide local anesthetics are broken down into inactive metabolites for excretion. In the liver, they

Do you now have, or have you ever had any of the following?

1.	Seizures	Yes/No
2.	Dental anxiety	Yes/No
3.	Diagnosed mental illness	Yes/No
4.	Obsessive-compulsive disorders	Yes/No
5.	Eating disorders	Yes/No
6.	Depression	Yes/No
7.	Treatment for chemical dependency	Yes/No
8.	Chronic pain	Yes/No
9.	Headaches or migraines	Yes/No
10.	Head injuries	Yes/No
11.	Temporary or permanent numbness (paresthesia)	Yes/No

■ **FIGURE 10–3** Assessment of the Nervous System.

compete for metabolic pathways with other drugs. This competition may result in significant drug interactions that influence the blood levels of the various drugs, as well as their half-lives and excretion patterns.

Metabolic issues play a key role in treatment planning for diabetics. Due to their daily schedule for meals and insulin, morning appointments are usually best. Before administering local anesthesia, blood sugar levels should be evaluated and patients should be questioned as to when they last ate and took their medication. The goal is to assess that the patient's blood sugar level is well controlled before local anesthesia is administered. This process may be especially critical in cardiac-compromised, brittle diabetics (ASA III) when epinephrine is being considered. These patients lack effective blood sugar control and swing frequently from hypo- to hyper-glycemic states. Epinephrine in these individuals can cause dangerous elevations in blood sugar (Little, Falace, Miller, & Rhodus, 2008).

Patients with hyperthyroidism have an increased risk of developing **thyrotoxicosis** which can result in what is known as **thyrotoxic crisis** or, more commonly, *thyroid storm*. Epinephrine is known to increase the risk of this life-threatening medical emergency. The nature of the relationship between hyperthyroidism and epinephrine is not entirely clear (Little et al., 2008; Herman, Joffe, Kalk, Panz, Wing, & Seftel, 1989). Although a higher-than-normal secretion rate of epinephrine has been suspected in thyrotoxicosis, studies have suggested that the signs and symptoms encountered in hyperthyroidism are not secondary to high secretion rates of epinephrine (Little et al., 2008; Herman et al., 1989).

Epinephrine is *absolutely contraindicated* for patients with poorly controlled or uncontrolled hyperthyroidism. It is important to note that it may not be possible to safely treat these individuals even without the use of epinephrine until their condition is controlled.

Examples of health history questions that focus on metabolic systems are presented in Figure 10–4 ■.

Do you now have, or have you ever had any of the following?

1.	Diabetes–Type I or Type II	Yes/No
2.	Liver condition (hepatitis, cirrhosis, jaundice)	Yes/No
3.	Hypothyroidism or hyperthyroidism	Yes/No

■ **FIGURE 10–4** Assessment of the Metabolic System.

> Do you now have, or have you ever had any of the following?
> 1. Kidney failure   Yes/No
> 2. Kidney dialysis treatment   Yes/No
> 3. Kidney transplant procedure   Yes/No
> 4. Other kidney conditions   Yes/No

■ **FIGURE 10–5**   Assessment of the Excretory System.

Excretory System

The kidneys are the primary excretory organs for local anesthetics. Suspected diminished function or kidney failure should be closely evaluated. Inadequate excretion of local anesthetics and their metabolic by-products may increase, possibly to toxic levels. Examples of health history questions that focus on the excretory system are presented in Figure 10–5 ■.

CONTRAINDICATIONS TO LOCAL ANESTHESIA

When patient assessment has determined that standard local anesthetic procedures are contraindicated, an appropriate course of care must be defined. Assessment results guide clinicians when determining the *extent* of the contraindications, which may be classified as either relative or absolute.

Some contraindications are permanent, such as hereditary medical conditions. Others may be temporary, such as recent cardiovascular events or pregnancies, which typically delay rather than prevent planned treatment.

Absolute and Relative Contraindications

Situations in which local anesthetic or vasoconstrictor drugs may not be administered safely are known as **absolute contraindications.** There are few absolute contraindications to the administration of local anesthetic agents. **Relative contraindications** for local anesthesia procedures are those in which local anesthetics may be given with caution.

There are a number of conditions that can be considered relative or absolute contraindications depending upon the *degree* of compromise. For example, if a patient has had a cerebrovascular accident (CVA), local anesthesia may be absolutely contraindicated for a minimum of 6 months. After a period of 6 months or an appropriate time determined by a physician, the administration of local anesthesia would be considered only a relative contraindication.

Relevant medical, pharmacological, and psychological conditions are discussed next. Refer to Appendices 10–3, 10–4, 10–5, and 10–6 for specific modifications related to medical and pharmacological factors.

Examples of Medical Compromise

Atypical Plasma Cholinesterase

Atypical plasma cholinesterase impairs a patient's ability to effectively metabolize ester-type local anesthetics in any form, injectible or topical. This condition is genetic (autosomal recessive) and has a frequency of approximately 1 in 3,000 patients (Malamed, 2004). Signs and symptoms of an ester local anesthetic overdose are more likely to occur when normal doses are administered. Since this condition is only a relative contraindication, esters may be administered with caution; however, the availability of excellent amide substitutes renders the point moot. Unless there is an absolute contraindication to amides or there are no amide injectables or topicals available, it is seldom necessary to use esters in these individuals.

Methemoglobinemia

Methemoglobinemia is a genetic or acquired condition that reduces the oxygen-carrying capacity of blood. Acquired methemoglobinemia has been reported following the administrations of benzocaine topical and injectable prilocaine and is a risk if greater-than-recommended doses of articaine have been administered (ASA, 2002; Knobeloch, Goldring, LeMay, & Anderson, 1994). Clinical anoxia may result from methemoglobin levels above 10 percent demonstrated by signs of reduced oxygenation and cyanosis

(Knobeloch et al., 1994) (see Box 10–7 and Box 10–8). Administering doses that exceed 4.0 mg/lb or 400 mg absolute maximum of prilocaine has been linked to the development of methemoglobinemia in adults (Knobeloch et al., 1994). This risk is increased in patients with known medical conditions involving enzyme deficiencies and for patients taking oxidant drugs such as sulfonamide, anti-malarial, acetaminophen, or nitrite-containing medications (Knobeloch et al., 1994) (see Box 10–9 and Box 10–10). An FDA Advisory, released April 2006, states that, ". . . patients with underlying breathing problems, such as asthma or emphysema, patients with heart disease, and those who smoke may be more susceptible" (FDA, 2006). Prilocaine and benzocaine should be administered with caution. For further discussions see Chapter 5, "Dental Local Anesthetic Drugs," Chapter 8, "Topical Anesthetics," and Chapter 17, "Local Anesthesia Complications and Management."

Liver or Kidney Dysfunction

Significant liver or kidney dysfunction in category ASA III is a relative contraindication for local anesthesia. Ester and amide local anesthetics can be used for these patients with caution. Articaine, particularly, in significant liver disease, may have an advantage over

---

| Box 10–8 | Signs and Symptoms of Methemoglobinemia |

Initial:

Bluish coloring (cyanosis) of the skin, buccal mucous membranes, lips, and nail beds

Severe:

Central cyanosis	Headache
CNS depression	Lethargy
Dizziness	Seizures
Dyspnea	Shock
Dysrhythmia	Syncope
Fatigue	

Source: Adapted from the Oraqix® product insert, Dentsply Pharmaceuticals, York, Pennsylvania

---

| Box 10–9 | Drug-Induced Methemoglobinemia |

In addition to benzocaine, prilocaine, and articaine, the following drugs may induce methemoglobinemia:

Acetaminophen; acetanilide; aniline dyes; chloroquine, dapsone; sulfonamides; naphthalene; nitrates and nitrites; nitrofurantoin; nitroglycerin; nitroprusside; pamaquine; para-aminosalicylic acid; phenacetin; phenobarbital; phenytoin; primaquine; and quinine.

Source: Adapted from the Oraqix® product insert, Dentsply Pharmaceuticals, York, Pennsylvania

---

| Box 10–7 | Detection of Methemoglobinemia |

Oxygen saturation of blood can be monitored during an appointment with a pulse oximeter attached to a patient's finger. In the Pennsylvania Patient Safety Advisory of April 2007, it was recommended that all facilities that routinely apply topical anesthetics use a pulse oximeter to detect methemoglobinemia (Pennsylvania Patient Safety Advisory, 2005).

This condition has been reported with the use of benzocaine and prilocaine in particular. If a patient's serum oxygen saturation is reduced, and other signs and symptoms of methemoglobinemia are detected, the patient should be transported to a hospital. If the blood methemoglobin concentration exceeds 30 percent, the patient will need an intravenous infusion of methylene blue to reverse this potentially lethal condition (Hegedus & Herb, 2005).

---

other drugs because it is packaged in dental cartridges (unlike the esters) and largely avoids liver metabolic pathways when used for oral injections (unlike the other amides). See the Chapter 5 section on articaine (Jastak, Yagiela, & Donaldson, 1995).

Cardiovascular Disease and Hyperthyroidism

Patients in category ASA III with cardiovascular disease and controlled hyperthyroidism may present as relative contraindications for high levels of vasoconstrictors.

Box 10–10   *Patient Education: Methemoglobinemia and Acetaminophen*

Acetaminophen is a widely consumed, over-the-counter drug that is used alone or in combination with other drugs. It has a known tendency to induce a potentially life-threatening anemia (methemoglobinemia) in animals (American Heart Association [AHA], 2007). Although not reported to have been observed in humans, literature from manufacturers cautions against the use of prilocaine when acetaminophen has been ingested (Oraqix, Dentsply Pharmaceuticals; EMLA Cream and Anesthetic Disc, Astra Pharmaceuticals) (ADA, 2007). Since there are suitable substitutes for acetaminophen, individuals may wish to avoid its use before, during, and after appointments.

In keeping with principles of informed consent, patients should be warned of these potential risks in order to make informed decisions before, during, and after therapy.

Box 10–11   *Differing Perspectives on Postmyocardial Infarction Local Anesthesia*

It is a generally accepted practice in dentistry to avoid all treatment within six months of an MI (an absolute contraindication). Recent literature, however, suggests that this time period may be excessive for less severe and uncomplicated MIs and reduced from six months to four-to-six weeks. Consultation with a patient's physician and a detailed risk assessment are recommended in making such a determination for elective dental care.

In more complicated cases, such as when there has been postinfarction disability or heart failure, a delay of elective treatment for at least six months or even longer may be recommended due to significant risks.

Source: Little et al., 2008.

Vasoconstrictors may be used in these individuals but at very low levels (no more than 0.04 mg of epinephrine or 0.2 mg of levonordefrin per appointment) or plain anesthetics without vasoconstrictors may be selected.

Myocardial Infarct

While controversial, some experts have stated that a recent cardiovascular event such as a myocardial infarct within the previous six months is an absolute contraindication to local anesthesia and to elective dental treatment, for that matter (Malamed, 2004). The first six months following a severe cardiovascular event are the most critical. It is within this period that the patient is at greatest risk for a repeat attack (Malamed, 2004). During this time, the patient is considered ASA IV and elective dental care is contraindicated. Local anesthesia (and treatment) should be postponed until medical evaluation determines that the individual's risk has returned to acceptable levels. Other experts have stated that six months may be excessive in many cases (see Box 10–11) (Little et al., 2008).

Cardiovascular Accident (CVA) and Transient Ischemic Attacks (TIA)

In the event of a stroke (CVA) or TIA, current recommendations suggest that dental treatment be deferred for six months. Within the first six months, dental care is absolutely contraindicated due to the high risk of suffering a subsequent stroke. Despite a lowering of that risk after six months, it has been reported that 14 percent of cases will suffer a recurrent stoke or TIA within one year. This statistic should be considered when treating these individuals even after the initial six months has passed following a CVA or TIA (Little et al., 2008).

Hypertension

High blood pressure increases the risk of medical complications following the administration of local anesthesia. Many patients are unaware that they have hypertension or are unaware of its consequences to their overall health. If the patient is not seeing a physician and their hypertension is uncontrolled, elective treatment should be deferred until control has been established. The decision to perform elective dental treatment on patients with significant hypertension must be based on several factors including consultation with the patient's

Table 10–1	Guidelines for Local Anesthesia Management in Hypertension
Blood Pressure Values	**Treatment and Referral Actions**
>120/80 but <160/100	No contraindications for treatment, suggest medical referral
≥160/100	Treatment may be initiated with monitoring, prompt medical referral
>180/110	Defer treatment, immediate medical referral

Source: Little et al., 2008.

physician, physiological status including past medical and dental history, and psychological status.

A reasonable course of action can be found in the recommendations of Little, Falace, Miller, and Rhodus (Little et al., 2008). For patients with ASA II blood pressure values, there is no contraindication for dental treatment; however, patients are encouraged to see a physician. When blood pressure values are at described ASA III levels, recommended dental treatment may be initiated provided that intraoperative monitoring of blood pressure for upper levels is considered and patients are referred to physicians promptly (within one month). For blood pressure values >180/110, all elective treatment should be deferred and patients should be referred to a physician as soon as possible, or immediately, if symptomatic. For a summary of these guidelines see Table 10–1 ■ and Appendix 10–1.

Allergies

Allergies to specific local anesthetic drugs or to bisulfite preservatives are absolute contraindications to their use. When considering alternative local anesthetic selections, clear knowledge of the specific allergen is necessary. If a patient has a documented allergy to an ester, an amide may be used safely. If a patient is allergic to any esters, all esters must be avoided. If there is an allergy to one amide, other amides may be used but only after appropriate allergy testing to confirm their safety.

These conditions apply regardless of whether or not these drugs are injected or topically applied. If a patient is allergic to esters, benzocaine and tetracaine topical may not be used but amides such as lidocaine and prilocaine topical can be used.

All local anesthetics drugs with vasoconstrictors contain bisulfite preservatives. These agents are also used as preservatives in foods and drinks (such as lettuce in salad bars and most wines). When there is a documented allergy to bisulfites, all drugs containing vasoconstrictors are absolutely contraindicated. Bisulfite sensitivity is more common in patients with asthma. Asthmatics should be questioned specifically about their tolerance to bisulfites in food products prior to the use of local anesthetics containing vasoconstrictors. If patients report any sensitivity to bisulfites, vasoconstrictors should not be used. In these patients, 3% mepivacaine is an excellent alternative.

Some patients report a previous *allergy to epinephrine.* Since synthetic epinephrine (exogenous) is identical to endogenous epinephrine, true allergies are impossible. Reactions to the administration of epinephrine instead are classified as *nonallergic* **adverse drug events (ADR),** such as heart palpitations, hypertension, anxiety, and general agitation.

Pregnancy

Healthy pregnant patients are classified as health status ASA II (see Appendix 10–1). Pregnancy poses a temporary and relative contraindication to local anesthetics that may require treatment modifications. Clinical judgment should be exercised prior to local anesthesia administration that includes the results of medical consultation. During the first trimester, the embryo is at greatest risk of injury from exposure to medications. The second trimester is considered to be the safest period for both the fetus and mother. Toward the end of the third trimester, some mothers may have difficulty metabolizing drugs. For specific information on the safe selection of local anesthetics during pregnancy, clinicians should consult the Food and Drug Administration list of Pregnancy Categories for local anesthetic agents (see Chapter 5, Table 5–4).

Alzheimer's Disease and Dementia

Alzheimer's disease and dementia are considered to be conditions of medical compromise; however, concerns for the use of local anesthetic agents are not of a medical origin. According to the Alzhiemer's Associaton, "Patients with middle to later stage dementia are *not* good candidates for local or regional anesthesia because they have difficulty cooperating, understanding directions and keeping still."

Examples of Pharmacological Compromise

Many prescribed drugs and other substances can affect the pharmacology of local anesthetics. Local anesthetics, in turn, can alter the actions and metabolism of a number of medications and other substances. Some effects are relatively mild when typical doses of local anesthetics are administered, such as the slightly increased toxicity of lidocaine when it is given on top of cimetidine, which competes with lidocaine for sites of metabolism (Malamed, 2004). Others can be dramatic and potentially life threatening, such as those that can occur when vasoconstrictors are administered to an individual who is high on methamphetamine.

When these compromises are present, they are referred to as interactions or considerations. A few examples of interactions are found in this section. A more extensive list may be found in Appendix 10–5.

Nonselective Beta-Blockers

Propranolol (Inderal), nadolol (Corgard), and timolol (Blocadren) are examples of prescribed nonselective beta blockers. When local anesthetic drugs containing vasoconstrictors are administered in the presence of these drugs there can be an increased risk of a serious hypertensive episode along with reflex bradycardia due to their unopposed α-adrenergic stimulation. Unless vasoconstriction is necessary, avoid both epinephrine and levonordefrin. When vasoconstriction is necessary, limited doses may be used with caution. Additionally, propranolol may interfere with lidocaine metabolism. This represents an additional relative contraindication for lidocaine use with propranolol. With the availability of excellent substitutes, it is easy to avoid concurrent lidocaine and propranalol administrations.

"Street Drugs"

Although this discussion is not inclusive of all street drugs, two of great concern with the use of local anesthetic and vasoconstrictor drugs, cocaine and methamphetamines, will be highlighted.

Cocaine

Unlike most local anesthetic drugs, cocaine is a potent vasoconstrictor and exhibits significant indirect-acting adrenergic stimulating effects. The administration of a vasoconstrictor on top of cocaine significantly increases the risk of hypertensive crisis, stroke, and myocardial infarction. Although less of an issue, as a local anesthetic drug, cocaine is also a CNS depressant. The addition of other local anesthetics can increase any existing CNS depression from cocaine. Consumed amounts might already have resulted in toxic blood levels prior to administering local anesthetic drugs with or without vasoconstrictors.

As an ester, cocaine is relatively quickly biodegraded. Peak blood levels of cocaine are typically reached within 30 minutes of consumption and are dissipated within 2 hours due to cocaine's rapid cholinesterase metabolism (Little et al., 2008). Nevertheless, *do not* administer local anesthetics with vasoconstrictors for a minimum of *6 hours after* cocaine use and monitor for local anesthetic drug overdoses (Little et al., 2008).

Little et al. state that solutions with epinephrine or levonordefrin should not be used for a "6-hour waiting period after cocaine administration," while Malamed suggests that a longer waiting period of 24 hours is more appropriate (Malamed, 2004). Any clinical decision regarding when to treat an individual who has consumed cocaine should also take into account the reliability of the information the patient is providing. Caution might suggest, whenever the information provided is suspect, that a longer versus a shorter waiting period might be more appropriate.

Methamphetamines

Administration of vasoconstrictors in the presence of **methamphetamines** may result in hypertensive crisis, stroke, and myocardial infarction. *Do not* administer local anesthetics with vasoconstrictors for a minimum of *24 hours after* methamphetamine use.

For a summary of restrictions to these and other concomitant drugs of concern see Appendix 10–6.

Examples of Psychological Compromise

Anxiety and fear can produce both psychological and physiological changes in the body that can affect the ability to administer local anesthesia and the effectiveness of the local anesthetic (Bourassa & Baylard, 1994; Gutmann,

DeWald, Solomon, & McCann, 1997; Newton, Allen, Coates, Turner, & Prior, 2006; Peretz & Mann, 2000; Simon, Peliier, Chambers, & Dower, 1994).

Based on psychological tolerance, stress reduction protocols may be used for anxious patients and can be effective at preventing psychogenically generated adverse events during treatment (see Appendix 10–2). For specific strategies for management of psychological factors of anxiety and fear see Chapter 18.

CASE MANAGEMENT: Carlos Martinez

Several factors suggest caution when treating Mr. Martinez. The selection of local anesthetic drug and vasoconstrictor as well as their observed maximum doses per appointment are most important. When there are multiple relative contraindications to the use of a drug, it may be considered an absolute contraindication or, in some instances, a strong relative contraindication.

Achieving adequate pain control is important in determining the need for vasoconstrictors, for example. Using at least minimal volumes of local anesthetic drugs for effective nerve block and infiltration anesthesia is also important.

Drug doses and appointments should be limited for Mr. Martinez in order to avoid vasoconstrictor interactions and local anesthetic drug toxicity. Some drugs will have less effect on areas of compromise while others will have greater effects. This does not mean that only those with least effect may be used, but it means that those with greatest effect should be used more cautiously. For example, 2% lidocaine with 1:100,000 epinephrine is not as safe as 4% articaine with 1:200,000 epinephrine for this patient. In lower doses and with shorter appointments, however, it is perfectly acceptable. Only 5 to 10 percent of articaine is metabolized in the liver, while lidocaine is entirely metabolized in the liver. While articaine provides a somewhat greater margin of safety when considering significant liver damage, lidocaine is safe to use, particularly in the volumes used in dentistry. Appointments should be limited regardless of the drug in order to limit the total doses of local anesthetic and vasoconstrictor drugs. In addition, articaine is available in a much more diluted concentration of epinephrine, which will limit the effects on blood sugar elevation.

Epinephrine and levonordefrin are relatively contraindicated in this patient due to the potential for serious hypertensive episodes and reflex bradycardia in the presence of Corgard. Prilocaine and benzocaine are relative contraindications as well, due to the family history of methemoglobinemia and Mr. Martinez's smoking habit. While their use is not absolutely contraindicated, both prilocaine and benzocaine are easily avoided rather than limited. Excellent substitutions are readily available and include 2% lidocaine with 1:100,000 epinephrine, 4% articaine with 1:200,000 epinephrine, and 3% mepivacaine plain. Of these three, none is ideal but all will work well with caution. Articaine with 1:200,000 epinephrine, for example, is superior from the standpoint of limiting hepatic interaction (compared with both lidocaine and mepivacaine), elevations in blood sugar (compared with lidocaine only), and interactions with the nonselective beta blocker, nadalol (compared with lidocaine only). It has been linked to methemoglobinemia, however, in excessive doses. Lidocaine has more epinephrine and hepatic pathways of metabolism and can be used as long as quantities administered are limited. Mepivacaine plain has no interactions with the beta-blocker or blood sugar levels but has a slower metabolic pathway through the liver compared with lidocaine. Due to its shorter durations and the lack of epinephrine, it is generally the least effective in infiltration procedures compared with lidocaine and articaine.

On occasion, when long durations are necessary, 0.5% bupivacaine with 1:200,000 epinephrine may also be used. It provides a vasoconstrictor challenge identical to articaine's (1:200,000 epinephrine) and less challenge to the liver's detoxification system compared with lidocaine and mepivacaine, due to the decreased quantity of drug (0.5% solution compared with 2% and 3% solutions).

Diabetics are best treated in the morning. When well-nourished and blood sugar is stable, short morning appointments are recommended.

Case Discussion: Mr. Martinez presents with several challenges when considering dental treatment, but treatment is indicated to eliminate disease and improve his oral health, especially as it contributes to his systemic health. The links between diabetes, periodontal disease, and cardiovascular health have been clearly established. An improvement in his periodontal health and elimination of his dental disease are necessary for him to achieve optimal oral health.

Blood pressure values above 120/80 but less than 160/100 do not present contraindications to treatment. Since Mr. Martinez is already being treated for his hypertension, there is no need for referral, which would be suggested otherwise.

Significant liver damage from hepatitis C, which is a chronic disease, would suggest caution when using local anesthetic drugs that are metabolized in the liver. Liver damage of this nature can increase the toxicity of local anesthetics by prolonging their biodegradation.

Smoking is a mild contraindication to certain drugs that may impair oxygenation, such as prilocaine, benzocaine, acetaminophen, and articaine in very large doses.

Insulin-resistant diabetes, or brittle diabetes, places Mr. Martinez at risk of experiencing epinephrine-elevated blood sugar levels. Epinephrine use should be minimized.

Corgard, or nadalol, is a nonselective beta-blocker. When vasoconstrictors are administered concomitantly, serious spikes in blood pressure and what is known as reflex bradycardia can result. In light of previous precautions already discussed with the use of vasoconstrictors, they should be used only with the utmost caution.

Finally, this case illustrates that procedural modifications (short appointments with more limited treatment areas per appointment) can be as important as the selection of drugs when planning safe experiences.

CHAPTER QUESTIONS

1. The delivery of local anesthesia requires both medical and technical skills. Which *one* of the following is *not* one of the six elements of the ASA Medical Components of Care associated with regional anesthesia?
   a. Pre-anesthetic evaluation of the patient
   b. Comprehensive tooth charting
   c. Remain present during the course of the anesthesia
   d. Providing indicated postanesthesia care

2. The ASA (American Society of Anesthesiologists) Physical Status Classification System categorizes patients based on their overall health. Classification P3 describes which *one* of the following?
   a. Normal Healthy Patient
   b. Severe Systemic Disease
   c. Moribund Patient
   d. Severe Systemic Disease (constant threat to life)

3. Which of the following is *not* considered a main tool for patient assessment when planning for local anesthesia?
   a. The medical/dental questionnaire
   b. The clinical examination
   c. Drug MRDs
   d. Medical consultation

4. Which *one* of the following drugs is an absolute contraindication for patients with poorly controlled or uncontrolled hyperthyroidism?
   a. Lidocaine
   b. Bupivacaine
   c. Epinephrine
   d. Felypressin

5. Your patient has identified or you suspect that your patient has used methamphetamines approximately 20 hours ago. Which of the following would be the most appropriate action when considering the use of local anesthetics?
   a. Continue with procedures, as it has been more than 12 hours since the use.
   b. Restrict the dose of vasoconstrictors to 20 percent of standard dose.
   c. Consider postponing care for a full 24 hours.
   d. Use only bupivacaine as the local anesthetic agent.

6. For which *one* of the following medical conditions is it unnecessary to obtain a medical consultation from the patient's physician prior to dental treatment?
   a. Significant liver disease
   b. Myocardial infarction within three weeks
   c. Kidney dialysis patients
   d. Organ transplant patients

REFERENCES

Alzheimer's Association; www.alz-nca.org/caretips/anesthesia.php. Accessed January 4, 2009.

American Dental Association (ADA). *Infective endocarditis guidelines.* http://www.ada.org/prof/resources/topics/infective_endocarditis.asp. Accessed April 28, 2007.

American Dental Association (ADA) and American Academy of Orthopaedic Surgeons (AAOS). (2003, July). Antibiotic prophylaxis for dental patients with total joint replacements. Advisory statement. *Journal of the American Dental Association, 134,* 895–898.

American Heart Association. (2007, April). *Prevention of Infective Endocarditis.* Guidelines from the AHA Circulation.

American Society of Anesthesiologists (ASA) Statement on Regional Anesthesia. (2002). http://www.asahq.org/PublicationsAndServices/standards/26.pdf. Accessed June 29, 2007.

American Society of Anesthesiologists (ASA) Physical Status Classification System. (2006). www.asahq.org/clinical/physicalstatus.htm. Accessed June 29, 2007.

Antibiotic Prophylaxis. American Dental Association. http://ada.org/prof/resources/topics/antibiotic.asp. Accessed July 13, 2007.

Barclay, L., & Vega, C. (2004, June 15). Methemoglobinemia linked to topical benzocaine use. Medscape CME. www.medscape.com. Accessed April 27, 2007.

Biggs, Q. M., Kelly, K. S., & Toney, J. D. (2003, Spring). The effects of deep diaphragmatic breathing and focused attention on dental anxiety in a private practice setting. *Journal of Dental Hygiene, 77*(2), 105–113.

Bourassa, M., & Baylard, J. F. (1994, January). Stress situations in dental practice. *Journal of the Canadian Dental Association, 60*(1), 65–67, 70–71.

CBC News. (2006, November 24). *Anesthetic benzocaine carries risk of blood condition.* www.cbc.ca. Accessed: April 27, 2007.

Colgate World of Care. *Treatments and coping methods.* www.colgate.com/app/Colgate/US/OC/Information/Oral HealthBasics/CheckupsDent. Accessed July 13, 2007.

Corah, N. L. (1969). Development of a dental anxiety scale. *Journal of Dental Research 48,* 596. http://www.dentalfearcentral.org/media/dental_anxiety_scale.pdf

Dower, J. S., Jr., Simon, J. F., Peltier, B., & Chambers, D. (1995, September). Patients who make a dentist most anxious about giving injections. *Journal of the California Dental Association, 23*(9), 35–40.

FDA Patient Safety News Advisory on benzocaine sprays and methemoglobinemia: Show #50, April 2006. Available at: http://www.accessdata.fda.gov/scripts/cdrh/cfdocs/psn/printer.cfm?id=4

Guggenheimer, J., Orchard, T., Moore, P., Myers, D. E., & Rossie, K, M. (1998). Reliability of self-reported heart murmur history: Possible impact on antibiotic use in dentistry. *Journal of the American Dental Association, 129*(7), 861–866.

Gutmann, M. E., DeWald, J. P., Solomon, E. S., & McCann, A. L. (1997, September–October). Dental and dental hygiene students' attitudes in a joint local anesthesia course. *Probe, 31*(5), 165–170.

Hegedus, F., & Herb, K. (2005, Winter). Benzocaine-induced methemoglobinemia. *Journal of the American Dental Society of Anesthesia, 52*(4), 136–139.

Herman, V. S., Joffe, B. I., Kalk, W. J., Panz, V., Wing, J., & Seftel, H. C. (1989). Clinical and biochemical responses to nadolol and clonidine in hyperthyroidism. *Journal of Clinical Phamacology, 29,* 1117–1120.

Humphris, G. M., Morrison, T., & Lindsay, S. (1995). The modified dental anxiety scale: Validation and United Kingdom norms. *Community Dental Health, 12,* 143–150.

Ibuprofen. University of Maryland Medical Center. http://www.umm.edu/altmed/drugs/ibuprofen-066400.htm. Accessed July 13, 2007.

Jastak, J. T., Yagiela, J. A., & Donaldson, D. (1995). *Local anesthesia of the oral cavity.* Philadelphia: Saunders.

Kan, M., Ishikawa, T., & Nagasaka, N. (1999, January–February). A study of psychological stress created in dentists by children during pediatric treatment. ASDC *Journal of Dentistry for Children, 66*(1), 41–48, 12–13.

Kaufman, E., Goharian, S., & Katz, Y. (2000, Winter). Adverse reactions triggered by dental local anesthetics: A clinical survey. *Journal of the American Dental Society of Anesthesia, 47*(4), 134–138.

Knobeloch, L., Goldring, J., LeMay, W., & Anderson, H. (1994, September 9). Prilocaine-induced Methemoglobinemia—Wisconsin, 1993. *MMWR Weekly, 43*(35), 655–657. www.cdc.gov. Accessed April 27, 2007.

Little, J. W., Falace, D. A., Miller, C. S., & Rhodus, N. L. (2008). *Dental management of the medically compromised patient* (7th ed.). St. Louis: Mosby Elsevier.

Malamed, S. F. (2004). Handbook of local anesthesia (5th ed.). St. Louis: Elsevier Mosby.

Malamed, S. F. (2007). Medical emergencies in the dental office (6th ed.). St. Louis: Elsevier Mosby.

Medical history questionnaire. www.dental.pacific.edu.

Medical history questionnaire. www.metdental.com.

Meechan, J. G. (2005, Summer). Differences between men and women regarding attitudes toward dental local anesthesia among junior students at a United Kingdom dental school. *Journal of the American Dental Society of Anesthesia, 52*(2), 50–55.

Miller, C. S., Egan, R. M., Falace, D. A., Rayens, M. K., & Moore, C. R. (1999). Prevalence of infective endocarditis in patients with systemic lupus erythematosus. *Journal of the American Dental Association, 130*(3), 387–392.

Moore, R., & Brodsgaard, I. (2001, February). Dentists' perceived stress and its relation to perception about anxious patients. *Community Dentistry and Oral Epidemiology, 29*(1), 73–80.

Montebuglioni, L., & Pelliccioni, G. A. (1990, May–June). Evaluation of cardiac function in dentists during professional activity. *Prevenzione & Assistenza Dentale, 16*(3), 11–14.

Muzyka, B. C. (1999). Atrial fibrillation and its relationship to dental care. *Journal of the American Dental Association, 130*(7), 1080–1085.

Newton, J. T., Allen, C. D., Coates, J., Turner, A., & Prior, J. (2006, April 22). How to reduce the stress of dental practice: The need for research into the effectiveness of multifaceted interventions. *British Dental Journal, 200*(8), 437–440.

Newton, J. T., & Buck, D. J. (2000). Anxiety and pain measures in dentistry: A guide to their quality and application. *Journal of the American Dental Association, 131*(10), 1449–1457.

Nield-Gehrig, J. S., & Willman, D. E. (2008). *Foundations of periodontics for the dental hygienist* (2nd ed.). Philadelphia: Lippincott Williams & Wilkins.

Oral Sedation. Dental Fear Central – Your Hub for Dental Phobia Information. www.dentalfearcentral.org/oral_sedation.html. Accessed July 13, 2007.

O'Shea, R. M., Corah, N. L., & Ayer, W. A. (1984, July). Sources of dentists' stress. *Journal of the American Dental Association, 109*(1), 48–51.

Pennsylvania Patient Safety Advisory Vol. 2. No.1. (March 2005). *Topical anesthetic-induced methemoglobinemia.* www.psa.state.pa.us. Accessed April 27, 2007.

Peretz, B., & Mann, J. (2000, August). Dental anxiety among Israeli dental students: A 4-year longitudinal study. *European Journal of Dental Education, 4*(3), 133–137.

Pickett, F. A., & Terezhalmy, G. T. *Dental drug reference with clinical applications.* (2006). Baltimore: Lippincott Williams & Wilkins.

Roberts, H. W., & Redding, S. W. (2000). Coronary artery stents: Review and patient management recommendations. *Journal of the American Dental Association, 131*(6), 797–801.

Sachdeva, R., Pugeda, J. G., Casale, L. R., Meizlish, J. L., & Zarich, S. W. (2003). Benzocaine-induced methemoglobinemia—A potentially fatal complication of transesophageal echocardiography. *Texas Heart Institute Journal, 30*(4), 308–310.

Schwam, S. J., Gold, M. I., & Craythorne, U. W. G. (1982, September). American Society of Anesthesiologists (ASA) physical status classification: A revision. *Anesthesiology, 57*(3), Supp: A439.

Simon, J. F., Peltier, B., Chambers, D., & Dower, J. (1994, September). Dentists troubled by the administration of anesthetic injections: Long term stresses and effects. *Quintessence International, 25*(9), 641–646.

Tong, D. C., & Rothwell, B. R. (2000). Antibiotic prophylaxis in dentistry: A review and practice recommendations. *Journal of the American Dental Association, 131*(3), 366–374.

Wilburn-Goo, D., & Lloyd, L. M. (1999). When patients become cyanotic: Acquired methemoglobinemia. *Journal of the American Dental Association, 130*(6), 826–831.

Wilder, R. *The premedication predicament.* www.dimensiosofdentalhygiene.com. Accessed April 28, 2007.

ASA Physical Status Classification: Examples of Diseases and Conditions

ASA Classification	Health Status	
ASA I	**NORMAL AND HEALTHY PATIENT**	
	Healthy:	• Well-balanced whole body health, physiological systems not compromised, main organs healthy
	Lifestyle Conditions:	• Nonsmoker, minimal to nondrinker
	TREATMENT GUIDELINES	
	• Routine dental treatment • Recheck blood pressure in 6 months • Implement SRP** if patient is anxious	
ASA II	**MILD SYSTEMIC DISEASE OR CONDITION (WELL-CONTROLLED)**	
	Healthy with:	• Allergies, pregnancy, Age 60 + years
	Psychological:	• Dental anxiety
	Cardiovascular:	• High blood pressure (140–159 mm Hg syst 90–94 mm Hg diast)
	Respiratory System:	• Asthma • Short-term upper respiratory tract infection (cold)
	Nervous System:	• Epilepsy, seizure disorders
	Metabolic System:	• Diabetes—type 2 (non–insulin dependent) • Hyperthyroid or hypothyroid disorders
	Lifestyle Conditions:	• Smoker, > than minimal drinker
	• Recheck BP during three consecutive appointments • Advise patient to monitor blood pressure at home or at the pharmacy • Medical Consult recommended if three consecutive blood measurements are in this range • Dental treatment with careful patient observation—measure BP after local anesthesia administration • Implement SRP as needed	
ASA III	**SEVERE SYSTEMIC DISEASE OR CONDITION (UNCONTROLLED)**	
	Unhealthy:	• Significant limits to activity but not incapacitated
	Cardiovascular:	• History of myocardial infarction, cerebral vascular accident, transient ischemic attacks more than 6 months prior to the dental appointment with no residual signs and symptoms

ASA Classification	Health Status	
		• Congestive heart failure—orthopnea and ankle edema
		• Angina pectoris (stable)
		• High blood pressure (160–199 mm Hg systolic and/or 95–114 mm Hg diastolic)
	Respiratory:	• Emphysema, chronic bronchitis, chronic obstructive pulmonary disease
		• Asthma—exercise induced
	Nervous System:	• Epilepsy (less well controlled)
	Metabolic System:	• Diabetes—type 1 (insulin dependent, well controlled)
		• Hyperthyroid or hypothyroid (patient is symptomatic)
	Lifestyle Conditions:	• Smoker w/one or more of above, > minimal drinker
	• Recheck in 5 minutes • Medical Consult before dental treatment if blood pressure still elevated • Implement SRP as needed	
ASA IV	**SEVERE SYSTEMIC DISEASE OR CONDITION THAT IS A CONSTANT THREAT TO LIFE UNCONTROLLED**	
	Cardiovascular:	• Heart attack (myocardial infarction) less than 6 months prior to the dental appointment
		• Brain attack (stroke) within the past 6 months
		• Severe heart failure or COPD (requiring O_2 supplementation or confinement in a wheelchair)
		• Angina pectoris—unstable
		• High blood pressure—greater than 200 mmHg systolic or 115 mmHg diastolic
	Respiratory:	• Severe COPD (requiring O_2 supplementation or confinement in a wheelchair)
	Nervous System:	• Epilepsy—uncontrolled
	Metabolic:	• Diabetes—type 1 (uncontrolled, hx of hospitalization)
	• Recheck in 5 minutes • Medical Consult before dental treatment if blood pressure still elevated • Implement SRP as needed	
ASA V	**MORIBUND PATIENT NOT EXPECTED TO SURVIVE WITHOUT AN OPERATION TERMINAL SYSTEMIC DISEASES OR CONDITIONS**	
	Moribund:	• All end-stage diseases
	• Recheck in 5 minutes • Medical checkup immediately • **DO NOT** deliver dental treatment until BP corrected • Consider arranging transportation for the patient	
ASA VI	**CLINICALLY DEAD PATIENTS BEING MAINTAINED FOR HARVESTING OF ORGANS**	

Adapted from: ASA (American Society of Anesthesiologists) Physical Status Classification System, 2006, www.asahq.org/clinical/physicalstatus.htm, and Malamed, S. F..: *Medical Emergencies in the Dental Office*, 6th edition, 2007, pp. 50–53.

SRP: Stress Reduction Protocols for Anxious Patients

ASA Classification	Strategies for Stress Reduction	
ASA I *HEALTHY W/ ANXIETY*	**Communication:**	Establish trust, using empathy and effective communication skills Recognize the patient's level of anxiety Determine the cause of the patient's anxiety
	Anxiety Reduction:	Premedicate the evening before the dental appointment, as needed Premedicate immediately before the dental appointment, as needed
	Scheduling:	Schedule the appointment early in the day (patient will be well rested and will not worry all day about the appointment) Minimize the patient's waiting time Short appointments
	Suggestions to Patient:	Try to avoid additional stress by getting enough sleep, eat a well-balanced meal before the appointment, and allow enough travel time to get to the appointment
	Anxiety and Pain Control during the Appointment:	Consider sedation during therapy (nitrous oxide) Administer adequate pain control during therapy Obtain frequent feedback, giving the patient a sense of control and caring
	Postoperative Care:	• Follow up with postoperative pain and anxiety control • Telephone the highly anxious or fearful patient later that same day that treatment was delivered
ASA II, ASA III *MEDICAL COMPROMISE W/ ANXIETY*	**APPLY STRATEGIES FOR ASA 1 PATIENT WITH THE FOLLOWING ADDITIONAL PROCEDURES:**	
	Pre-Appointment Procedures:	• Recognize the patient's level of medical risk • Complete medical consultation, as needed
	Procedures during the Appointment:	• Monitor and record preoperative and postoperative vital signs
	Scheduling:	• Arrange the appointment for the highly anxious or fearful, moderate-to-high-risk patient during the first few days of the week when the office is open for emergency care and the treating doctor is available.

Modifications to Local Anesthesia for Common Medical Conditions

Condition	Local Anesthetic Considerations	Vasoconstrictor Considerations	Modifications
Diabetes	None of Significance	Epinephrine opposes the action of insulin Minute amounts used in dentistry do not raise blood levels significantly	Use epinephrine with **caution** when there is significant cardiovascular disease &/or uncontrolled diabetes.
Glaucoma	None of Significance	Vasoconstrictors cause increased ocular pressure	**Avoid** vasoconstrictors
Hypertension	None of Significance	Vasoconstrictors can increase the risk of hypertensive episodes; however the *lack* of profound anesthesia can increase levels of endogenous epinephrine *Controversial topic*	Clinical **judgment** and medical **consult** advised **Note**: Uncontrolled hypertensives either *should not be treated or treated with* **caution**, depending upon severity See Table 10–1
Hyperthyroidism *A—Controlled*	None of Significance	Hyperthyroidism *appears* to increase tissue sensitivity to epinephrine	When there is *obvious evidence* of hyperthyroidism **avoid** epinephrine
Hyperthyroidism *B—Uncontrolled*	None of Significance	Risk of seriously increased tissue sensitivity to epinephrine	**Avoid** *all treatment* until condition is under control
Hypothyroidism *A—Controlled* *B—Uncontrolled*	Generally Safe	Generally Safe	Hypothyroid patients tend to be sensitive to CNS depressants Mild **caution** with LA drug dosing
Myasthenia Gravis	Esters and articaine compete for diminished supplies of acetyl choline	None of Significance	**Avoid** esters and articaine

Medical Predispositions That May Require Modifications

Condition	Local Anesthetic Considerations	Vasoconstrictor Considerations	Modifications
Significant Hepatic Disease	Amides are primarily metabolized in the liver	Cholinesterase is primarily manufactured in the liver, although there are extrahepatic sources	**Caution** with use of amides Articaine is the preferred amide but *appointments* should be *shorter* with *reduced dosages* administered If other amides are used, **limit** even further
Atypical Cholinesterase	Amides are not affected	None of Significance	**Avoid** esters & articaine
Significant Renal Dysfunction	All drugs cleared more slowly, with increased risk of overdose	All drugs cleared more slowly, with increased risk of overdose	Medical **consult** advised **Limit** doses of all drugs depending upon severity
Methemoglobinemia	Increased risk with prilocaine and benzocaine	None of Significance	**Substitute** other amides for prilocaine and other topicals for benzocaine **Avoid** prilocaine or benzocaine when excessive doses of acetaminophen are used
Malignant Hyperthermia	Local anesthetic agents safe for MH patients: articaine bupivacaine lidocaine mepivicaine prilocaine	None of Significance	Medical **consult** is recommended When treating these patients, follow the **MHAUS*** *guidelines*

*MAUS: Malignant Hyperthermia Association of the United States

Modifications to Local Anesthesia for Common Concomitant Drug Therapy

Medications Examples: Proprietary (generic)	Local Anesthetic Considerations	Vasoconstrictor Considerations	Modifications
Anticonvulsants Klonopin (clonazepam) Dilantin (phenytoin) Depakote (valproic acid) Topamax (topiramate)	Anxiety reduction requires effective local anesthesia Sensitive to CNS depressants	None of Significance	**Avoid** higher doses of local anesthetic drugs
Antipsychotics Zyprexa (olanzapine) Seroquel (quetiapine) Risperdal (risperidone)	Increased sensitivity to CNS depressants	None of Significance	**Avoid** higher doses of local anesthetic drugs
Anxiolytics Valium (diazepam)	CNS depressant effect of local anesthetics may be additive	None of Significance	**Limit** dosages
Glucocorticoids Nasonex (mometasone) Entocort (budesonide) Advair (fluticasone) Aristocort (triamcinolone)	Stress associated with local anesthesia is considered to be low	Stress associated with local anesthesia is considered to be low	**Consider** supplemental stress reduction such as nitrous oxide or IV sedation
Histamine H$_2$ Receptor Blockers Tagamet (cimetidine) Zantac (ranitidine)	Tagamet competes with lidocaine for liver isoenzymes Slows lidocaine metabolism increasing the risk of overdose Zantac and others do not have this effect	None of Significance	Use **caution** with large doses of lidocaine particularly **in the presence** of significant congestive heart failure
Monamine Oxidase Inhibitors Nardil (phenylzine) Parnate (tranylcypromine) Marplan (isocarboxacid)	None of Significance	None of Significance	None
Nonselective β-blockers Inderal (propranolol) Corgard (nadolol) Blocadren (timolol)	With propranolol, minimal doses of lidocaine are recommended	Increases risk of hypertensive episode and reflexive bradycardia	Unless vasoconstriction is necessary, **limit or avoid** vasoconstrictors

Medications Examples: Proprietary (generic)	Local Anesthetic Considerations	Vasoconstrictor Considerations	Modifications
Phenothiazides Thorazine (chlorpromazine) Mellaril (thioridazine)	None of Significance	Hypotension, possibly severe, is the primary effect of epinephrine with these drugs	**Observe** cardiac **limit** of vasoconstrictors (0.04 mg). **Do not use 1:50,000** epinephrine
Tricyclic Antidepressants Elavil (amitriptyline) Tofranil (imipramine)	None of Significance	Increases risk of hypertensive episode by opposing the reuptake of norepinephrine	**Limit** doses of **epinephrine** (observe cardiac dose limits) **Avoid levonordefrin**

Illegal ("Recreational") Drug Use*

Drug	Local Anesthetic Considerations	Vasoconstrictor Considerations	Modifications
Methamphetamine	None of Significance	Administration of vasoconstrictors may result in hypertensive crisis, stroke, or myocardial infarction	**Do not** administer local anesthetics with vasoconstrictors for a minimum of **24 hours after** methamphetamine use
Cocaine	Cocaine is a strong CNS depressant; local anesthetics compound CNS depression and administration should be **avoided**	Administration of vasoconstrictors significantly increases the risk of hypertensive crisis, stroke, or myocardial infarction	**Do not** administer local anesthetics with vasoconstrictors for a minimum of **6 hours after** cocaine use
Alcohol	May decrease the effectiveness of local anesthetics	None of Significance	Use **caution** to avoid overdose

*If a patient is under the influence of a drug or alcohol, any informed consent taken may be invalid as the patient may not be "competent" to give consent.

**For all drugs not on this list, it is prudent to consult a drug index prior to administering all local anesthetic drugs.

APPENDIX REFERENCES

1. Aldrete, J. A., & Narang R. (1975). Deaths due to local analgesia in dentistry. *Anaesthesia, 30,* 685–686.
2. Aldrete, J. A., Narang, R., Liem, S., Sada, T., & Miller, G. P. (1975). Untoward reaction to local anaesthetics via reverse intracarotid flow. *J Dent Res, 54,* 145–148.
3. Little, J. W., Falace, D. A., Miller, C. S., & Rhodus, N. L. (2008). *Dental management of the medically compromised patient* (2nd ed.). St. Louis: Mosby.
4. Malamed, S. F. (2004). *Handbook of local anesthesia* (5th ed.). St. Louis: Mosby.
5. Paarman, C. P., & Royer, R. (2008). *Pain control for the dental practitioner*. Philadelphia: Wolters Kluwer / Lippincott Williams & Wilkins.
6. Pickett, F. A., & Terezhalmy, G. T. (2006). Dental drug reference with clinical implications. Baltimore: Lippincott Williams & Wilkins.
7. Tetzlaff, J. E. (2000). *Pharmacology of local anesthetics* (pp.177–178). Woburn, MA: Butterworth-Heinemann.
8. Nield-Gehrig, J. S., & Willman, D. E. (2008). *Foundations of periodontics for the dental hygienist* (2nd ed.). Philadelphia: Lippincott Williams & Wilkins.

Chapter 11

Fundamentals for Administration of Local Anesthetic Agents

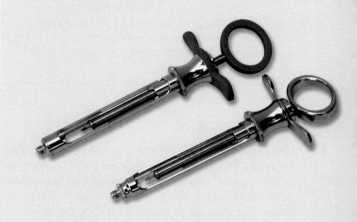

OBJECTIVES

- Define and discuss the key terms in this chapter.
- Identify and discuss the general principles and elements of informed consent.
- Identify and discuss key factors that impact the successful delivery of local anesthetic agents.
- Identify and discuss stress and anxiety factors that impact both patients and clinicians during the delivery of local anesthetic injections.
- Discuss the impact of clinician/patient communications before, during, and after the delivery of local anesthetic injections.
- Differentiate between the three basic types of injections.
- List and describe the basic steps involved in the delivery of local anesthetic injections.
- Identify and discuss the general principles of ergonomics during the delivery of local anesthetic injections.

KEY TERMS

aspiration test **202**
cumulative trauma disorders **204**
deposition site **194**
false negative aspiration **202**
field block **194**
informed consent **195**
local infiltration **194**
needle pathway **194**

negative aspiration **202**
nerve block **194**
penetration site **194**
positive aspiration **202**
supportive communication **197**
supraperiosteal injection **194**

CASE STUDY: HECTOR MELENDEZ

Hector Melendez, a 45-year-old social worker, related that during his most recent dental visit, the "shots" were given to him within what seemed like only seconds of sitting down and they were fast and painful. Before they started, he was told to raise his hand if he "needed a break" and he had done so after the pain became intense but was told that it was almost over.

While the actual treatment had been comfortable, he had decided to try out a new office and then asked if there were a way to have his dental treatment accomplished without novocaine.

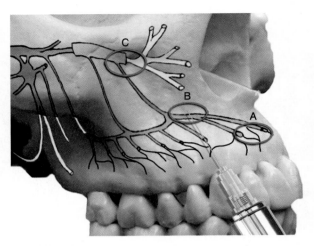

FIGURE 11–1   Types of Injections Defined. A—Local infiltration involves deposition directly at or near small terminal nerve endings in the immediate area of treatment. B—Field block injections involve depositions near larger terminal nerve branches. C—Nerve block injections involve depositions near major nerve trunks at a greater distance from the area of treatment, which provide wider areas of anesthesia.

INTRODUCTION

Basic skills necessary for the safe and comfortable delivery of all local anesthetic injections will be discussed in this chapter. In addition to technical and procedural skills, informed consent, ergonomic awareness, and patient and clinician perspectives will be discussed.

Few will argue that injections represent one of the most if not *the* most stressful aspect of dental appointments (Dionne, Gordon, McCullagh, & Phero, 1998; Rissolati, Fadiga, Gallese, & Fagassi, 1996). In order to reduce stress and provide both safe and comfortable environments for injections, the development of specific strategies and clinical skills is necessary. Local anesthetic procedures should take into account the need for good pain control both during and after injections. They are perhaps most successful when all components of the process have been considered.

BASIC INJECTION GUIDELINES

Injection Definitions

There are three basic types of intraoral injections: **local infiltrations, field blocks,** and **nerve blocks** (Evers & Haegerstam, 1981; Lipp, 1993; Malamed, 2004; U.S. Department of Labor, 2002) (see Figure 11–1 ■). A local infiltration involves the deposition of local anesthetic drug directly at or near small terminal nerve endings in the immediate area of treatment. Fields block injections, also referred to as **supraperiosteal injections,** involve deposition of anesthetic drugs near larger terminal nerve branches for treatment of areas usually near or a small distance away from the site of the injection. Nerve block injections usually involve depositions near major nerve trunks at greater distances from the areas of treatment, which provide wider areas of anesthesia. In dentistry, field block and nerve block injections are used most frequently to provide pulpal as well as soft tissue anesthesia. These injections are identified by the nerve branches to be anesthetized; for example, the inferior alveolar nerve block will anesthetize the inferior alveolar nerve. Box 11–1 discusses common usage of the terms infiltration and nerve block injection.

With all injection types, it is necessary to consider each step in the process prior to delivery, similar to a pilot's "preflight" check. Proper functioning of the plane and its equipment helps to ensure the safety of the flight. Basic pre-injection checks are intended to ensure safe injections, proper functioning of armamentarium, and optimal access.

Key terms relevant to the basic injection steps for local anesthesia include **penetration site, needle pathway,** and **deposition site.** The penetration site is the specific location where a needle first pierces mucosa. Locating this site for each technique requires inspection

Box 11–1 Infiltrations vs. Nerve Blocks

While the terms *infiltration, supraperiosteal injection* (field block), and *nerve block injection* (regional nerve block) accurately apply to all local anesthetic techniques in this chapter, common usage limits dental local anesthetic injections to either nerve blocks or infiltrations. Nerve blocks refer to injections that involve deposition of anesthetic near major trunks of nerves, usually at a significant distance from the treatment area, and to injections that provide anesthesia to multiple teeth via a single deposition site regardless of the distance to the nerve. Infiltrations refer to most other injections regardless of whether they anesthetize soft, hard, or pulpal tissue.

of the oral cavity and visual identification of key landmarks. Needle pathway refers to the route a needle travels as it advances to what may be referred to as a target site. The deposition site may be defined as the anatomical location at which a drug is deposited. Establishing these locations for each technique requires an understanding of head and neck anatomy (see Box 11–2).

A summary of the key elements for each basic injection discussed in the following chapters is provided in Appendices 12–1, 13–1, and 14–1. Target structures, needle gauges, penetration sites, injection angles, depths of insertion, and suggested drug doses are available for quick reference. Suggested drug volumes are provided for both soft tissue and pulpal anesthesia.

Box 11–2 Penetration and Deposition Site—Technique Considerations

The greater the distance from the penetration to the deposition site, the greater the potential for deviation of the needle tip. For example, the distance from the site of penetration to the deposition site in most infiltrations is usually only a few millimeters, while the penetration site for a nerve block injection may be as much as 16 to 27 millimeters or more from its deposition site. Close attention to proper landmarks and maintaining appropriate barrel angles during injections will reduce these deviations.

Basic Injection Guidelines

Successful development of strategies and skills necessary for the administration of local anesthetics involves following a framework of fundamental steps (Evers & Haegerstam, 1981; Lipp, 1993; Malamed, 2004; Robinson, Ford, & McDonald, 2000). The sequence of basic steps, which incorporates various schools of thought, will be discussed.

Steps in the Administration of Local Anesthesia

Ten basic steps serve as standard operating procedures (SOPs) for monitoring safe injection technique, patient comfort, documentation, and follow-up. These 10 steps are individually discussed in the following section and summarized in Appendix 11–1.

Step 1: Pre-injection Patient Assessment

Thorough patient evaluation determines individual local anesthetic needs based on the factors discussed in Chapter 10, "Patient Assessment for Local Anesthesia." After consideration of all precautions, contraindications, and necessary modifications, appropriate injection techniques and anesthetic drugs are selected.

Step 2: Informed Consent

Discussions with patients to obtain **informed consent** should include the nature of and need for any intended treatment and specific discussions regarding the use of local anesthesia, when anticipated (American Medical Association [AMA], 2007; Malamed, 2004; University of Washington [UW] School of Medicine, 1999). This discussion should include an explanation that local anesthesia involves the delivery of an injection ("shot") that results in the temporary numbing of an area from the effects of the local anesthetic drug. Patients must be advised of the specific risks associated with the delivery of injectable local anesthetic drugs. See Box 11–3 for a summary of the elements of informed consent and some specific risks.

Step 3: Assemble Appropriate Armamentarium

Prior to the delivery of an injection, assembly of the appropriate armamentarium and confirmation of the proper function of local anesthetic delivery devices is required. The cartridge is properly loaded when the

Box 11–3   Elements of Informed Consent

Obtaining *informed consent* requires communication *before* proceeding with any treatment.

This communication should:

1. be discussed in a language patients can understand
2. provide patients with opportunities to ask questions
3. explain the procedures that have been recommended and explain the need for each
4. clarify the risks and rewards of the recommended treatment, including the risks of failing to treat
5. provide acceptable alternatives to the recommended treatment

Patients should understand that the topical placement and injection of local anesthetic agents induce temporary numbness of specific areas of the mouth and, although rarely encountered, there are significant risks associated with their use. These risks may include but are not limited to swelling, bruising, temporary muscle tightening, prolonged temporary or permanent tingling or numbness, localized pain and soreness, allergic and overdose reactions, and short-term racing of the heart.

Source: AMA, 2007; Malamed, 2004; UW School of Medicine, 1999.

harpoon is fully engaged into the rubber stopper. This will allow the piston to be retracted when performing aspiration tests. The cartridge should remain fully visible throughout the injection in order to reconfirm that the correct drug has been loaded into the syringe, to confirm the results of aspiration tests, and to monitor the drug dose and the rate at which it is delivered (see Figure 11–2 ■). Window orientation does not apply when using plastic syringes with clear barrels.

Once the syringe has been properly loaded, the needle is attached and the bevel orientation is checked (if bevel orientation adjustment is appropriate for the particular injection). To adjust the bevel, recap and rotate the needle in the desired direction until the bevel is properly aligned (see Box 11–4).

The final step in armamentarium preparation is to confirm that all safety controls are in place. These controls must include appropriate personal protective

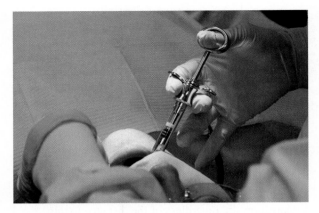

■ FIGURE 11–2   Syringe Cartridge View. Keep the large window in full view to accurately monitor the outcome of aspiration, delivery rate, and the dose of drug deposited.

Box 11–4   *Point of View: Bevel Orientation*

Although some clinicians consider it unimportant, others believe that the needle bevel should be oriented toward bone when bony landmarks may be encountered during injection. Orienting the bevel of the needle toward bone lessens the likelihood of discomfort and trauma to the periosteum when or if bone is contacted. In the event of inadvertent contact, needles tend to glance off bone rather than pierce periosteum when bevels are oriented to face the bone. Withdrawing needles from tissue in order to reposition them is not recommended, since it can result in unnecessary tissue trauma. Bevel orientation does not affect success rates.

Source: Malamed, 2004.

equipment (PPE) for both clinician and patient, and must focus special attention on the safe handling of needles. It is the clinician's responsibility to comply with all Centers for Disease Control and Prevention (CDC) and Occupational Safety and Health Administration (OSHA) guidelines for dental healthcare providers related to the handling of needles and other sharps. This is required in order to assure not only clinician safety but that of patients and co-workers. Appropriate procedures and devices for recapping needles must be available and functioning properly.

See Appendix 9–1 and Appendix 9–2 for CDC guidelines. Needle recapping will be discussed in Step 9—Completion of Injection, and a variety of techniques are shown in Appendix 9–4, "Needle Recapping."

Step 4: Pre-injection Preparation

Placing patients in supine positions during injections puts them in a "head-lower-than-heart" position, which provides physiological support during stress and is the primary position recommended for management of medical emergencies. Ideally, a patient's head should be positioned for the clinician's direct vision of the penetration site. Attention to the principles of proper ergonomics should be applied for all injections. Further discussion of proper ergonomics is presented at the end of this chapter (see Box 11–8).

Supportive Communication and PREP

Supportive communication begins during the pre-injection period. Efforts to reduce stress from the beginning to the end of the injection are enhanced by maintaining positive, supportive communication as a central focus. Providing reassurance and gaining trust can allay anxiety and fears. As discussed in Chapter 2, "Fundamentals of Pain Management," the PREP strategy and steps (Prepare, Rehearse, Empower, and Praise), along with a debriefing session, can further build trust and reassurance. To review these steps, see Chapter 2, Box 2–2, "PREP to Minimize Patient Anxiety and Fear."

It is helpful to establish safe strategies for patients to enable them to communicate anxiety or discomfort during injections. This protects both patients and clinicians from surprise movements while at the same time allowing patients to have a sense of control. As discussed in Chapter 2, patients may raise their hands when they feel unable to cope. It is important to designate which hand to raise to avoid interference with injections. For the highly anxious patient, taking a moment to pause during the procedure can give them time to regain control and allow them to proceed.

In most cases, keeping the syringe out of the patient's sight is a valuable stress reduction strategy. Impulses from the image of the syringe travel to the brain and can trigger a number of possible responses, including unanticipated anxiety, voluntary withdrawal, and autonomic recoil. For anxious or fearful patients, the "show-tell-do" strategy can be valuable when preparing them for what is actually going to happen (Milgrom, Weinstein, & Getz, 1995).

Once the specific injections have been determined, establish effective soft tissue retraction (see Figure 11–3 ■). Palpating the areas adjacent to the penetration site (see Figure 11–4 ■) will identify anatomical variations that are not visible. Anatomical variations can interfere with the basic injection technique and may

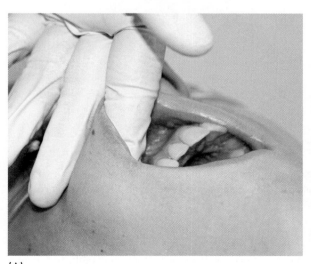
(A)

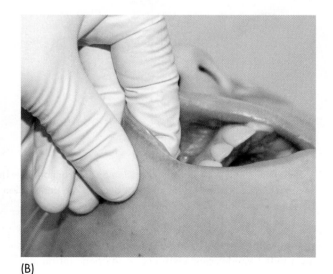
(B)

■ **FIGURE 11–3**   Pre-insertion Soft Tissue Retraction. A—The first step of a safe injection is to establish a firm but gentle grasp of the soft tissue. B—Then fully retract the lip for vision and control during the injection.

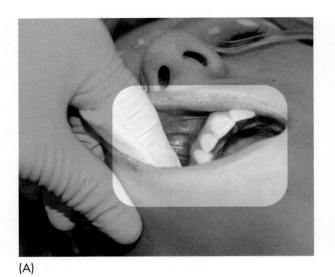

(A)

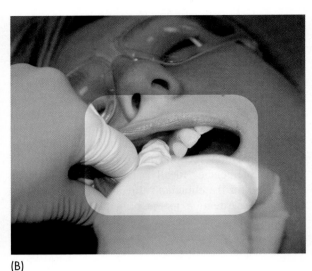

(B)

■ **FIGURE 11–4** Injection Step: View & Palpate. A—Once stable retraction has been accomplished, establish a clear view of the selected penetration site by positioning the patient ergonomically. B—Gently palpate the site for any anomalies that could interfere with the injection.

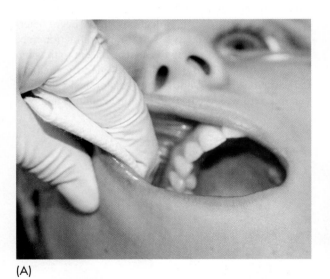

(A)

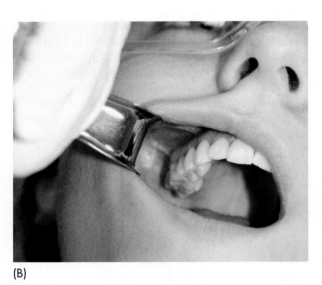

(B)

■ **FIGURE 11–5** Injection Penetration Site Retraction. A—The use of gauze aids in the control of "slippery" tissues, is used to remove gross debris from the site and to dry the penetration site prior to placing topical anesthetic. B—Retraction can also be established with a mouth mirror or metal retractor.

require adjustment. To proceed, reestablish retraction. This will provide clear visibility of the penetration site (see Figure 11–5 ■) and allow the clinician to view the needle throughout the injection as demonstrated in Figure 11–6 ■.

Step 5: Prepare Injection Site

With adequate soft tissue retraction established, gently dry the mucosa with gauze prior to the placement of topical. Drying tissue with gauze will reduce dilution and spread of the topical agent and improve its uptake into

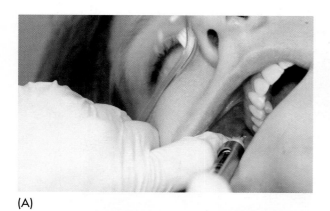

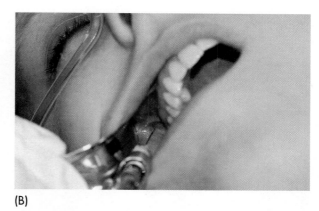

(A)
(B)

■ **FIGURE 11-6** Soft Tissue Retraction During the Injection. A—Retraction is provided manually. B—Retraction is provided by a retraction device.

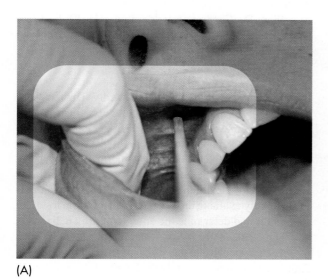

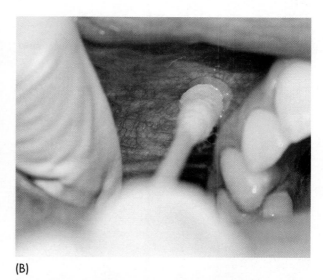

(A)
(B)

■ **FIGURE 11-7** Injection Step: Rehearse & Topical. A—Begin by visualizing the angle of the injection and rehearse the approach with a cotton swab. B—Maintaining this angle, place topical anesthetic at the penetration site.

the mucosal tissue. It also serves as a debridement step by removing gross and microscopic debris from the site. Using a cotton-tipped applicator, apply a small amount of an appropriate topical anesthetic agent at the site of penetration (see Figure 11–7 ■). Consult the manufacturer's directions for the appropriate onset time. Most agents will reach peak effectiveness in about 1 minute.

The preparation time can also be viewed as the "rehearsal" time for the injection (see Figure 8–7). This is an ideal time for clinicians to mentally review the injection technique and reevaluate the patient for any factors that may require adjustments to the planned technique.

Before proceeding with the injection, test the site for effective onset of topical anesthesia (Figure 11–8 ■). If the patient expresses that the site is not numb, allow more time for the topical to be effective. This step may reduce patient anxiety surrounding initial needle penetration. The tip of a cotton swab, periodontal probe, or other instrument works well for testing topical effectiveness.

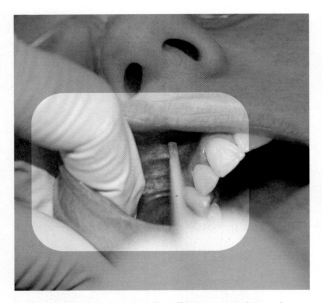

■ **FIGURE 11-8** Testing for Effective Topical Anesthesia.

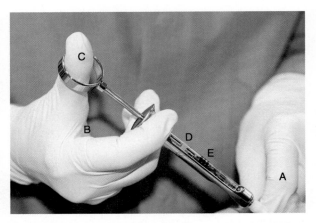

■ **FIGURE 11-10** Injection Technique: Initial Approach. Key elements of a safe injection: A—Stable retraction; B—"Palm up" grasp; C—Thumb positioned for effective aspiration; D—Confirm cartridge drug color ID; E—Clear vision of large window and rubber stopper (showing "½ cartridge").

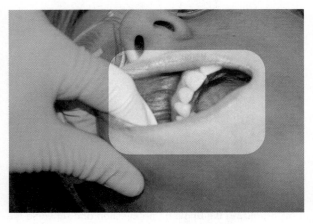

■ **FIGURE 11-9** Establish Retraction. Retract and gently pull the mucosa "taut."

Step 6: Initiate Injection

Maintain supportive communication with the patient while keeping the syringe out of the patient's view as much as possible. With adequate retraction established, gently pull the mucosa "taut" (see Figure 11-9 ■), which will ease penetration of the needle and then establish a point of stability for the syringe. Avoid using the patient's body for stability. Establishing syringe stability on the patient's shoulders or chest increases the risk of

trauma if the patient moves unexpectedly. The most stable position for the syringe is a "palm up" grasp. Stability can be increased with the index finger extended onto the barrel for support (see Figure 11-10 ■, Box 11-5, and Appendix 11-2). The large window of the syringe should face the clinician and the length of the cartridge should remain visible throughout the procedure in order to accurately evaluate the outcome of aspiration tests and to monitor and determine the amount of drug delivered.

Once clear vision and a stable fulcrum have been established, penetrate the mucosa to a depth of 1 to 2 millimeters (approximately the length of the bevel) with the bevel oriented toward bone (see Figure 11-11 ■). A few drops of solution are usually deposited because even gentle contact with the thumb on the front inner surface of the thumb ring will cause a few drops of anesthetic to be deposited ahead of the needle. Note that this does not require visible advancement of the stopper and no separate action is required other than to proceed slowly. The total volume administered in this manner should be less than 0.2 ml (the volume displaced by 1 stopper length).

Slowly advance the needle to the desired depth and angle for delivery at the deposition site (see Figure 11-12 ■). Throughout the injection, observe and communicate with the patient, monitoring for signs of discomfort, distress, and adverse reactions.

Box 11–5   Stability vs. Fulcrum

Safe delivery of injections requires clinicians to have constant control of the syringe. As with other dental instrumentation, this can be accomplished with well-placed, extra-oral finger fulcrums. Those with small hands may not be able to achieve stable fulcrums using only the fingers on the hand that is holding the syringe. When this is the case, a variety of methods may be used, some of which include two-handed fulcrums. Others do not use fulcrums at all but nevertheless allow for *stability* of the syringe during injection. For example, stability can be achieved through arm-to-body, barrel-to-retraction-finger, secondary finger-to-finger, elbow-stabilized-on-leg, and many other methods, each of which may be as unique as the clinician. The goal of stability is to maintain both constant control of the syringe and a position that supports musculoskeletal health. Appendix 11–2 shows a number of useful strategies for creating stability during local anesthetic injections.

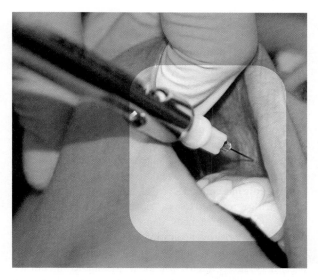

■ **FIGURE 11–11**   Initiate Penetration. Penetration is made slowly, at the height of the mucobuccal fold. Deliver a few drops of anesthetic solution after penetration and ahead of needle pathway.

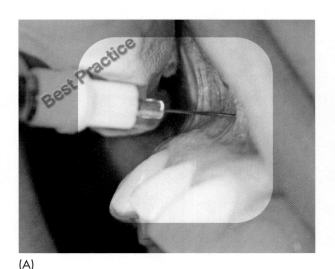

(A)

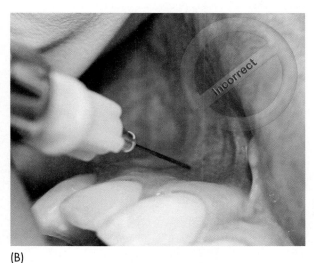

(B)

■ **FIGURE 11–12**   Penetration Site: Correct/Incorrect. A—CORRECT: angle and height of penetration at the mucobuccal fold. B—INCORRECT: the angle is somewhat steep and the height of penetration is too low. This injection is likely to encounter premature contact with alveolar bone below the apex of the tooth.

Step 7: Aspiration

One of the two *most important safety steps* in the delivery of local anesthetic agents is the **aspiration test** (slow delivery is the other). This test reduces the risk of inadvertent deposition of a drug directly into the bloodstream.

Once the needle is advanced to the appropriate deposition site for a specific injection, and *before* depositing solution, perform an aspiration test by applying gentle, brief back pressure on the upper inside surface of the thumb-ring. This action changes the pressure inside the cartridge from positive to negative (see Figure 11–13 ■). If the needle has entered a vessel, blood will be drawn into the cartridge, referred to as a "positive aspiration." *Do not* under any circumstances deposit drug in the *specific* location of a positive aspiration.

Responding to the outcomes of aspiration tests is a primary safety factor for local anesthetic injections. Failure to aspirate or appropriately respond can result in toxic overdose or injury.

A **negative aspiration,** one in which no blood is drawn into the cartridge, requires no corrective action. A clinician may continue with the injection and deposit the indicated volume of drug.

Despite performing this step correctly, it is still possible to have **false negative aspirations** at times. This can occur when a bevel is in contact with a vessel wall. During an aspiration test, negative pressure can retract the vessel wall into the lumen of the needle blocking the flow of blood through the needle into the cartridge. To check for false negative responses, rotate the syringe slightly, which will reposition the bevel away from the vessel wall. This step is encouraged for all injections in which there is a greater risk of positive aspiration.

A **positive aspiration** in which blood is visible in the cartridge (see Figure 11–14 ■) requires an immediate response. If the aspiration test results in a small trickle of blood or "wormlike" thread into the cartridge and does not obstruct clear vision of a subsequent aspiration, the needle can be repositioned slightly and aspiration can be repeated. After a second test that is negative, the clinician may continue with the injection and deposit the drug. If the aspiration test results in a burst of blood, creating a "cloudy and reddened" solution in the cartridge (see Figure 11–14) or if the clinician for any reason is concerned about the ability to see aspiration results clearly, the needle should be withdrawn, the cartridge replaced, and the needle flushed or replaced before reinitiating the injection.

Re-aspiration is also necessary whenever the depth or angle of the needle changes at any time during deposition. It may be performed any time a clinician determines another "safety check" is warranted. It may also be used to pace the rate of deposition of a drug solution. The best practice is to perform an aspiration in two planes, rotating the syringe slightly to reorient the bevel to a new position.

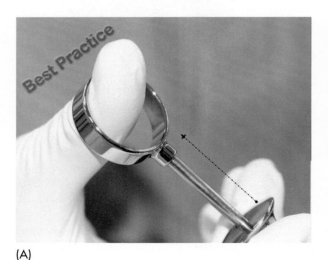

(A)

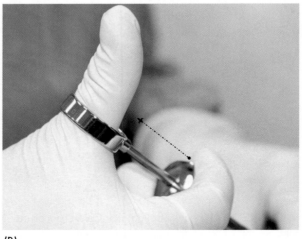

(B)

■ **FIGURE 11–13** *Aspiration Best Practice: Thumb Position.* A—*Ideal position* of the thumb ring. This position during aspiration tests allows for a full range of backward motion. B—*Restricted position* of the thumb ring. This position may create difficulty for small hands and limits the range of "back-pull" motion.

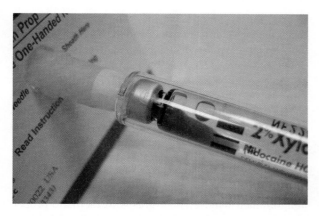

■ **FIGURE 11-14**   Positive Aspiration. Blood backflowing into the cartridge following a positive (+) aspiration test.

Following any positive aspiration, even though a subsequent aspiration tested negative and solution was deposited, evaluate the injection site immediately after completion. Observe for signs of local complications, such as swelling, and monitor the patient for any systemic effects. If there are no immediate complications, it is acceptable to continue with the planned treatment. The patient should be advised according to the significance of the situation and monitored following treatment as indicated. Follow-up for a positive aspiration includes management of hematomas and will be discussed in Chapter 17, "Local Anesthesia Complications and Management."

If there are repeated positive aspirations at the same injection site, rescheduling treatment should be considered. Bleeding at the deposition site may result in an inability to determine a subsequent positive aspiration. Repeated penetrations and the development of an inflammatory response may diminish the effectiveness of the local anesthetic agent. Clinicians may also have other concerns such as the development of hematomas and postoperative pain or trismus.

It is important to maintain supportive communication at all times during the injection process, especially during aspiration tests to educate patients that these simple tests and the responses to them are necessary in order to practice safely.

Step 8: Deposition and Rate

Avoid delivering too much solution en route to the deposition site. Once at the optimum deposition site, the *most important step* in the administration of a safe injection is the rate of delivery (Malamed, 2004). Slow delivery of the drug reduces the risk of overdose and complications even if the drug is inadvertently injected into the bloodstream.

Slow deposition of solution also increases the likelihood of having a comfortable experience by preventing tearing of tissue due to the pressure of the solution being injected. This recommendation is not always followed by clinicians. In some cases, rapid injection is suspected to be the cause of unwanted complications following local anesthesia injections. A safe and more comfortable rate of deposition allows for the delivery of 1 milliliter of solution per minute, which means it requires about 2 minutes to deposit a 1.8 milliliter cartridge of anesthetic drug. Malamed states that "a more realistic time span in a clinical situation however is 60 seconds for a full 1.8 ml cartridge" (Malamed, 2004). Specific exceptions to this guideline are discussed in Chapter 13, "Injections for Palatal Pain Control."

Time-consuming injections are more likely to stimulate anxiety in patients. A useful strategy to relieve this anxiety is to report the progress of the injection such as "¼ done, ½ done, ¾ done, complete." For others, distractions may be more useful.

Step 9: Completion of Injection

Upon completion of the injection, withdraw the syringe slowly. The final safety step is to properly manage and recap the needle. It is safest if the person performing the injection completes the recapping. This reduces the number of individuals who come into contact with the syringe and needle and reduces the potential for accidental injury. After the needle has been protected, communicate with the patient to observe and monitor for any adverse effects. Once it is confirmed that the patient tolerated the procedure well, begin to evaluate for onset and effectiveness of anesthesia prior to beginning treatment. Onset of anesthesia will usually occur within 3 to 10 minutes depending on the type of drug, the injection technique, and the accuracy of the location of the deposition site.

Step 10: Documentation of Local Anesthetics

As part of a patient's medico-legal record, key elements of an injection procedure should be properly documented.

The patient's record must include:

1. date of administration
2. type of drug(s) administered (both topical and injectable)
3. injection(s) administered (or area of delivery when topical alone is used)

4. total volume of drug(s) administered
5. results of aspiration, recorded as "positive" (+) or negative (−)

The volume of drug administered can be noted in terms of the total number of cartridges, the total milliliters of solution, or the total milligrams of a specified drug and concentration. If a vasoconstrictor was delivered, the type and dilution should also be recorded. The specific format of the record is based on professional judgment and workplace policy. If it is the policy of the workplace, include the gauge of any needles used. In addition to recording positive aspirations, if they occur, adverse reactions must be recorded along with the details of the responses to them (their management) (see Box 11–6).

ERGONOMICS FOR INJECTION ADMINISTRATION

Safe practice for the administration of local anesthetics involves ergonomics in addition to drug factors and patient issues. A discussion of the basic steps for administration of injectable local anesthetics is not complete without commenting on *ergonomics*. Previously, very little attention was placed on ergonomics during local anesthetic delivery. Attention was focused on hand and body positions for syringe stability and visibility as well as access to the site of injection. The effects of nonergonomic positions on the development of **cumulative trauma disorders**

(CTDs) during procedures, including anesthetic procedures, can be significant over a period of years and are all too common among dental healthcare personnel (Andrews & Vigoren, 2002; Stabbe, 2006; U.S. Department of Labor, 2005; Wann & Canull, 2003) (see Box 11–7).

Basic principles of ergonomics (see Box 11–8) suggest that clinicians at least consider nontraditional approaches to the delivery of injections that otherwise require reaching over the patient, twisting the trunk, hyperextending the neck, and angling the wrist in an awkward manner. Nontraditional approaches include repositioning the clinician and/or the patient, as well as nondominant hand syringe grasps to facilitate proper ergonomic positions of the back, neck, shoulders, arms, wrists, and hands. These approaches can provide ergonomically correct positions for local anesthetic administration. They can also be challenging, especially for novices who may wish to wait until they are more adept at the local anesthesia process before attempting nondominant hand techniques. Others may find them easy to accomplish from the outset. Applying updated ergonomic approaches to the administration of local anesthetics can reduce musculoskeletal trauma linked to the development of MSDs and CTDs, and possibly reduce the impact of this trauma on existing disorders.

Operatory design can significantly impact the ability to apply alternative ergonomic positions to the administration of local anesthetics. Having the ability to

---

Box 11–6   Sample Chart Documentation for Local Anesthetics

Date	Procedures
02/14/07	20% benzocaine topical, R-PSA, MSA, ASA, 2 cart (3.6 ml) lidocaine 2% (72 mg)* w/ epi 1:100 (0.036 mg), (−) aspirs., no complications. Signature = Identifiable Name
03/17/07	5% lidocaine topical, R-IA, LB, 1 cart (1.8 ml) mepivacaine 2% (36 mg) w/ levo 1:20 (0.09 mg), (+) aspir., visible hematoma, pressure/ice 15 minutes, monitor 30 min, no further swelling. Treatment complete w/o complication. Patient to call if any further problem. Signature = Identifiable Name
03/18/07	T/W Patient no further complications from hematoma, will call if changes. Signature = Identifiable Name
09/06/07	Vibraject, R-PSA, AMSA, 2 cart (3.6 ml) Articaine 4% (144 mg) w/ epi 1:200 (0.018 mg), (−) aspirs., no complications. Signature = Identifiable Name

*Total drug volumes are noted in ( ); this format may be preferred by some clinicians.

approach patients from either side of a chair greatly improves ergonomic positioning; however, the close physical design of some operatories can make this difficult. Taking time to determine if it is possible to swivel the chair on the base can improve nondominant side access.

A New Look at Ergonomics for Local Anesthetic Administration

The posterior superior alveolar, middle superior alveolar, anterior superior alveolar, inferior alveolar, Gow-Gates, buccal, and mental/incisive injections when delivered with the clinician's arm extending across the patient's body, forces the clinician into awkward arm, neck, and wrist positions to access the injection site (see Figure 11–15 ■ and Figure 11–16 ■), while maintaining

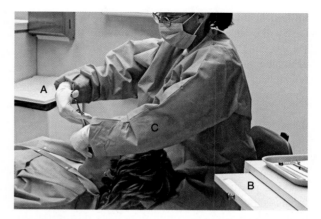

■ **FIGURE 11–15**   Ergonomics: Poor Practices 1. Example of poor ergonomics: A—Wrist is not in neutral position. B—Location of armamentarium requires clinician to twist and reach across the patient's trunk. C—Arms and elbows are above 30 degree angle.
Source: Courtesy of Kimberly A. Stabbe, R.D.H., M.S.

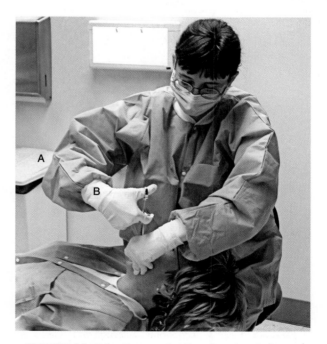

■ **FIGURE 11–16**   Ergonomics: Poor Practices 2. Example of poor ergonomics: A—Elbow is above 30 degree angle. B—Wrist is significantly bent, not in a neutral position.
Source: Courtesy of Kimberly A. Stabbe, R.D.H., M.S.

limited vision. It is easy for clinicians to assume that they will be in awkward positions for only brief periods, yet over the course of careers these brief periods can produce significant "trauma." This long-term trauma is referred to as a *cumulative effect* (Stabbe, 2006; U.S. Department of Labor, 2005; Wann & Canull, 2003).

The following are examples of corrective actions that will improve clinician ergonomics and reduce traumas that can lead to MSDs and CTDs for the inferior alveolar and posterior superior alveolar injections. Note that each suggestion places the clinician in a "neutral" working position, minimizing stress and trauma to the wrists, shoulders, and neck. Clinicians are encouraged to consider basic ergonomic principles during the administration of injections (see Box 11–8) that include alternative body positions (see Figure 11–17 ■) and nondominant hand techniques (see Figure 11–18 ■).

The posterior superior alveolar injection may be administered with either the dominant or nondominant hand, from the side of the injection (see Figure 11–18 and

Figure 11–19 ■). For example, a right-handed clinician can give this injection with his or her dominant hand while seated at the patient's right side for a right PSA. For the left PSA, the injection could also be given with the left hand while seated on the patient's left side. Many clinicians find it *surprisingly* easy to use their nondominant hand, appreciate the improved view and angle, and feel more stable and comfortable throughout the injection.

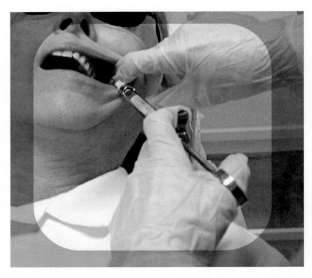

■ **FIGURE 11–18** Ergonomic Alternative 2. Ergonomic position for left nondominant hand delivery of a left PSA, from the left side.
Source: Courtesy of Kimberly A. Stabbe, R.D.H, M.S.

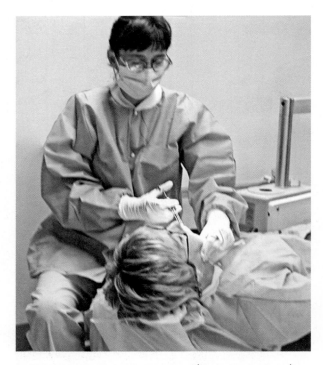

■ **FIGURE 11–17** Ergonomic Alternative 1. Good ergonomic position for right-dominant hand delivery of a right IA nerve block, from the patient's left side. Wrist neutral, elbows below 30 degrees, "arm-to-body" fulcrum.
Source: Courtesy of Kimberly A. Stabbe, R.D.H., M.S.

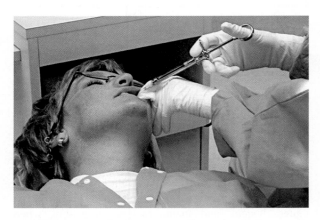

■ **FIGURE 11–19** Ergonomic Alternative 3. Ergonomic position for right-dominant hand delivery of a left PSA injection, from the left side.
Source: Courtesy of Kimberly A. Stabbe, R.D.H., M.S.

The inferior alveolar and Gow-Gates blocks can be administered with the clinician seated opposite the side where the injection is being given. Either the dominant or nondominant hand may be used (see Figure 11–19). This modified clinical position offers ergonomic positioning that reduces twisting of the trunk, lowers the arm, enables the elbows to stay within 30 degrees from the clinician's body, and keeps the wrist in a neutral position. Standing during administration of these blocks can also facilitate good ergonomic balance when the patient cannot be positioned easily (see Figure 11–20 ■).

A View from "Outside the Box"

The dental operatory provides a classic "box" for practice. It is easy for dental professionals to become *comfortable* with the *uncomfortable* and to believe and even accept that work practices will fit only one approach in the workspace, becoming complacent with sometimes physically harmful work practices. Clinicians are encouraged to "think outside the box" and develop ways to improve the ergonomics of work spaces and work practices for all chairside procedures.

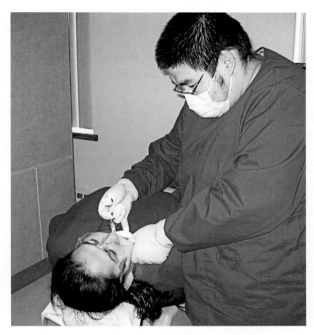

■ **FIGURE 11–20** Ergonomic Alternative 4. Ergonomic position for right-dominant hand, standing delivery, of a right IA from the right side.

CASE MANAGEMENT: Hector Melendez

It was explained to Mr. Melendez that the treatment he needed could not be accomplished comfortably without local anesthesia. While waiting for the topical anesthetic to take effect, the anesthetic procedure was explained as well as the reason it would be a slower experience compared with his previous one. After about 2 minutes, an infiltration over #5 was administered slowly with a couple of drops of solution administered ahead of the very slow advance of the needle. Once the target site was reached and negative aspiration confirmed, solution was deposited at a rate of 6 to 7 seconds per stopper (0.2 ml), which is equal to 1 minute when an entire cartridge is administered.

Case Discussion: Following basic steps promotes safety and comfort. Reassurance during preliminary steps prior to administering local anesthesia is useful. Rationale for taking those steps can help ease patient fears and provide some sense that the current experience will not be a repeat of previous experiences.

Mr. Melendez was apprehensive because his expectations for a satisfactory experience, one in which there was minimal to no pain, had not been met on a previous occasion. Importantly, he had no reason for altering his expectations in the current situation until it was provided to him. Local anesthesia procedures do not have to begin with "raise your hand" statements that are meaningless when they are subsequently ignored but can begin instead with soothing words, followed by brief explanations and assurances that contracts (to respond to hand signals, for example) will not be broken.

CHAPTER QUESTIONS

1. A technique that deposits anesthetic solution near larger terminal nerve branches for treatment near the site of an injection is called:
   a. an infiltration injection.
   b. a ligamental injection.
   c. a field block injection.
   d. a nerve block injection.

2. Which *one* of the following describes the target site for local anesthetic solutions?
   a. Needle pathway
   b. Deposition site
   c. Penetration site
   d. Aspiration site

3. The first step in the administration of local anesthetic solutions is to:
   a. assemble the armamentarium.
   b. obtain informed consent.
   c. assess the patient before proceeding.
   d. make sure that solution is able to exit the needle.

4. A primary benefit of orienting needle bevels toward bone during injections is that it:
   a. reduces trauma to the periosteum when bone is contacted.
   b. deflects the needle away from the bone during penetration.
   c. prevents false negative aspirations within a vessel.
   d. reduces discomfort from the advancing needle.

5. Which *one* of the following is the most appropriate local anesthesia chart entry?
   a. 10/21/2002: Review Health History. BP 120/80. 2 cartridges 2% lidocaine, 1:100,000 epi, no complications
   b. Review Health History. BP 120/80. 2 cartridges 2% lidocaine, w/1:100,000 epi, Rt IA, LB
   c. Review Health History. BP 120/80. 72 mg of 2% lidocaine w/ 0.036 mg 1:100,000 epi, IA, LB
   d. 10/21/2002: Review Health History. BP 120/80. 2 cartridges 2% lidocaine (72 mg) w/1:100,000 epi (0.036 mg), Rt IA, LB, (–) aspiration. No adverse reactions.

6. When is it safe to deposit local anesthetic solution?
   a. After a negative aspiration, where no blood is drawn into the cartridge.
   b. After a negative aspiration, following a positive aspiration where blood was visible in the cartridge only as a small trickle of blood or "worm-like" thread.
   c. Following a positive aspiration that obscures the results of subsequent aspirations.
   d. A & B

7. The *most* important safety step(s) during a local anesthetic injection is (are):
   a. to aspirate before depositing.
   b. to administer local anesthetics slowly.
   c. to direct the bevel away from bone.
   d. to aspirate before depositing and to administer drugs slowly.

8. Upon completion of an injection, the most important *subsequent* step is to:
   a. rinse the patient's mouth.
   b. calculate the volume of drug delivered.
   c. make the needle safe with a one-handed technique.
   d. determine if the patient experienced discomfort.

REFERENCES

American Medical Association, Office of the General Counsel, Informed Consent, Last updated: May 07, 2007. Available at: http://www.ama-assn.org. Accessed June 14, 2007.

Andrews, N., & Vigoren, G., (2002, March). Ergonomics: Muscle fatigue, posture, magnification, and illumination. *Compendium, 23*(3), 261–264, 266, 268, 270, 272, 274.

Branson, B. G., Williams, K. B., Bray, K. K., McIlnay, S. L., & Dickey, D. (2002, Fall). Validity and reliability of a dental operator posture assessment instrument (PAI). *Journal of Dental Hygiene, 76*(4), 255–261.

Dionne, R. A., Gordon, S. M., McCullagh, L. M., & Phero, J. C. (1998, February). Assessing the need for anesthesia and sedation in the general population. *Journal of the American Dental Association, 167–173.*

Evers, H., & Haegerstam, G. (1981). *Handbook of dental local anaesthesia.* Copenhagen: Schultz.

Haas, D. A. (2002). An update of local anesthetics in dentistry. *Journal of the Canadian Dental Association, 68,* 546–551.

Lipp, M. D. W. (1993). *Local anesthesia in dentistry.* Carol Stream, IL: Quintessence.

Little, J. W., & Falace, D. A. (1997). *Dental management of the medically compromised patient* (5th ed.). St. Louis: Mosby.

Malamed, S. F. (2004). *Handbook of local anesthesia* (5th ed.). St. Louis: Mosby.

Milgrom, P., Weinstein, P., & Getz, T. (1995). Treating fearful dental patients: A patient management handbook (2nd ed.). Seattle, WA: University of Washington Continuing Dental Education.

Rizzolati, G., Fadiga, L., Gallese, V., & Fagassi, L. (1996). Premotor cortex and the recognition of motor actions. *Cognitive Brain Research, 3,* 131–141.

Robinson, P. D., Ford, T. R. P., & McDonald, F. (2000). Local anesthesia in dentistry. London: Wright.

Stabbe, K. A. (2006, March). Maintaining ergonomic positioning during local anesthetic administration. *Journal of Practical Hygiene, 15*(2), 8.

University of Washington School of Medicine, Ethics in Medicine, Informed Consent. Last modified: February 22, 1999. Available at http://depts.washington.edu/bioethx/topics/consent.html. Accessed June 14, 2007.

U.S. Department of Labor—Bureau of Labor Statistics (2002). Lost-working injuries and illnesses: Characteristics and resulting days away from work. Available at: http://www.bls.gov/news.release/osh2.nr0.htm. Last modified: March 30, 2005. Accessed November 14, 2005.

Wann, O., & Canull, B. (2003, May). Ergonomics and dental hygienists. *Contemporary Oral Hygiene,* 16–22.

10 Basic Steps in the Administration of Local Anesthesia

Step 1: **Patient Assessment**
- Assess the patient's medical history, treatment plan, and individual pain control needs
- Identify alterations, precautions, or contraindications to care
- Implement appropriate injection(s) and anesthetic drug(s) to be delivered

Step 2: **Obtain Informed Consent**
- Review the intended treatment plan, including the delivery of any anesthetic agents, with the patient and obtain proper Informed Consent as indicated for care

Step 3: **Assemble Armamentarium**
- Assemble appropriate armamentarium and confirm proper function of delivery devices
  - Harpoon engaged and device able to aspirate
  - Cartridge is fully visible and the correct drug is loaded
  - The needle bevel is oriented toward the bone during injection
  - Safe needle recapping controls are in place and functioning properly

Step 4: **Pre-Injection Preparation**
- Position patient supine for visibility and support during stress
- Position patient's head for good visibility
- Assume an ergonomic position to support musculoskeletal health
- Employ positive, supportive communication
- Establish effective retraction for visibility and needle penetration
- Palpate site for anatomical anomalies

Step 5: **Prepare Injection Site**
- Gently dry mucosa with gauze
- Apply controlled amount of topical agent to dry tissue at injection site
  - Ideally no less than 1 minute to assure effectiveness
- Visualize best injection angle
- Evaluate for effective onset of topical agent at penetration site

Step 6:   **Initiate Injection**
- Keep the syringe out of the patient's sight as much as possible throughout
- Maintain positive, supportive communication with the patient
- Retract the soft tissues for good visibility of penetration site
  - Gently make mucosa "taut" to ease needle penetration
- Establish a fulcrum or point of stability for the syringe during the injection
- Penetrate the mucosa 1–2 millimeters, deposit a few drops of anesthetic
- Gently advance the needle to the desired depth and angle for deposition

Step 7:   **Aspiration**
Aspirate at deposition site BEFORE depositing solution
- Aspirate in two planes for highly vascular areas
- Re-aspirate if depth changes during injection
- Re-aspirating can help pace injection if needed
- NEGATIVE aspiration: continue with injection
- POSITIVE aspiration:
  - Employ positive, supportive communication to explain situation to patient
  - Assess signs of positive aspiration
    - Small trickle of blood in cartridge—re-aspirate, if negative continue with deposition
    - Cartridge clouded with blood—replace cartridge, replace or flush needle and reinitiate injection
  - Evaluate post-injection for complications and advise patient as indicated

Step 8:   **Deposition and Rate**
SLOWLY deposit the specified anesthetic dose (1.8 ml over 1 to 2 min.)

Step 9:   **Completion**
Completion: CAREFULLY withdraw the needle
- Make the needle safe with an accepted recapping technique
- Observe and evaluate patient for adverse reactions

Step 10:   **Documentation**
Document injection specifics and complications in patient chart

Suggested Fulcrum Positions

Each clinician should determine the ergonomic position that best establishes stability during injection procedures. The following figures suggest a variety of fulcrums and supplemental supports for balance.

A. Rest the back of the dominant hand (with syringe) gently against the patient's shoulder. To use this rest safely, the clinician must be alert to the possibility of sudden patient movements and must be able to respond to them quickly.
B. A "palm-up" grasp provides stability.
C. The thumb of the nondominant (retraction) hand is placed on the barrel of the syringe.

A. Keep the arm low and close to the body.
B. A "palm-up" grasp provides stability.
C. The third finger of the dominant hand is placed against the barrel of the syringe to enhance stability. Along with a "palm-up" grasp, this increases stability.

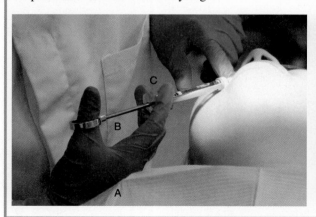

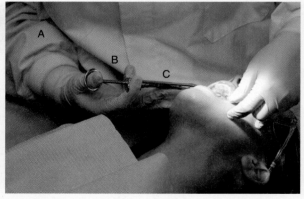

A. Place a finger of the dominant hand on the patient's chin, along with a "palm-up" grasp position to provide stability.

A. Keep the arm low and close to the body and rest the back of the dominant hand gently against the patient's shoulder.

B. Place a finger of the dominant hand on the patient's chin when able, along with a "palm-up" grasp position to provide stability.

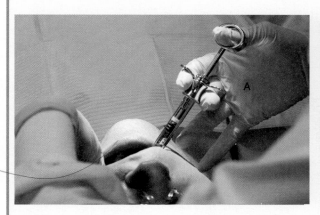

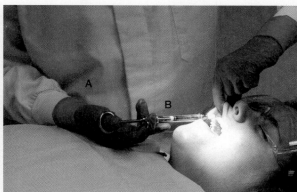

A. Keep the arm close to the body, along with a "palm-up" grasp position to provide stability.

B. The thumb of the nondominant (retraction) hand is placed against a finger of the dominant hand to create a "bridge" of stability.

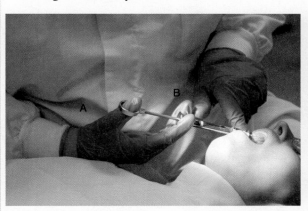

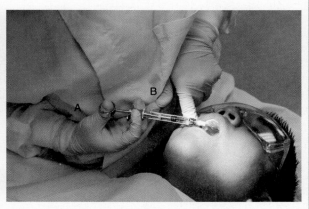

Section IV

Clinical Administration of Local Anesthesia

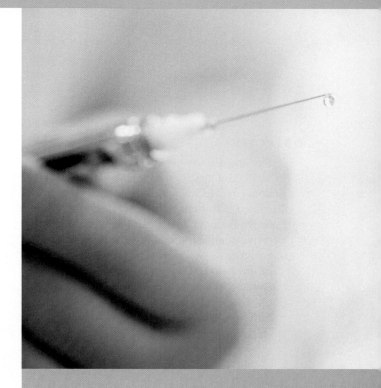

Chapters 11,12,13, and 14 include discussions of anatomical factors relevant to each injection technique and assume clinicians have a basic knowledge of head and neck anatomy.

Appendix I: Anatomical review provides a general discussion of head and neck anatomy, with on anatomical structures and landmark anesthesia.

Chapter 12

Injections for Maxillary Pain Control

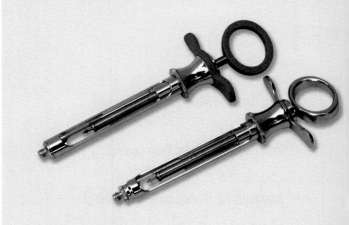

OBJECTIVES

- Define and discuss the key terms in this chapter.
- Describe and discuss the indications, relevant anatomy, and technique features of the injections discussed in this chapter.
- Describe the basic technique steps for safe and effective administration for the following injections:
  - Infiltrations
  - Anterior superior alveolar nerve block (ASA or ASANB)
  - Middle superior alveolar nerve block (MSA or MSANB)
  - Infraorbital nerve block (IO or IONB)
  - Posterior superior alveolar nerve block (PSA or PSANB)

KEY TERMS

anterior superior alveolar (ASA) nerve block **221**

cross-innervation **223**

dental plexus **217**

deposition site **217**

hematoma **221**

infiltration injection **217**

infraorbital (IO) nerve block **227**

middle superior alveolar (MSA) nerve block **224**

needle pathway **217**

penetration site **217**

posterior superior alveolar (PSA) nerve block **232**

CASE STUDY: Elena Gagarin

Elena Gagarin needed restorative treatment on her right maxillary anterior teeth. Despite an ASA nerve block, she was uncomfortable when cavity preparation was commenced with a high-speed handpiece on #8. Despite a repeat ASA injection, #8 remained uncomfortable.

INTRODUCTION

Anatomic landmarks and considerations for each maxillary injection technique discussed in this chapter will be presented in reference to a **penetration site, needle pathway,** and **deposition site** as described in Chapter 11, "Fundamentals for Administration of Local Anesthetic Agents." The penetration site will be related to hard and soft tissue landmarks. The needle pathway will be described in terms of the types of tissue that will be penetrated by or located in the vicinity of the needle, including mucosa, superficial fascia, muscle, vessels, nerves, and bone. The deposition site will be described in terms of the tissues at or near the target and in relation to specific landmarks.

Note that injection techniques in this and the following chapters may describe nerve blocks in several ways. Full descriptive phrases may be used, such as superior alveolar nerve blocks. Acronyms followed by descriptive phrases may be used, such as the PSA nerve block. Full acronyms may be used, such as an PSANB. Regardless of the description, all are equivalent in meaning.

MAXILLARY INJECTION TECHNIQUES

This chapter will discuss nonpalatal maxillary injection techniques commonly used in dentistry. Even though they are also maxillary techniques, palatal injections will be discussed separately due to common modifications specific to the sensitive and less flexible tissues in the palate (Chapter 13, "Injections for Palatal Pain Control"). Key factors for each maxillary injection discussed in this chapter are summarized in Appendix 12–1. Common variations and precautions will be discussed where applicable (Blanton & Jeske, 2003; Fehrenbach & Herring, 2007; Jastak, Yagiela, & Donaldson, 1995; Malamed, 2004; Wong, 2001).

INFILTRATION INJECTION

Infiltration injections are indicated when procedures are confined to one or two teeth or to tissue in a limited area. Infiltration injections are among the simplest and safest local anesthesia techniques to learn. They are relatively easy to execute, have a high rate of success, and have wide margins of safety.

Field of Anesthesia

Structures affected by infiltrations include the **dental plexus** of the injected site (the pulp of the tooth and facial areas of the gingiva, periodontal ligament, and alveolus). Additionally, due to the diffusion of anesthetic solution, some terminal branches of the facial nerve (VII) are affected. All or a portion of the upper lip, cheek, and lower nose are anesthetized with anterior infiltration injections (see Figure 12–1 ■ and Appendix 12–2).

Anatomical Factors

Small terminal nerve endings of the posterior superior, middle superior, and anterior superior alveolar nerve branches form the maxillary dental neural plexus. This plexus innervates the pulps of the teeth and facial periodontium as previously described. The facial bone of the maxilla is relatively thin and permeable. Local anesthetic solutions diffuse easily through this bone anesthetizing the nerves of the dental plexus. This allows for high success rates when administering infiltrations on the maxillary arch.

Technique Factors

The following information describes key factors for successful infiltration injections.

Penetration Site

The optimum site of penetration for infiltration injections is at the height of the mucobuccal fold closest to the apex of the tooth to be anesthetized. A bony ridge, or eminence, can usually be palpated in the mucosa overlying the facial root of most maxillary teeth. This eminence serves as a landmark for visualizing the long axis of the tooth and locating the apex of the tooth for the penetration site (see Figure 12–2 ■).

Examining radiographs for root lengths and inclinations, as well as assessing crown–root ratios can be helpful when determining optimum penetration and deposition sites for infiltration injections (see Figure 12–3 ■).

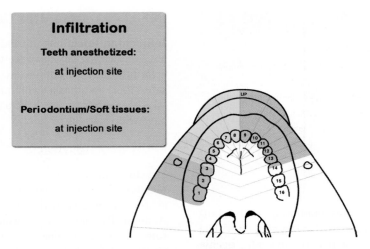

■ **FIGURE 12–1** Field of Anesthesia for Infiltration Injections. Anesthesia will occur in a small, confined area close to the site of deposition.

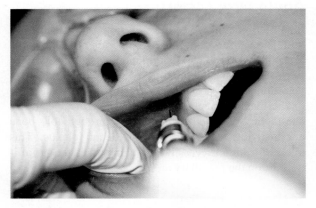

■ **FIGURE 12–2** Penetration Site for Infiltration Injections. The penetration site for infiltration injections will be near the apex of a single tooth or in a small, confined area of tissue.

Needle Pathway

The needle generally parallels the long axis of the tooth and the slope of the alveolus in maxillary infiltrations. The needle passes through thin mucosal tissues to superficial fascia containing loose connective tissue, small vessels and microvasculature, and nerve endings.

Deposition Site

The deposition site is slightly above the apex of the root of the tooth being anesthetized. Contact with bone is unnecessary and should be avoided for comfort (see Figure 12–4 ■).

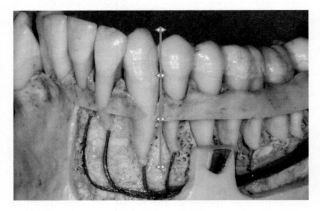

■ **FIGURE 12–3** Height of Penetration for Infiltration Injections. Average *crown-to-root ratios* can be used to select the height of penetration near the apex of a tooth for infiltration injections.

Technique Steps

Apply the basic injection steps outlined in Chapter 11 and summarized in Appendix 11–1.

Needle Selection

The selection of needle gauge for infiltrations is made based upon clinical judgment. Either a 27 or 25 gauge short needle is appropriate for infiltrations. Based on the low risk of positive aspiration (1 percent or less), and the shallow depths of penetration, many clinicians choose to

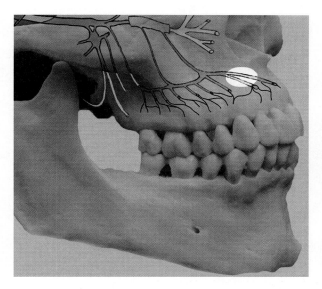

■ **FIGURE 12–4** Deposition Site for Infiltration of a Single Tooth. Deposition for an infiltration will be near the apex of a single tooth or in a small, confined area of tissue.

use a 27 gauge short needle. Some prefer to use 30 gauge needles out of concern for comfort, although increased discomfort with larger diameter needles has not been demonstrated (Hamburg, 1972; Malamed, 2004).

Injection Procedure

Gain access to the penetration site by retracting the lip, pulling the tissue taut with the thumb and index finger (see Figure 12–5 ■). Locate the appropriate penetration site. In order to achieve proper angulations, align the barrel of the syringe parallel to the long axis of the tooth, following the contour of the maxilla (see Figure 12–6 ■). The depth of penetration (to the site of deposition) is based on the location of the apex of the tooth and is usually achieved within 3 to 6 mm.

Following negative aspiration, deposit an adequate volume of an appropriately selected local anesthetic drug to achieve anesthesia. When performing maxillary infiltrations, a generally accepted minimum volume of anesthetic is 0.6 ml (1/3 of a cartridge). Adequate volumes will vary regardless of the technique, depending on a variety of patient and pharmacological factors as well as the length of planned procedures. For example, procedures with longer durations will require a greater pool of anesthetic in the deposition area to provide a longer-term supply of base molecules. Some

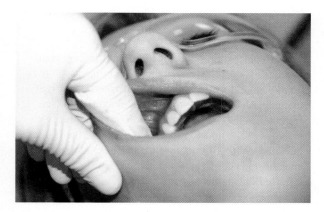

■ **FIGURE 12–5** Tissue Retraction. Retract the tissue tautly to improve ease of insertion and increase the visibility of the penetration site.

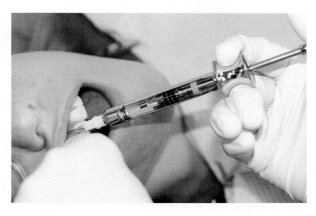

■ **FIGURE 12–6** Syringe Angulations for Infiltration of a Single Tooth. Align the syringe barrel parallel to the long axis of the tooth, along a plane parallel to the slope of the maxilla.

patients will require greater volumes even for relatively short procedures.

Confirming Anesthesia

Subjective signs of anesthesia for infiltration injections include a sense of numbness of the gingival and labial tissues at the site of injection. Objective signs include a lack of response to gentle stimulation with an instrument and no pain during the procedure at the site of injection. For a general discussion on confirming anesthesia, see Box 12–1.

Box 12–1 Confirming Anesthesia

Prior to performing any procedures, it is important to assess for effective anesthesia (numbness) in the area of injection. This can be confirmed objectively using an electronic pulp testing device (EPT) (see Figure 12–7 ■) or the application of cold (see Figure 12–8 ■ and Figure 12–9 ■) on the teeth in question. With all injection techniques, adequate anesthesia is confirmed when there is no pain reported during procedures.

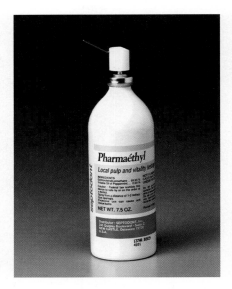

■ **FIGURE 12–8** Cold Stimulation to Confirm Anesthesia— "Freeze" Method. Pain stimuli can be initiated with the use of a cryo-anesthetic ("cold spray") to test for anesthesia similar to the use of an EPT.
Source: Courtesy of Septodont USA.

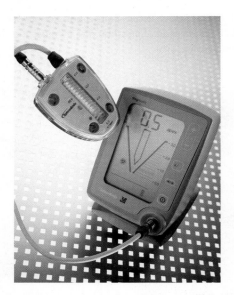

■ **FIGURE 12–7** Electric Pulp Tester (EPT) to Confirm Anesthesia. An EPT can provide objective feedback to determine whether or not patients are profoundly anesthetized.
Source: Courtesy of Sybron Dental—Analytic-Endodontics.

Common Causes of Injection Failure

The most common causes of failure after infiltrations include deposition of solution too far from the apex of a tooth and inadequate volumes of solution. Other causes of failure include inflammation or infection in the area of deposition, inadequate diffusion of solution to the palatal roots of molars due to dense bone, and accessory innervations.

Troubleshooting

When infiltrations are unsuccessful, it is helpful to reevaluate by visualizing, palpating, checking radiographs,

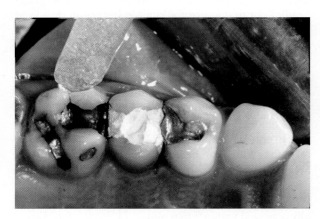

■ **FIGURE 12–9** Cold Stimulation to Confirm Anesthesia— "Icicles" Method. In addition to EPT devices and cryo-anesthetics, pain stimuli can be initiated with the use of small "icicles" to test for anesthesia.
Source: Courtesy of Albert "Ace" Goerig DDS, MS.

reassessing syringe angulations and depths of penetration, and reconsidering volumes of solution deposited. Failure of infiltration anesthesia occurs most commonly when solution is deposited too far from the apex of a tooth (see Box 12–2). In some instances, adequate diffusion of solution is impossible due to anatomic obstructions. In these

> ### Box 12–2   Deposition Site Errors
>
> Failure to consider needle angulations and penetration depths can result in deposition of solution that is too far away from the apex of a tooth or target site. This can occur when deposition is too far from targets in one or more than one of the following orientations:
>
> - superior   - anterior   - lateral
> - inferior   - posterior   - medial

instances, nerve blocks (discussed later in this chapter) or supplemental techniques, such as periodontal ligament injections, may be indicated (discussed in Chapter 15, "Injections for Supplemental Pain Control").

Occasionally, medially-displaced branches of the PSA nerve and/or branches of the greater palatine nerve provide sensory innervation to the palatal roots of maxillary molars and premolars. In these instances, solution may not diffuse far enough palatally through the bone to reach these branches. To anesthetize these branches, a supplemental greater palatine nerve block can be administered (Blanton & Jeske, 2003).

Technique Modifications and Alternatives

In some situations, it is apparent during initial patient evaluation that standard injection techniques will not be successful. In these instances, technique modifications or alternate approaches will be necessary. This is often related to anatomical variances, which may include hard and soft tissue obstructions, and accessory or aberrant innervations.

Large facial bony eminences, exostoses, and skeletal variations can interfere with syringe angulations requiring modifications or alternate techniques to infiltration injections. A modification appropriate for these situations is to position the syringe at an angle that will bypass the bony obstruction and still allow access to the deposition site. When adaptive angulations are not possible or are ineffective, an alternative injection technique(s) may be indicated.

When infiltrations are unsuccessful, alternative injections may be considered. To anesthetize incisors, canines, and premolars, alternatives include:

1. anterior superior alveolar (ASA) nerve blocks
2. infraorbital (IO) nerve blocks

3. anterior middle superior alveolar (AMSA) nerve blocks
4. palatal anterior superior alveolar (P-ASA) nerve blocks

For molars, alternatives include:

1. posterior superior alveolar (PSA) nerve blocks

Supplemental greater palatine (GP) nerve blocks may be indicated if anesthesia is not profound. Periodontal ligament (PDL) injections are also appropriate alternatives to all of the infiltration injections described previously. Each of these injections will be discussed in this text.

Complications

The risk of complications following infiltration injection techniques is minimal. These may include postoperative pain at the site of injection, postoperative edema, and rarely, **hematoma** (bleeding in tissue spaces surrounding injured vessels). For further discussion see Chapter 17, "Local Anesthesia Complications and Management."

ANTERIOR SUPERIOR ALVEOLAR NERVE BLOCKS

The **anterior superior alveolar (ASA) nerve block** is a common technique, similar to the basic anterior infiltration technique. Unlike infiltrations, the ASA avoids multiple needle penetrations when anesthesia is needed for more than one maxillary anterior tooth in the same quadrant.

Field of Anesthesia

The ASA nerve block will anesthetize structures innervated by the ASA nerve. They include the pulps of the maxillary central incisor through the canine on the injected side and their facial periodontium. Additionally, due to diffusion of anesthetic solution, some terminal branches of the facial nerve are affected. All or a portion of the upper lip, cheek, and lower nose may be anesthetized (see Figure 12–10 ■ and Appendix 12–2).

Anatomical Factors

The ASA nerve is the internal terminal branch of the maxillary division of the trigeminal nerve. It branches from the infraorbital nerve within the infraorbital canal 6 to 10 mm prior to the infraorbital foramen (Malamed, 2004).

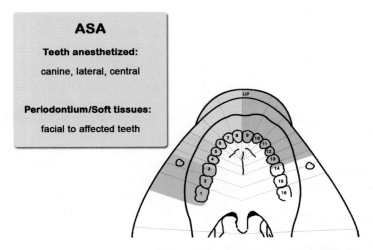

■ **FIGURE 12–10** Field of Anesthesia for ASA Nerve Blocks. The field of anesthesia for ASA nerve blocks is indicated by the shaded area.

The ASA nerve descends through the anterior wall of the maxillary sinus to supply sensation to the dental plexus of the canine and lateral and central incisors. As previously discussed, the facial bone of the maxilla is relatively thin and permeable. Local anesthetic solution diffuses easily through the bone anesthetizing the ASA nerve.

Technique Factors

The following information describes key factors for successful ASA nerve block injections.

Penetration Site

The optimal site of penetration for an ASA injection is at the height of the mucobuccal fold anterior to the canine eminence. This area is called the canine fossa (see Figure 12–11 ■).

Needle Pathway

The needle pathway parallels the long axis of the canine, passing through thin mucosal tissues to superficial fascia containing loose connective tissue, small vessels and microvasculature, and nerve endings.

Deposition Site

The deposition site is above the apical area of the canine at the height of the canine fossa (see Figure 12–12 ■).

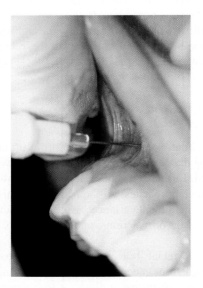

■ **FIGURE 12–11** Penetration Site for ASA Nerve Blocks. The penetration site for ASA Nerve Blocks is indicated by the needle.

Contact with bone is unnecessary and should be avoided for comfort.

Technique Steps

Apply the basic injection steps outlined in Chapter 11 and summarized in Appendix 11–1.

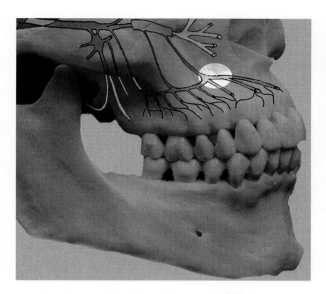

■ **FIGURE 12-12** Deposition Site for ASA Nerve Blocks. The deposition site for ASA nerve blocks is indicated in the spotlighted area.

Needle Selection

A 27 or 25 gauge needle is recommended for this technique. Similar to infiltrations, a 27 gauge short needle is most commonly used and is consistent with the shallow depth of penetration and the low rate of positive aspiration (1 percent) although some clinicians prefer a 25 or 30 gauge needle.

Injection Procedure

Gain access to the penetration site by retracting the lip, pulling the tissue taut with the thumb and index finger (see Figure 12–5). Locate the appropriate penetration site. In order to achieve proper angulations, align the barrel of the syringe parallel to the long axis of the canine, following the contour of the maxilla (see Figures 12–11 and 12–13 ■). The depth of penetration to the site of deposition is based on the location of the apex of the tooth and is usually achieved within 3 to 6 mm. Following negative aspiration, deposit an adequate volume of an appropriately selected local anesthetic drug to achieve anesthesia. A generally accepted minimum volume of anesthetic to accomplish this is 0.9 ml (1/2 of a cartridge). Adequate volumes will vary regardless of the technique depending on a variety of patient and pharmacological factors as well as planned procedures.

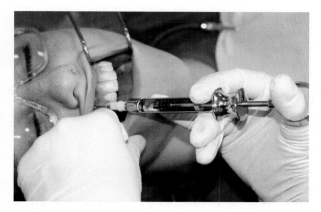

■ **FIGURE 12-13** Syringe Angulations for ASA Nerve Blocks. Correct syringe barrel angulations for ASA nerve blocks parallel the long axes of the canines, following the contour of the maxilla.

Confirming Anesthesia

Subjective signs of anesthesia for ASA injections include a sense of numbness of the gingival and labial tissues from the distal of the canine through the mesial of the central incisor. Objective signs include a lack of response to gentle stimulation with an instrument and no pain during procedures in the expected field of anesthesia (see Box 12–1).

Common Causes of Injection Failure

As with infiltration techniques, the most common causes of anesthetic failure in the ASA technique include deposition of solution too far from the target (see Box 12–2) and inadequate volumes of solution. Other causes include inflammation or infection in the area of deposition and inadequate diffusion of solution.

Troubleshooting

Similar to infiltrations, when ASA nerve blocks are unsuccessful, it is helpful to reevaluate by visualizing, palpating, checking radiographs, reassessing syringe angulations and the depth of penetration, and the volumes of solution deposited. In some instances, adequate diffusion of solution is impossible due to anatomic obstructions.

Incomplete anesthesia with ASA nerve blocks can also be attributed to what is known as **cross-innervation** or overlap of terminal fibers of the contralateral side

ASA nerve at the midline of the maxilla. When this is the case, teeth in one anterior segment of the maxilla will receive sensory innervation from the ASA nerve on the contralateral side. To achieve adequate anesthesia in these instances, an infiltration over the same side central incisor is necessary.

Technique Modifications and Alternatives

Large facial bony eminences, exostoses, and other skeletal variations can interfere with syringe angulations, requiring modifications or alternate techniques. Positioning the syringe at an angle that bypasses bony obstructions may allow access to the deposition site. When adaptive angulations are not possible, alternate injection techniques may be indicated.

Nerve blocks that may be effective when ASA nerve blocks are unsuccessful include the infraorbital (IO), anterior middle superior alveolar (AMSA), and palatal anterior superior alveolar (PASA). PDL injections may also be used (see Chapter 15).

Complications

The risk of complications following ASA nerve block injections is minimal. These may include postoperative pain at the site of injection and, rarely, hematoma and postoperative edema.

MIDDLE SUPERIOR ALVEOLAR NERVE BLOCKS

Middle superior alveolar (MSA) nerve blocks are often used in combination with other maxillary nerve blocks. The MSA injection is indicated for pain management of both premolars in one quadrant.

Field of Anesthesia

The MSA nerve block will anesthetize structures innervated by the MSA nerve, when present, and its terminal branches, to include the pulps of the maxillary first and second premolars and their facial gingiva, periodontal ligament, and alveolar bone. In some individuals, the MSA nerve also innervates the mesiobuccal root of the first molar. Due to diffusion of anesthetic solutions, some terminal branches of the maxillary and facial nerves that innervate the cheek and upper lip may be affected (see Figure 12–14 ■ and Appendix 12–2).

Anatomical Factors

The MSA nerve separates at varying points from the infraorbital branch of the maxillary nerve within the infraorbital canal. It supplies sensation to the dental plexus of the first and second premolars and, in some individuals, the mesiobuccal root of the maxillary first molar.

Studies have reported the *absence* of an MSA nerve branch in somewhere between 50 to 72 percent

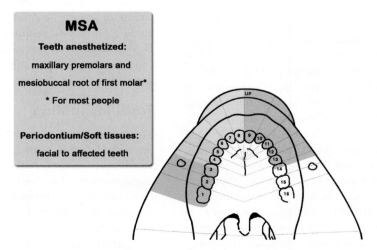

■ FIGURE 12–14   Field of Anesthesia for MSA Nerve Blocks. The field of anesthesia for MSA nerve blocks is indicated by the shaded area.

of individuals. In the absence of an MSA nerve, branches of the anterior superior alveolar and/or the posterior superior alveolar nerve innervate the first and second premolars and the mesiobuccal root of the first molar (Jastak et al., 1995; Loestscher & Walton, 1988).

An anatomical variation that can complicate MSA nerve blocks is the presence of a large zygomaticoalveolar crest. This excessive bony processes may obstruct access to the apices of the maxillary second premolars (Blanton & Jeske, 2003; Jastak et al., 1995).

In general, the presence or absence of MSA nerves in an individual is unknown. Despite uncertainties over innervation, profound anesthesia of the maxillary first molars can nevertheless be determined using electric pulp testers. When these devices are not readily available, it is common practice to administer local anesthetics with the presumption that MSA innervation exists in order to avoid unnecessary pain (see Box 12–3).

Technique Factors

The following information describes key factors for successful MSA nerve block injections.

Penetration Site

The optimum site of penetration is at the height of the mucobuccal fold over the maxillary second premolar (see Figure 12–15 ■).

Needle Pathway

The needle advances parallel to the long axis of the second premolar through thin mucosal tissue to superficial fascia consisting of loose connective tissue, microvasculature, and nerve endings.

Deposition Site

The deposition site is *well above* the apex of the second premolar. In order to be certain that both first and second premolars are anesthetized, solution must be deposited superior to the branching of the nerve to the first premolar. A deposition site inferior to the branching would anesthetize only the second premolar; therefore, solution must be deposited well above the apex of the second premolar. Contact with bone should be avoided for comfort (see Figure 12–16 ■).

Box 12–3   Anesthesia of the Mesiobuccal Roots of Maxillary First Molars

Anatomically, nerves tend to follow what have been termed *patterns of innervation*. The right posterior superior alveolar nerve, for example, can be expected to provide innervation to the maxillary right molars, and the right middle superior alveolar nerve can be expected to provide innervation to both right premolars. Because the middle superior alveolar nerve is absent more often than it is present, in anywhere from 50 to 72% of individuals, there is a known deviation in these patterns. Even when present, the MSA nerve may or may not provide innervation to the mesiobuccal root of the maxillary first molar. It is possible that fibers from one or any combination of the MSA, ASA, and PSA nerves may provide innervation to the mesiobuccal root of the maxillary first molar.

From a practical standpoint, the issue of which fibers innervate the mesiobuccal root of maxillary molars is irrelevant. To overcome uncertainty regarding the source of its innervation, clinicians routinely administer an infiltration over the mesiobuccal root of the maxillary first molar in addition to a PSA nerve block. If infiltration techniques alone are planned for the maxillary first molar, an infiltration over each facial root is recommended due to the distance between the roots, the uncertainties of diffusion, and the extent of MSA, ASA, and PSA innervation.

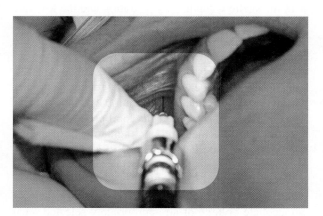

■ **FIGURE 12–15** Penetration Site for MSA Nerve Blocks. The penetration site for MSA nerve blocks is indicated by the needle.

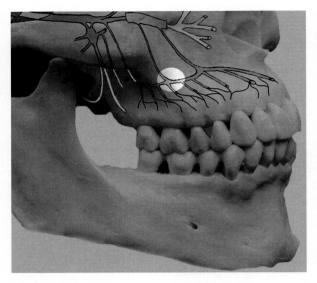

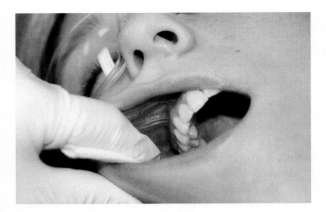

■ **FIGURE 12–17** Tissue Retraction for the MSA Nerve Block. Align the syringe barrel along the contour of the maxilla.

■ **FIGURE 12–16** Deposition Site for MSA Nerve Blocks. The deposition site for MSA nerve blocks is indicated in the spotlighted area.

Technique Steps

Apply the basic injection steps outlined in Chapter 11 and summarized in Appendix 11–1.

Needle Selection

A 27 or 25 gauge short needle is recommended for this technique. A 27 gauge short needle is used most commonly for the MSA nerve block, which is consistent with the shallow depths of penetration and the low rate of positive aspiration (1 percent). A 25 gauge needle is also frequently used for this injection.

Injection Procedure

Gain access to the penetration site by retracting the lip, pulling the tissue taut with the thumb and index finger (see Figure 12–17 ■). Locate the appropriate penetration site. In order to achieve proper angulations, follow the contour of the maxilla (see Figure 12–18 ■). The depth of penetration to the site of deposition is based on the location of the apex of the tooth and is usually achieved within 5 to 8 mm. Following negative aspiration, deposit an adequate volume of an appropriately selected local anesthetic drug to achieve anesthesia. A generally accepted minimum volume of anesthetic to accomplish this is 0.9 to 1.2 ml (1/2 to 2/3 of a cartridge). Adequate

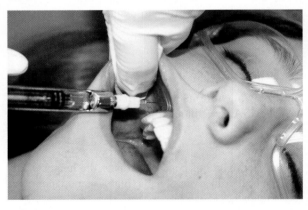

■ **FIGURE 12–18** Syringe Angulations for MSA Nerve Blocks. Align the syringe barrel along the contour of the maxilla.

volumes will vary regardless of the technique depending on a variety of patient and pharmacological factors, and procedures that are planned.

Confirming Anesthesia

Subjective signs of anesthesia for MSA injections include a sense of numbness of the gingival and labial tissues from the distal of the second premolar through the mesial of the first premolar. Objective signs include a lack of response to gentle stimulation with an instrument and no pain during the procedure in the expected field of anesthesia (see Box 12–1).

Common Causes of Injection Failure

Similar to both infiltration techniques and anterior superior alveolar nerve blocks, the most common causes of anesthesia failure for the MSA technique include deposition of solution too far from the target (see Box 12–2) and inadequate volumes. Other causes include inflammation or infection in the areas of deposition and inadequate diffusion of solutions, due to anatomic (fascial plane) deflection of solution away from target sites.

Troubleshooting

As is true for most other injections, when MSA nerve blocks are unsuccessful it is helpful to reevaluate by visualizing, palpating, checking radiographs, reassessing syringe angulations, and depths of penetration as well as to reconsider volumes of solution deposited. As previously noted, when adequate diffusion of solution is impossible due to anatomic obstructions, such as the presence of a large zygomaticoalveolar crest, alternate nerve blocks or supplemental techniques are indicated. These include PDL injections (see Chapter 15).

Occasionally, medially-displaced branches of the PSA nerve and sometimes branches of the greater palatine nerve provide pulpal innervation to the palatal roots of maxillary molars and accessory innervation to the premolars. Solution deposited for infiltrations and blocks of premolars and molars may not diffuse far enough lingually to reach these branches. In this situation, a supplemental greater palatine nerve block will anesthetize palatal branches (Blanton & Jeske, 2003).

Technique Modifications and Alternatives

As with infiltration injections and anterior superior alveolar nerve blocks, large facial bony eminences, exostoses, and skeletal variations can interfere with syringe angulations requiring modifications or alternate techniques to MSA injections. Positioning the syringe at an angle that will bypass the bony obstruction will allow access to the deposition site. When adaptive angulations are not possible, an alternative injection technique(s) may be indicated.

Alternate injection techniques for MSA injections include the anterior superior alveolar (ASA), the infraorbital (IO), the anterior middle superior alveolar (AMSA), and the palatal anterior superior alveolar

(P-ASA) nerve blocks. Periodontal ligament (PDL) injections are also appropriate alternatives.

Complications

The risk of complications following MSA nerve block injections is minimal. These may include postoperative pain at the site of injection and, rarely, hematoma and postoperative edema.

INFRAORBITAL NERVE BLOCKS

The infraorbital nerve is a continuation of the maxillary nerve within the infraorbital groove and canal located in the portion of the inferior orbit formed by the maxilla. It branches into the middle superior and anterior superior alveolar nerves within the maxilla (Fehrenbach & Herring, 2007). The terminal branches of the infraorbital nerve enter the maxilla at the infraorbital foramen and provide sensory innervation to the upper lip, lateral portion of the nose, and the lower eyelid on one side. The discussion of the infraorbital (IO) nerve block can be confusing because, like the ASA nerve block, it also anesthetizes the ASA nerve. The ability to discuss the ASA and IO nerve blocks as distinctly different techniques is explained in Box 12–4. A major distinction is that, in addition to the area of anesthesia provided by the ASA nerve block, the IO nerve block typically provides conduction blockage of a large portion of the face, the premolars on the same side as the injection, and some percentage of the time, the mesiobuccal root of the maxillary first molar on the same side.

The IO nerve block is indicated for pain management of anterior and premolar teeth in one quadrant. A benefit of the IO nerve block is that smaller volumes of local anesthetics are needed to accomplish the same field of anesthesia compared with administering both an anterior superior alveolar and a middle superior alveolar nerve block, or multiple infiltrations. This injection technique also avoids multiple needle penetrations required when separate anterior and middle superior alveolar nerve blocks or infiltrations are administered.

Field of Anesthesia

The IO nerve block will affect structures innervated by the anterior and middle superior alveolar and IO nerves. Areas anesthetized include the pulps of the maxillary central incisors through the canine, and premolars, and

---

Box 12–4   Injection Comparison:
IO vs. ASA Nerve Blocks

The infraorbital nerve block technique and the anterior superior alveolar nerve block technique are distinctly different in the following ways:

1. *Penetration site:* The penetration site for an IO nerve block is located over the first premolar, whereas the penetration site for the ASA nerve block is located over the canine.
2. *Deposition site:* The deposition site for an IO nerve block is located at the infraorbital foramen, whereas the deposition site for the ASA nerve block is located at the apex of the canine in the canine fossa.
3. *Nerves anesthetized:* The IO nerve block anesthetizes the ASA, MSA, and IO nerves, whereas the ASA nerve block typically anesthetizes only the ASA nerve.
4. *Effect by diffusion through bone:* Only the ASA nerve block requires diffusion through bone.
5. *Effect by direct contact with nerve:* The IO nerve block directly bathes the nerve with anesthetic solution at the IO foramen and in the IO canal. It does not require diffusion through bone.
6. *Success rates:* The ASA nerve block demonstrates a much higher rate of success, which may be due to clinician inexperience with IO nerve blocks.

---

their facial periodontium, the lower eyelid, lateral aspect of nose, and upper lip. In some individuals, the mesiobuccal root of the maxillary first molar is also anesthetized (see Figure 12–19 ■ and Appendix 12–2).

Anatomical Factors

As previously discussed, the maxillary nerve segment within the IO groove and canal is called the infraorbital nerve. The anterior and middle superior alveolar nerves branch from the IO nerve within the infraorbital canal. The IO nerve then exits the infraorbital foramen and further divides to provide innervation to areas of the upper lip, cheek, nose, and lower eyelid (Blanton & Jeske, 2003).

The height of the mucobuccal fold and the position of the IO foramen vary, based on facial size, vestibular depth, and age. In a typical adult, for example, the IO foramen is located approximately 8 to 10 mm below the IO ridge. This is a safe distance from the orbit. In children and adolescents, however, the vertical growth of the facial skeleton is incomplete. Incomplete growth results in a shorter distance between the IO foramen and the IO ridge compared with adults. These differences warrant caution in these individuals (see Figure 12–20 ■).

Technique Factors

The following information describes key factors for successful IO nerve block injections.

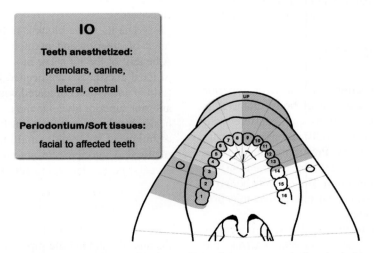

■ FIGURE 12–19 Field of Anesthesia for IO Nerve Blocks. The field of anesthesia for IO nerve blocks is indicated by the shaded area.

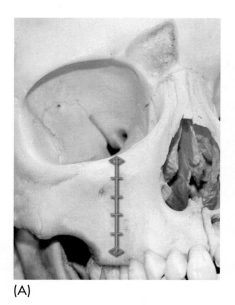 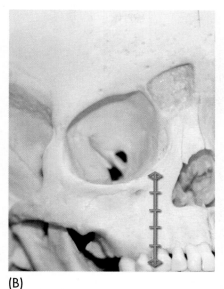

(A)   (B)

■ **FIGURE 12–20** Comparison of Adult and Child IO Foramen. A—In a typical adult, the IO foramen is located approximately 8 to 10 mm below the IO ridge. B—Due to incomplete vertical growth of the facial skeleton in children and adolescents, this distance is shorter.

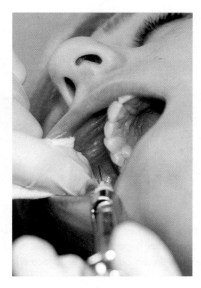

■ **FIGURE 12–21** Penetration Site for IO Nerve Blocks. The penetration site for IO nerve blocks is indicated by the needle.

Penetration Site

The typical penetration site is at the height of the mucobuccal fold directly over the first premolar (see Figure 12–21 ■).

Needle Pathway

The needle advances through thin mucosal tissue to superficial fascia consisting of connective tissue, microvasculature, and nerve endings to the infraorbital foramen.

Deposition Site

The deposition site is anterior to or superficial to the infraorbital foramen at a depth adequate to reach the foramen (see Figure 12–22 ■). The foramen is located inferior and slightly medial to the infraorbital notch.

Although not crucial to success, some sources recommend contact with bone at the height of the infraorbital foramen to assure adequate depth of penetration (Malamed, 2004).

Technique Steps

Apply the basic injection steps outlined in Chapter 11 and summarized in Appendix 11–1.

Needle Selection

A 27 or 25 gauge needle is recommended for this technique. A 27 gauge short needle is used most commonly for the IO nerve block which is consistent with the

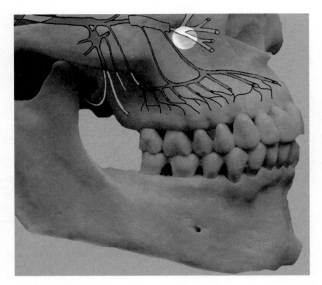

■ **FIGURE 12–22** Deposition Site for IO Nerve Blocks. The deposition site for IO nerve blocks is indicated in the spotlighted area.

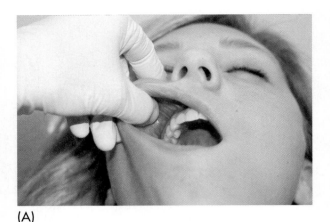

(A)

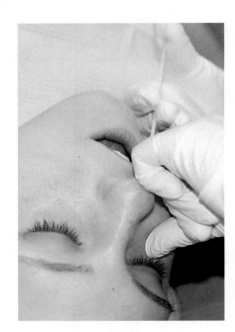

(B)

■ **FIGURE 12–23** Retraction. A—To gain access to the site of penetration, lift the lip, pulling the tissue taut with the thumb and index finger, lifting the tissues away from the maxilla. B—The thumb or forefinger is located over the IO foramen to assist in establishing tissue retraction, and is maintained at that site during the injection

shallow to moderate depths of penetration and the low rate of positive aspiration (less than 3 percent) (Malamed, 2004). In some cases, a 27 gauge long or a 25 gauge short or long needle may be preferred.

Injection Procedure

To gain access to the site of penetration, lift the lip, pulling the tissue taut with the thumb and index finger (see Figures 12–23A ■ and 12–23B ■). After locating the foramen (see Box 12–5), the angle of insertion is oriented toward the foramen along a line parallel to the pupil of the eye on the side of injection (see Figure 12–24 ■ and Figure 12–25 ■). Following a negative aspiration, deposit a minimum of 0.9 ml (1/2 of a cartridge) of an appropriately selected local anesthetic drug. An important step after deposition is to apply finger pressure over the deposition site for 1 to 2 minutes to enhance diffusion of the anesthetic solution into the infraorbital canal. It is customary to maintain a finger position on the infraorbital notch throughout the injection to avoid overinsertion of the needle as shown in Figure 12–23B. Following the administration of the anesthetic, pressure is applied at this same spot, over the deposition site as shown in Figure 12–23B and Figure 12–26 ■.

Confirming Anesthesia

Subjective signs of anesthesia for IO injections include a sense of numbness of the gingival and labial tissues from the distal of the second premolar through the mesial of the central incisor. In addition, numbness

The success of IO injections is improved when the
infraorbital foramen is correctly located. This landmark is easily identified inferior to the infraorbital
ridge by palpating the infraorbital rim on the side of
injection and locating the IO notch. From the notch,
move the finger inferiorly along a line parallel to
the pupil of the eye approximately 10 mm. Typically, the rim of the foramen can be palpated at this
site (see Figure 12–26).

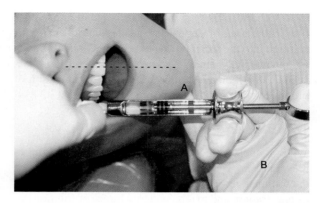

■ **FIGURE 12–25** Syringe Angulations for IO Nerve
Blocks. Align the syringe barrel toward the foramen along
a line parallel to the pupil of the eye on the side of injection.
Note the stable fulcrum on the chin (A) and the palm-up
grasp (B) to aid stability.

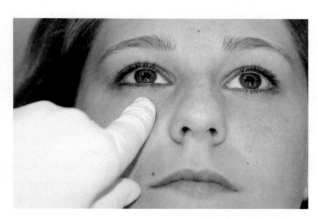

■ **FIGURE 12–26** Locating the Infraorbital Foramen.
The infraorbital foramen is easily located inferior to the
infraorbital ridge by palpating the infraorbital rim and
locating the IO notch.

occurs in the facial tissues from the lip to the lower
eyelid, including the side of the nose. Objective signs
include a lack of response to gentle stimulation with an
instrument and no pain during procedures.

Common Causes of Injection Failure

The most common causes of anesthetic failure include
deposition of solution too inferior to the infraorbital
foramen or too superficial to the bone, and inadequate
volumes of solution.

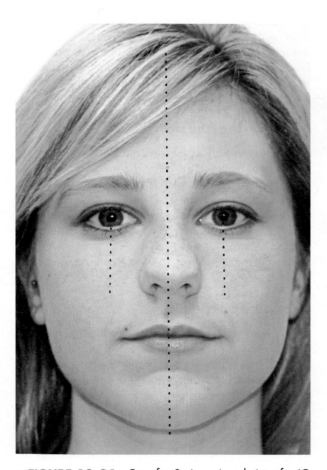

■ **FIGURE 12–24** Cues for Syringe Angulations for IO
Nerve Blocks. To establish syringe angulations, visualize a
line parallel to the midsagittal plane and to the pupil of the
eye on the side of injection.

Other causes may include inflammation or infection in the area of deposition, inadequate diffusion of solution into the foramen due to anatomical factors such as an unusually small foramen and technical factors such as insufficient duration or incorrect application of pressure following the injection.

Troubleshooting

When IO nerve blocks are unsuccessful, it is helpful to reevaluate by visualizing and palpating the location of the foramen, reassessing syringe angulations and depths of penetration, and to reconsider volumes of solution deposited. When necessary, repeat the injection, paying close attention to these factors.

In some instances, the postinjection pressure applied is adequate; however, the location of the foramen is incorrectly assessed. In others, the foramen is correctly located but the depth of penetration is inadequate, the needle direction is incorrect, or pressure is applied for too short a period of time or ineffectively (see Box 12–6).

Some foramina are quite small and do not accept solutions readily. Whenever IO injections prove to be ineffective repeatedly, choose an alternate technique.

Technique Modifications and Alternatives

In some instances, an ideal pathway is not possible due to anatomical factors such as restrictive musculature and tissue inflexibility. In these cases, a more anterior penetration and pathway may be necessary or an alternative technique selected.

Alternative injections can include anterior superior alveolar nerve blocks, along with middle superior alveolar, anterior middle superior alveolar, and palatal anterior superior alveolar nerve blocks, multiple infiltrations, and PDL injections (see Chapter 15).

Complications

The risk of complications following IO nerve block techniques is minimal. These may include postoperative pain at the site of injection, hematoma, and transient numbness of peripheral nerve fibers of the facial nerve.

POSTERIOR SUPERIOR ALVEOLAR NERVE BLOCKS

Posterior superior alveolar (PSA) nerve blocks are indicated for pain management of multiple molar teeth in one quadrant. Alternate names for PSA nerve blocks include *tuberosity* or *zygomatic* blocks. Some clinicians refer to the PSA as a "maxillary block," which is not entirely accurate since a true maxillary, or *division 2* block is a specific and different technique that anesthetizes an entire hemi-maxilla (maxillary blocks are not introduced in this text).

Field of Anesthesia

Anesthesia will affect the structures innervated by the PSA nerve, including pulps of the maxillary first, second, and third molars, and the facial periodontium on the injected side (see Figure 12–27 ■ and Appendix 12–2). In some individuals, the mesiobuccal root of the maxillary first molar will not receive its entire innervation, or any innervation, from the PSA nerve, and a PSA block would not provide profound anesthesia for the entire tooth.

Anatomical Factors

The PSA nerve branches from the maxillary nerve in the pterygopalatine fossa prior to the maxillary nerve's entrance into the infraorbital canal. The PSA nerve then enters the maxillary tuberosity on its infratemporal surface. Generally, there are two or more posterior superior alveolar branches. One branch traverses downward along the external surface of the posterior maxilla and innervates the facial gingiva and mucosa of the molars. One or more internal branches typically divide further and the nerve fibers enter the maxilla through small foramina located on the posterior surface of the tuberosity of the maxilla. These nerve fibers serve the dental plexuses of the molar teeth with the common exception of the

---

Box 12–6 Ergonomics for IO Injections

To reduce repetitive stresses on clinicians' hands, it is helpful to ask patients to apply extraoral pressure over the foramen following deposition of solution and needle withdrawal. Patients should be reminded, if they agree to this task, that pressure must be applied in a specified direction and in a steady, constant manner over the entire 1- to 2-minute period.

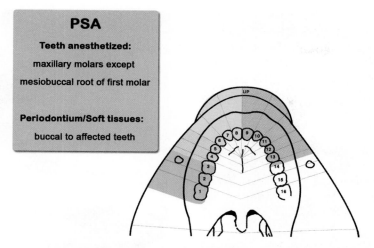

PSA

Teeth anesthetized:

maxillary molars except

mesiobuccal root of first molar

Periodontium/Soft tissues:

buccal to affected teeth

■ **FIGURE 12–27**   Field of Anesthesia for PSA Nerve Blocks. The field of anesthesia for PSA nerve blocks is indicated by the shaded area.

mesiobuccal root of the first molar. The innervation of the mesiobuccal root is further discussed in Box 12–3.

The area posterior to the infratemporal surface of the maxilla contains the infratemporal and pterygopalatine fossae. The infratemporal fossa contains the maxillary artery and its branches, the pterygoid plexus of veins, and branches of the mandibular nerve. The maxillary nerve traverses the superior area of the fossa. Branches of the maxillary artery and the maxillary nerve continue into the pterygopalatine fossa, which is located anterior and medial to the infratemporal fossa.

Technique Factors

The following information describes key factors for successful PSA nerve block injections.

Penetration Site

The penetration site is at the height of mucobuccal fold, posterior to the zygomatic process of the maxilla and generally superior to the distobuccal root of the maxillary second molar (see Figure 12–28 ■).

Needle Pathway

The needle advances through thin mucosal tissue, superficial fascia consisting of loose connective tissue, vessels, and nerve endings to a location close to the PSA nerve(s) on the posterior surface of the maxilla.

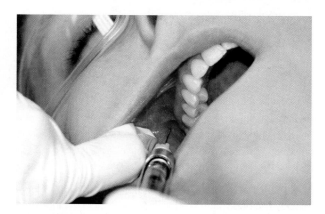

■ **FIGURE 12–28**   Penetration Site for PSA Nerve Blocks. The penetration site for PSA nerve blocks is indicated by the needle. At "minimum penetration" nearly the entire length of the needle shaft is visible.

Deposition Site

The deposition site is adjacent to the foramina for the PSA nerve branches on the posterior surface of the maxilla (see Figure 12–29 ■).

Technique Steps

Apply the basic injection steps outlined in Chapter 11 and summarized in Appendix 11–1.

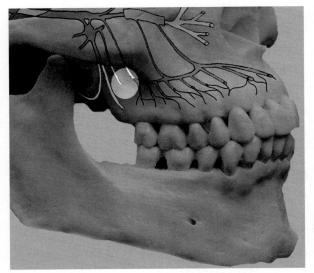

(A)

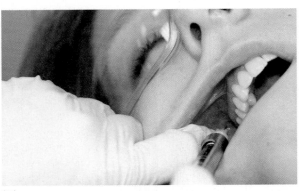

(B)

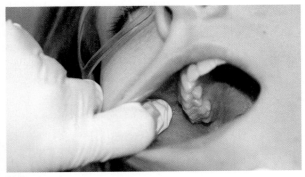

(A)

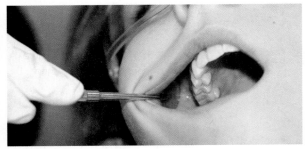

(B)

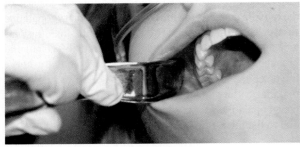

(C)

■ **FIGURE 12–29** A—Deposition Site for PSA Nerve Blocks. The deposition site for PSA nerve blocks is indicated in the spotlighted area. B—At optimum "depth and angle" only approximately 9 mm of the needle shaft will be visible beyond the needle hub.

Needle Selection

A 25 or 27 gauge needle is recommended for this technique. A 27 gauge short is most commonly used, which is consistent with the low rate of positive aspiration (slightly greater than 3 percent) (Malamed, 2004). Some clinicians prefer to use a long needle for a PSA nerve block. Others prefer 25 gauge short or long needles due to the moderate penetration depths necessary in this technique.

Injection Procedure

To gain access to the site of penetration, retract the lip upward and outward, lifting the buccal mucosa laterally as

■ **FIGURE 12–30** Retraction for PSA Nerve Blocks. Retracting the soft tissues both upward and outward provides for direct access to the penetration site and allows for the "upward" and "inward" pathway. A—Retraction can be provided manually or B—with the use of a mirror or C—tissue retractor.

demonstrated in Figure 12–30 ■ and Figure 12–31 ■. The angle of needle insertion is *upward* (at a 45 degree angle to the occlusal plane of the maxillary teeth), *inward* behind the maxillary tuberosity (at a 45 degree angle to the midsagittal plane), and then must be advanced *backward* behind the posterior aspect of the maxilla. To achieve this, the barrel of the syringe must be angled

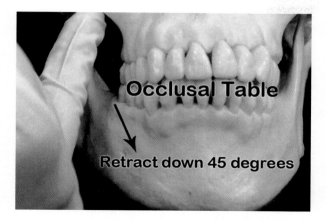

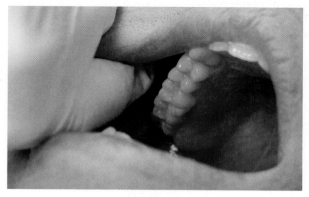

■ **FIGURE 12–31** Retraction for PSA Nerve Blocks—To establish access, first retract the lip downward to reduce pressure on the barrel from the lower lip.

downward from the occlusal table and outward from the patient's midsagittal plane (see Box 12–7). The optimum depth of insertion is 16 mm (9 mm from the hub of an average 25 mm short needle) (see Figure 12–29B); however, clinicians should allow for anatomical variances contributing to the depth of insertion, which can range from 10 to 16 mm. At depths greater than 16 mm the risk of hematoma increases. Deposit anywhere from 0.9 ml to 1.8 ml (½ to 1 cartridge) after negative aspiration. For further discussion on depth, see Box 12–8.

Aspirations in more than one plane are recommended when administering PSA injections due to the presence of the pterygoid plexus of vessels.

Confirming Anesthesia

Subjective signs of anesthesia for PSA injections include a sense of numbness of the gingiva and, in some cases, extending into the buccal mucosa from the distal

---

Box 12–7 Terminology for Needle Pathway for the PSA Nerve Block Injection

The pathway of the needle for the PSA nerve block has frequently been described as an *upward, inward,* and *backward* movement. This can be confusing to visualize and understand. It may be easier to consider this pathway in terms of the motion of the hand and syringe during the injection.

The *upward* needle pathway is achieved when the clinician angles the syringe barrel *downward* at a 45 degree angle, away from the occlusal plane of the maxillary teeth (see Figure 12–31). The *inward* needle pathway is achieved when the clinician angles the syringe barrel *outward* laterally at a 45 degree angle, away from the patient's midsagittal plane (see Figure 12–32 ■). The *backward* movement simply refers to the *advancement* of the needle to the deposition site. In short, the syringe will be moved "down and out" before advancing to depth.

It can be helpful to ask patients to close their mouth half way and shift their mandibles to the side of injection. This improves visibility and access for syringe angulations in order to achieve upward, inward, and backward movements. Using the thumb on the retraction hand can add stability to manage any pressure from the lower lip; this is demonstrated in Figure 12–33 ■.

Additional visual cues for achieving optimal angulations for PSA nerve blocks are provided in Figure 12–34 ■. Figure 12–35 ■ demonstrates ideal, acceptable, and incorrect angulations.

---

of the third molar through the first molar. It is not uncommon for patients to report no sensations of numbness. Objective signs include a lack of response to gentle stimulation with an instrument and no pain during the procedure in the expected field of anesthesia.

Common Causes of Injection Failure

The most common causes of anesthetic failure include deposition of solution too far from the PSA foramina (too inferior, posterior, or lateral) and inadequate volumes of solution.

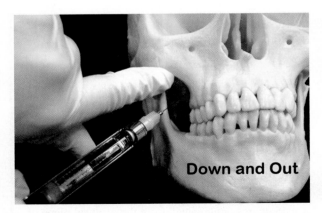

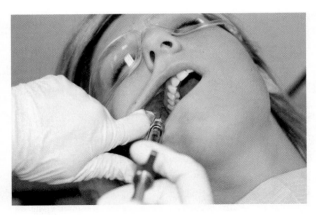

■ **FIGURE 12–32** Angulation for PSA Nerve Blocks—The "upward" needle pathway is achieved when the clinician angles the syringe barrel down and away from the occlusal plane. The "inward" needle pathway is achieved when the clinician angles the syringe barrel outward laterally away from the patient's midsagittal plane.

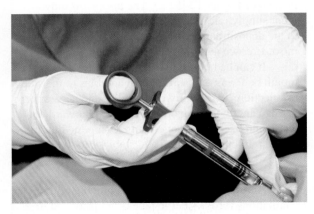

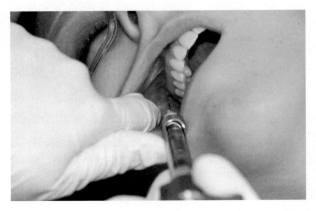

■ **FIGURE 12–33** Fulcrum and Access for PSA Nerve Blocks. Using the thumb on the retraction hand can add stability and manage pressure from the lower lip.

Other causes may include inflammation or infection in the area of deposition.

Troubleshooting

Occasionally, displaced branches of the PSA nerve and the greater palatine nerve may provide innervation to the palatal roots of maxillary molars and accessory innervation to the premolars. In this situation, a supplemental greater palatine nerve block will anesthetize these nerve branches (Blanton & Jeske, 2003).

Contact with bone is not expected. If contact occurs, the needle is touching the periosteum of the tuberosity. Withdrawing the needle and repenetrating at a more lateral site will avoid this obstruction. If an initial penetration site is too anterior to the ideal site, it is possible to contact the posterior surface of the zygomatic process, resisting further progress to the target site posterior to the tuberosity and causing discomfort. Withdrawing the needle and reassessing the posterior extent of the zygomatic process helps to establish a new penetration site that is posterior and/or lateral to the previous site.

Technique Modifications and Alternatives

The depth of penetration is reduced to prevent overinsertion in children and small adults. When skeletal anatomy prevents clinicians from establishing an initial insertion angle at 45 degrees to the midsagittal plane, it

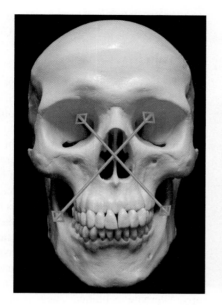

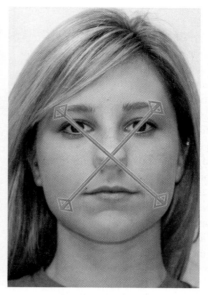

■ **FIGURE 12–34**   PSA Nerve Blocks—Visualizing the "Inward" Needle Pathway. Following an imaginary line that marks an "X" across the patient's face can provide a visual cue for the inward needle pathway that is achieved when the syringe barrel is angled outward 45 degrees laterally away from the patient's midsagittal plane.

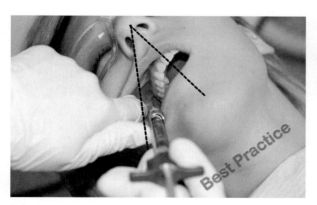

(A)

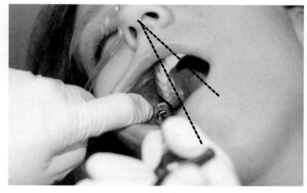

(B)

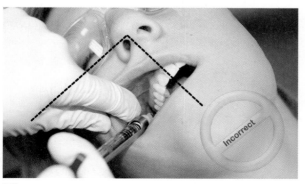

(C)

■ **FIGURE 12–35**   Evaluating Optimal Syringe Angulations. A—The ideal angulations for PSA nerve blocks create a needle pathway at a 45 degree angle to the midsagittal plane. B—In some situations it may be difficult to impossible to achieve this angle and a lesser angle, approximately 20 degrees, may be acceptable. Angulations less than 20 degrees (parallel to the midsagittal plane) are unacceptable. C—Angulations greater than 45 degrees outward are incorrect.

Alternatives include multiple infiltrations and PDL or intraosseous injections (see Chapter 15).

Box 12–8	PSA Nerve Block versus Infiltration

As with other procedures, there are accepted regional and professional philosophies of care. This also applies to variations in local anesthetic techniques. A number of variations for PSA anesthesia are taught, for example. One variation administers the PSA injection as a shallow infiltration, which is relatively successful for soft tissue procedures; however, it may be inadequate for pulpal anesthesia. Other terms used to describe PSA injection techniques include *deep infiltration* and *shallow block*.

It is important to note that in states where dental hygienists administer local anesthesia, a few states allow only infiltration techniques.

Complications

Due to its close proximity to the pterygoid plexus of veins and associated arteries, the PSA injection has the highest risk of postinjection hematoma compared with other intraoral techniques in this text (the maxillary or second division block, which is not discussed in this text, when administered from a tuberosity approach has a somewhat higher risk). The risk of hematoma is more likely if needles are inserted deeper into the pterygopalatine fossa than necessary. This risk also increases when needle penetrations are located too posterior to deposition sites on the posterior surface of the maxilla. Due to the higher risk of hematoma associated with PSA injections, the technique may be contraindicated in patients with clotting disorders or on anticoagulant therapy. Alternate techniques, such as multiple infiltrations, may be safer in these instances (see Chapter 17).

may be helpful to begin the injection with the syringe oriented parallel to the maxilla before establishing ideal angles as the needle is advanced.

CASE MANAGEMENT: Elena Gagarin

An infiltration was administered over #8 to supplement the ASA block and treatment was finished in comfort.

Case Discussion: Cross-innervation from the opposite side ASA nerve prevented an otherwise effective ASA block from providing complete anesthesia of #8. This very common pattern of accessory innervation in the maxillary anterior area is easily remedied with an infiltration above the apex of the central incisor on the side on which anesthesia is desired.

CHAPTER QUESTIONS

1. Which *one* of the following statements best describes the needle pathway for an infiltration injection technique?
   a. The needle is parallel to the long axis of the tooth, passing through thin mucosal tissues to superficial fascia containing loose connective tissue, and past small vessels and microvasculature, and nerve endings.
   b. The needle is distal to the long access of the tooth, passing through thin mucosal tissue to deep fascia of connective tissues, and past small vessels, alveolar bone, and nerve endings.
   c. The needle is parallel to the long axis of the tooth, passing through thin mucosal tissues to superficial tissue, and past small vessels, nerves, and bone.
   d. The needle is perpendicular to the long axis of the tooth, passing through thick mucosal tissue, dense connective tissues, muscle, and vessels, and past microvasculature and nerve endings.

2. When infiltration injections are unsuccessful it may be helpful to:
   a. change the length of the needle and repeat the injection.
   b. visualize, palpate, check radiographs, and reassess the technique.
   c. establish contact with bone before administering one cartridge of anesthetic solution.
   d. repeat the same injection and deposit more solution.

3. The middle superior alveolar nerve is absent in approximately 28%–50% of individuals.
   a. True
   b. False

4. In a typical adult patient, the infraorbital foramen is approximately 8 to 10 mm below the infraorbital ridge.
   a. True
   b. False

5. Which *one* of the following provides the *most accurate* description of the field of anesthesia in a PSA injection?
   a. Pulps of the maxillary premolars and molars, and their facial gingiva, periodontal ligament, and alveolar bone on the side injected
   b. Pulps of the maxillary and mandibular molars on the side injected
   c. Pulps of the maxillary teeth to the midline, and their facial gingiva, periodontal ligament, and alveolar bone on the side injected
   d. Pulps of the maxillary molars, except sometimes the mesiobuccal root of the first molar, and their facial gingiva, periodontal ligament, and alveolar bone on the injected side

6. Which *one* of the following is most likely to increase the risk of hematoma following a PSA nerve block?
   a. The needle is inserted too deep or too posterior to the deposition site on the posterior surface of the maxilla.
   b. The needle is inserted too inferior to the posterior surface of the maxilla.
   c. The porous bony surface of the maxilla allows the needle to penetrate the maxilla-piercing blood vessels.
   d. A long needle is inserted, contacting the bony periosteum on the surface of the maxilla.

REFERENCES

Blanton, P., & Jeske, A. (2003, June). The key to profound local anesthesia—neuroanatomy. *Journal of the American Dental Association, 134,* 755–756.

Fehrenbach, M. J., & Herring, S. W. (2007). *Illustrated anatomy of the head and neck* (3rd ed.). St. Louis: Saunders Elsevier.

Hamburg, H. L. (1972). Preliminary study of patient reaction to needle gauge. *New York State Dental Journal, 38,* 425–426.

Jastak, J. T., Yagiela, J. A., & Donaldson, D. (1995). *Local anesthesia of the oral cavity.* Philadelphia: Saunders.

Loestscher, C. A., & Walton, R. E. (1988). Patterns of innervation of the maxillary first molar: A dissection study. *Oral Surgery Oral Medicine Oral Pathology, 65,* 86–90.

Malamed, S. F. (2004). *Handbook of local anesthesia* (5th ed.). St. Louis: Elsevier Mosby.

Shimada, K., & Gasser, R. F. (1989). *The Anatomical Record: Advances in Integrative Anatomy and Evolutionary Biology, 224*(1), 177–122.

Wong, J. A. (2001). Adjuncts to local anesthesia: Separating fact from fiction. *Journal of the Canadian Dental Association, 67,* 391–397.

Summary of Maxillary Injections

Nerve Block	Needle	Penetration Site	Deposition Site		Dose*	Field of Anesthesia See Appendix 12-2
			Depth of Insertion	**Angle of Insertion**		
Anterior Superior Alveolar (ASA)	Short 25/27 gauge	Height of mucobuccal fold above canine See Figure 12–11	Variable, needle tip inserted to a point above apex of canine.	Needle directed 25 degrees medially bevel toward bone	0.9–1.2 ml	***Teeth anesthetized:*** Canine, lateral, central
			Target			***Periodontium/Soft tissues:*** Facial to affected teeth
			Above apex of canine. See Figure 12–12			
			Depth of Insertion	**Angle of Insertion**		
Middle Superior Alveolar (MSA)	Short 25/27 gauge	Height of mucobuccal fold above the second premolar See Figure 12–14	Variable, needle tip inserted to a point well above apex of second premolar	Needle directed 20 degrees medially bevel toward bone	0.9–1.2 ml	***Teeth anesthetized:*** Maxillary premolars and mesiobuccal root of first molar* *For most people
			Target			***Periodontium/Soft tissues:*** Facial to affected teeth
			Well above apex of second premolar. See Figure 12–16			
			Depth of Insertion	**Angle of Insertion**		
Infraorbital (IO)	Short or Long 25/27 gauge	Height of mucobuccal folder above first premolar See Figure 12–21	Variable, needle tip inserted to a point lateral to the infraorbital foramen	Needle parallel to long axis of tooth bevel toward bone	0.9–1.2 ml	***Teeth anesthetized:*** Premolars, canine, lateral, central
			Target			***Periodontium/Soft tissues:*** Facial to affected teeth
			Infraorbital foramen See Figure 12–22			

(Continued)

		Depth of Insertion	Angle of Insertion	0.9–1.8 ml	Teeth anesthetized:
Posterior Superior Alveolar (PSA)	Short 25/27 gauge	Height of mucobuccal fold above second molar See Figure 12–28	Needle advanced along a path 45 degrees medially to midsaggital plane, 45 degrees superior to occlusal plane		Maxillary molars except mesiobuccal root of first molar
		Target			**Periodontium/Soft tissues:**
		Slightly above and distal to distobuccal root of last molar, second or third if present See Figure 12–29A			Buccal to affected teeth
		Depth of Insertion	Angle of Insertion	0.6 ml	Teeth anesthetized:
Local infiltration injections	Extra-Short or Short 25/27/30 gauge	Height of mucobuccal fold buccal to tooth See Figure 12–2	Approximately 20 degrees to long axis of tooth, directed toward apex of tooth bevel toward bone		At injection site
		Target			**Periodontium/Soft tissues:**
		Selected soft tissue, gingival or apex of tooth See Figure 12–4			At injection site

*Dose volumes provided are minimum recommendations for pulpal anesthesia.
Modified from: 1) Malamed SF, Handbook of local anesthesia, ed 5, St Louis, 2004, Mosby; 2) Jastak JT, Yagiela JA, Donaldson D, Local anesthesia of the oral cavity. Philidelphia, 1995 W.B. Saunders; 3) Daniels SJ, Harfst SA, Wilder RS, Dental hygiene: concepts, cases and competencies, 2nd edition, St Louis, 2007, Mosby

Field of Anesthesia

Maxillary Injections

ASA

Teeth anesthetized:
canine, lateral, central

Periodontium/Soft tissues:
facial to affected teeth

MSA

Teeth anesthetized:
maxillary premolars and
mesiobuccal root of first molar*
* For most people

Periodontium/Soft tissues:
facial to affected teeth

PSA

Teeth anesthetized:
maxillary molars except
mesiobuccal root of first molar

Periodontium/Soft tissues:
buccal to affected teeth

IO

Teeth anesthetized:
premolars, canine,
lateral, central

Periodontium/Soft tissues:
facial to affected teeth

Infiltration

Teeth anesthetized:
at injection site

Periodontium/Soft tissues:
at injection site

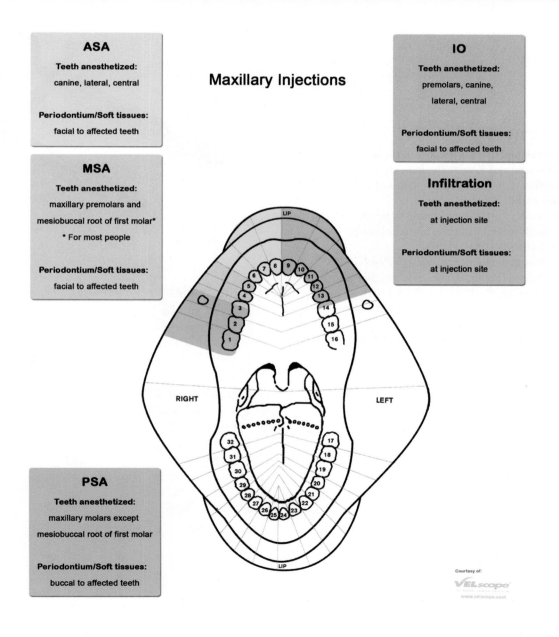

Courtesy of:

VELscope
www.velscope.com

Chapter 13

Injections for Palatal Pain Control

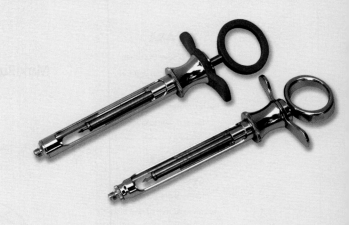

OBJECTIVES

- Define and discuss the key terms in this chapter.
- Describe and discuss the indications, relevant anatomy, and technique features of the injections discussed in this chapter.
- Describe the basic technique steps for safe and effective administration of the following injections:
  - Nasopalatine nerve block (NP or NPNB)
  - Palatal (approach) anterior superior alveolar nerve block (P-ASA or PASANB)
  - Anterior middle superior alveolar nerve block (AMSA or AMSANB)
  - Greater palatine nerve block (GP or GPNB)

CASE STUDY: Elena Gagarin

Elena Gagarin was appointed for two-and-one-half hours to treat the maxillary right quadrant. She needed a combination of restorative and dental hygiene therapy and had opted to have it completed in one appointment due to difficulty in arranging her appointments. Anesthesia was necessary for the entire quadrant, including the palate. There were notes of her previous requests that palatal injections be minimized or avoided and that, when necessary, she would require nitrous oxide.

She had required so many shots the last time she was in, she stated, that she had almost canceled today's appointment. She also had to speak in her daughter's classroom immediately following her appointment and was concerned that her lips would be numb. She even reminded the office staff on arrival that she wanted fewer shots and hoped that the numbing would work better this time. The office staff checked the record and verified that five infiltrations on the left maxilla, including two on the palate, had been administered during her last appointment.

INTRODUCTION

Anatomic landmarks and considerations for each palatal injection technique will be presented in reference to the **penetration site, needle pathway,** and **deposition site** as described in Chapter 11. The penetration site will be related to hard and soft tissue landmarks. The needle pathway will be described in terms of the types of tissue that will be penetrated by or located in the vicinity of the needle, including mucosa, superficial fascia, muscle, vessels, nerves, and bone. The deposition site will be described in terms of the tissues at or near the target and in relation to specific landmarks.

PALATAL INJECTION TECHNIQUES

This chapter will discuss palatal injection techniques. Palatal injections are true maxillary injections, usually discussed with other maxillary techniques. They are separated in this text because there are common technique considerations that apply to all palatal procedures that do not apply to nonpalatal maxillary techniques. Some of these considerations address the pain that is often associated with administering palatal anesthesia. Others address unique challenges presented by palatal anatomy. These considerations and challenges have direct impacts on the safety and success of palatal techniques. Key elements for each injection discussed are summarized in Appendix 13–1. Common variations and precautions will be discussed where applicable.

NASOPALATINE NERVE BLOCK

Nasopalatine nerve blocks (NPNBs) are indicated for pain management of palatal soft and osseous tissue in the anterior third of the palate, approximately from canine to canine. The NP nerve occasionally provides pulpal anesthesia to the central incisors, and the NP block is sometimes needed when traditional methods of anesthetizing the central incisors fail to provide profound anesthesia (Blanton & Jeske, 2003). The NP nerve block is also known as an *incisive* or *sphenopalatine* nerve block.

Field of Anesthesia

Anesthesia will affect the structures innervated by the nasopalatine nerves bilaterally. This field includes structures located in the anterior one-third of the palate (see Figure 13–1 ■ and Appendix 13–2).

Anatomical Factors

The nasopalatine nerve is the longest branch of the posterior superior nasal branch of the maxillary nerve. It passes along the nasal septum and descends to the anterior portion of the maxilla. Both the right and left nasopalatine nerves exit the maxilla through the incisive foramen. The fibers innervate the mucosa and osseous tissue of the anterior hard palate and palatal gingiva to the mesial aspects of the first premolars or slightly posterior to that location due to some degree of overlap with fibers of the right and left greater palatine nerves. The nasopalatine nerves occasionally provide pulpal innervation to central incisors, as well. When this pattern is present, it is frequently necessary to anesthetize the nasopalatine nerves in order to provide profound anesthesia of the central incisors (Blanton & Jeske, 2003).

Technique Factors

The following information describes key factors for successful NP nerve block injections.

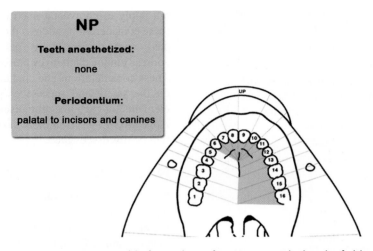

■ **FIGURE 13–1**   Field of Anesthesia for NP Nerve Blocks. The field of anesthesia for NP nerve blocks is indicated by the shaded area.

Penetration Site

The optimum site of penetration for the NP nerve block is the palatal mucosa lateral to the widest anteroposterior dimension of the incisive papilla (see Figure 13–2 ■).

Needle Pathway

The needle advances under the incisive papilla through dense mucosal tissues to contact the opposite wall of the incisive canal near its entrance.

Deposition Site

The deposition site is near the wall of the incisive canal (see Figure 13–3 ■).

Technique Steps

Apply the basic injection steps outlined in Chapter 11 and summarized in Appendix 11–1.

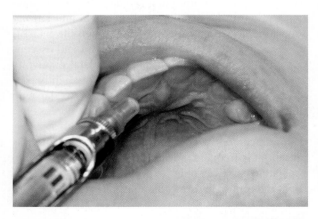

■ **FIGURE 13–2**   Penetration Site for NP Nerve Blocks. The penetration site for NP nerve blocks is indicated by the needle.

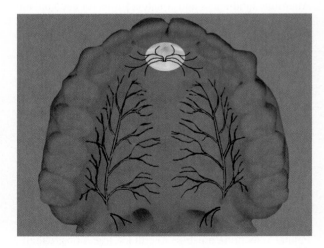

■ **FIGURE 13–3**   Deposition Site for NP Nerve Blocks. The deposition site for NP nerve blocks is indicated in the spotlighted area.

Needle Selection

A 27 gauge short needle is recommended and consistent with the minimal penetrations depths required and the low rate of positive aspiration (less than 1 percent) (Malamed, 2004). Some clinicians prefer to use a 30 gauge short or x-short needle in the palate.

Injection Procedure

Palatal injections have a reputation for causing discomfort. They can be administered more comfortably if a technique alteration known as pre-injection anesthesia, also referred to as **pre-anesthesia,** is used. Pre-anesthesia may be defined as anesthesia that is already in effect from previous injections in the area (see Figure 13–4 ■)

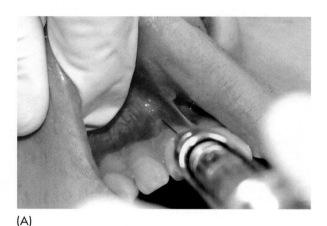

(A)

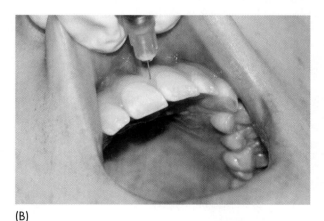

(B)

■ **FIGURE 13–4**   Pre-anesthesia Infiltration. A—Step 1, Infiltrate labial mucosa. B—Step 2, Infiltrate "through" the interdental papilla tissue. These steps are followed by the penetration under the incisive papilla.

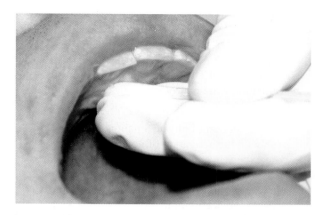

■ **FIGURE 13–5**   Pre-anesthesia—Topical Anesthetic and Pressure.

or a two-step topical method that includes an initial 1 minute application of topical followed by firm pressure for a subsequent minute (see Figure 13–5 ■).

The pressure can be applied to the tissue with a cotton swab (used to place the topical) or with a smooth, blunt-ended instrument handle, until blanching is observed at the penetration site.

Pressure anesthesia to deeper tissues will develop, enhancing patient comfort during needle penetration. It is important to apply constant pressure to the site for a full minute in order to achieve profound pressure anesthesia of deeper tissues.

This two-step method reduces the potential for pain when penetrating sensitive palatal tissues. A number of other strategies for decreasing or eliminating discomfort during palatal injections may also be quite useful. Most of these rely on what is known as the **Gate Control Theory** of Pain Perception, which states that there are certain locations or *gates* within the spinal nervous system. When flooded with impulses from less painful stimuli, impulses generated from more painful and subsequent stimuli, such as needle penetrations, can be blocked (see Box 13–1).

Topical anesthetic patches can also be useful for injection site preparation in palatal techniques. Some may provide a 4 to 6 mm depth of penetration compared with 2 to 4 mm for standard topical agents.

To gain access to the site of penetration, ask the patient to tip his or her head up and slightly away, with the mouth wide open. Penetrate lateral to and at the base of the broadest aspect of the incisive papilla (see Figure 13–2). Continue penetrating at a 45 degree angle

Box 13–1 The Gate Control Theory of Pain Perception

The Gate Control Theory of Pain Perception suggests that there are neurological gates that can block signals to the brain. This theory asserts that:

1. The perception of physical pain is not based solely on the activation of nociception.
2. The experience of pain is a modulation between activation of large non–pain transmitting (non-nociceptive) nerve fibers and small pain transmitting (nociceptive) nerve fibers.
3. The activation of large non-nociceptive fibers can interfere with signals from small nociceptive fibers.
4. If the stimulation of non-nociceptive fibers is greater than the stimulation of nociceptive fibers, pain will be inhibited or blocked.

Pressure anesthesia administered by holding a cotton-tipped applicator or smooth instrument handle against the tissues can eliminate or nearly eliminate pain from needle puncture. In addition to providing a decrease in sensitivity due to temporary anoxia, dull pressure from the applicator or handle floods gates with less painful stimuli compared with needle penetration.

A device that makes use of Gate Control desensitization by means of what is referred to as an analgesic syringe clip, the VibraJect (see Figure 13–6 ■) purportedly " . . . blocks pain from injections based on the Gate Control Theory. A battery operated motor attaches to a conventional syringe which when activated causes very rapid vibrations. The high vibration of the needle stimulates the nerve endings and blocks the transmission of pain feelings to the brain."

Sources: Chudler, http://faculty.washington.edu/chudler/pain.html; Deardorff, www.spine-health.com/conditions/chronic-pain/modern-ideas-gate-control-theory-chronic-pain; VibraJect LLC, http://www.vibraject.com/patients.html.

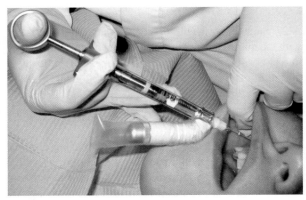

(A)

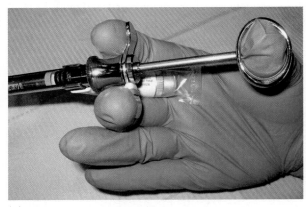

(B)

■ **FIGURE 13–6** VibraJect. A—Device attached near needle adaptor. B—Device attached near finger grip and obscured from view in larger hand.

under the papilla as demonstrated in Figure 13–7 ■. Advance slowly until the opposite wall of the incisive canal is contacted. Once bone is contacted, withdraw the needle ~1 mm. The depth of insertion ranges from 4 to 7 mm. Following negative aspiration, deposit a minimum of 0.4 ml (a little less than 1/4 of a cartridge) of

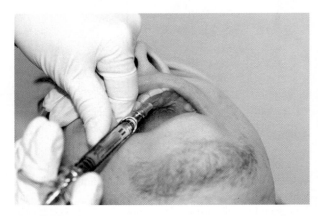

■ **FIGURE 13–7** Syringe Angulations. Align the syringe barrel at a 45 degree angle to the palate.

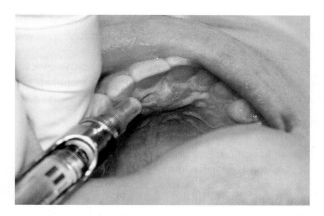

■ **FIGURE 13–8**   Blanching from the NP Nerve Block. As solution is deposited, blanching will occur, extending laterally and lingually to the anterior teeth.

an appropriately selected local anesthetic drug (the tissue will usually blanch to a region extending to the lingual aspects of the anterior teeth) (see Figure 13–8 ■).

Deposition Rate

In order to avoid discomfort, the rate of deposition should be reduced to 0.4 ml over 40 seconds. This rate is significantly slower than the previously mentioned standard injection rate of approximately 1.8 ml over 1 minute (0.4 ml over about 13 to 14 seconds) and may be thought of as a *palatal* rate (3 minutes per cartridge). Very slow rates for NP blocks and other palatal injections may seem tedious but the dense tissues of the palate resist deposition and do not accommodate solution easily. In addition to providing increased comfort, slow rates also avoid unnecessary tissue trauma.

Confirming Anesthesia

Subjective signs of anesthesia for NP injections include a sense of numbness of the gingiva on the anterior palate. Objective signs include a lack of response to gentle stimulation with an instrument and no pain during the procedure in the expected field of anesthesia.

Common Causes of Injection Failure

The most common causes of anesthetic failure include inadequate depth of penetration and inadequate volumes of solution deposited.

Other causes include inflammation or infection in the area of deposition, inadequate diffusion of solution, and overlapping innervation by the greater palatine nerve.

Troubleshooting

When NP injections are unsuccessful, it is helpful to reevaluate by visualizing and reassessing syringe angulations and depths of penetration as well as volumes of solution deposited.

The NP block may result in unilateral anesthesia if the opposite wall of the canal is not contacted. This may be the desired outcome if teeth in only half the anterior maxilla are being treated. When the NP nerve block injection technique is followed, bilateral anesthesia will develop. If this is desired but fails to occur, repeat the procedure, making sure to meet resistance on the opposite side of the incisive canal.

Technique Modifications and Alternatives

An alternate method for administering the NP injection uses a multiple injection technique. This is sometimes helpful when patients are afraid of palatal injection pain. It is first necessary to infiltrate and deposit about 0.3 ml of anesthetic near the facial midline (see Figure 13–4A). After the tissues in the midline are anesthetized, penetration is made through the interdental papilla known as an *interpapillary injection* (from the facial to the lingual aspect) (see Figure 13–4B), administering a few drops of solution ahead of the needle until the palatal tissues have been initially numbed. After an appropriate pause for soft tissue anesthesia to be effective (30 seconds), a standard NP injection is administered.

Computer-controlled local anesthetic devices (CCLADs) are ideal for this type of injection because they provide electronically regulated, slow rates of injection recommended for all palatal techniques and accomplish this without causing hand fatigue.

When administering 4 percent solutions, the total volume delivered should be reduced by half due to concerns of neurotoxicity. This does not affect the rate of deposition. For further discussion of CCLADs, see Chapter 9, "Local Anesthetic Delivery Devices."

Complications

The risk of complications following NP injections is minimal. Complications may include postoperative pain at the site of injection, hematomas, and postoperative edema. If 1:50,000 concentrations of epinephrine are used, there is an increased risk of necrosis due to the vigorous vasoconstriction it provides, depriving the tissues of oxygen for extended periods.

PALATAL ANTERIOR SUPERIOR ALVEOLAR NERVE BLOCK

Palatal anterior superior alveolar nerve blocks (P-ASANBs) were defined by Friedman and Hochman in the 1990s as "palatal approach—anterior superior alveolar nerve blocks" and will be discussed as palatal anterior superior alveolar nerve blocks (PASANB or P-ASANB). They are indicated for pain management of maxillary anterior sextants and are especially useful in cosmetic procedures that involve perioperative assessment of "smile lines" and when public speaking is anticipated after appointments because they do not result in labial numbness or motor disturbances (Friedman & Hochman, 1999; Malamed, 2004).

Field of Anesthesia

Anesthesia will affect the structures innervated by the right and left nasopalatine nerves and the anterior branches of the ASA nerves, to include the facial and palatal soft and hard tissues associated with the teeth and the pulps of the teeth in the sextant (see Figure 13–9 ■ and Appendix 13–2), although pulpal anesthesia of the canines is more questionable (Malamed, 2004). Results of one study published in 2004 determined that the success rate of the P-ASA when using 2% lidocaine with 1:100,000 epinephrine for any of the anterior teeth resulted in a disappointing 32 to 58 percent. Even lesser results were achieved with 3% mepivacaine at 22 to 38 percent (Burns, Reader, Nusstein, Beck, & Weaver, 2004). As is true of other techniques with low published success rates, such as the AMSA and IO nerve blocks, clinicians who are more familiar with this technique often experience much higher rates of success.

Anatomical Factors

The right and left anterior superior alveolar nerves and vessels travel together through the nasopalatine canal. The canal provides a pathway for nerves and vessels that supply the entire anterior palate. Access to the superior portion of the canal is through the incisive foramen.

Technique Factors

The following information describes key factors for successful P-ASA nerve block injections.

This injection is performed similar to the NP technique, with an important exception. Rather than deposit solution shortly after meeting resistance on the opposite wall of the canal, the barrel is adjusted to a steep angle relative to the wall once contact has been confirmed (see Figure 13–6). The needle is then advanced up the canal approximately 6 to 10 mm, parallel to the inclination of the roots of the central incisors using the opposite wall as a guide.

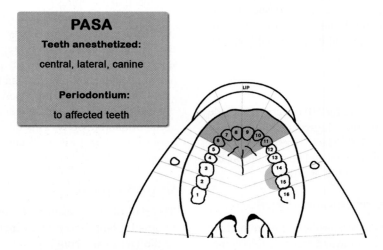

PASA

Teeth anesthetized:

central, lateral, canine

Periodontium:

to affected teeth

■ **FIGURE 13–9** Field of Anesthesia for P-ASA Nerve Blocks. The field of anesthesia for P-ASA nerve blocks is indicated by the shaded area.

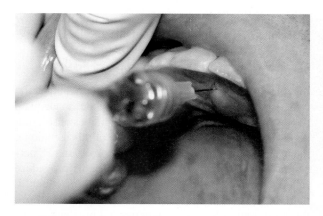

■ **FIGURE 13–10** Needle Pathway for P-ASA Nerve Blocks. The needle pathway for P-ASA nerve blocks is indicated by the needle.

Penetration Site

The optimum site of penetration for the P-ASA is the palatal mucosa lateral to the widest anteroposterior dimension of the incisive papilla (see Figure 13–2).

Needle Pathway

The needle advances under the incisive papilla through dense mucosal tissue, to contact the opposite wall of the incisive canal just below the foramen. From this point, the needle advances superiorly into the canal until penetrated to depth (see Figure 13–10 ■).

Deposition Site

The deposition site is within the incisive canal at a penetration depth of approximately 6 to 10 mm (Malamed, 2004) (see Figure 13–11 ■).

Technique Steps

Apply the basic injection steps outlined in Chapter 11 and summarized in Appendix 11–1.

Needle Selection

A 27 gauge short needle is recommended. This is consistent with the moderate penetration depths required and the low rate of positive aspiration (assumed to be less than 1 percent) in P-ASA nerve blocks (Malamed, 2004). Some clinicians prefer a 30 gauge x-short needle although extra-short needles may lack sufficient length to reach the target area.

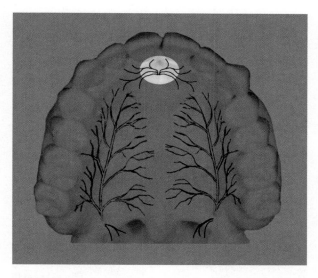

■ **FIGURE 13–11** Deposition Site for P-ASA Nerve Blocks. The deposition site for P-ASA nerve blocks is indicated in the spotlighted area.

Injection Procedure

Discomfort associated with palatal injections can be significantly reduced when pre-anesthesia is used. This can be achieved by applying a topical drug followed by physical pressure. Follow the two-step method, beginning with a 1 minute application of topical anesthetic. Topical patches may have added benefit when used with P-ASA nerve blocks due to the significant sensitivity often experienced in this area of the mouth.

To gain access to the site of penetration, ask patients to tip the head up and slightly away, opening the mouth wide. The penetration site is lateral to the incisive papilla. The angle of penetration should be adjusted to one that is parallel to the roots of the central incisors after initial bony contact on the opposite wall of the canal. The angle of insertion is approximately 45 degrees to the palate on a line that will enter the nasopalatine canal (see Figure 13–12A ■). Advance the needle slowly, 1 to 2 mm every 4 to 6 seconds, to an insertion depth of 6 to 10 mm (see Figure 13–12B ■). Following a negative aspiration at the deposition site, deposit a minimum of 1.4 ml (a little over 2/3 of a cartridge) of an appropriately selected local anesthetic drug.

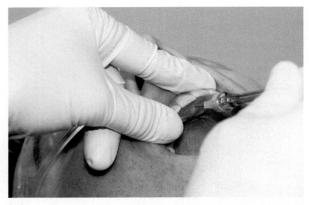

(A)

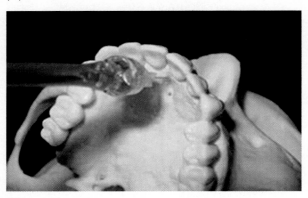

(B)

■ **FIGURE 13–12** A—Syringe Angulations. Align the syringe barrel approximately 45 degrees to the palate. B—Insertion into the Incisive Foramen. Prior to deposition for P–ASA nerve blocks, the needle is advanced into the incisive foramen.

Deposition Rate Modification

The rate of deposition is modified for this injection to 0.5 ml over 60 seconds (Malamed, 2004). Note that this rate is even *slower* than the previously described palatal injection rate of approximately 1.8 ml over 3 minutes.

Confirming Anesthesia

Subjective signs of anesthesia for P-ASA injections include an immediate sense of tightness and numbness of the gingiva on the anterior palate following injection. Objective signs include a lack of response to gentle stimulation with an instrument and no pain during the procedure in the expected field of anesthesia.

Common Causes of Injection Failure

In addition to a lack of familiarity with the technique, the most common causes of failure include inadequate depths of penetration and inadequate volumes of solution deposited. In one study of the efficacy of this technique, the results were quite disappointing, approaching 58 percent at best (Burns et al., 2004). While this procedure failed to provide profound anesthesia more frequently than any other technique described in this text, those more familiar with it have experienced greater rates of success.

Other causes of failure include inflammation or infection in the area of deposition, inadequate diffusion of solution, and overlapping innervation by the greater palatine nerve.

Troubleshooting

When P-ASA injections are unsuccessful, it is helpful to reevaluate by visualizing and reassessing syringe angulations and depths of penetration, and by reconsidering volumes of solution deposited.

Technique Modifications and Alternatives

The use of a CCLAD is ideal for this type of injection because it provides a controlled, continuous, and slow rate of deposition.

When administering 4 percent solutions in the palate, the maximum volume delivered should be reduced to half of what is normally deposited with other drugs, but never more than one-half of a cartridge, due to concerns of nerve injury resulting in paresthesia. The *rate* of deposition is also important. A 4 percent solution should be administered no faster than half the rate of any 2 or 3 percent solution (note that this represents the total milligrams of drug administered per minute, compared with 2 percent solutions). This means that a maximum of *one-half* of a cartridge of 4% articaine, compared to *one* cartridge 2% lidocaine, should be administered no faster than over a *full 3 minutes* in the palate, regardless of the technique.

Alternatives to the P-ASA include bilateral ASA blocks, bilateral IO blocks with an NP injection, and bilateral AMSA blocks (Malamed, 2004).

Complications

The risk of complications following P-ASA injections is minimal. These may include postoperative pain at the site of injection, hematoma, infection, and edema. When high concentrations of vasoconstrictors are used, necrosis is possible.

ANTERIOR MIDDLE SUPERIOR ALVEOLAR NERVE BLOCK

Anterior middle superior alveolar nerve blocks (AMSANBs) are indicated for pain management of the incisors, canine, and premolars on the side anesthetized as well as palatal tissue from the midline through the molars and the buccal periodontium of the pulpally affected teeth (Friedman & Hochman, 1998; Malamed, 2004). A significant benefit of this technique is that it reduces the number of injections and therefore the total volumes of solution necessary to achieve the same field of anesthesia as traditional ASA/IO, MSA, NP, and GP approaches. In addition, the lack of labial anesthesia in AMSA blocks allows for normal patterns of speech and facial expression (Friedman & Hochman, 2001).

In 2004, one study concluded that the AMSA nerve block was more successful when a computer controlled device was used (35 to 58 percent) versus a conventional syringe (20 to 42 percent) (Lee, Reader, Nusstein, Beck, & Weaver, 2004). While critical to the degree of relative success in this study, the choice of syringe did not significantly alter the disappointing overall success rate determined by the study. Two other studies published in the same year, however, reported promising efficacy when using the technique for periodontal therapy (Loomer & Perry, 2004; Sculean, Kasaj, Berakdar, &Willershausen, 2004). As with other less familiar techniques, success rates often improve dramatically following review and repetition. Reports from clinicians who have been administering the AMSA for several years are generally very positive. The benefits of AMSA nerve blocks over other techniques are summarized in Table 13–1 ■.

Field of Anesthesia

Anesthesia will affect the structures innervated by the ASA nerve, the MSA nerve, the palate, and terminal branches to include the pulps of the central and lateral incisors, canine, and premolars on the anesthetized side. It is important to note that the AMSA injection does not provide labial anesthesia (Friedman & Hochman, 2001) (see Figure 13–13 ■, Appendix 13–2, and Box 13–2).

Anatomical Factors

The median palatine suture and its overlying raphe appear to prevent solution from flowing to the opposite side of the palate. Palatal bone is porous and has multiple nutrient canals through which solution easily diffuses to the **dental plexus** of the ASA and MSA nerves (Malamed,

Table 13–1	Benefits of the AMSA Technique
Quadrant Procedures	
Traditional Approach	***AMSA Approach***
Requires 4 to 5 injections *Option 1:* ASA, MSA, PSA, NP, GP 5 penetrations *Option 2:* IO, PSA, NP, GP 4 penetrations	Requires 2 injections PSA, AMSA 2 penetrations
Anesthesia to associated labial tissues	No anesthesia to associated labial tissues *Useful for cosmetic dental procedures (does not interfere with "smile line")*
Total drug dose varies 2 to 3 cartridges	Total drug dose varies 1⅔ to 2 cartridges *Reduce total local anesthetic and vasoconstrictor drugs administered*
Significant post-op labial anesthesia	Minimal to no residual post-op labial anesthesia *Important to patients in public speaking roles*

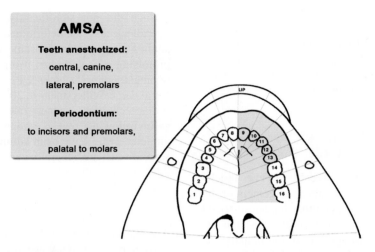

■ **FIGURE 13–13** Field of Anesthesia for AMSA Nerve Blocks. The field of anesthesia for AMSA nerve blocks is indicated by the shaded area.

Box 13–2 Innervation of Maxillary Labial Soft Tissues

Neither the ASA nor MSA nerve provides labial soft tissue innervation. Sensory innervation of the maxillary labial tissues is provided by terminal branches of the infraorbital (upper lip) and zygomaticofacial nerves (skin of the cheek). These are also branches of the maxillary (V2) division of the trigeminal (V) nerve and are usually anesthetized when other injection techniques, such as infiltrations and ASA or MSA nerve blocks, are used to anesthetize the maxillary teeth.

2004). The region of the maxillary plexus is demonstrated in Figure 13–14 ■. Diffusion through porous palatal bone is enhanced by gentle hydraulic pressure that develops when solution is deposited within tightly bound palatal tissues (Fehrenbach & Herring, 2007).

Technique Factors

The following information describes key factors for successful AMSA nerve block injections.

Penetration Site

The optimum site of penetration for AMSA injections is located between the premolars approximately halfway along an imaginary line drawn from the median palatine

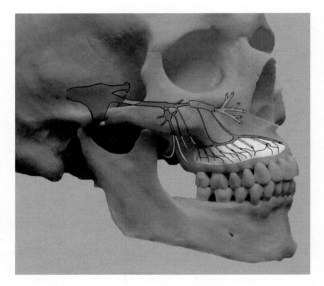

■ **FIGURE 13–14** Maxillary Dental Plexus. The maxillary dental plexus is highlighted along the apices of the maxillary teeth.

raphe to the gingival margin on the side to be anesthetized. This can also be described as the junction between the vertical and horizontal aspects of the palate directly above the free gingival margin between the maxillary premolars on the side to be anesthetized (see Figure 13–15 ■).

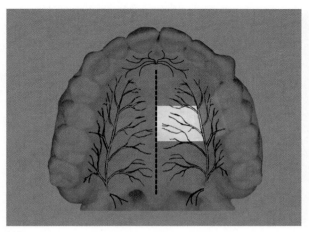

(A)

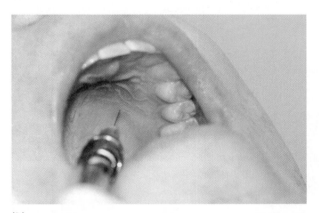

(B)

■ **FIGURE 13-15** Penetration Site for AMSA Nerve Blocks. The penetration site for AMSA nerve blocks is at the junction of the horizontal and vertical aspects of the palate (A) and is indicated by the needle (B).

Needle Pathway

The needle pathway is very short, through dense palatal tissue directly to bone.

Deposition Site

The deposition site is near the junction of the vertical alveolar process and the horizontal palatal process (see Figures 13–15 and 13–16 ■). Note that if the ideal site does not have enough tissue thickness to accommodate solution, a nearby site with greater thickness may be chosen. This can be determined by probing the chosen area with a cotton swab (see Figure 13–17 ■).

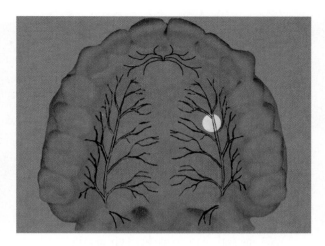

■ **FIGURE 13-16** Deposition Site for AMSA Nerve Blocks. The deposition site for AMSA nerve blocks is indicated in the spotlighted area.

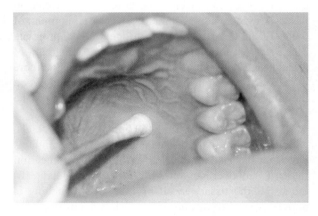

■ **FIGURE 13-17** Determining Tissue Thickness at AMSA Deposition Site. Adequate tissue thickness to accommodate solution can be determined by probing the chosen area with a cotton swab.

Technique Steps

Apply the basic injection steps outlined in Chapter 11 and summarized in Appendix 11–1.

Needle Selection

A 27 gauge needle is recommended (Malamed, 2004). A 27 gauge short needle is most commonly used although some clinicians prefer a 30 gauge x-short. Considering the limited depths of penetration required as well as the low risk of intravascular injection (positive aspiration less than 1 percent), 30 gauge x-short needles are appropriate.

Injection Procedure

As previously discussed with the NP and P-ASA nerve blocks, discomfort associated with palatal injections can be significantly reduced with the use of pre-anesthesia. This can be achieved by applying the two-step method of topical anesthesia already discussed. Some clinicians prefer topical patches for injection site preparation for AMSA injections.

Ask the patient to tip the head up and slightly away, opening the mouth wide. The angle of insertion is approximately 45 degrees to the palate with the syringe barrel positioned over the opposite side of the mouth and the bevel facing bone. This is demonstrated in Figure 13–18 ■. Advance slowly until resistance is met (contact with bone). The insertion depth is variable, often no more than enough penetration to bury the bevel of the needle in tissue. After a negative aspiration, deposit a minimum of 0.9 to 1.2 ml (1/2 to 2/3 of a cartridge) of an appropriate 2 or 3 percent local anesthetic drug over a minimum of 3 minutes. When administering a 4 percent drug, no more than 0.7 to 0.9 ml of solution should be deposited over a minimum of 3 minutes to lessen the risk of toxicity to the nerves (Malamed, 2004).

The rate of deposition is 0.5 ml over 60 seconds, which translates to a little under 1.8 ml over 3 minutes. Note that this rate is *slower* than the standard injection rate of 1.8 ml over 3 minutes for most other palatal techniques. If the tissues swell or excessive blanching is noticed (a *stark white* appearance), slow deposition rates even more until no swelling and only pale blanching are seen (see Box 13–3).

Confirming Anesthesia

Subjective signs of anesthesia for AMSA injections include an immediate sense of tightness and numbness of the palatal tissues and periodontium from the central incisors through the second molar on the side of injection and a numb sensation in the teeth from the central incisor to the second premolar on the same side. Objective signs include a lack of response to gentle stimulation with an instrument and no pain during procedures in the expected field of anesthesia.

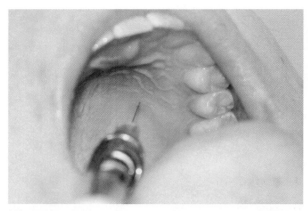

(A)

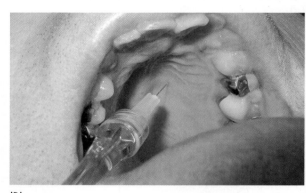

(B)

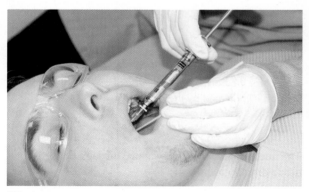

(C)

■ **FIGURE 13–18** Insertion Angulations for AMSA Nerve Blocks. The angle of insertion is approximately 45 degrees to the palate with the syringe barrel over the opposite side of the mouth. A—Penetration with a standard, manual syringe. B—Penetration with a CCLAD and Wand handpiece. C—For access, ask the patient to tip the head up and slightly away, opening the mouth wide.

Box 13–3 Deposition Rate & Blanching for the AMSA Nerve Block

It is not uncommon to modify deposition rates for the administration of local anesthetics in some situations. In the AMSA nerve block, for example, a large volume of solution must be deposited into tightly bound, fibrous palatal tissues. These tissues resist the volumes sometimes necessary to achieve profound anesthesia. While the minimum deposition rate of 1.8 ml in most locations has been described as 1 minute (60 seconds), in the AMSA technique this rate is slowed to ≥3 minutes (see Figure 13–19 ■). When 4 percent solutions are administered, only 0.7 ml (or half the volume) to up to a maximum of 0.9 ml (about 1/3 to 1/2 of a cartridge), should be delivered over a 3 minute time period.

The previously described rate should be regarded as a starting point in determining the ideal rate of deposition for each individual AMSA block. To determine the actual rate for an individual patient in a specific area of the palate, it is necessary to determine whether or not solution is being deposited too quickly by observing for tissue bulging and excessive blanching. If either occurs, continue with the deposition *only after* pausing to allow for diffusion and absorption of the solution from areas of swelling and a return to normal coloration from a stark white appearance when there is excessive blanching. This reduces tissue damage from stretching and allows normal blood flow to return to the area. In either instance, when deposition resumes, the rate should be slowed from the previous rate (less than one cartridge per 3 minutes).

While excessive blanching should be avoided, it is important to observe light blanching in the palate because it confirms that the resisting tissues are nearing their limit for accommodating solution (see Figure 13–20 ■). This gently forces the solution in medial, lateral, anterior, and posterior directions, and, importantly, into the palatal bone. Deposited solution thereafter will be diffusing through bone at the deposition site, into the maxillary dental plexus, and progressing throughout the soft tissues of the entire half of the palate overlying the affected side of the maxillary bone.

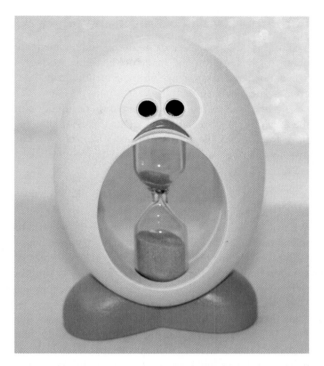

■ **FIGURE 13–19** Deposition Rate for AMSA Nerve Blocks. While the standard deposition rate has been described previously as 1.8 ml over a period of 1 minute (60 seconds), in the AMSA technique this rate is increased to 3 minutes (approximately the time lapsed on a standard egg timer).

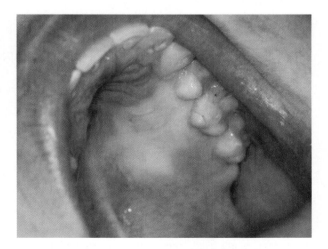

■ **FIGURE 13–20** Blanching with AMSA Nerve Blocks. This pattern of blanching followed the delivery of 1.2 ml of local anesthetic agent for an AMSA nerve block. Note the limited anterior blanching.

Common Causes of Injection Failure

The most common causes of failure include inadequate depths of penetration and inadequate volumes of solution deposited. Inexperience with the technique also decreases success rates, initially.

Other causes include inflammation or infection in the area of deposition and inadequate diffusion of solution. Inadequate anesthesia of the incisors may occur due to overlapping innervation by the contralateral ASA nerve.

Troubleshooting

When AMSA injections are unsuccessful, it is helpful to reevaluate by visualizing and reassessing syringe angulations and depths of penetration, as well as volumes of solution deposited. Penetration site selection is slightly more variable compared with most other techniques. Understanding this variability can be crucial to success. Sites that provide adequate tissue thickness, for example, can accommodate solution much more readily than supposedly ideal sites. If an ideal site appears to lack adequate thickness, an adjacent site that is thicker is not only acceptable but preferable.

Inadequate anesthesia of incisors may occur due to overlapping fibers of the contralateral ASA nerve. An infiltration over the same side central incisor will anesthetize these overlapping fibers.

If solution is flowing in only one direction from the penetration site, posteriorly for example, it may be necessary to allow the diffusion to reach the molars in that case (see Figure 13–20) (follow the blanching to confirm) and then withdraw and choose a slightly more anterior penetration site. Once negative aspiration has been confirmed, blanching should be seen progressing anteriorly.

Technique Modifications and Alternatives

Computer-controlled local anesthetic devices (CCLADs) are ideal for this type of injection because they provide controlled, continuous, and slow rates of deposition. At least one study has indicated higher success rates when these devices are used compared with conventional syringes (Lee et al., 2004).

When administering 4 percent solutions, the total volume delivered should be reduced to no more than 0.9 ml due to the potential for paresthesia (Malamed, 2004). This does not affect the rate of deposition (no less than 3 full minutes for 1/2 cartridge of any 4 percent drug).

Excessive blanching, such as that seen more commonly when administering higher concentrations of epinephrine (1:50,000), should be avoided. Failure to notice and respond to the color of the tissue as it lightens can result in postoperative pain and possible necrosis.

The AMSA may be used as an alternative to the ASA (or IO), MSA, GP, and NP nerve blocks, as well as multiple infiltrations.

Complications

The risk of complications following AMSA injections is minimal. These may include postoperative pain at the site of injection, hematoma, and postoperative edema. When high concentrations of vasoconstrictors are used, necrosis is possible. Some individuals experience an intense burning sensation during deposition of AMSA blocks, regardless of the drug used. This reaction contraindicates the use of AMSA nerve blocks in those individuals.

GREATER PALATINE NERVE BLOCK

Greater palatine nerve blocks (GPBs), also referred to as anterior palatine nerve blocks, are indicated for pain management of palatal soft and osseous tissues distal to the canine in one quadrant.

Field of Anesthesia

Anesthesia will affect the structures innervated by the greater palatine nerve and its terminal branches to include the posterior portion of the hard palate and its overlying soft tissues, anteriorly as far as the first premolar and medially to the midline (Malamed, 2004) (see Figure 13–21 ■ and Appendix 13–2).

Anatomical Factors

The greater palatine nerve branches from the maxillary nerve within the pterygopalatine fossa before traveling inferiorly through the pterygopalatine canal. It exits the canal through the greater palatine foramen on the hard palate of the maxilla. The foramen is located at the junction of the alveolar process of the maxilla and the palatine bone. The greater palatine nerve innervates one side of the posterior portion of the hard palate and its overlying soft tissues. It travels anteriorly as far as the first

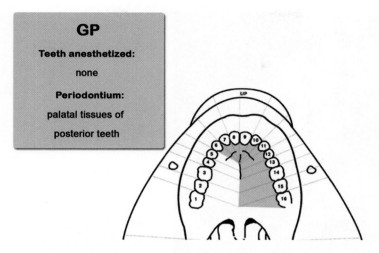

■ FIGURE 13-21   Field of Anesthesia for GP Nerve Blocks. The field of anesthesia for GP nerve blocks is indicated by the shaded area.

premolar and medially to the midline. Terminal fibers overlap the nasopalatine nerve anteriorly.

The location of the greater palatine foramen is variable but can usually be noted palatal to the apices of the second and third maxillary molars, depending on the size and age of the patient. The position may be more posterior than commonly expected. In children, it is often found anterior to typical adult locations, close to the second primary molar.

Anesthesia of the soft palate is not uncommon because the lesser palatine nerve and foramen are located immediately posterior to the greater palatine foramen and may be anesthetized inadvertently when the GP nerve is anesthetized.

Technique Factors

The following information describes key factors for successful GP nerve block injections.

Penetration Site

The optimal penetration site for GP nerve blocks is in the palatal soft tissue slightly anterior to the greater palatine foramen, at the anterior border of the *depression* formed by the foramen. The angle of insertion is perpendicular to the palatal bone at the foramen, with the syringe barrel near the lower lip (see Figure 13–22 ■).

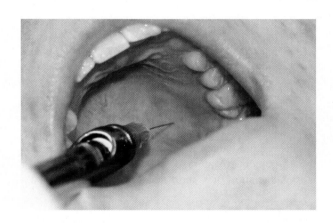

■ FIGURE 13-22   Penetration Site for GP Nerve Blocks. The penetration site for GP nerve blocks is indicated by the needle.

Needle Pathway

The needle advances slowly for 4–10 mm through dense mucosal tissue to make gentle contact with bone. Small vessels and capillaries are present in the tissue.

Deposition Site

The deposition site is anterior to the opening of the anterior palatine foramen (see Figure 13–23 ■).

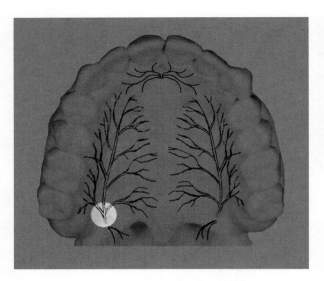

■ **FIGURE 13-23** Deposition Site for GP Nerve Blocks. The deposition site for GP nerve blocks is indicated in the spotlighted area.

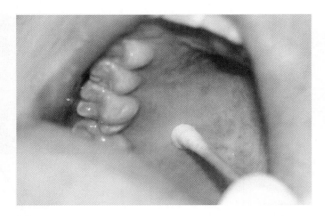

■ **FIGURE 13-24** Locate the Optimum GP Nerve Block Penetration Site. Use a cotton swab to gently palpate the posterior palate near the apices of the second molar. This site will be a soft spongy depression over the greater palatine foramen.

Technique Steps

Apply the basic injection steps outlined in Chapter 11 and summarized in Appendix 11–1.

Needle Selection

A 27 gauge short needle is recommended for this injection, which is consistent with the minimal penetration depths required and a low positive aspiration rate (less than 1 percent) (Malamed, 2004). A 27 gauge short or a 30 gauge short or x-short needle is commonly used.

Injection Procedure

As previously discussed with all palatal injections, discomfort associated with palatal injections can be significantly reduced with the use of pre-anesthesia. Apply the two-step method of topical anesthesia.

To gain access to the site of penetration, ask the patient to tip the head up and slightly away, opening the mouth wide. To locate the penetration site (a soft spongy depression over the greater palatine foramen) use a cotton swab to gently palpate the posterior palate near the apices of the second molar (see Figure 13–24 ■). The penetration site is located at the anterior aspect of the depression. Advance slowly until bone is contacted. Once resistance has been met, withdraw the needle 1 mm. The depth of insertion ranges from 4 to 6 mm and sometimes up to 10 mm. Following a negative aspiration, deposit a minimum of 0.45 ml (1/4 of a cartridge) of an appropriately selected local anesthetic drug (blanching and palatal "sweating" around the needle are common during deposition).

Deposition Rate

The rate of deposition for this injection is 0.4 ml over 30 seconds or approximately 1.8 ml over 2 minutes.

Confirming Anesthesia

Subjective signs of anesthesia for GP nerve block injections include an immediate sense of tightness and numbness of the gingiva on the same side posterior palate following injection. Objective signs include a lack of response to gentle stimulation with an instrument and no pain during the procedure in the expected field of anesthesia.

Common Causes of Injection Failure

The most common causes of anesthetic failure include deposition of solution that is too shallow, too lateral, or too medial to the foramen as well as inadequate volumes of solution.

Other causes include inflammation or infection in the area of deposition.

Troubleshooting

When adequate anesthesia is not achieved, reevaluation is indicated. Start by visualizing, palpating, and reassessing syringe angulations and depths of penetration, as well as volumes of solution deposited. Repeating the injection is almost always sufficient if profound anesthesia is not established.

Technique Modifications and Alternatives

Although rarely administered in young children, when a decision is made to perform the GP in children, the foramen will be located posterior to all the erupted teeth if only primary teeth are present.

Alternatives include the AMSA, palatal infiltrations, PDL injections around the teeth to be treated, and maxillary blocks (which are not described in this text).

Complications

The risk of complications is minimal with this technique. Postprocedural lesions such as herpes are more common in the palate but more frequent in anterior areas. Hematomas are possible, although infrequent, and tend to be minimal when they occur. Although infrequent, ischemia and necrosis occur with greater frequency in the palate than elsewhere in the mouth. They usually require no more than palliative therapy.

CASE MANAGEMENT: Elena Gagarin

Due to her prior experience, a PSA block was administered along with an AMSA nerve block during nitrous oxide administration. 2.8 ml of 2% lidocaine with 1:100,000 epinephrine were administered for both (56 mg of lidocaine and 0.028 mg of epinephrine).

Case Discussion: Diffusion of anesthetic solutions through maxillary bone is usually quite effective but is not as efficient in some individuals. This was the case for Ms. Gagarin. PSA nerve blocks, because they directly expose the nerve membranes to anesthetic solutions, are excellent alternatives to infiltrations for anesthesia of maxillary molars. The AMSA block provides pulpal and periodontal anesthesia of the rest of the teeth in the quadrant as well as nearly all palatal tissues in the quadrant. The number of injections is reduced in this plan because only two are necessary to provide equivalent anesthesia to other combinations of infiltrations or blocks of a hemi-maxilla. Ms. Gagarin was pleased afterward that her speech was unaltered because neither the PSA nor AMSA blocks typically anesthetizes the labial tissues.

CHAPTER QUESTIONS

1. Which *one* of the following statements best describes the deposition site for a nasopalatine nerve block?
   a. The deposition site is within the nasopalatine canal.
   b. The deposition site is near the wall of the incisive canal.
   c. The deposition site is anterior to the opening of the anterior palatine foramen.
   d. The deposition site is near the junction between the vertical alveolar process and the horizontal palatal process.

2. The most common cause of failure for palatal injection techniques is:
   a. Solution is deposited too far from the associated bone or foramen.
   b. Inadequate volumes of solution are deposited.
   c. B only.
   d. Both A and B.

3. The AMSA technique can provide anesthesia for areas traditionally anesthetized by which *one* of the following groups of injections?
   a. ASA, MSA, PSA, NP, and GP
   b. ASA, MSA, NP, and GP
   c. PSA and GP
   d. NP and MSA

4. Which *one* of the following statements is true of NP nerve blocks?
   a. They have the highest rate of positive aspiration in the palate.
   b. They have the second-highest rate of positive aspiration in the palate.
   c. They provide more durable anesthesia compared with other palatal techniques.
   d. They provide bilateral anesthesia.

5. Which *one* of the following is an important consideration in all palatal LA procedures?
   a. Always apply topical anesthetic for 1 to 2 minutes.
   b. Always administer solutions slowly.
   c. Always use patch anesthetics.

6. AMSA nerve blocks provide bilateral anesthesia of palatal tissues at least 20 percent of the time.
   a. True
   b. False

REFERENCES

Blanton P., Jeske A. (2003, June). The key to profound local anesthesia—Neuroanatomy. *Journal of the American Dental Association, 134,* 755–756.

Burns, Y., Reader, A., Nusstein, J., Beck, M., & Weaver, J. (2004). Anesthetic efficacy of the palatal-anterior superior alveolar injection. *Journal of the American Dental Association, 135*(9), 1269–1276.

Chudler, C. H. Pain and why it hurts. Neuroscience for Kids. Available at http://faculty.washington.edu/chudler/pain.html.

Deardorff, W. W. (2007). Modern ideas: The gate control theory of chronic pain. Available at http://www.spine-health.com/conditions/chronic-pain/modern-ideas-gate-control-theory-chronic-pain.

Fehrenbach, M. J., & Herring, S. W. (2007) *Illustrated anatomy of the head and neck* (3rd ed.). St. Louis: Saunders Elsevier.

Friedman, M. J., & Hochman, M. N. (1998). The AMSA injection: A new concept for local anesthesia of maxillary teeth using a computer-controlled injection system. *Qunitessence International, 29*(5), 297–303.

Friedman, M. J., & Hochman, M. N. (1999). P-ASA block injection: A new palatal technique to anesthetize maxillary anterior teeth. *Journal of Esthetic Dentistry, 11*(2), 63–71.

Friedman, M. J., & Hochman, M. N. (2001). Using AMSA and P-ASA nerve blocks for esthetic restorative dentistry. *General Dentistry, 49*(5), 506–511.

Jastak, J. T., Yagiela, J. A., & Donaldson, D. (1995) *Local anesthesia of the oral cavity.* Philadelphia: Saunders.

Lee, S., Reader, A., Nusstein, J., Beck, M., & Weaver, J. (2004). Anesthetic efficacy of the anterior middle superior alveolar (AMSA) injection. *Journal of the American Dental Society of Anesthesia, 51*(3), 80–89.

Loomer, P. M., & Perry, D. A. (2004). Computer-controlled delivery versus syringe delivery of local anesthetic injections for therapeutic scaling and root planing. *Journal of the American Dental Association, 135*(3), 358–365.

Malamed, S. F. (2004). *Handbook of local anesthesia* (5th ed.). St. Louis: Elsevier Mosby.

Sculean, A., Kasaj, A., Berakdar, M., & Willershausen, B. (2004). A comparison of the traditional injection and a new anesthesia technique (the Wand® for non-surgical periodontal therapy). *Periodontal Practice Today, 1*(4), 363–368.

Shimada, K., & Gasser, R. F. (1989). *The Anatomical Record: Advances in Integrative Anatomy and Evolutionary Biology, 224*(1), 177–122.

Wong, J. A. (2001). Adjuncts to local anesthesia: Separating fact from fiction. *Journal of the Canadian Dental Association, 67,* 391–397.

Summary of Palatal Injections

Nerve Block	Needle	Penetration Site	Deposition Site — Depth of Insertion	Deposition Site — Angle of Insertion	Deposition Site — Target	Dose*	Field of Anesthesia See Appendix 13–2
Nasopalatine (NP)	Extra-Short or Short 30/27 gauge	Just lateral to incisive papilla at widest aspect see Figure 13–2	Infiltration: 3–5 mm Block: 6–10 mm	Approach at 45 degrees to anterior palate bevel toward palate	Incisive foramen beneath incisive papilla see Figure 13–3	≤0.4 ml	*Teeth anesthetized:* None *Periodontium:* Palatal to incisors and canines
Palatial Anterior Superior Alveolar (PASA)	Extra-Short or Short 30/27 gauge	Infiltration: just lateral to incisive papilla Block: center of papilla on midline see Figure 13–10	6–10 mm	Approach at 45 degree angle bevel toward palate	Beneath incisive papilla, slightly into incisive foramen see Figure 13–11	1.4–1.8 ml	*Teeth anesthetized:* Central, lateral, canine *Periodontium:* To affected teeth
Anterior Middle Superior Alveolar (AMSA)	Extra-Short or Short 30/27 gauge	At the junction of the horizontal & vertical aspects of the palate, inline with the bisection of the free gingival margin of the premolars. MUST have adequate tissue thickness see Figure 13–15	4–7 mm	From opposite side of mouth at right angle to alveolar process bevel toward palate	Above apex, between premolars on the palatal side see Figure 13–16	0.9–1.8 ml w/ 4% solutions 0.7–0.9 ml	*Teeth anesthetized:* Central, lateral, canine, premolars *Periodontium:* To incisors and premolars, palatal to molars

		Depth of Insertion	Angle of Insertion		Teeth anesthetized:
Greater Palatine (GP)	Extra-Short or Short 30/27 gauge	In the anterior depression of the GP foramen, at junction of palatine bone and alveolar process above and lingual to second molar. see Figure 13-21	From opposite side of mouth at right angle to target area bevel toward palate	0.4-0.6 ml	None
		Target Greater palatine foramen see Figure 13-22			**Periodontium:** Palatal tissues of posterior teeth
		Depth of Insertion	**Angle of Insertion**		**Teeth anesthetized:**
Local infiltration injections	Extra-Short or Short 30/27 gauge	In palatal mucosa lingual to tooth	Directed toward apex of tooth bevel toward bone	0.2-0.4 ml	None
		Target Selected soft tissue, gingival or apex of tooth			**Periodontium:** At injection site

*Dose volumes provided are minimum recommendations for pulpal anesthesia.
Modified from: 1) Malamed SF, Handbook of local anesthesia, ed 5, St Louis, 2004, Mosby; 2) Jastak JT, Yagiela JA, Donaldson D. Local anesthesia of the oral cavity. Philidelphia, 19.

Field of Anesthesia

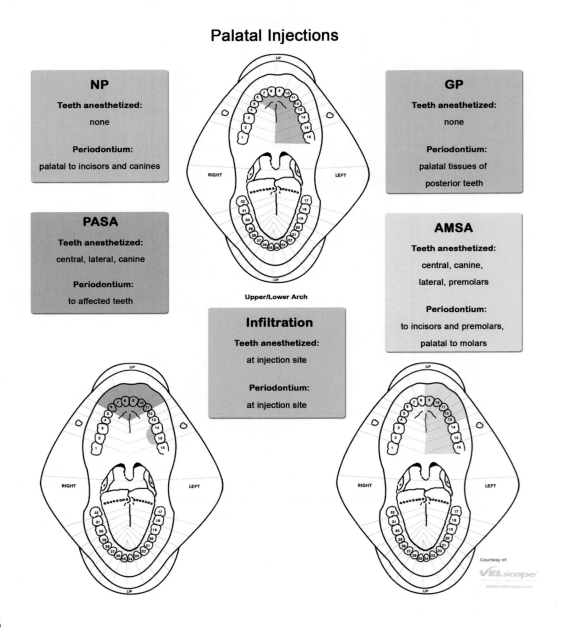

Palatal Injections

NP

Teeth anesthetized:
none

Periodontium:
palatal to incisors and canines

GP

Teeth anesthetized:
none

Periodontium:
palatal tissues of
posterior teeth

PASA

Teeth anesthetized:
central, lateral, canine

Periodontium:
to affected teeth

AMSA

Teeth anesthetized:
central, canine,
lateral, premolars

Periodontium:
to incisors and premolars,
palatal to molars

Infiltration

Teeth anesthetized:
at injection site

Periodontium:
at injection site

Upper/Lower Arch

Courtesy of:
VELscope
www.velscope.com

Chapter 14

Injections for Mandibular Pain Control

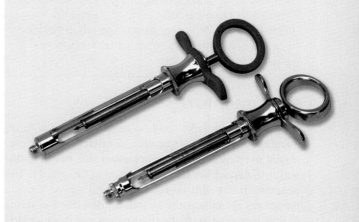

CASE STUDY: Lee Chung

Lee Chung is a healthy mother of five who wanted both sides of her lower jaw treated at the same appointment due to her hectic schedule. It had been explained to her that this might cause considerable alteration of function but she had insisted that she did not have time to return to the office for another appointment. All other treatment had been completed on previous visits. The first premolar and anterior teeth on the right mandible, which had been treated previously, required follow-up with local anesthesia. The left mandible was the only untreated quadrant and it also required local anesthesia.

INTRODUCTION

Anatomic landmarks and considerations for each mandibular injection technique discussed will be presented in reference to the **penetration site, needle pathway,** and **deposition site** as described in Chapter 11. The penetration site will be related to hard and soft tissue landmarks. Needle pathway will be described in terms of the types of tissue that will be penetrated by or located in the vicinity of the needle, including mucosa, superficial fascia, muscle, vessels, nerves, and bone. The deposition site will be described in terms of the tissues at or near the target and in relation to specific landmarks.

MANDIBULAR INJECTION TECHNIQUES

This chapter will discuss mandibular injection techniques commonly used in dentistry. Key elements for each mandibular injection discussed are summarized in Appendix 14–1. Common variations and precautions will be discussed where applicable.

INFERIOR ALVEOLAR NERVE BLOCK

Inferior alveolar nerve blocks (IANBs), also referred to as mandibular or lower blocks, are indicated for pain management of mandibular teeth in one quadrant.

Field of Anesthesia

IA nerve blocks anesthetize the structures innervated by the IA nerve and typically the lingual nerve on the injected side, to include the mandibular teeth to the midline, soft tissues of the inferior portion of the ramus and body of the mandible, the lower lip and buccal periodontium of the premolars and incisors, the lingual soft tissues and periodontium, the floor of the mouth, and the anterior two-thirds of the tongue (see Figure 14–1 ■). Box 14–1 provides further discussion on lingual nerve anesthesia.

Anatomical Factors

The inferior alveolar nerve is the largest branch of the mandibular division of the trigeminal nerve. It branches from the posterior division of the mandibular nerve in the

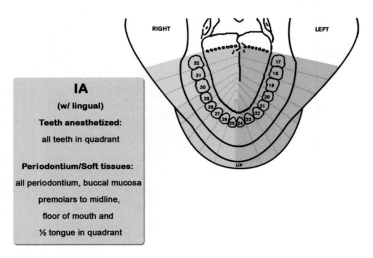

■ FIGURE 14–1 Field of Anesthesia for Inferior Alveolar Nerve Blocks. Anesthesia will occur in hard and soft structures of half the mandible with the exception of the buccal tissues in the molar region.

infratemporal space, then travels medial to the lateral pterygoid muscle and passes through the pterygomandibular space between the sphenomandibular ligament and the medial surface of the ramus of the mandible. It then enters the mandibular foramen and canal.

The infratemporal and pterygomandibular spaces also contain arteries and veins. The maxillary artery, the terminal branch of the external carotid artery, traverses the infratemporal space either superficial or deep to the lateral pterygoid muscle and divides into several branches, including the inferior alveolar artery. The inferior alveolar artery descends through the pterygomandibular space anterior to the nerve and enters the mandibular foramen along with the inferior alveolar nerve. The inferior alveolar vein travels within the mandibular canal with the inferior alveolar artery and inferior alveolar nerve. It exits through the mandibular foramen, and travels medioanteriorly to the inferior alveolar artery, through the pterygomandibular and infratemporal spaces and drains into the pterygoid plexus of veins located in the infratemporal space.

There are three key intraoral landmarks for successful IA injections, the *pterygomandibular raphe,* the *coronoid notch* on the anterior border of the ramus of the mandible, and the *internal oblique ridge* on the medial surface of the mandible close to the molars and continuing posteriorly. The purpose of locating these landmarks is to limit the areas into which penetrations are made. This allows the tips of needles to end up as close to inferior alveolar nerves as possible, once solution is deposited.

The mucosa of the pterygomandibular fold overlies the **pterygomandibular raphe,** which is the attachment of the buccinator muscle to the superior constrictor muscle of the pharynx. The significance of the raphe is that it represents the *medial* extent of the area into which penetration is made. In other words, penetration must be made slightly lateral to the raphe. Penetration that is medial to the raphe is likely to result in an injection that places the needle tip too far *posterior* to the ideal site for depositing solution. The appearance of the raphe (observed under the fold) will vary significantly among patients. It can appear quite distinct in some individuals and nearly nonexistent in others. It can appear to be nondistinct but can then become more obvious when patients open wide. The raphe is easier to visualize when individuals open their mouths, although in some individuals the raphe is barely detectable, regardless (see Figure 14–2 ▪). The architecture of the raphe and the

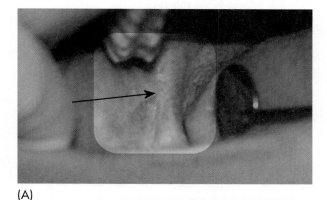

(A)

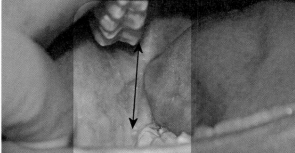

(B)

▪ **FIGURE 14–2** The Pterygomandibular Raphe. A—The arrow identifies the pterygomandibular raphe (observed under the fold). B—The pterygomandibular raphe represents the medial extent of the penetration site and the pterygomandibular triangle.

thickness of the mucosa overlying it are primarily responsible for obscuring the raphe when it is not clearly visible.

The second key intraoral feature is the **coronoid notch** of the mandible. The significance of the notch is that it defines the *height* of the injection. The ideal height is slightly higher than the deepest concavity of the notch. In other words, penetrations that are above or below this point are likely to place the tips of needles too far *superior* or *inferior* to the ideal site for depositing solution. This landmark is used to identify a height of penetration that allows for advancement of the needle to a site *directly above* the mandibular foramen (Fehrenbach & Herring, 2007; Jastak et al., 1995; Malamed, 2004). It should be noted that deposition of solution below this site results in more failures compared with deposition above the site.

The term *coronoid notch* is used in dentistry to define the concavity on the anterior border of the ramus of the mandible (see Figure 14–3 ■). It extends inferiorly from the external oblique ridge to the coronoid process superiorly. The greatest concavity of the coronoid notch is located approximately 6 to 10 mm superior to the mandibular occlusal plane. See Box 14–2 for further discussion on the term *coronoid notch*.

The third key intraoral landmark for IA nerve block injections is the **internal oblique ridge.** The significance of the ridge is that it represents the *lateral* extent of the area into which penetration is made. By penetrating well medial to this landmark, premature contact of the tip of the needle with the bone of the mandible is avoided (see Figure 14–4 ■). Not only can premature contact be uncomfortable but it prevents further penetration to the ideal site for depositing solution. It also risks barbing the needle. The internal oblique ridge is a posterior and superior extension of the mylohyoid line, forming the medial border of the retromolar triangle (see Figure 14–5 ■). It represents the most *medial* surface of the mandible at the inferior aspect of the pterygomandibular sulcus (see Figure 14–6 ■). Penetrating too far lateral can result in premature contact with bone. Figures 14–7 ■ and Figure 14–8 ■ contrast an ideal penetration and a penetration too far lateral.

Box 14–2 **Terminology: Origin and Use of the Terms *Coronoid* and *Coronoid Notch***

The origin of the word *coronoid* relates to its Greek root meaning *crown* or *shaped like a crown*, which describes this bony feature of the mandible (*Taber's Cyclopedic Medical Dictionary* [*Taber's*], 2005).

In dentistry, reference to the *coronoid notch* is frequently made in relation to IA injections. Interestingly, the term coronoid notch is used primarily in dentistry. Medical references define the region containing the notch as the anterior border of the ramus of the mandible without making specific reference to its notch feature.

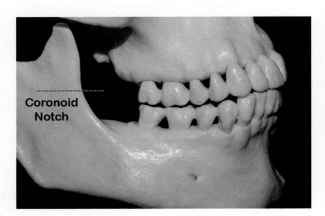

■ FIGURE 14–3 The Coronoid Notch. Slightly above the deepest concavity of the notch on the anterior border of the mandible identifies the approximate height of the mandibular foramen.

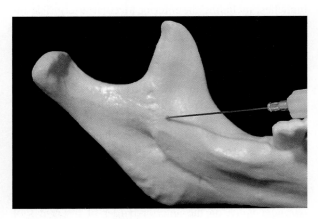

■ FIGURE 14–4 Premature Contact Near the Internal Oblique Ridge. Premature contact of the tip of the needle with the bone of the mandible, slightly superior and posterior to the internal oblique ridge. The needle needs to be relocated in order to penetrate to the mandibular foramen.

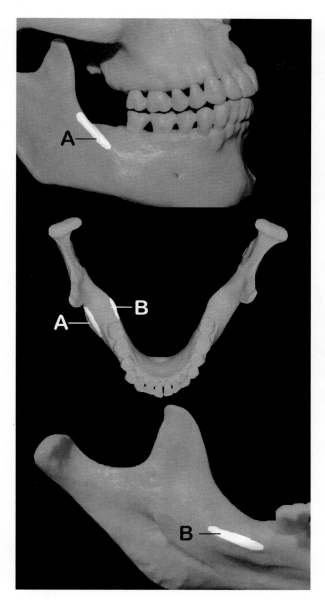

■ **FIGURE 14–5** Bony Landmarks: Internal and External Oblique Ridges. Palpating these structures provides guidance to the location of the correct penetration site. A—The external oblique ridge. B—The internal oblique ridge.

Finally, the location of the mandibular foramen is variable and it may be located at, below, or above the mandibular molar occlusal plane. Panoramic radiographs can be helpful when locating the mandibular foramen (Blanton & Jeske, 2003; Malamed, 2004).

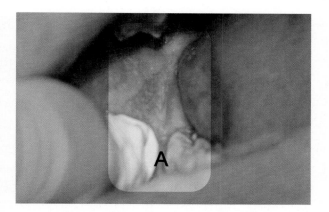

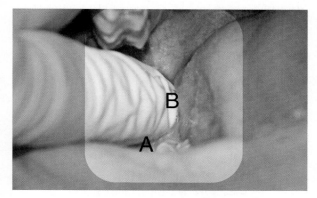

■ **FIGURE 14–6** Soft Tissue Landmarks: External and Internal Oblique Ridges. A—Palpation of the external oblique ridge. B—Palpation of the internal oblique ridge.

Technique Factors

The following information describes key factors for successful IA nerve blocks.

Penetration Site

The penetration site for an IA nerve block can be described as *slightly* lateral to the pterygomandibular raphe (see Figure 14–7) at a height that is *2 to 3 millimeters* superior to the greatest concavity of the coronoid notch, and *well* medial of the internal oblique ridge.

Needle Pathway

The needle advances along the lateral aspect of the pterygomandibular raphe through thin mucosal tissue and fibers of the buccinator muscle into the pterygomandibular

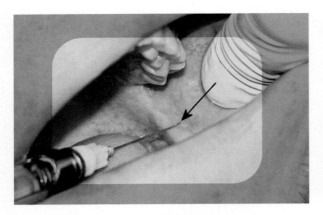

■ **FIGURE 14–7** Penetration Site for IA Nerve Blocks. The optimal penetration site for IANB is *slightly* lateral to the pterygomandibular raphe, at the depth of the pterygomandibular sulcus.

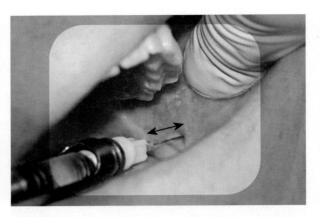

■ **FIGURE 14–8** Penetration Site Too Far Lateral. Penetration sites too far lateral to the pterygomandibular raphe can result in premature contact on the medial surface of the ramus.

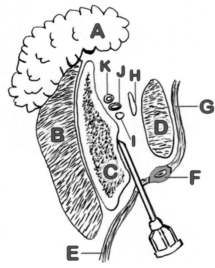

(A)

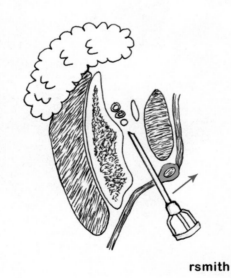

rsmith

(B)

■ **FIGURE 14–9** Needle Pathway for IA Nerve Blocks. A—Demonstrates premature bony contact. B—Demonstrates an optimal needle pathway. Key: A—parotid gland, B—masseter muscle, C—ramus of mandible, D—medial pterygoid muscle, E—buccinator muscle, F—pterygomandibular raphe, G—superior constrictor muscle, H—sphenomandibular ligament, I—lingual nerve, J—inferior alveolar nerve, K—inferior alveolar artery/vein.

space. The needle passes lateral to the medial pterygoid muscle, lingual nerve, and sphenomandibular ligament, and superior to the lingula and mandibular foramen (see Figure 14–9 ■).

Deposition Site

The deposition site is 1 mm lateral to the medial aspect of the ramus and above the mandibular foramen (see Figure 14–10 ■ and Figure 14–11 ■).

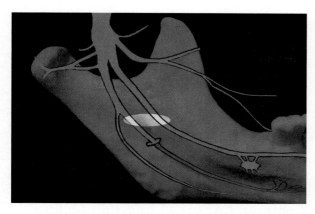

■ **FIGURE 14–10**   Deposition Site for IA Nerve Blocks—Medial View. The deposition site for IA nerve blocks is indicated by the spotlight.

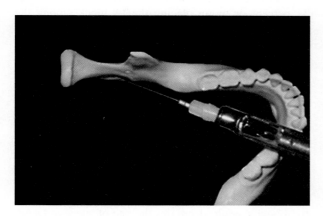

■ **FIGURE 14–11**   Deposition Site for IA Nerve Blocks—Superior View. The deposition site for IA nerve blocks is superior to the mandibular foramen as indicated by the needle. Note the barrel of the syringe is over the contralateral premolars.

Technique Steps

Apply the basic injection steps outlined in Chapter 11 and summarized in Appendix 11–1.

Needle Selection

A 25 gauge long needle is recommended, consistent with the significant depths of penetration required and the high rate of positive aspiration (10 to 15 percent) in IA nerve blocks. A 27 gauge long needle is acceptable and is used most commonly for this injection (see Box 14–3).

Box 14–3   Needle Selection for IANB (25 Gauge vs. 27 Gauge Needles)

Needles in dentistry are flexible. The higher the gauge of a needle, the greater its flexibility and deflection in tissues (Jastak et al., 1995). In areas where tissues are more fibrous or in which greater depths must be penetrated in order to place solution close to nerves, the risk of needle deflection increases. A 25 gauge needle will deflect less compared with a 27 gauge needle, which will deflect less than a 30 gauge needle.

Despite increased deflection, a majority of clinicians select 27 gauge needles out of concern for patient comfort even though increased discomfort with larger diameter needles has not been demonstrated (Hamburg, 1972; Malamed, 2006). Nevertheless, 27 gauge needles are perfectly acceptable as evidenced by the long-term safety record of dental local anesthesia, including a majority of inferior alveolar blocks having been administered with 27 gauge needles. The probability of deflection is an even greater issue in Gow-Gates mandibular nerve blocks (described later in this chapter) where typical penetration depths are equal to or greater than the depths for inferior alveolar nerve blocks (Malamed, 2004).

Injection Procedure

Gain access to the site of penetration by retracting the cheek laterally, avoiding overly aggressive retraction, which can displace soft tissue landmarks, particularly the penetration site. Hold the mucosa taut by keeping the index finger or thumb on the anterior border of the ramus at the depth of the coronoid notch (see Figure 14–12 ■) or on the internal oblique ridge. If the internal oblique ridge is selected as the location of the finger or thumb, it is important to avoid needle contamination and needlestick injury, which are more likely to occur whenever fingers remain in close proximity to penetration sites (see Box 14–4).

The syringe barrel is positioned at the labial commissure over the premolars on the contralateral side of the mouth. The barrel remains parallel to and above the occlusal plane of the mandibular molars throughout the injection (see Figure 14–12). After gentle needle

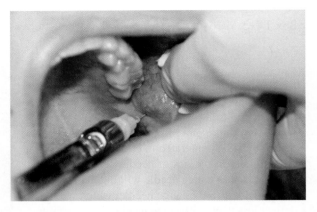

■ FIGURE 14–12　Retraction and Syringe Angulations for IA Nerve Block. To establish firm retraction, hold the mucosa taut by keeping the index finger or thumb on the anterior border of the ramus at the depth of the coronoid notch. The syringe barrel is positioned at the labial commissure over the premolars on the contralateral side of the mouth. The barrel remains parallel to and above the occlusal plane of the mandibular molars throughout the injection.

Box 14–4　Needlestick Safety Consideration

The risk of needlestick injury is greater whenever the finger is held on the internal oblique ridge. Selecting a site at the depth of the coronoid notch on the ramus can decrease this risk by providing more clearance during initial needle approach. Alternative retraction techniques may be applied once an optimum penetration site is determined. See Chapter 12, "Injections for Maxillary Pain Control," Figure 12–30 for examples.

---

contact with bone, which confirms the deposition site near the medial aspect of the ramus, withdraw 1 mm. Following negative aspiration, slowly deposit a minimum of about 1.5 ml (3/4 of a cartridge) of any appropriately selected local anesthetic drug over no less than 1 minute. Depositing too much solution ahead of the needle prior to reaching the deposition site should be avoided. After depositing the solution, slowly withdraw the needle parallel to the pathway of insertion to avoid soft tissue trauma. See Box 14–5 for further discussion of drug doses for the IA nerve blocks injection.

Confirming Anesthesia

Subjective signs of anesthesia for IA nerve blocks include a sense of numbness on the injected side, including soft tissues of the inferior portion of the ramus and body of the mandible, the lower lip, and the buccal periodontium of the premolars and incisors. Typically, patients will report anesthesia of the lingual soft tissues and anterior two-thirds of the tongue as well.

Objective signs include a lack of response to gentle stimulation with an instrument and no pain during the procedure for soft tissues or mandibular teeth.

Common Causes of Injection Failure

IA nerve blocks are considered by some to be among the most difficult injections from a technical standpoint. Published failure rates support this and vary from 10 to 31 percent or more, placing the IA block among the highest failure rates in dentistry, regardless of whether figuring from the high or low end of the failure range (Blanton & Jeske, 2003; Hamburg, 1972; Jastak et al., 1994; Malamed, 2004).

There are several causes of failure of IA nerve blocks. Greater anatomical variation and the need for deeper needle penetrations are key factors to understanding these failures. The most common specific failures are technique-related such as depositing solution too far away from the foramen (too shallow, too medial, too posterior, and, especially, *too inferior*). Shallow deposition of solution (less than 20 to 25 mm for a typical adult) decreases the rate of success. Deposition medial to soft tissue barriers such as the sphenomandibular ligament can block diffusion of solution to the IA nerve.

Most variations in anatomical form can be accommodated with an understanding of basic technique. Figure 14–13 ■ demonstrates premature contact on the lingula; needle penetration more medial or slight medial deflection of the pterygomandibular raphe with needle insertion can help to avoid or clear this obstruction.

Other anatomic factors also contribute to failure, including accessory, aberrant, and ectopic innervations. These are discussed in detail in Chapter 16, "Troubleshooting Inadequate Anesthesia." Among these, midline overlapping of branches of incisive, mental, and mylohyoid nerves is a common occurrence that provides additional innervation of the incisor teeth and associated soft tissue from the side opposite the injection (Blanton & Jeske, 2003). This is an example of what is

Box 14–5   Considerations of Drug
Volumes for IANB

The inferior alveolar nerve is the largest division of the trigeminal nerve. As a large, heavily myelinated nerve, greater volumes of solution are required to flood enough length of its membrane in order to temporarily disable saltatory conduction. In other words, if an insufficient length of the IA nerve is flooded with solution, impulses will have enough energy to pass through several nodes (even if those particular nodes are effectively anesthetized) to the first nodal area of the IA nerve that is not affected by the anesthetic solution. Drug volumes in IA nerve blocks are greater compared with many other techniques. The following factors are helpful to consider when determining volumes to administer:

Factor 1: Nerve Anatomy
The large diameter of the IA nerve at the site of deposition requires a minimum of 1.5 ml of solution to provide adequate diffusion through the nerve and profound anesthesia for the typical patient.

Factor 2: "Budgeting" for the Buccal Nerve Block
Following the recommended dose of anesthetic drug for an IA nerve block, 1.5 ml, about 0.3 ml of solution remains in the cartridge. This is an adequate volume to complete a buccal nerve block when needed, if the needle has not barbed. If the needle appears to be barbed on withdrawal, it should be replaced before proceeding with the buccal nerve block.

Factor 3: Multiple Cartridges as Initial Dose
Long procedures or past patient experience may establish a need for additional initial volumes of anesthetic solution. Despite the effectiveness of this initial dose, some clinicians administer more than one cartridge for IA nerve blocks every time, regardless of the length of procedure or past experience. Malamed recommends that clinicians ". . . *minimize drug doses and use the smallest clinically effective dose*" (Malamed, 2004).

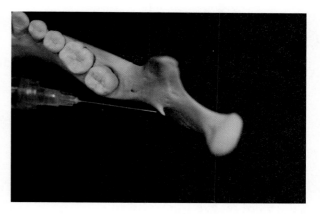

■ **FIGURE 14–13** Impact of Anatomical Variations. Premature contact on the lingula requires redirection of the needle and may have been prevented by needle penetration more medial or by slightly deflecting the pterygomandibular raphe medially.

actually be considered less of a deviation and more of a variation.

In some individuals, the medial aspect of the penetration site for IA nerve blocks may be difficult to identify due to an obscure pterygomandibular raphe. This can lead to inaccurate assessments of the penetration site and inadequate anesthesia. For further discussion on anatomical variations of consequence in IA nerve blocks, see Box 14–6 and Chapter 16.

Troubleshooting

When IA nerve blocks are unsuccessful, it is helpful to reevaluate by visualizing, palpating, and checking radiographs and to reassess syringe angulations and depths of penetration. Safe increases in the volume of solution administered should also be considered.

In some instances, adequate diffusion of solution is impossible due to anatomic obstructions. Alternate nerve blocks (discussed later in this chapter) or supplemental techniques, such as the periodontal ligament injection, are indicated when this is the case (see Chapter 15, "Injections for Supplemental Pain Control") because their success is not restricted by these barriers.

If anatomical variances are encountered, documenting them as well as any modifications that were implemented to overcome them can be helpful at subsequent appointments.

known as accessory innervation, which is an expected pattern of innervation that deviates from what is considered normal. Midline overlapping of fibers in the mandible is fairly common, so much so that it could

Absence of a Pterygomandibular Raphe

At least one study demonstrates a complete absence of the pterygomandibular raphe in a significant percentage of individuals. In 36 percent of raphes reviewed, there was a continuation of the buccinator and superior pharyngeal constrictor muscles with no obvious presence of a pterygomandibular raphe (Malamed, 2006).

Cervical Nerve Innervation to Mandibular Teeth

Cervical nerves have been described as providing accessory innervation to mandibular teeth in the past. A more recent study demonstrated that accessory cervical innervation of the molars and premolars is unlikely, however still possible. The controversy remains unresolved (Blanton & Jeske, 2003).

Bifid and Ectopic IA Nerves

Only 60 of 6,000 panoramic radiographs studied identified the presence of bifid IA nerves and ectopic mandibular canals (Jastak et al., 1995; Langlais, Broadus, & Glass, 1985). This relatively rare variation was found to be both unilateral and bilateral.

Sensory fibers of the mylohyoid nerve, an efferent nerve to the mylohyoid and anterior digastric muscles, can provide a small portion of the pulpal innervation of mandibular teeth, especially the mandibular molars (Stein, Brueckner, & Milliner, 2007). A **mylohyoid nerve block** can be a useful supplement to IA blocks that appear to be profound but prove to be inadequate (see Box 14–7, Figure 14–14 ■).

Technique Modifications and Alternatives

Due to variations in anatomical landmarks, slight technique adjustments are frequently necessary. One common technique challenge occurs when premature contact is made with bone on the medial surface of the ramus, prior to reaching the optimum deposition site. This is referred to as **premature contact** (see Figure 14–13).

If bony resistance is met immediately after penetration, it is probable that penetration was too low and/or too lateral to the pterygomandibular raphe. If this occurs, withdraw the needle completely, re-evaluate the anatomical landmarks, and proceed by repenetrating at the adjusted site.

If premature contact with bone occurs at less than one-half the penetration depth, withdraw the needle to a more superficial depth and reposition the syringe barrel anteriorly over the contralateral canine or lateral incisor before re-advancing the needle. If no further resistance is encountered, reposition the syringe barrel back over the premolars and advance the needle until contact with bone (resistance) occurs at optimum depth.

When no contact is encountered with bone at the target depth, withdraw the needle at least halfway and reposition the syringe barrel posteriorly over the molars. Advance until bone is contacted. If bone is not encountered after this adjustment, *do not* deposit anesthetic. Withdraw the needle and consider alternate techniques to achieve inferior alveolar nerve anesthesia.

Examples of variations in the form of the mandible are demonstrated in Figure 14–15 ■, Figure 14–16 ■, and Figure 14–17 ■.

Alternatives for IA nerve blocks include Gow-Gates nerve blocks (GG), Akinosi (Vazirani-Akinosi) nerve blocks (VA), periodontal ligament (PDL) and intraosseous injections, and incisive nerve blocks (if treatment is

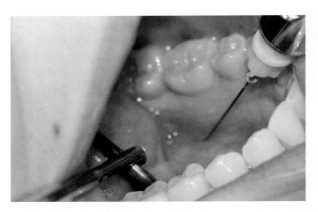

■ **FIGURE 14–14** Penetration Site for Mylohyoid Nerve Blocks. The penetration site for mylohyoid nerve blocks is indicated by the needle.

Box 14–7   Mylohyoid Nerve Blocks

Mylohyoid nerve blocks are indicated for supplemental pain management during procedures involving mandibular molars when IA blocks fail to provide profound anesthesia (Malamed, 2004).

Field of Anesthesia

The mylohyoid nerve is primarily an efferent nerve although it has been recognized that it frequently provides sensory fibers to mandibular teeth (Stein et al., 2007). The sensory innervation of the mylohyoid nerve is an accessory innervation, the extent of which is limited to providing only a minor portion of the innervation of these teeth (Stein et al., 2007). The nerve is frequently blocked during inferior alveolar blocks but anesthetic solution may be prevented from reaching the mylohyoid nerve due to the location of its branching from the mandibular nerve and due to anatomic obstructions such as the pterygomandibular fascia and sphenomandibular ligament (Stein et al., 2007).

Anatomical Factors

The mylohyoid nerve is a branch of the third division of the trigeminal nerve, providing efferent fibers to the mylohyoid muscle and the anterior belly of the digastric.

Technique Factors

The following information describes key factors for successful mylohyoid nerve blocks.

Penetration Site

The penetration site is located in the lingual mucosa below the apex of the tooth immediately posterior to the tooth in question (see Figure 14–14).

Needle Pathway

The needle advances through thin mucosal tissues to the apical area of the tooth just posterior to the one in question.

Deposition Site

The deposition site is at the mesiolingual apex of the tooth just posterior to the one in question.

Technique Steps

Apply the basic injection steps outlined in Chapter 11 and summarized in Appendix 11–1.

Needle Selection

A 25 or 27 gauge long needle is common following IA injections. If administered separately, a 27 gauge short may be used.

Injection Procedure

To gain access to the site of penetration, retract the tongue and approach from the opposite side. Penetrate below the apex of the tooth immediately posterior to the tooth in question and advance until resistance is met (bony contact). The insertion depth is anywhere from 3 to 5 mm. Following a negative aspiration, slowly (20 seconds) deposit a minimum of 0.6 ml of solution (1/3 of a cartridge).

Confirming Anesthesia

Subjective signs of anesthesia for mylohyoid nerve blocks include a sense of numbness of the tissues lingual to the mandibular molars. Objective signs include a lack of response to gentle stimulation with an instrument and no pain during procedures involving pulpal tissues of the mandibular molars (when performed after IA nerve blocks).

Common Causes of Injection Failure

Mylohyoid nerve block failures are rare and occur primarily due to operator error in assessing depths of penetration and deposition sites.

Troubleshooting

Mylohyoid nerve blocks have little purpose in dental local anesthesia other than as supplements to IA blocks. Although failure is therefore not a particular issue, reassessment of the penetration and deposition sites and of the volumes of solution used may be helpful.

Technique Modifications and Alternatives

Alternatives to mylohyoid nerve blocks are essentially alternatives to inferior alveolar blocks, including Gow-Gates nerve blocks, Vazirani-Akinosi blocks, and intraosseous injections, including the PDL.

Complications

Complications following mylohyoid nerve blocks are rare and include bleeding, hematoma, and postoperative discomfort.

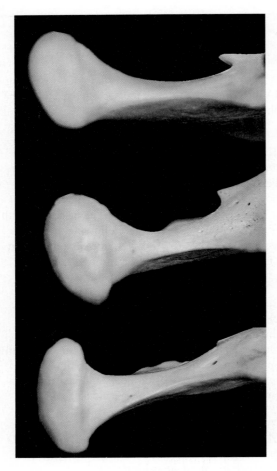

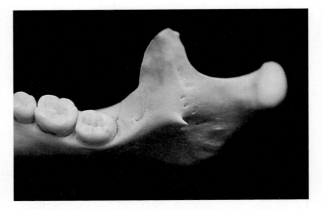

■ **FIGURE 14–16** Anatomical Variances of the Ramus—Medial View. When viewed from medial and superior view, the prominence of the internal oblique ridge and the lingula are clearly evident.

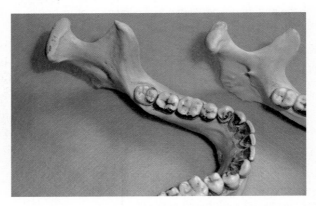

■ **FIGURE 14–15** Anatomical Variances of the Ramus—Superior View. Premature contact can be related to prominence of the medial surface of the ramus at the internal oblique ridge and variations in the flare of the lingula anterior to the deposition site. Note the increasing flare and prominence of the lingula from the bottom up.

■ **FIGURE 14–17** Anatomical Variances—Flare of the Ramus. Variations in the flare of the mandible can impact angulations for IA nerve blocks. Note the differences in both the overall size of the examples and the degree of lateral flare. Insertion angulations may need to be adjusted to reach the optimum deposition site.

limited to teeth located anterior to the mental foramen), or mental nerve blocks (if treatment is limited to buccal soft tissues anterior to the mental foramen). Infiltration injections for incisors may provide pulpal anesthesia depending on the density and thickness of the cortical bone over each tooth. The intraosseous and periodontal ligament injection techniques are discussed in Chapter 15.

Complications

The IA injection has a 10 to 15 percent positive aspiration rate. This is the highest rate of all injections described due to the presence of the inferior alveolar artery and veins at the mandibular foramen and the frequent presence of the maxillary artery in the lower pterygomandibular space. When present in this inferior location, the maxillary artery has been demonstrated to be located, at times, immediately above the level of the mandibular foramen (Blanton & Jeske, 2003). Some authorities recommend avoiding higher deposition sites on the medial ramus for this reason while others recommend these higher locations because they are related to increased rates of success (Blanton & Jeske, 2003; Wong, 2001).

Post-injection muscle soreness or limitation of mandibular movement can occur due to localized injury to muscle fibers at the site of injection. This is referred to as **trismus.** The risk of trismus increases with the number of needle penetrations.

Paresthesia (prolonged anesthesia) can occur following IA nerve blocks but it is usually transient. Studies of the risks of paresthesia have suggested many causes but have largely failed to identify any specific causes.

If anesthetic solution is inadvertently deposited into the body of the parotid gland, it is possible to anesthetize branches of the facial nerve (VII). Drooping of the upper lip and inability to close the eyelid on the injected side are signs of facial nerve anesthesia, which usually lasts only as long as the anesthetic effect on other tissues. In some individuals, branches of the facial nerve lie directly in the insertion pathway for IA nerve blocks and facial nerve anesthesia in those instances is unavoidable (Jastak et al., 1995).

Postoperative soft tissue self-injury (lip/cheek biting) may occur following appointments where anesthesia was used. It is important to remind patients, especially small children and their caretakers, to monitor for postanesthetic lip chewing. See Chapter 17, "Local Anesthesia Complications and Management," for additional discussion and management protocol.

LINGUAL NERVE BLOCK

Lingual nerve blocks (LNBs) are indicated for pain management during procedures that involve the lingual soft tissues of the mandible.

Field of Anesthesia

The lingual nerve provides anesthesia to the lingual soft tissues, the floor of the mouth, and the anterior two-thirds of the tongue (to the midline) (see Figure 14–18 ■).

Anatomical Factors

The lingual nerve is located in close proximity to the inferior alveolar nerve and is usually located medial and anterior to it.

Technique Factors

The following information describes key factors for successful lingual nerve blocks.

A separate injection is usually not necessary in order to anesthetize the lingual nerve. Due to its typical location anterior and medial to the inferior alveolar nerve, it is routinely anesthetized when the inferior alveolar nerve is anesthetized.

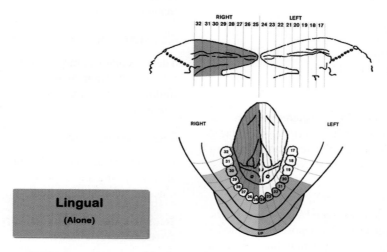

Lingual
(Alone)

■ **FIGURE 14–18** Field of Anesthesia for Lingual Nerve Blocks. The field of anesthesia for lingual nerve blocks is indicated by the shaded area.

Techniques to anesthetize the lingual nerve all have significant similarities and include:

1. while depositing solution for IA nerve blocks
2. as a supplemental injection after depositing solution for IA nerve blocks
3. as a single injection not associated with IA nerve blocks; for lingual-only anesthesia (when there is no need to anesthetize buccal soft tissues, buccal periodontium, or mandibular teeth)

Penetration Site

The penetration site for lingual nerve blocks is the same as for IA nerve blocks (see Figure 14–7) and is slightly lateral to the pterygomandibular raphe and medial to the internal oblique ridge at a height that approximates a few millimeters above the deepest concavity of the coronoid notch.

Needle Pathway

The needle advances along the lateral aspect of the pterygomandibular raphe through thin mucosal tissue and fibers of the buccinator muscle into the pterygomandibular space. The needle then passes lateral to the medial pterygoid muscle to the lingual nerve (see Figure 14–9).

Deposition Site

The path of the lingual nerve varies. Deposition at a point half-way between the ramus and the penetration site will usually allow sufficient diffusion for profound anesthesia (see Figure 14–19 ■).

Technique Steps

Apply the basic injection steps outlined in Chapter 11 and summarized in Appendix 11–1.

Needle Selection

For lingual nerve injections, 25 or 27 gauge long needles are recommended when administered in conjunction with IA nerve blocks. When administered alone, a 25 or 27 gauge *short* needle may be preferred.

Injection Procedure

When performed in conjunction with IA nerve blocks, the needle is withdrawn half-way after deposition for the IA block and, after negative aspiration, a minimum of 0.2 ml (1/9 of a cartridge or one stopper) of solution is deposited. When administered as a separate injection, a long needle is penetrated in the same manner as for the IA nerve block

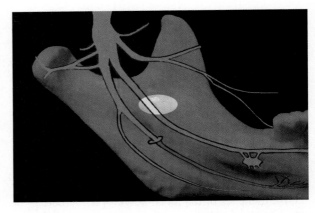

■ **FIGURE 14–19**   Site for Lingual Nerve Blocks. The deposition site for lingual nerve blocks is indicated by the spotlight.

but is advanced only 10 to 13 mm. If a short needle is used, the length of the shank showing after optimum penetration is about 8 to 11 mm (see Figure 14–20 ■).

Confirming Anesthesia

Subjective signs of anesthesia for lingual nerve blocks include a sense of numbness of the lingual soft tissues and half of the anterior two-thirds of the tongue. Objective signs include a lack of response to gentle stimulation with an instrument and no pain during procedures involving soft tissues lingual to the mandibular teeth.

Common Causes of Injection Failure

These techniques rarely fail to provide profound anesthesia of the lingual soft tissues except perhaps in the midline where fibers from the contralateral lingual nerve may overlap.

Troubleshooting

If lingual anesthesia is not achieved, reevaluate by visualizing the site and depth of penetration as well as volumes of solution deposited.

Technique Modifications and Alternatives

The Gow-Gates nerve block is an excellent alternative for achieving lingual anesthesia because it anesthetizes the trunk of the IA nerve before the branching of the

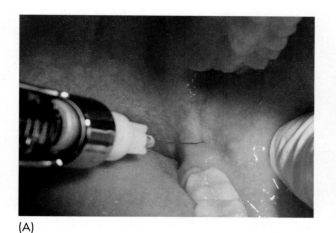

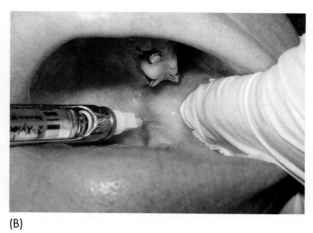

(A)   (B)

■ **FIGURE 14–20** Depth of Penetration for Lingual Nerve Blocks. The depth of penetration for lingual nerve blocks is ~1/3 to 1/2 the length of a long needle (~10 to 13 mm). A—Depth of penetration for lingual nerve blocks. B—Depth of penetration for IA nerve blocks.

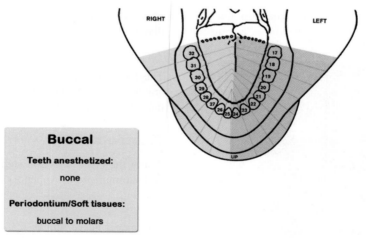

■ **FIGURE 14–21** Field of Anesthesia for Buccal Nerve Blocks. The field of anesthesia for buccal nerve blocks is indicated by the shaded area.

lingual nerve and not only anesthetizes the lingual nerve but it also largely avoids lingual nerve injury. Solution is deposited from 5 to 10 millimeters away from the nerve, as well, so the nerve is rarely in danger of being touched by a needle.

Complications

The lingual nerve is one of the most frequently injured nerves during dental injections. The symptoms associated with these injuries range from transient "electric shocks" to permanent paresthesias. See Chapter 17 for further discussion on nerve injuries and paresthesia.

BUCCAL NERVE BLOCK

Buccal nerve blocks (BNBs) are indicated for pain management during procedures involving the buccal soft tissue along the molar teeth in the mandibular region. BNBs are also referred to as long buccal and buccinator nerve blocks (Jastak et al., 1995; Malamed, 2004).

Field of Anesthesia

The buccal nerve and its terminal branches provide innervation to the soft tissue and periodontium buccal to the mandibular posterior teeth, primarily the molars (see Figure 14–21 ■).

Anatomical Factors

The buccal nerve crosses the coronoid notch of the ramus at the level of the occlusal plane. It then divides into several branches, one of which penetrates the buccinator muscle to innervate the buccal mucosa and gingiva of the mandibular molars and occasionally of the premolars.

Technique Factors

The following information describes key factors for successful buccal nerve blocks.

Penetration Site

The penetration site is located in the buccal fold just distal and buccal to the most posterior molar for which soft tissue anesthesia is required (see Figure 14–22 ■).

Needle Pathway

Due to the thinness of the mucosa in the area and the limited depths of penetration, the needle is advanced

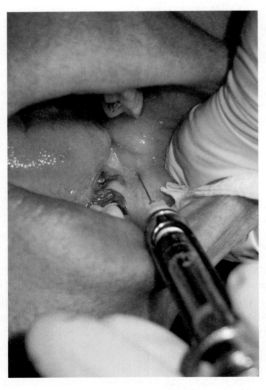

■ **FIGURE 14–22** Penetration Site for Buccal Nerve Blocks. The penetration site for buccal nerve blocks is indicated by the needle.

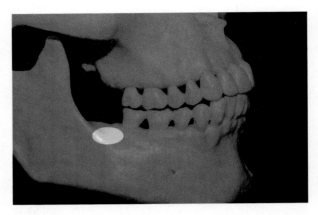

■ **FIGURE 14–23** Deposition Site for Buccal Nerve Blocks. The deposition site for buccal nerve blocks is indicated by the spotlighted area.

very slowly until the bevel is fully inserted, to avoid discomfort.

Deposition Site

The deposition site is at the buccal aspect of the ramus, lateral to the external oblique ridge as the nerve passes over the anterior border of the ramus (see Figure 14–23 ■).

Technique Steps

Apply the basic injection steps outlined in Chapter 11 and summarized in Appendix 11–1.

Needle Selection

For buccal nerve blocks, 25 or 27 gauge long needles are common following IA injections. When administered alone, a 27 gauge short is recommended, consistent with the shallow depth of penetration and the low rate of positive aspiration (less than 1 percent) (Jastak et al., 1995).

Injection Procedure

To gain access to the site of penetration, retract the lip and cheek laterally, pulling the tissue taut (see Figure 14–22). The penetration site is located in the buccal fold just distal and buccal to the most posterior molar in the arch or just posterior to the most posterior molar requiring treatment or rubber dam clamp placement. The angle of insertion is parallel to the occlusal plane on the side of injection as demonstrated in Figure 14–22. The insertion depth is about 3 to 4 mm. Following a negative aspiration, begin depositing 0.2 to 0.3 ml (1/9 to 1/6 cartridge) of an appropriately selected local anesthetic drug. This injection has a high tendency to cause discomfort if solution is administered too rapidly.

The bevel must be fully inserted into the tissue. If penetration is initiated in an area with *inadequate* tissue thickness, resistance may be met, preventing complete bevel insertion. If this occurs, withdraw and penetrate more laterally, away from the ramus. To confirm proper bevel insertion after aspiration, observe for backflow at the penetration site while depositing. If this occurs, the solution will leak into the patient's mouth (the patient may experience a bitter taste from the solution).

Confirming Anesthesia

Subjective signs of anesthesia for BNBs include a sense of numbness of the buccal soft tissues of the mandibular molars. Objective signs include a lack of response to gentle stimulation with an instrument and no pain during procedures involving soft tissues buccal to the mandibular molars.

Common Causes of Injection Failure

BNB failures are rare and occur primarily due to operator error. Failure to reserve adequate volumes after IA nerve blocks or to fully insert the bevel into the tissue, can result in the deposition of inadequate volumes of solution.

Troubleshooting

When reevaluating failed buccal anesthesia, it is useful to consider the following factors:

1. Adequate retraction is critical. If the tissue is not held taut during penetration it can be difficult to achieve full bevel penetration. Additionally, if retracted tissues are allowed to slump over the penetration site, it may seem that bevels are inserted when they actually are not.
2. If the site of penetration is too medial, the tissue may be too thin and fibrous for adequate penetration. The needle may even contact bone on the lateral surface or retromolar region of the ramus, preventing adequate bevel insertion and causing sharp pain. Locating a more lateral penetration site in more loosely attached mucosa can provide greater success and comfort.

Technique Modifications and Alternatives

Alternatives to buccal nerve blocks are rarely needed due to their high rate of success. Localized infiltrations can be administered for site specific anesthesia. Additionally, buccal nerve anesthesia is usually achieved with the administration of Gow-Gates nerve blocks, and PDL injections are effective as well.

Complications

Complications following BNBs are rare and include bleeding, hematoma, and postoperative discomfort.

MENTAL NERVE BLOCK

Mental nerve blocks (MNBs) are administered for procedures requiring pain management of the buccal soft tissues in the mandible anterior to the mental foramen (Jastak et al., 1995; Malamed, 2004).

Field of Anesthesia

Anesthesia of the mental nerve will affect the buccal mucous membrane and skin of the lower lip and chin anterior to the mental foramen to the midline (see Figure 14–24A ■ and Figure 14–24B ■).

Anatomical Factors

The mental nerve exits the mandible on the anterolateral surface through the mental foramen, usually between the apices of the first and second premolars.

Technique Factors

The following information describes key factors for successful mental nerve blocks.

Penetration Site

The penetration site varies with the location of the mental foramen. It is helpful to locate the foramen before selecting the penetration site. This can be accomplished with the aid of radiographs and by gentle palpation in the buccal vestibule beginning with the first molar and moving anteriorly until the foramen is located, most typically in relationship to the apices of the first or second premolars. The foramen may appear as a small depression, a "crater," or a rough elevation or ledge. Gentle pressure applied over the area of the foramen frequently elicits a slight achy discomfort

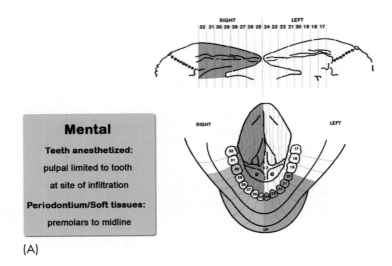

Mental

Teeth anesthetized:

pulpal limited to tooth

at site of infiltration

Periodontium/Soft tissues:

premolars to midline

(A)

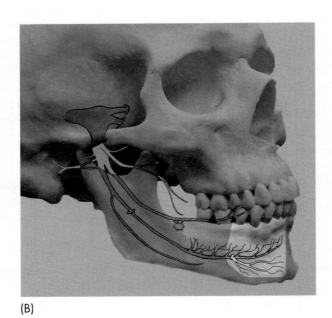

(B)

■ **FIGURE 14–24**   Field of Anesthesia for Mental Nerve Blocks. A—The field of anesthesia for mental nerve blocks is indicated by the spotlighted area. B—Field of Anesthesia Limitations. Note that the field of anesthesia for mental nerve blocks does not include the teeth, only the soft tissue anterior to the mental foramen.

or tingling sensation. Patients can be asked to confirm this as the vestibular area is palpated, by raising their hands when they feel these sensations. The site of penetration is in the depth of the mucobuccal fold superior to the foramen (see Figure 14–25 ■). An alternative site is in the mucobuccal fold anterior to the foramen. This alternate penetration site will be described in Technique Modifications and Alternatives toward the end of this topic.

Needle Pathway

The needle passes through thin mucosal tissues to superficial fascia containing loose connective tissue, small vessels and microvasculature, and nerve endings.

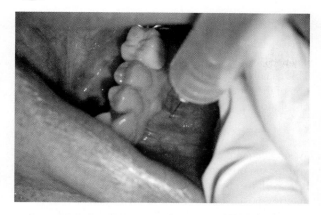

■ **FIGURE 14–25** Penetration Site for Mental Nerve Blocks. The penetration site for mental nerve blocks is indicated by the needle.

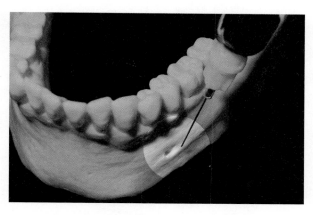

■ **FIGURE 14–27** Deposition Site for Mental Nerve Blocks—Superior Lateral View.

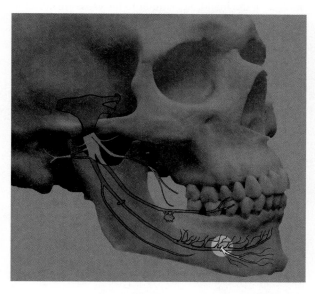

■ **FIGURE 14–26** Deposition Site for Mental Nerve Blocks. The deposition site for mental nerve blocks is indicated by the spotlighted area.

Deposition Site

The deposition site is just superior to the mental foramen for both techniques discussed (see Figure 14–26 ■ and Figure 14–27 ■).

Technique Steps

Apply the basic injection steps outlined in Chapter 11 and summarized in Appendix 11–1.

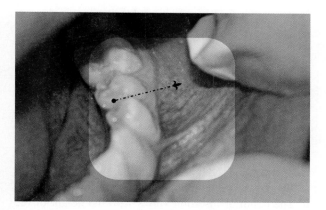

■ **FIGURE 14–28** Tissue Retraction for Mental Nerve Blocks. Establish gentle lateral retraction to make the tissue taut for ease of penetration and accuracy of depth of insertion.

Needle Selection

A 25 gauge needle is recommended for this injection, consistent with its relatively high rate of positive aspiration (nearly 6 percent) (Jastak et al., 1995). A 27 gauge needle is most commonly used and is also recommended.

Injection Procedure

To gain access to the site of penetration, the clinician is seated at a posterior position. Begin by retracting the lip and cheek laterally, pulling the tissue taut at the mucogingival junction (see Figure 14–28 ■). After asking the patient to close his or her eyes, the syringe is aligned vertically with the patient's cheek to approach

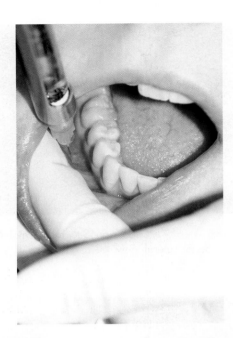

■ **FIGURE 14-29** Vertical Approach to Needle Insertion. For this technique, align the syringe vertically to approach the penetration site. The clinician will be seated at the 12:00 position.

the penetration site (see Figure 14–29 ■). Following initial penetration, advance the needle tip at an angle directly vertical to the foramen to a depth just superior to it. The depth of insertion varies with the height of the alveolar process and the angle of tissue retraction but is typically about 4 to 6 mm.

Following negative aspiration, slowly deposit a minimum of 0.6 ml (1/3 of a cartridge) of an appropriately selected local anesthetic drug. This injection can be quite uncomfortable if adequate topical has not been applied, if solution is administered too rapidly, or if bone is inadvertently contacted.

Confirming Anesthesia

Subjective signs of anesthesia for mental nerve blocks include a sense of numbness on the injected side, including the buccal soft tissues of the chin and lower lip, and of the premolars and incisors.

Objective signs include a lack of response to gentle stimulation with an instrument and no pain during procedures involving soft tissues overlying the premolars and incisors.

Common Causes of Injection Failure

This injection is highly successful. Failure to achieve anesthesia of the buccal tissues in the area of the MNB is rare. This usually involves failure to correctly identify the location of the foramen, which results in insufficient diffusion of solution or inadequate volumes of solution deposited.

Troubleshooting

When adequate anesthesia is not achieved, reassess the volume of solution deposited and the deposition site, as it may have been located too far superior, inferior, anterior, posterior, or lateral to the foramen.

Incomplete anesthesia after mental nerve blocks can frequently be attributed to what is known as cross-innervation or overlap of terminal fibers of the nonanesthetized or contralateral mental nerve, at the midline of the mandible, similar to the cross-innervation that occurs with the ASA nerve as discussed in Chapter 12, "Injections for Maxillary Pain Control."

When this is the case in the mandible, tissues of the anterior segment of the mandible will receive sensory innervation from the mental nerve on the nonanesthetized side. To achieve adequate anesthesia in these instances, an infiltration over the apex of the central incisor is necessary (see Figure 14–30 ■). (Note: Other than the difference in anatomic location, the technique for performing a mandibular anterior infiltration is the same as the technique for a maxillary anterior infiltration.)

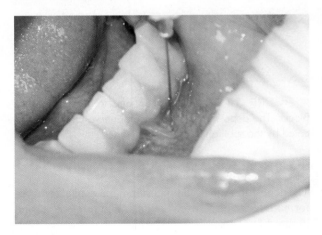

■ **FIGURE 14-30** Infiltration to Supplement Mental-Incisive Injections. Incomplete anesthesia due to cross-innervation at the midline is easily managed by infiltration injection of the central incisor.

Technique Modifications and Alternatives

An alternative to the technique previously described is to approach the penetration from an anterior position, with the angle of insertion parallel to the occlusal plane on the side of injection (see Figure 14–31 ■). This is considered by many to be a less "threatening" approach because it is easier to keep the syringe out of the patient's line of sight.

For situations in which bilateral soft tissue anesthesia is desired but where pulpal anesthesia of one of the two posterior segments is not needed, many clinicians administer mental nerve blocks on the side where soft tissue anesthesia only is needed, in conjunction with a contralateral IA nerve block. This approach can also be useful when there are overlapping branches of the contralateral mental nerve. In these situations, the clinician will typically use the same 25 or 27 gauge long needle that was used for IA nerve blocks.

Complications

Complications following mental nerve blocks are infrequent and can include bleeding, hematoma, and postoperative discomfort.

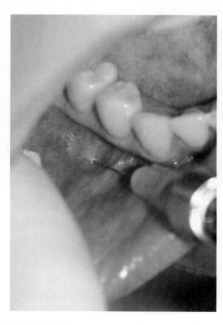

■ **FIGURE 14–31** Horizontal Approach to Needle Insertion. For this technique, align the syringe horizontally, parallel to the occlusal place, to approach the penetration site. The clinician will be seated at the 8:00 position.

INCISIVE NERVE BLOCK

Incisive nerve blocks (INBs) are administered for procedures requiring pain management in the mandible anterior to the mental foramen. This injection is nearly identical to the mental nerve block. Unlike the mental nerve block, the incisive nerve block incorporates an additional step in order to achieve pulpal anesthesia. Some clinicians refer to this injection as a "mental incisive" nerve block because it is impossible to deliver an incisive nerve block without also anesthetizing the mental nerve. Conversely, mental nerve block techniques alone do not reliably anesthetize incisive nerves.

Field of Anesthesia

When the incisive nerve is anesthetized, the distributions of both the mental and incisive nerves will be affected including the buccal mucous membrane and skin of the lower lip and chin, and the pulps and facial periodontium of the teeth anterior to the mental foramen, to the midline (see Figure 14–32 ■ and Figure 14–33 ■).

Anatomical Factors

The incisive nerve travels within the mandibular canal from the mental foramen to the midline, and terminal fibers frequently innervate contralateral incisors.

Technique Factors

The following information describes key factors for successful incisive nerve blocks.

Penetration Site

Similar to mental nerve blocks, penetration sites vary with the locations of mental foramina. It is helpful to locate the foramen before selecting the penetration site. As with the mental block, it can be accomplished with the aid of radiographs and by gentle palpation in the buccal vestibule beginning with the first molar and moving anteriorly until the foramen is located, most typically in relationship to the apices of the first or second premolars. It may feel like a small depression, or "crater," or a rough elevation, or ledge. Gentle pressure applied over the area of the foramen frequently elicits a slight discomfort or tingling sensation.

The site of penetration is in the mucobuccal fold superior to the foramen or alternately in the mucobuccal fold anterior to the foramen (see Figure 14–25). This

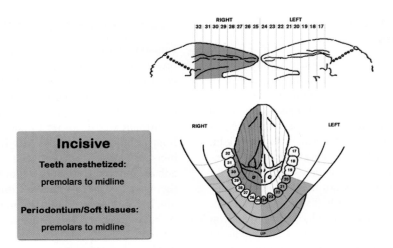

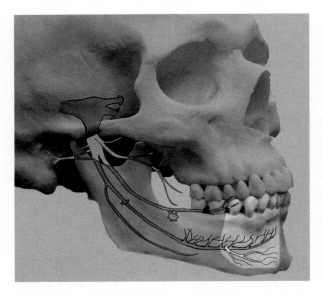

FIGURE 14–32 Field of Anesthesia for Incisive Nerve Blocks. The field of anesthesia for incisive nerve blocks is indicated by the shaded area.

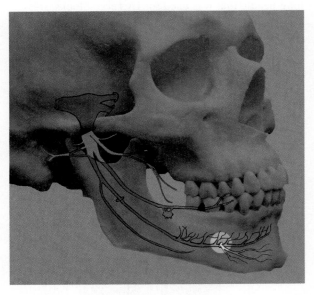

FIGURE 14–33 Field of Anesthesia Limitations. Note that the field of anesthesia for incisive nerve blocks includes the soft tissue anterior to the mental foramen.

FIGURE 14–34 Deposition Site for Incisive Nerve Blocks. The deposition site for incisive nerve blocks is indicated by the the spotlighted area.

alternate penetration site will be further discussed in Technique Modifications and Alternatives toward the end of this topic.

Needle Pathway

The needle passes through thin mucosal tissues to superficial fascia containing loose connective tissue, small vessels and microvasculature, and nerve endings.

Deposition Site

The deposition site is just superior to the mental foramen for both techniques discussed (see Figure 14–34 ■).

Technique Steps

Apply the basic injection steps outlined in Chapter 11 and summarized in Appendix 11–1.

Needle Selection

A 25 gauge needle is recommended for incisive nerve blocks due to the high rate of positive aspiration (nearly 6 percent) (Jastak et al., 1995). A 27 gauge needle is more commonly used and is also recommended.

Injection Procedure

To gain access to the site of penetration, the clinician is seated at a posterior position and begins by retracting the lip and cheek laterally, pulling the tissue taut at the mucogingival junction (see Figure 14–28). After asking the patient to close his or her eyes, the syringe is aligned vertically near the patient's cheek to approach the penetration site (see Figure 14–29). Following initial penetration, advance the needle tip at an angle directly vertical to the foramen to a point just superior to it. The depth of insertion varies with the height of the alveolar process and the angle of tissue retraction. This is typically about 4 to 6 mm.

Following negative aspiration, slowly deposit a minimum of 0.6 ml (1/3 of a cartridge) of an appropriately selected local anesthetic drug. Once the full dose of solution is delivered, tissue at the injection site will bulge. Unlike mental nerve blocks, the incisive nerve block requires that gentle pressure be exerted over the bulge of solution in the direction of the mental foramen, in order to force solution through the foramen to flood the incisive nerve (see Figure 14–35 ■). Pressure can be applied either intra- or extra-orally by the clinician or

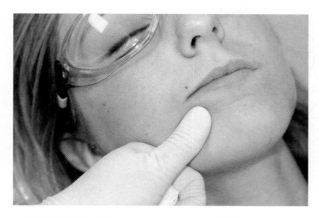

■ **FIGURE 14–35** Key Step to Successful Incisive Nerve. Gently apply pressure over the bulge of solution in the direction of the mental foramen to force solution through the foramen to flood the incisive nerve.

patient. It is important to remind patients, if they are applying the pressure, that it must be applied directly and steadily over the foramen and maintained for at least 1 full minute for reliable success. This injection can be uncomfortable if adequate topical has not been applied, if inadvertent contact with bone occurs, or if solution is administered too rapidly.

Confirming Anesthesia

Subjective signs of anesthesia for the incisive (mental incisive) nerve block include a sense of numbness on the injected side, including the buccal mucous membrane, skin of the lower lip and chin, and the pulps and periodontium anterior to the mental foramen to the midline. Objective signs include a lack of response to gentle stimulation with an instrument and no pain during procedures involving the premolars, canine, and incisors.

Common Causes of Injection Failure

This injection is highly successful. Failure to achieve anesthesia of the incisive and mental nerves is uncommon. This usually involves failure to correctly identify the location of the foramen, which results in insufficient diffusion of solution into it. This can also result from anatomical factors such as unusually small foramina or technical factors such as insufficient duration or incorrect location of pressure over the foramen following the injection. Other causes may include inflammation or infection in the area of deposition.

Troubleshooting

When inadequate anesthesia occurs, reassess the deposition site for proximity to the foramen. It is also possible that the direction or duration of the post-injection pressure was inadequate or that insufficient volumes were deposited preventing successful passage of the solution through the foramen.

Technique Modifications and Alternatives

As with mental nerve blocks, the deposition site may be approached from an anterior position, with the angle of insertion parallel to the occlusal plane on the side of injection. This is considered by many to be a less "threatening" approach, as the syringe may be below the patient's line of sight (see Figure 14–31).

For situations in which bilateral anesthesia is desired, but posterior anesthesia of one of the quadrants of the mandible is not needed, many clinicians administer incisive nerve blocks on the side where posterior anesthesia is not needed in conjunction with contralateral IA nerve blocks. This approach can also be useful when there are overlapping branches of the contralateral incisive nerve. In these situations, the clinician will typically use the same 25 or 27 gauge long needle that was used for the contralateral IA nerve block.

Complications

Following incisive nerve blocks, complications are infrequent and can include bleeding, hematoma, and postoperative discomfort.

GOW-GATES MANDIBULAR NERVE BLOCK

Similar to IA nerve blocks, **Gow-Gates Mandibular Nerve Blocks (GGMNBs)** are indicated for pain management of multiple teeth in one quadrant. Unlike IA blocks, GG mandibular nerve blocks are "true" mandibular blocks because they routinely anesthetize the full extent of a mandibular quadrant (Jastak et al., 1995; Malamed, 2004; Gow-Gates & Watson, 1977).

Field of Anesthesia

GG nerve blocks routinely anesthetize structures innervated by the inferior alveolar, mental, incisive, lingual, mylohyoid, and auriculotemporal nerves to the midline. Unlike IA nerve blocks, GG nerve blocks anesthetize the buccal nerve 75 percent of the time (see Figure 14–36 ■) (Malamed, 2004).

Anatomical Factors

As previously discussed, the inferior alveolar nerve is the largest branch of the mandibular division of the trigeminal nerve. It is important to note that it branches from the posterior division of the mandibular nerve within the infratemporal space, then travels medial to the lateral pterygoid muscle and passes through the pterygomandibular space between the sphenomandibular ligament and the medial surface of the ramus of the mandible. It then enters the mandibular foramen and travels through the mandibular canal (Fehrenbach & Herring, 2007; Hamburg, 1972; Jastak et al., 1995).

Numerous arteries and veins are also located within infratemporal and pterygomandibular spaces. The maxillary artery traverses the infratemporal space either superficial or deep to the lateral pterygoid muscle. The middle meningeal artery branches from the maxillary artery within the space while several other arteries, including the inferior alveolar, branch off afterward.

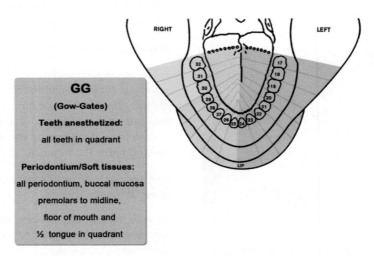

GG
(Gow-Gates)
Teeth anesthetized:
all teeth in quadrant

Periodontium/Soft tissues:
all periodontium, buccal mucosa
premolars to midline,
floor of mouth and
½ tongue in quadrant

■ **FIGURE 14–36** Field of Anesthesia for GG Nerve Blocks. The field of anesthesia for GG nerve blocks is indicated by the shaded area.

The inferior alveolar vein travels within the mandibular canal along with the inferior alveolar artery and nerve. It exits through the mandibular foramen, travels medioanteriorly with the inferior alveolar artery, through the pterygomandibular and infratemporal spaces and drains into the pterygoid plexus of veins located in the infratemporal space.

Importantly, although the deposition site of local anesthetic solution in a GG mandibular nerve block is often at least 5 to 10 mm from the inferior alveolar nerve *trunk* (which includes the inferior alveolar, lingual, and 75 percent of the time, the buccal nerve), the relatively structure-free upper portion of the pterygomandibular space does not restrict the downward, anterior, and medial movement of solution. In fact, the initial volume of solution recommended (about 1.8 ml or more) nearly fills the pterygomandibular space at that level.

Technique Factors

The following information describes key factors for successful GG nerve blocks.

Penetration Site

The penetration site is located in the buccal mucous membrane, directly posterior to the maxillary second molar, at the level of its mesiolingual cusp. The precise location, however, is variable and must be established using extra-oral landmarks, in addition to the intraoral landmarks. The existence of both intra- and extra-oral landmarks makes the GG block somewhat unique (see Figure 14–37 ■).

Needle Pathway

The needle passes through thin mucosal tissues and limited amounts of superficial fascia that contains loose connective tissue, small vessels and microvasculature, large vessels, and nerve endings. Typically, less resistance to forward movement is encountered in the upper portion of the pterygomandibular space because it is relatively free of blocking fascia.

Deposition Site

The deposition site is on the anterolateral surface of the neck of the condyle, just below the insertion of the lateral pterygoid muscle. The deposition site for GG nerve blocks is at the highest point in the pterygomandibular space of all three mandibular block techniques, IANB (lowest), VANB (intermediate), and GGNB (highest) (see Figure 14–38 ■ and Figure 14–45).

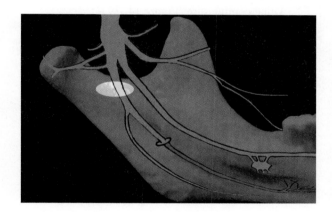

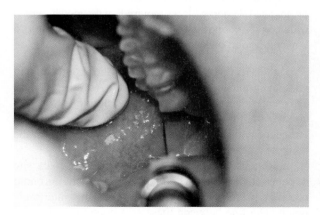

■ **FIGURE 14–37**   Penetration Site for GG Nerve Blocks. The penetration site for GG nerve blocks is indicated by the needle.

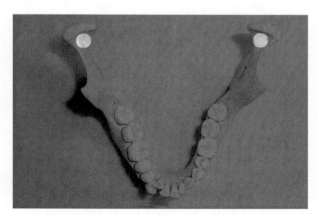

■ **FIGURE 14–38**   Deposition Site for GG Nerve Blocks. The deposition site for GG nerve blocks is indicated by the spotlighted area.

Technique Steps

Apply the basic injection steps outlined in Chapter 11 and summarized in Appendix 11–1 and figue 127.

Needle Selection

A 25 gauge long needle is recommended, consistent with the depth of penetration, which is equal to or greater than the depth for an IA block for the same individual. The rate of positive aspiration is considered to be relatively low (2 percent) but some sources have placed this rate much higher, reinforcing the recommendation of 25 gauge needles (Watson, J. E., 1992).

Injection Procedure

In preparing for GG nerve blocks, there are two key landmarks to observe:

1. a line visualized from the intertragic notch to the labial commissure (Figure 14–39 ■)
2. the height or most occlusal aspect of the mesiolingual cusp of the second molar (Figure 14–40 ■)

The flare of the tragus of the ear is also important because it can provide confirmation regarding the location of the barrel of the syringe (see Figure 14–39). While not a critical landmark (the flare of the ramus can also be assessed by visualization and external palpation of the posterior mandible and condyle), the flare of the tragus is nevertheless useful in confirming barrel location (see Figure 14–39 and Figure 14–41 ■). The significance of all landmarks will be explained in the following discussion.

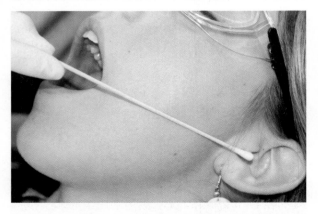

■ **FIGURE 14–39** GG Nerve Blocks: Key Landmarks 1. A line visualized from the intertragic notch to the labial commissure is indicated by the cotton swab. This is the angle of the needle pathway. Observing the flare of the tragus can indicate the corresponding flare of the ramus of the mandible.

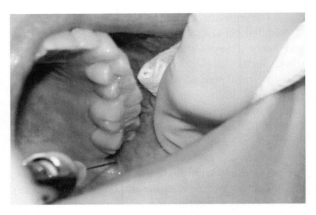

■ **FIGURE 14–40** GG Nerve Blocks: Key Landmarks 2. The optimum height of penetration is indicated by the height or most occlusal aspect of the mesiolingual cusp of the second molar.

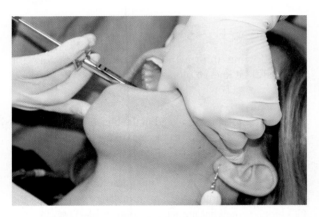

■ **FIGURE 14–41** GG Nerve Blocks: The "Wide Open" Technique. GG nerve blocks require that the mouth remain wide open during the entire procedure, including a 2 minute period after completion of the injection.

GG nerve blocks require that the mouth remain wide open during the entire procedure (see Box 14–8). This anterior orientation of the mandible allows the condyle to remain fully translated over the articular eminence and provides needle access to the neck of the condyle (see Figure 14–41).

Retract the cheek laterally to gain access to the site of penetration. While keeping the thumb on the coronoid process, place the index finger over the intertragic notch. The line between these two points provides the upward orientation angle of the syringe for this injection (see Figure 14–41).

Unlike IA nerve blocks, the barrel orientation to the molars is more variable. The orientation of the barrel

Critical to the success of GG nerve blocks, patients must remain in *wide open* positions throughout procedures, and approximately 2 minutes following deposition. It can be helpful to place a bite block in the mouth as soon as the needle has been withdrawn. Another key to success is to seat the patient upright immediately following the injection, to facilitate diffusion toward the nerve.

Closure at any time during a Gow-Gates procedure can prevent the needle from reaching the target. Closure immediately upon completion of the injection and failure to upright the patient can cause diffusion of solution away from the nerve.

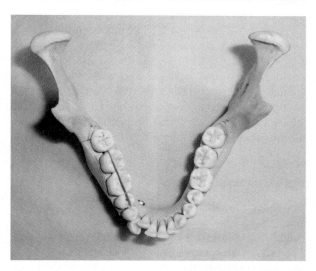

■ **FIGURE 14–42** Variations of Syringe Angulations for the GG Nerve Block. The barrel orientation to the molars is variable with the GG nerve block. The orientation of the barrel is dependent on the flare of the ramus and condyle. Note the unilateral differences in the flare of the ramus of this mandible.

is dependent on the flare of the ramus and condyle. See Figure 14–42 ■ for an example of asymmetrical flare of the condyles on the same mandible. Each side would require different angulations. Dr. Gow-Gates observed that the flare of the tragus of the ear roughly corresponded to the barrel orientation over the lower dentition. A tragus that arises from the side of the face at a right angle suggests a more posterior location of the

barrel of the syringe, over the molars. One that is flush with the face suggests a more anterior location of the barrel, over the canine and incisors. A tragus at a 45 degree angle to the face suggests a barrel orientation that is initially over the premolars. It is important to note that these are typical starting points, and adjustments may be necessary.

Advance slowly until gentle contact with bone is made, confirming that the tip of the needle has reached the condylar neck (see Figure 14–38). If contact is not made and the needle is nearly fully inserted, it is likely that medial deflection has occurred. To adjust for this deflection, withdraw the needle slightly, reposition the barrel of the syringe posteriorly, and reinsert until contact is made.

In practical terms, the deposition site is confirmed by gently contacting bone at the neck of the condyle. The insertion depth is variable, although typically it is about 25 mm. It has been described as being the same to somewhat greater than the penetration depth of IA nerve blocks for the same individual.

Once contact has been established, withdraw the needle 1 mm and, following negative aspiration, deposit a minimum of 1.8 ml (one cartridge) of an appropriately selected local anesthetic drug.

Confirming Anesthesia

Subjective signs and symptoms of anesthesia for GG nerve blocks include a sense of numbness on the injected side, which includes the buccal and lingual mucous membranes, the skin of the tongue, lower lip, chin, and ramus of the mandible, and the pulps and periodontium of the teeth as well as the distributions of the mylohyoid, buccal (75 percent of the time), lingual, and auriculotemporal nerves. Objective signs include a lack of response to gentle stimulation with an instrument and no pain during procedures involving the molars, premolars, and incisors.

Common Causes of Injection Failure

As with any technique, failures may occur due to lack of experience. This seems particularly true for GG nerve blocks due to the use of both intra- and extra-oral landmarks and the importance of postprocedural protocols. In addition, Dr. Gow-Gates used cartridges that contained greater volumes of solution (2.2 ml) compared to cartridges containing 1.8 ml. Volumes higher than 1.8 ml may be necessary at times in order to provide reliable and profound anesthesia due to the distance from deposition site to target. Onset is also much slower compared to many other techniques (estimated at anywhere from 5 to up to 10 minutes, although frequently closer to 10). Due to slow onset times, less familiar clinicians may declare failure prematurely.

As previously mentioned, failure to upright patients after making the needle safe and to instruct them to remain in wide open positions both during and after the procedure, can cause solution to diffuse away from the nerve.

Troubleshooting

When inadequate anesthesia occurs, reassess the deposition site, the flare of the tragus, the line from the intratragic notch to the angle of the mouth, the barrel orientation, the ability of the patient to maintain a "wide open" position during and following the injection, prompt uprighting, and the volumes of solution deposited.

Modifications may include the selection of more lateral or more medial penetration sites, slightly higher or lower penetration sites, and the use of more concentrated drugs such as 4% articaine, 4% prilocaine, and 3% mepivacaine. Greater volumes of solution may also be effective, particularly if 1.8 ml fails repeatedly to achieve profound anesthesia in a particular patient.

Technique Modifications and Alternatives

Alternatives include IA nerve blocks, PDL injections, VA nerve blocks, incisive nerve blocks, and intraosseous techniques.

Complications

Injury can occur from injection into the temporomandibular joint capsule and otic ganglion. The most reliable way to prevent injury to these structures is to confirm that the needle is at the neck of the condyle by making gentle contact with bone.

Although the rate of positive aspiration with GG nerve blocks is reportedly low, there are major vessels in the pathway of this injection. The large and prominent maxillary artery and a major branch, the middle meningeal artery, are located in the superior portion of the pterygomandibular space.

Possible temporary paralysis of cranial nerves III (oculomotor), IV (trochlear), and VI (abducens) may occur on occasion and will resolve as soon as the anesthetic effect diminishes (Malamed, 2004; Fish,

McIntire, & Johnson, 1989). This may have occurred due to missing the target area or failure to adequately aspirate prior to injection (Johnson & Badovinac, 2007). Hematomas and trismus of the lateral pterygoid muscle have also occurred with typical uneventful healing (Malamed, 2006; Budenz & Osterman, 1995).

An interesting and rare postoperative complication affecting the middle ear was reported in 2001. It was concluded that the effects were likely the result of inflammation or occult (concealed) hematoma formation or both (Brodsky & Dower, 2001).

VAZIRANI-AKINOSI NERVE BLOCK

Vazirani-Akinosi Nerve Blocks (VANBs) are ideal for pain management of the mandibular teeth in a single quadrant when the ability to open the jaw is limited, either due to physiologic, pathologic, or phobic circumstances. This injection is also referred to as the Akinosi or "closed-mouth" technique (Jastak et al., 1995; Malamed, 2004).

VA nerve blocks may also be of use in initiating anesthesia in fearful patients who will not open wide enough for IA nerve blocks. In this situation, Akinosi blocks can be used to provide profound anesthesia of the structures through which the needle passes in IA nerve blocks. The IA nerve block can then be administered comfortably.

Field of Anesthesia

Due to their location, VA nerve blocks can provide wider areas of anesthesia compared to IA nerve blocks and slightly more limited areas compared to GG nerve blocks. The inferior alveolar, mental, incisive, lingual, mylohyoid, and frequently buccal nerves are all affected (see Figure 14–1, Figure 14–18, and Figure 14–21).

Anatomical Factors

Relative to IA and GG nerve blocks, Vazirani-Akinosi nerve blocks are administered in an intermediate position in the pterygomandibular space. Their location actually places them closer to target nerve trunks. Tissue resistance is minimal due to the relative lack of fascia that might deflect needles or solutions.

Technique Factors

The following information describes key factors for successful VA nerve blocks.

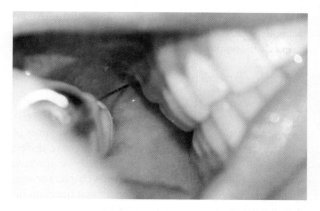

■ **FIGURE 14–43**   Penetration Site for VA Nerve Blocks. The penetration site for VA nerve blocks is indicated by the needle.

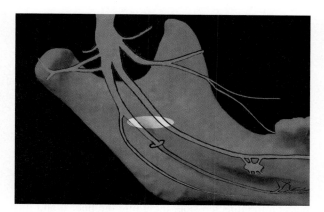

■ **FIGURE 14–44**   Deposition Site for VA Nerve Blocks. The deposition site for VA nerve blocks is indicated by the spotlighted area.

Penetration Site

The site of penetration is in the soft tissue medial to the ramus, directly adjacent to the maxillary tuberosity at the height of the mucogingival junction of the maxillary molars (see Figure 14–43 ■).

Needle Pathway

The needle advances slowly through thin mucosal tissue parallel to the mandibular molar teeth and passes lateral to the medial pterygoid muscle, lingual nerve, and sphenomandibular ligament, well superior to the lingula and mandibular foramen.

Deposition Site

The deposition site is well above the mandibular foramen on the medial surface of the ramus in the pterygomandibular space (see Figure 14–44 ■). Figure 14–45 ■ shows the deposition site in comparison to both the IA and GG nerve blocks.

Technique Steps

Apply the basic injection steps outlined in Chapter 11 and summarized in Appendix 11–1.

Needle Selection

Both 25 and 27 gauge long needles are recommended, consistent with penetration depths which do not exceed 25 mm. Moderate aspiration rates between 5 to 10 percent have been observed with this technique (Malamed, 2004; Johnson & Badovinac, 2007).

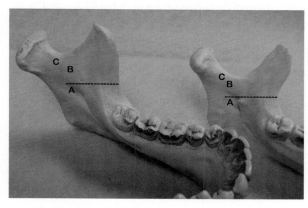

■ **FIGURE 14–45**   Deposition Site Differences: IANB, GGNB, VANB. Note the differences in the deposition site of each of these nerve blocks: A—Inferior alveolar, B—Vazirani-Akinosi, C—Gow Gates. The height of the coronoid notch is indicated by the dotted line.

Injection Procedure

With the patient's teeth in a comfortably closed position (not maximum intercuspation), gain access to the site of penetration by retracting the cheek laterally.

Penetrate in the soft tissue medial to the ramus, directly adjacent to the maxillary tuberosity at the height of the mucogingival junction of the maxillary molars (see Figure 14–43). The angle of insertion is parallel to the mandibular molar teeth.

Advance slowly to the deposition site medial to the ramus and well superior to the mandibular foramen to a depth of *not more than* 25 mm (Malamed, 2004). This depth is approximately one-half the anteroposterior dimension of the ramus in the area. Contact with bone is unusual and is not desired in this injection. Although minimal, there is a tendency for deflection away from the nerve with VA nerve blocks; therefore, it is advised that bevels be oriented medially to encourage lateral deflection toward the ramus. Following negative aspiration, deposit 1.8 ml (one full cartridge) of an appropriately selected local anesthetic drug and seat the patient upright after withdrawal.

Confirming Anesthesia

Subjective signs and symptoms of anesthesia for Vazirani-Akinosi nerve blocks include a sense of numbness on the injected side, including the buccal and lingual mucous membranes, the tongue, skin of the lower lip and chin, the ramus of the mandible, and the pulps and periodontium of the teeth on the side of injection as well as the distribution of the mylohyoid nerve. Objective signs include a lack of response to gentle stimulation with an instrument and no pain during procedures involving the molars, premolars, and incisors.

Common Causes of Injection Failure

As with any injection, failures may occur due to lack of experience with the technique. This seems particularly true for VA nerve blocks. Although Akinosi claimed a success rate of 93 percent with his technique, many have been frustrated (Johnson & Badovinac, 2007). Whether this is due to the lack of specific landmarks, or to a lack of comfort with the closed position or both, is not known.

In the event of medial deflection of the needle, solution may be deposited medial to the sphenomandibular ligament, which may prevent it from reaching the nerve. When penetration is too low, the deposition will be at a further distance from the nerve due to the flare of the ramus. Over- or under-insertion may place the solution too far from the nerve. Since there is no confirming contact with bone, the location of the tip of the needle is more speculative compared to IA and GG blocks.

Troubleshooting

When VA nerve blocks are unsuccessful, it may be helpful to reevaluate by visualizing, and palpating, and to reassess syringe angulations, depths of penetration, and volumes of solution deposited. In some instances, anatomy differs markedly from typical patterns and may make alternate nerve blocks (discussed previously in this chapter) or supplemental techniques such as the periodontal ligament injection more successful (see Chapter 15).

Technique Modifications and Alternatives

Modifications to the technique are necessary for individuals in whom the anteroposterior dimension of the ramus is considerably smaller. Penetration depth must be adjusted accordingly.

Alternatives for VA nerve blocks include GG nerve blocks, IA nerve blocks, incisive nerve blocks, infiltrations, and supplemental techniques such as PDL injections.

The VA block can be particularly useful in children and adults who are reluctant to open. Since it is a closed mouth technique, when administered in this position it will anesthetize all the structures through which the needle passes in IA nerve blocks. The IA can then be performed comfortably.

Complications

Complications are rare and include hematomas, trismus, and postoperative soreness.

CASE MANAGEMENT: Lee Chung

A left IA nerve block was administered to Lee Chung along with a buccal nerve block followed by a mental incisal nerve block on the right side. Interpapillary injections between #27, 28, and 29 were also administered to provide anesthesia of the lingual gingiva of these teeth (these injections do not anesthetize the tongue on the right side).

Case Discussion: Bilateral mandibular anesthesia, while not contraindicated, should be avoided where possible due to the considerable alteration of function that follows. Numbing the entire tongue, in particular, places patients at risk both during treatment and afterward due to the loss of normal protective feedback mechanisms. These mechanisms may remain operable under local anesthesia but they require sensation for initiation. Foreign substances and injurious substances such as hot liquids will not be sensed and can result in everything from inhalation of foreign objects to local tissue damage and an inability to speak coherently. A unilateral block of the tongue will provide more reasonable feedback.

CHAPTER QUESTIONS

1. The rate of positive aspiration in the inferior alveolar nerve block is the highest of all techniques and approximates which *one* of the following?
   a. 2 to 5 percent
   b. 5 to 10 percent
   c. 10 to 15 percent
   d. 15 to 20 percent

2. Which *one* of the following techniques is an alternative to nearly all mandibular anesthetic techniques?
   a. Gow-Gates
   b. Vazirani-Akinosi
   c. PDL
   d. Infiltrations

3. Which *one* of the following result(s) in pulpal anesthesia?
   a. Buccal nerve block
   b. Mental nerve block
   c. A and B
   d. Neither A nor B

4. When administering a Gow-Gates mandibular nerve block, *all* of the following are essential, *except:*
   a. performing one or more aspirations.
   b. meeting bony resistance.
   c. determining the site, height, and depth of penetration as well as the syringe barrel orientation.
   d. having the client remove all ear jewelry before administering.

5. Palpating anatomy prior to all mandibular anesthetic procedures is:
   a. an unnecessary step in anesthesia techniques.
   b. helpful in some techniques and useless in others.
   c. the least important aspect of anesthetic assessment.
   d. critical to the success of these techniques.

6. Which *one* of the following is the correct order, from inferior to superior location, of the mandibular techniques listed in relation to the pterygomandibular space?
   a. IA, Gow-Gates, Akinosi
   b. IA, Akinosi, Gow-Gates
   c. Gow-Gates, IA, Akinosi
   d. Akinosi, IA, Gow-Gates

REFERENCES

Blanton, P., & Jeske, A. (2003). The key to profound local anesthesia—Neuroanatomy. *Journal of the American Dental Association, 134,* 755–756.

Brodsky, C. D., & Dower, J. S. (2001). Middle ear problems after a Gow-Gates injection. *Journal of the American Dental Association, 132*(10), 1420–1423.

Budenz, A. W., & Osterman, S. R. (1995). A review of mandibular nerve block techniques. *Journal of the California Dental Association, 23,* 27–34.

Fehrenbach, M. J., & Herring, S. W. (2007). Illustrated anatomy of the head and neck (3rd ed.). St. Louis: Saunders Elsevier.

Fish, L. R., McIntire, D. N., & Johnson, L. (1989). Temporary paralysis of cranial nerves III, IV, and VI after a Gow-Gates injection. *Journal of the American Dental Association, 119,* 127–130.

Gow-Gates, G. A., & Watson, J. E. (1977). The Gow-Gates mandibular block: Further understanding. *Journal of the American Dental Society of Anesthesia, 24,* 183–189.

Hamburg, H. L. (1972). Preliminary study of patient reaction to needle gauge. *New York State Dental Association, 38,* 425–426.

Jastak, J. T., Yagiela, J. A., & Donaldson, D. (1995). *Local anesthesia of the oral cavity.* Philadelphia: Saunders.

Johnson, T. M., & Badovinac, R. (2007). Teaching alternatives to the standard alveolar nerve block in dental education: Outcomes in clinical practice. *Journal of Dental Education, 71*(9), 1145–1152.

Langlais, R. P., Broadus, R., & Glass, B. J. (1985). Bifid mandibular canals in panoramic radiographs, *Journal of the American Dental Association, 110*(6), 923–926.

Levy TP: An assessment of the Gow-Gates mandibular block for third molar surgery. *Journal of the American Dental Association, 103,* 37–41.

Malamed, S. F. (2004). *Handbook of local anesthesia* (5th ed.). St. Louis: Elsevier Mosby.

Malamed, S. F. (2006). *Anesthesia & medicine in dentistry.* Presentation to the Spokane District Dental Society and Eastern Washington University, Department of Dental Hygiene, July 21, 2006.

Montagnese, T. A., Reader, A., & Melfi, R. (1984). A comparative study of the Gow-Gates technique and a standard technique for mandibular anesthesia. *Journal of Endodontics, 10,* 158–163.

Quinn, J. (1998, August) Clinical directions, *Journal of the American Dental Association, 129,* 1147–1148.

Robertson, W. D. (1979). Clinical evaluation of mandibular conduction anesthesia. *General Dentistry, 27,* 49–51.

Shimada, K., & Gasser, R. (1989). *The Anatomical Record: Advances in Integrative Anatomy and Evolutionary Biology, 224*(1), 177–122.

Stein, P., Brueckner, J., & Milliner, M. (2007). Sensory innervation of mandibular teeth by the nerve to the mylohyoid: Implications in local anesthesia. *Clinical Anatomy, 20*(6), 591–595, 2007.

Taber's Cyclopedic Medical Dictionary (20th ed.). (2005). Philadelphia: F. A. Davis Company.

Watson, J. E., (1992). Incidence of positive aspiration in the Gow-Gates mandibular block. Anesthesia & Pain Control in Dentistry, 1(2),73–6.

Wong, J. A. (2001). Adjuncts to local anesthesia: Separating fact from fiction, *Journal of the Canadian Dental Association, 67,* 391–397.

Summary of Mandibular Injections

Nerve Block	Needle	Penetration Site	Deposition Site			Dose*	Field of Anesthesia See Appendix 14–2
			Depth of Insertion	**Angle of Insertion**			
Inferior alveolar (IA) w/ Lingual	Long 25/27 gauge	Medial to internal oblique ridge, lateral to pterygomandibular raphe, at or above height of coronoid notch see Figure 14–7	⅔ to ¾ length of needle, until contact with bone, bevel toward bone	⅔ to ¾ length of needle, until contact with bone, bevel toward bone		1.5–1.8 ml	***Teeth anesthetized:*** All teeth in quadrant
			Target				
			On medial surface of ramus, slightly superior to mandibular foramen see Figure 14–10				***Periodontium/Soft tissues:*** All periodontium, buccal mucosa premolars to midline, floor of mouth and ½ tongue in quadrant (not soft-tissues buccal to molars)
			Depth of Insertion	**Angle of Insertion**			
Buccal	Short* or Long** 25/27 gauge * When given alone ** Usually given following IA	Mucous membrane distal and lateral to most posterior molar see Figure 14–22	≤4 mm, bevel under tissue, bevel toward bone	Syringe parallel to occlusal plane, lateral to teeth, bevel toward bone see Figure 14–23		0.2–0.3 ml* * Width of rubber stopper	***Teeth anesthetized:*** None
			Target				
			Supraperiosteal, distal, and buccal to most posterior molar				***Periodontium/ Soft tissues:*** Buccal to molars
			Depth of Insertion	**Angle of Insertion**			
Mental (M) Incisive (I)	Short 25/27 gauge	Mucobuccal fold at or just anterior to mental foramen see Figure 14–25	5–6 mm	Approximately 20 degrees to long axis of premolars, bevel toward bone		0.6 ml	***Teeth anesthetized:*** (M) pulpal limited to tooth at site of infiltration (I) premolars to midline
			Target				
			Slightly superior to mental foramen, Note: (I) Keep pressure over foramen for 1 minute after injection see Figure 14–26				***Periodontium/Soft tissues:*** Premolars to midline

		Depth of Insertion	Angle of Insertion			Teeth anesthetized:
Gow-Gates (GG)	Long 25/27 gauge	Distal to maxillary second molar at height of mesiolingual cusp see Figure 14–37	½ to ¾ length of needle, MUST contact bone	Barrel of syringe in corner of mouth on opposite side. Proceed on a parallel line from corner of mouth to tragus	1.8 ml	All teeth in quadrant
			Target			**Periodontium/Soft tissues:**
			Lateral side of condylar neck Note: Patient should keep mouth open for 1–2 minutes after injection, mouth prop recommended see Figure 14–38			All periodontium, buccal mucosa premolars to midline, floor of mouth and ½ tongue in quadrant
		Depth of Insertion	**Angle of Insertion**			**Teeth anesthetized:**
Local infiltration injections	Extra-Short or Short 25/27/30 gauge	Mucobuccal fold buccal to tooth see Figure 14–30	3–6 mm to apex	Approximately 20 degrees to long axis of tooth, directed toward apex of tooth, bevel toward bone	0.6 ml	At injection site
			Target			**Periodontium/Soft tissues:**
			Selected soft tissue, gingival or apex of tooth			At injection site

Field of Anesthesia

IA
(w/ lingual)

Teeth anesthetized:

all teeth in quadrant

Periodontium/Soft tissues:

all periodontium, buccal mucosa

premolars to midline,

floor of mouth and

½ tongue in quadrant

Buccal

Teeth anesthetized:

Periodontium/Soft tissues:

buccal to molars

Mandibular Injections

GG
(Gow-Gates)

Teeth anesthetized:

all teeth in quadrant

Periodontium/Soft tissues:

all periodontium, buccal mucosa

premolars to midline,

floor of mouth and

½ tongue in quadrant

Infiltration

Teeth anesthetized:

at injection site

Periodontium/Soft tissues:

at injection site

Incisive

Teeth anesthetized:

premolars to midline

Periodontium/Soft tissues:

premolars to midline

Mental

Teeth anesthetized:

pulpal limited to tooth

at site of infiltration

Periodontium/Soft tissues:

premolars to midline

Lingual
(Alone)

Tongue - Lateral View

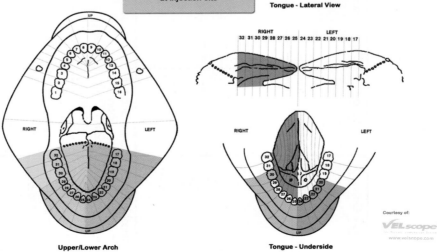

Upper/Lower Arch

Tongue - Underside

Courtesy of:

VELscope
www.velscope.com

Chapter 15

Injections for Supplemental Pain Control

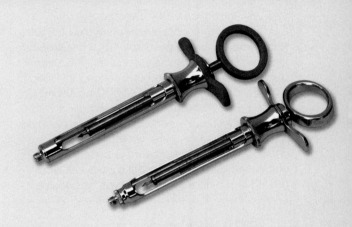

OBJECTIVES

- Define and discuss the key terms in this chapter.
- Describe and discuss the indications, relevant anatomy, and technique features of the injections discussed in this chapter.
- Describe the basic technique steps for safe and effective administration for the following injections:
  - Periodontal ligament (PDL)
  - Intraosseous
  - Intraseptal
  - Intrapulpal

KEY TERMS

backflow **305**
blanching **306**
cancellous bone **310**
computer controlled local anesthetic device (CCLAD) **304**
cortical plate **310**
dental plexus **310**
deposition site **304**
intraligamentary **304**

intraosseous **304**
intrapulpal **317**
intraseptal **315**
needle pathway **304**
paresthesia **317**
penetration site **304**
peridental **304**
periodontal ligament (PDL) injection **304**
spongy bone **310**

John Jones, a 45-year-old male presented for treatment at a university clinic for a restorative procedure on tooth #4. As he was being seated, he stated that he had dreaded this appointment because no one had ever been able to numb #4. "It's the only tooth they can't numb," he said to the student. Significantly, he remembered the tooth's number.

An infiltration using 2% lidocaine with 1:100,000 epinephrine was attempted but failed to provide any signs or symptoms of anesthesia in the area, not even in the soft tissues. The student decided to use articaine but a second infiltration with 4% articaine with 1:100,000 epinephrine yielded no better results. A third infiltration with articaine, where the penetration site was located as high as possible in the vestibule, resulted in widespread anesthesia over the buccal surface of the tooth and upper lip but a pulp test quickly proved that pulpal anesthesia was inadequate.

INTRODUCTION

Anatomic landmarks and considerations for each supplemental injection technique discussed will be presented in reference to the **penetration site, needle pathway,** and **deposition site** as described in Chapter 11. The penetration site will be related to hard and soft tissue landmarks. The needle pathway will be described in terms of the types of tissue that will be penetrated by or located in the vicinity of the needle, including mucosa, superficial fascia, muscle, vessels, nerves, and bone. The deposition site will be described in terms of the tissues at or near the target and in relation to specific landmarks.

SUPPLEMENTAL INJECTION TECHNIQUES

This chapter will discuss supplemental injection techniques that are used primarily in special situations in dentistry. Key elements for each of these injections are summarized in Appendix 15–1. Common applications, variations, and precautions will be discussed where applicable.

PERIODONTAL LIGAMENT INJECTION

Perhaps the most universal of the supplemental injections is the **periodontal ligament (PDL) injection.** This technique is indicated as a primary method of anesthesia for single teeth, for supplemental anesthesia of individual teeth when other techniques have failed to provide profound anesthesia, when widespread anesthesia is contraindicated, and when total doses need to be minimized (Blanton & Jeske, 2003). It can also be beneficial for individuals with bleeding disorders and when needle insertions into vascular regions may be a risk and, in some very specific applications, may provide widespread anesthesia when inferior alveolar blocks have failed to provide it. The PDL is also referred to as an **intraligamentary** or **peridental** technique. PDL injections are classified as **intraosseous** techniques because they rely on diffusion of solution through *bone* in order to achieve anesthesia.

A standard dental syringe can be used to administer PDL injections. Specialized syringes for administering these injections have been available for over a century and provide for easier delivery of anesthetic solution. As discussed in Chapter 9, "Local Anesthetic Delivery Devices," these syringes require less hand pressure. **Computer controlled local anesthetic devices (CCLADs)** eliminate manual pressures altogether, and regulate the rate of delivery of anesthetics electronically.

Field of Anesthesia

PDL injections anesthetize individual teeth at the sites of injection and their associated periodontium. The field of anesthesia is minimal. Individual teeth can be profoundly anesthetized along with their lingual and buccal mucosa without any anesthesia of the tongue or cheek.

Occasionally, more widespread anesthesia can develop from PDL injections in the mandible providing anesthesia to all of the teeth on one side (discussed in Box 15–1), or when 4% articaine is used, which has reportedly provided wider areas of anesthesia (Quinn, 1998; Reitz, Reader, Nist, Beck, & Meyers, 1998a) (see Figure 15–1 ■).

Anatomical Factors

PDL injections deposit anesthetic solution under pressure into the periodontal ligament, forcing the drug through alveolar bone to the apex of a tooth. Solution

Box 15–1   *PDL Techniques to Supplement IA Blocks*

Symptomatic verification of anesthesia following IA nerve blocks has been problematic. Despite confirmation that the teeth, lip, and chin "feel" numb prior to treatment, pain is sometimes experienced. This can occur due to what is referred to as accessory innervation where fibers from other sources provide at least some of the innervation to the teeth in question. See Chapter 16, "Troubleshooting Inadequate Anesthesia" for a more complete description of accessory innervation. This can also occur due to incomplete IA blocks which are estimated to be 80 to 85% successful (Malamed, 2004). Even after negative pulp tests have confirmed pulpal anesthesia, pain can be experienced during treatment.

When accessory innervation from afferent fibers of nonprimary nerves provides pulpal sensations to teeth, techniques that address those fibers can provide profound anesthesia. For example, when afferent fibers of the mylohyoid nerve provide pulpal sensation to mandibular molars, mylohyoid nerve blocks can provide profound anesthesia. See Box 15–7, "Mylohyoid Nerve Block" in Chapter 14, "Injections for Mandibular Pain Control," for a description of the mylohyoid nerve block technique.

When the difficulty arises due to inadequate IA blocks rather than accessory innervation, techniques to block accessory sources of innervation will not provide profound anesthesia. Instead, individual teeth can be anesthetized using PDL injections. PDL injections can provide profound

anesthesia even when accessory sources are innervating the teeth, because PDLs are effective at the apical regions of teeth, blocking impulse conduction in all directions from that location.

Some clinicians have observed profound inferior alveolar nerve anesthesia developing after administering PDL injections around all four aspects of the mandibular second molar (ML, DL, DB, MB). The location of the mandibular canal in close proximity to the apices of the roots of the mandibular second molar may provide insight into the efficacy of this approach.

No lingual anesthesia is provided with this series of PDL injections (other than in the vicinity of the lingual surface of the second molar) and the duration of the block is usually no greater than 60 minutes. The failed IANB usually provides adequate soft tissue anesthesia in the area of the PDL injections. If the soft tissues are not adequately anesthetized, pre-anesthesia using a lingual and/or buccal nerve block will allow the PDLs to be administered comfortably.

Once PDL anesthesia is in effect, patients frequently touch their *chins* and say, "It's really getting numb now." The increased symptoms of anesthesia in the chin are a good indication that core bundles of the IA nerve have been flooded with sufficient anesthetic to provide profound anesthesia. While the durations are short compared with traditional IA nerve blocks, probably due to the limited volumes of solution administered, onset is rapid and usually sufficient to complete treatment in comfort.

---

does not diffuse through the dense, fibrous periodontal ligament. In order to arrive at the apical region of a tooth, solution follows the *path of least resistance,* which includes the thin, porous layer of alveolar bone proper and the spongy underlying bone surrounding the ligament and tooth. To better appreciate this difference in resistance, imagine creating a pool of anesthetic solution over a sheet of dense, fibrous periodontal ligament versus creating the same pool over porous alveolar bone. The bone will absorb the solution much more readily. In order to diffuse through bone, solution must

be fully surrounded by and enclosed within the dense fibers of the periodontal ligament and the root of the tooth. If the solution enters the sulcus, it will leak out, following the path of least resistance. Solution will then **backflow** or leak into the patient's mouth rather than diffuse through bone.

Technique Factors

Key factors for successful PDL injections are discussed as follows.

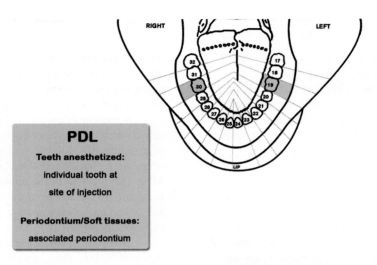

■ **FIGURE 15–1** Field of Anesthesia for Periodontal Ligament Injections. The field of anesthesia for PDL injection is indicated by the shaded areas.

Penetration Site

The penetration site for a PDL injection is within the sulcus that surrounds a tooth. Multiple sites are often necessary in order to achieve profound anesthesia. The easiest areas to approach are the mesial and distal gingival aspects. In single rooted teeth, selecting up to two sites is usually adequate, while in multiple rooted teeth, selecting three to four sites is more typical (see Figures 15–2 ■ and 15–4).

Needle Pathway

The needle first enters the sulcus and then penetrates the junctional epithelium. With the tooth root as a guide, it is then advanced within the periodontal ligament to a point of resistance.

Deposition Site

The deposition site for a PDL injection is any point in which the tip of the needle is wedged between the root of a tooth and within the periodontal ligament (see Figure 15–3 ■). This is typically no more than enough tissue to "bury" the bevel, or 3 to 4 mm beyond the attachment. Functionally, this means that the needle is at an adequate depth to prevent backflow of anesthetic solution and to note light **blanching** or paling of the attached gingiva when depositing solution. If solution flows out of the sulcus or light blanching is not seen, slightly deeper penetration within the periodontal ligament to a new site is usually necessary for successful deposition. Box 15–2 discusses how to observe for adequate blanching.

Technique Steps

Establishing soft tissue anesthesia ("pre-anesthesia") is necessary before attempting any intraosseous technique. Since the rationale for performing intraosseous anesthesia is to control pain, anesthetizing the tissues first with a different technique is a logical and mandatory first step.

PDL injections are comfortably administered supplemental to other injection techniques where soft tissue anesthesia already exists. In the absence of pre-existing anesthesia, an infiltration or nerve block technique (such as a buccal nerve block) may be used to pre-anesthetize the soft tissues around a tooth or teeth.

When using CCLADs, such as the STA Single Tooth Anesthesia System™ and CompuDent/Wand® Instruments, pre-anesthesia may be beneficial but is not always required, according to the manufacturer of these devices (Milestone Scientific, Livingston, New Jersey), because the technique establishes an "anesthesia pathway" providing comfort during penetration.

Needle Selection

Needles for PDL injections vary. Standard syringe needles of all gauges may be used including ultra-short 30 gauge needles, which are designed specifically for limited penetration injections such as the PDL. Some CCLAD systems provide their own needles, which do not fit

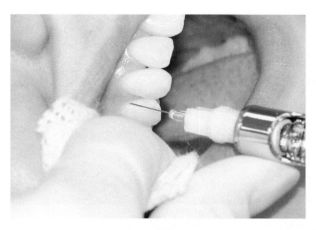

■ **FIGURE 15–2** Penetration Site for PDL Injections. The penetration site for a PDL injection is indicated by the needle.

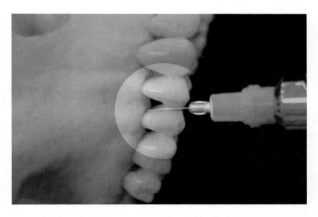

■ **FIGURE 15–3** Deposition Site for PDL Injections. The deposition site for a PDL injection is indicated by the needle in the spotlighted area.

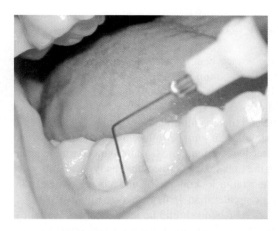

■ **FIGURE 15–4** Bending Needles for Access in PDL Injections. Enhanced visibility and access using a bent needle for a PDL injection. Factors related to bending needles for PDL injections are discussed in Box 15–3.

Box 15–2 Blanching & Deposition in PDL Injections

It is important to observe light blanching in the attached gingiva of the tooth being anesthetized because it confirms that solution is being retained in the tissues (not exiting via the sulcus) and that the resisting tissues are nearing their limit for accommodating solution. The deposition time period (the 20 second count) begins only after there is no observed backflow and blanching is observed (the accommodation limit is reached). Deposited solution thereafter will be diffusing through bone.

Light blanching may be described as pale pink in color with visibly less color compared with adjacent tissues. Stark, white blanching should be avoided and, if it occurs, the depth of penetration should be increased slightly.

---

standard syringes and are available only in 27 and 30 gauge diameters.

Successful PDL injections have been performed using 25, 27, and 30 gauge standard and specialized needles. Since there is a negligible rate of positive aspiration and the penetration depth is minimal, safety is not compromised with 30 gauge needles. While these needles may be more convenient from the standpoint of access, some clinicians find their excessive flexibility to be awkward. Long needles can prove awkward as well, due to the difficulties encountered when positioning them for sulcular access in posterior areas of the mouth.

Accessing posterior sites, in general, can be challenging with standard needle angulations. Although not an ideal practice, this restriction can be eliminated by bending the needle to a 45 degree angle (see Figure 15–4 ■). Before attempting to bend a needle, see Box 15–3 for detailed information on bending needles and safety recommendations.

Box 15–3 *Factors for Bending Needles*

Needles are bent for ease of access every day. Many experts recommend bending needles in very specific circumstances (Jastak, Yagiela, & Donaldson, 1995; Malamed, 2004). If a decision is made to bend a needle and there is minimal risk that the needle will be lost within tissue, the following should be observed: a sterile technique; the least amount of torque placed on the hub/shaft interface; the ready availability of a hemostat or locking pliers; and a bend in the needle of no greater than 45 degrees (see Figure 15–4).

The bend should be made near the center of the needle shaft, *not* at the hub/shaft interface, in order to create a 45 degree angle and to avoid undue stress on the shaft (see Figure 15–5 ■). The needle must first be bent to *no more than* a 90 degree angle and then released, allowing it to "spring back" to a 45 degree angle or less, depending on the degree of the initial bend.

For optimal safety, commercially designed syringe adaptors with 45 degree angles are available and recommended (see Figure 9–33). These attachments eliminate the need for bending needles and their use does not compromise safety. OSHA regulations relating to work place safety do not prohibit bending *sterile* needles. Bending of *contaminated* needles, however, *is* prohibited except under certain "compelling circumstances." These devices are discussed in Chapter 9, "Local Anesthetic Delivery Devices."

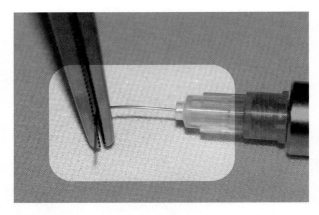

■ **FIGURE 15–5** Technique for Bending Needles. A one-handed technique for bending a needle with a sterile hemostat is illustrated, using a 90 degree bend and allowing the needle to spring back to a 45 degree final position relative to the shank.

Box 15–4 *Site Selection and Sequence of PDL Injections*

Ease of access is key to maintaining stability in PDL injections. Blanching and the absence of backflow confirm that the selected site readily accommodates solution and will likely result in success. Pre-anesthesia eliminates concerns that the injection is causing discomfort. A primary benefit of eliminating concerns of causing discomfort is clinician confidence when solutions are forced into ligamental areas under pressure. If patients react, clinicians typically "ease up" on the pressure.

The following guidelines recognize the importance of ease of access as well as ergonomics when administering PDL injections:

1. For maxillary teeth, select sites on the buccal
2. For mandibular teeth, select sites on the lingual
3. Observe blanching in subsequent sites before penetrating additional sites
4. When blanching is observed circumferentially, no more penetrations are necessary

Injection Procedure

Once pre-anesthesia has been established, PDL injections may be administered in comfort and with confidence. The selection of penetration sites around a tooth is based upon ease of access, penetrating within areas of existing anesthesia, and confirmation of diffusion through bone (no backflow and light blanching). If any of the three conditions is absent, a different site should be chosen (see Box 15–4).

Bevel orientation is irrelevant to the success of PDL injections. If bevels are oriented to face the roots of teeth, two useful purposes can be served. Easier penetration to depth is possible when the sharp tips of needles are kept away from root surfaces, and gouging can be minimized while needles are advancing.

Begin by slipping beneath the sulcular epithelium, through the periodontal ligament attachment, until resistance is met. At the point of resistance, start depositing solution. Aspiration is unnecessary because there is no significant risk of intravascular injection with this technique. Once the tissues blanch lightly and there is no backflow of solution, deposit 0.2 ml, at a rate of 0.2 ml (about one stopper) over a *full* 20 seconds. Slow timing is critical, remembering that the solution needs adequate time to diffuse through the alveolus. It may be helpful to count silently while depositing (1001, 1002, 1003 . . . 1020) to make sure that adequate time is allowed for diffusion of solution. In single-rooted teeth, 0.2 ml of solution is recommended in up to two different sites. In multiple-rooted teeth, three to four sites are usually necessary, or 0.6 to 0.8 ml (up to ~1/2 cartridge) of total solution.

Syringes designed specifically for PDL injections are discussed in Chapter 9 (see Figure 9–31). These devices are able to deliver controlled volumes of drug while tracking doses.

Confirming Anesthesia

Subjective signs of anesthesia for PDL injections are variable. Patients typically report a sense of numbness when biting down on the anesthetized tooth or teeth, and the soft tissues surrounding the tooth or teeth may feel somewhat numb. Typically, patients will report few signs or symptoms of anesthesia from this injection when used as a primary method of anesthesia compared with standard nerve blocks, for example. When given as a supplemental injection, patients typically report the rapid development of more profound numbness.

Objective signs include a lack of response to gentle stimulation with an instrument, a negative response to pulp testing, and no pain during procedures.

Common Causes of Injection Failure

Failures occur most frequently while clinicians are learning this technique, specifically when needles are not maintained securely in the PDL space, when solution backflows into the mouth, or when the deposition rate is accelerated (less than 20 seconds). Failures also occur when penetration sites do not allow solution to be deposited. There should be no hesitation to select a different site if solution will not flow out of the tip of the needle or blanching is not observed.

Troubleshooting

If anesthesia is inadequate, repeat the procedure in a different location around the tooth, making sure that there is no backflow and that pale pink blanching develops *before* depositing for the timed 20 second interval.

Technique Modifications and Alternatives

Since PDL injections are alternatives to nearly all other techniques, alternatives to PDLs include nearly all other techniques, depending on the location of the teeth in question. The choice of device also provides alternatives to the delivery of PDLs. This includes standard versus computer-controlled and specialized syringes (Blanton & Jeske, 2003).

It is important to read accompanying literature furnished with these devices because recommended volumes of solution and injection times vary significantly. For example, when using the STA Single Tooth Anesthesia System Instrument or CompuDent Instrument CCLAD (both manufactured by Milestone Scientific), it is recommended that a full 0.9 ml of any 2% or 3% solution be deposited for each penetration site. When administering 4% articaine, 0.45 ml is recommended by the manufacturer for PDL injections with the new STA Single Tooth Anesthesia System Instrument. If using the Comfort Control Syringe (Dentsply International, York, Pennsylvania), 0.2 ml per site is recommended, similar to other PDL injections, but the deposition rate slows from 20 to 30 seconds. These devices are discussed in Chapter 9; see Figures 9–37 and 9–38.

Complications

As may be true with other intraosseous techniques, patients occasionally experience slight postoperative soreness or sensitivity in the areas of injection.

Other complications are rare. Even though greater tissue damage can be expected following PDL injections compared with most nonintraosseous techniques, the damage has been described as reversible (Kanaa, Whitworth, Corbett, & Meechan, 2006). It may be helpful to caution patients that they may expect a little postoperative soreness around the specific tooth or teeth that were injected.

The use of PDL injections in two specific circumstances is controversial. Some sources suggest that primary teeth with underlying permanent successors should not be exposed to the pressures involved in PDL injections in order to avoid damage to developing teeth (Dudkiewicz, Schwartz, & Laliberte, 1987; Malamed, 2004; Replogle, Reader, Nist, Beck, Weaver, & Meyers, 1997). While this caution has not been fully substantiated due to ethical concerns, it has not been fully refuted, for the same reason. For further discussion, see Box 15–5.

As with all other intraosseous procedures, infective endocarditis and orthopedic premedication with antibiotics is recommended for those at highest risk. Local anesthetic injections, in general, are not considered invasive and therefore are not indications for antibiotic prophylaxis. All intraosseous injections, however, *are* considered invasive because they target medullary bone.

INTRAOSSEOUS TECHNIQUE

The primary benefit of intraosseous anesthesia is to provide anesthesia when other techniques have failed or when profound anesthesia of specific teeth is indicated (Blanton & Jeske, 2003; Brown, 2000; Coggins, Reader, Nist, Beck & Meyers, 1996; Replogle et al., 1997; Gallatin, Reader, Nusstein, Beck, & Weaver,

2003). Secondary benefits include minimizing bleeding when there are increased risks, limiting the extent of anesthetized areas, and decreasing total drug doses. Some have suggested that intraosseous injections are most successful when used as adjuncts for IA nerve blocks, particularly in molar areas (Dunbar, Reader, Nist, Beck, & Meyers, 1996; Reitz, Reader, Nist, Beck, & Meyers, 1998b). It has been reported that supplemental intraosseous injections improved the success rate of anesthesia in vital asymptomatic mandibular first molars up to 97 percent (Daniel, Harfst, & Wilder, 2008; Fehrenbach & Herring, 2007; Jastak et al., 1995; Malamed, 2004; Nusstein, Reader, Nist, Beck, & Meyers, 1998). While less frequently used in the maxilla, there have been occasions, particularly during endodontic therapy, where intraosseous injections have proven useful (Coggins et al., 1996).

Cancellous, spongy bone (the compressible bone between adjacent tooth sockets) was originally accessed with surgical round burs. In addition to round burs, several specialized devices are currently available which facilitate penetration of the thin, however dense, outer layer of bone in the jaw **(cortical plates).** These devices provide access to the spongy alveolar bone surrounding the **dental plexus.** Anesthesia provided by these devices is localized to one or two teeth.

Field of Anesthesia

The areas anesthetized are minimal and include the pulps of the teeth and their supporting structures immediately adjacent to the sites of deposition. Occasionally, more widespread signs and symptoms develop (see Figure 15–6 ■).

Anatomical Factors

Intraosseous techniques involve the same alveolar bone as the PDL injections. Unlike the PDL, it requires surgical access to spongy bone. A thin layer of highly-innervated connective tissue, the periosteum, covers and protects the bone, and also must be penetrated.

Technique Factors

Key factors for successful intraosseous injections are discussed as follows.

Devices for Intraosseous Injection

There are a number of devices available for intraosseous injection; they include: the Stabident® system (Fairfax Dental, Inc.); the X-Tip™ (Dentsply Maillefer); and

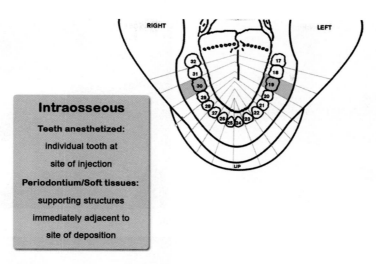

Intraosseous

Teeth anesthetized:

individual tooth at

site of injection

Periodontium/Soft tissues:

supporting structures

immediately adjacent to

site of deposition

■ **FIGURE 15–6** Field of Anesthesia for an Intraosseous Injection. The field of anesthesia for an intraosseous injection is indicated by the shaded area.

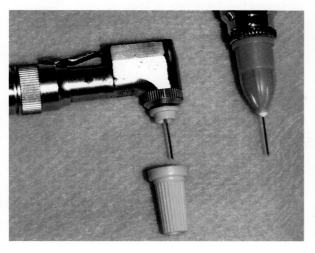

■ **FIGURE 15–7** Stabident Intraosseous Anesthesia Delivery System.

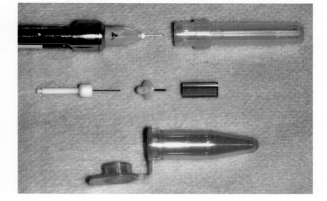

■ **FIGURE 15–8** X-Tip Intraosseous Anesthesia Delivery System.

Penetration Site

The optimal penetration site for an intraosseous injection is the most apical extent of the attached gingiva between adjacent teeth (see Figure 15–11A ■). While

the IntraFlow™ device (Pro-Dex Micro Motors). These devices are shown in Figure 15–7 ■, Figure 15–8 ■, Figure 15–9 ■, and Figure 15–10 ■.

penetration should occur within attached tissue, it should be located only barely within it, in an apical direction. Chapter 20, "Insights from Specialties: Oral Surgery, Periodontics, and Endodontics," provides alternate descriptions of this site.

In the molar region of the mandible, where cortical plate thickness is greatest, the crestal third of the alveolar process lies beneath the most apical extent of the attached gingiva and is the area where the cortical plate of bone is thinnest.

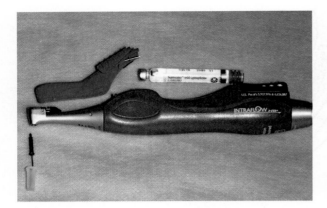

■ **FIGURE 15–9** IntraFlow Intraosseous Anesthesia Delivery System. Components of the IntraFlow device.

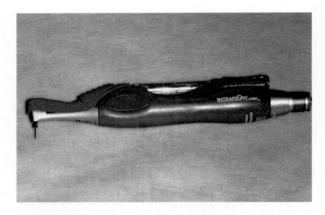

■ **FIGURE 15–10** Assembled IntraFlow Device.

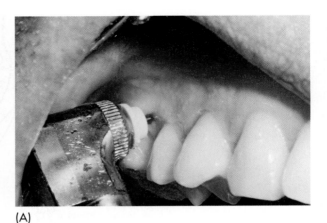

(A)

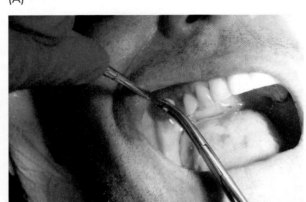

(B)

■ **FIGURE 15–11** A—Penetration Site for an Intraosseous Injection. The penetration site for an intraosseous injection is indicated by the perforator (Stabident). B—Removing the Perforator after Initial Penetration. The perforator is removed prior to needle insertion with a Stabident.

Source: Courtesy of Albert "Ace" Goerig DDS, MS.

The site chosen should be distal to the tooth to be anesthetized at an equal distance from the adjacent tooth. It should approximate the apical extent of the attached gingiva, which is approximately 2 mm below a line connecting the gingival margins of the teeth (Shimada & Gasser, 1989). Mesial penetration is acceptable but distal penetration is recommended.

After withdrawal of the perforator portion of the Stabident or X-Tip device, the needle is introduced into the perforation to deliver a local anesthetic drug into the periradicular medullary bone as demonstrated in Figure 15–12 ■. If an IntraFlow device is used, it is

not necessary to withdraw the perforator and insert a needle since the device contains both perforator and needle (see Figure 15–13 ■ and Box 15–6).

Needle Pathway

The needle follows the perforation through the cortical plate of bone into interproximal bone.

Deposition Site

The deposition site is the interproximal bone underlying the cortical plate. Once penetration through the cortical plate is "felt" by the clinician (for an alternate description

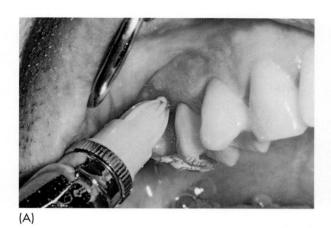

(A)

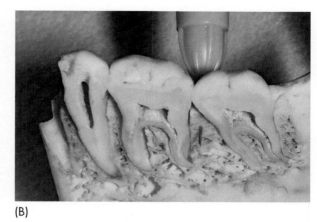

(B)

■ **FIGURE 15–12** Needle Insertion for Drug Delivery with a Stabident. After removal of the perforator portion the needle is introduced to deliver a local anesthetic drug. A—Needle inserted through perforation. B—Needle penetration demonstrated into spongy bone.

Source: Courtesy of Albert "Ace" Goerig DDS, MS.

of this sensation, see Chapter 20) the deposition site has been reached (see Figure 15–13A and Figure 15–13B).

Technique Steps

Apply the basic injection steps outlined in Chapter 11 and summarized in Appendix 11–1. Additionally, apply the guidelines listed in Box 15–6.

Periosteum overlying the mandible and maxilla is very sensitive and pre-anesthesia is recommended for comfort before performing any intraosseous technique.

Needle Selection

For intraosseous injections, needles and other armamentarium must be purchased for the specific system selected. All manufacturer instructions should be followed.

Injection Procedure

With pre-anesthesia in place, begin perforation (see Figure 15–11A, Figure 15–13A, and Figure 15–14 ■), avoiding the buildup of heat due to friction. Once the cortical plate has been perforated, insert the needle as

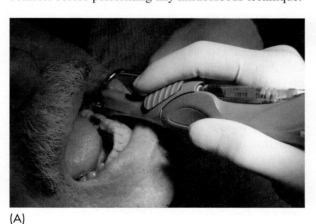

(A)

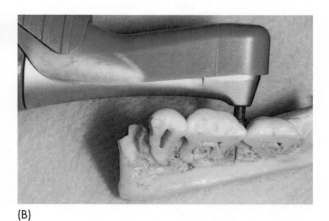

(B)

■ **FIGURE 15–13** Initial Penetration and Delivery with the IntraFlow. The initial penetration (A) is performed in the same manner as for Stabident and X-Tip devices. However there is no need to remove the perforator. The drug is delivered directly through the device into spongy bone (B).

Source: Courtesy of Albert "Ace" Goerig DDS, MS.

> ### Box 15–6   Guidelines for Administering an Intraosseous Injection
>
> - **Step 1**—If there is no previous existing anesthesia of soft tissue, anesthetize the attached gingiva first
> - **Step 2**—Mark the penetration site by blanching with a blunt-tipped instrument
> - **Step 3**—Perforate the cortical plate and deposit solution into cancellous bone (this is painless when Step 1 has been performed)
>
> *Note:* Avoid vasoconstrictors (these drugs enter the CVS rapidly) and observe all maximum dose recommendations.

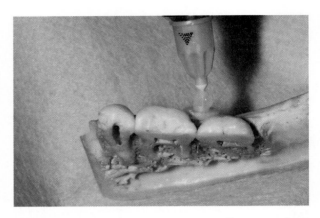

■ **FIGURE 15–16**   Needle Insertion Following Perforation using X-Tip System.

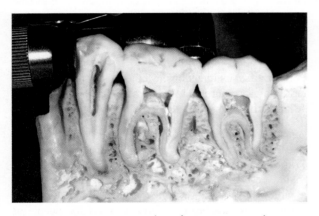

■ **FIGURE 15–14**   Initial Perforation Using the X-Tip System.

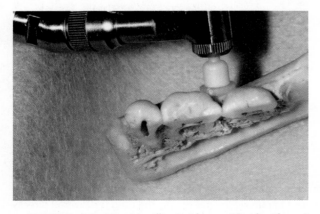

■ **FIGURE 15–15**   Needle Guide or "Guide Sleeve" Placed for X-Tip System.

recommended for the specific device being used (see Figure 15–12, Figure 15–13B, Figure 15–15 ■ and Figure 15–16 ■). As with the PDL injection, aspiration is not necessary. Box 15–7 provides suggested volumes of solutions when using the Stabident system, as an example. It is important to refer to manufacturers' instructions at all times for proper use of these devices. For an alternate description of this injection procedure see Chapter 20.

Confirming Anesthesia

Subjective signs of anesthesia for intraosseous injections are few. Patients may report a sense of numbness when biting down on the tooth or teeth anesthetized, or the soft tissues surrounding the tooth or teeth may feel somewhat numb. The absence of a response to electronic pulp testers (EPTs) or to the application of icy cold temperatures can confirm anesthesia. In Chapter 12, "Injections for Maxillary Pain Control" see Figure 12–7, Figure 12–8, and Figure 12–9.

Objective signs include a lack of response to gentle stimulation with an instrument and no pain during the procedure for soft tissues or teeth. The absence of pain is confirming.

Common Causes of Injection Failure

Inadequate cancellous bone in the central incisor region may not allow this technique to be performed. Solution is not able to diffuse easily through what is essentially a cortical "sandwich" of bone with no intermediate spongy layer.

Failures occur most frequently while clinicians are learning this technique. Studies have shown it to

---

> Box 15–7   Suggested Volumes for
> Intraosseous Injections
> (Stabident)
>
> *Mandible:*
>
> 1 tooth: 0.45–0.6 ml (mesial or distal to tooth)
>
> 2 teeth: 0.6–0.9 ml (between the two)
>
> 3 teeth: 0.9 ml (distal to the middle tooth)
>
> 6 anteriors: one injection on each side, between
>   canines and premolars 0.9 ml per side
>
> *Maxilla:*
>
> 1: 0.45 ml
>
> 2: 0.45 ml
>
> 4 adjacent teeth: midway between 0.9 ml
>
> Up to 8 teeth on one side: 1.8 ml midway between

Source: Malamed, 2004.

be nearly 100 percent successful once clinicians gain confidence and experience and *when it is used as an adjunctive technique.* When used as the initial approach to anesthesia, some studies have demonstrated only a 75 percent success rate (Gallatin, Stabile, Reader, Nist, & Beck, 2000). With practice, success rates, along with skill and confidence, tend to increase.

Troubleshooting

Penetration of the cortical plate *distal* to the tooth to be anesthetized is more successful compared with mesial sites when using these techniques. Choose alternate sites, including mesial areas, if none is acceptable distal to a tooth. If unable to perforate cortical bone *quickly* in any site, an alternate site should be chosen without hesitation. If no sites will allow easy perforation, choose an alternate technique.

Technique Modifications and Alternatives

In some situations, the mandibular molar region is difficult to penetrate due to thick cortical bone, which reduces the effectiveness of intraosseous injections. Alternatives to bone-perforating intraosseous injections include nonperforating intraosseous injections (PDLs), nerve blocks, and reappointing after providing appropriate medications.

Complications

As with all other intraosseous techniques, patients may experience postoperative soreness and sensitivity in the areas of injection.

Complications are rare and include root damage when adjacent teeth are very close to one another and preassessment failed to note this contraindication to the technique. Injury to the cortical plate is unique to intraosseous techniques. Fortunately, this damage has been shown to be reversible. Since the technique requires injury to bone regardless of the perforating system, the healing process is somewhat slow, although usually painless. Reported complications include pain and swelling at the injection site as well as bruising (Dudkiewicz et al., 1987).

Heart palpitations can be expected when vasoconstrictors are used. To avoid palpitations, use solutions without vasoconstrictors (Guglielmo, Reader, Nist, Beck, & Weaver, 1999). If vasoconstrictors are selected, use minimal volumes and greater dilutions, such as 1:200,000 dilutions. According to a 1993 comparison study, 85 percent of injections with the Stabident system and 93 percent with the X-Tip resulted in *perceived* increases in heart rate (Guglielmo et al.).

INTRASEPTAL TECHNIQUE

The **intraseptal** technique is used to provide anesthesia of the periodontium lingual to a tooth and can be particularly useful when palatal tissues require anesthesia and clinicians and/or patients wish to avoid palatal injections (Malamed, 1982).

This technique is also useful when soft tissue anesthesia and hemostasis are desired for periodontal procedures but PDL injections are contraindicated due to infection. It does not provide reliable pulpal anesthesia.

Field of Anesthesia

Anesthesia provided by the intraseptal technique involves the bone, soft tissues, and other structures of the tooth in the area in which it is administered. The anesthesia provided tends to be localized and specific to one or two teeth. This technique also provides significant hemostasis when a vasoconstrictor is administered. While some pulpal anesthesia may be provided on occasion, it tends to be unreliable or very short-term in nature (see Figure 15–17 ■).

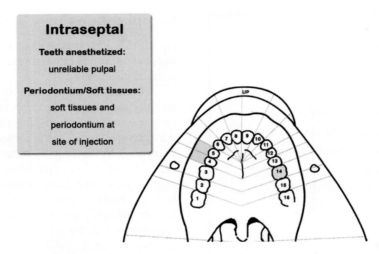

■ **FIGURE 15–17**   Field of Anesthesia for an Intraseptal Injection. The field of anesthesia for an intraseptal injection is indicated by the shaded area.

Anatomical Factors

The intraseptal technique involves alveolar bone, similar to the intraosseous and PDL injections. Unlike the PDL, intraosseous, and intrapulpal techniques, however, it does not provide reliable pulpal anesthesia.

Technique Factors

Key factors for successful intraseptal injections are discussed as follows.

Penetration Site

The penetration site is at the center of the interdental papilla adjacent to the tooth to be treated and below the *height* of the interdental papilla (about 2 mm) but *within* the attached gingiva (note: insufficient attached gingiva would preclude using this technique for any particular site). This is similarly represented by the penetration site for an intraosseous injection in Figure 15–11.

Needle Pathway

The needle advances through soft tissue until bone is contacted and then is gently forced deeper into the interdental bone.

Deposition Site

The deposition site is just inside the cortical plate of bone. Unlike an intraosseous injection (see Figure 15–16),

however, no perforation is made in the bone prior to needle insertion.

Technique Steps

Apply the basic injection steps outlined in Chapter 11 and summarized in Appendix 11–1. Pre-anesthetize the area if anesthesia is not already in effect at the penetration site. See Box 15–6 for a summary of steps.

Needle Selection

A 27 gauge needle (short) is recommended, which is consistent with the negligible rate of positive aspiration and the need for a needle with less flexibility compared with 30 gauge needles.

Injection Procedure

Once the area has been anesthetized using infiltration or any other technique, intraseptal injections can be delivered with comfort and confidence.

Insert the needle in the center of the interdental papilla, about 2 mm below the height of the attached gingiva but still within the attached tissue. Saadoun and Malamed recommend orienting the bevel toward the apex (Saadoun & Malamed, 1985). The orientation of the needle is 45 degrees to the frontal plane, at right angles to the soft tissue.

The needle is advanced until bony resistance is met, at which time pressure is applied to the syringe to force the needle just barely deeper into the interdental septum. Once within the septum, 0.2 to 0.4 ml of local anesthetic is administered (0.2 ml each over 20 seconds) against what should be considerable resistance, similar to that experienced in PDL and palatal injections. Backflow of solution and a failure to notice blanching when a vasoconstrictor is used indicate that the needle is not deep enough.

Confirming Anesthesia

Subjective signs of anesthesia for all intraosseous injections, including intraseptal injections, are few. The patient may report a sense of numbness in the soft tissues on the palatal aspects of the tooth or teeth where the intraseptal injection was delivered. Typically, patients will report few signs or symptoms of anesthesia.

Objective signs include a lack of response to gentle stimulation with an instrument and no pain during the procedure for the soft tissues. Significant blanching is the best indicator of success. The absence of pain during the procedure is often the only way to confirm anesthesia. If hemostasis is desired, decreased bleeding confirms successful procedures.

Common Causes of Injection Failure

Inadequate retention of solution and inadequate volumes of solution are the most common causes of injection failure. Failures occur most frequently as clinicians are learning this technique.

Troubleshooting

It may be necessary to repeat the injection if anesthesia fails. Alternate techniques may be necessary, such as intraosseous injections, PDL injections, AMSA nerve blocks, NP nerve blocks, GP nerve blocks, and palatal infiltrations.

Technique Modifications and Alternatives

Effectiveness is reduced for this technique in some situations. Mandibular molar regions, in particular, are more difficult to penetrate due to the presence of thicker cortical bone. Selecting penetration sites in this area can be challenging if there is unusually dense bone.

Complications

Complications are rare. As with other intraosseous techniques, patients may experience postoperative soreness or sensitivity in the area of injection.

The procedure may not be appropriate when the roots of adjacent teeth are very close to one another because roots may be inadvertently injured.

Injury to the cortical plate is unique to intraosseous techniques. Although more extensive injury has been demonstrated to occur compared with nonintraosseous techniques, damage tends to be reversible. Healing after intraseptal injections tends to be a slow, painless process but somewhat faster compared with intraosseous techniques that use cortical perforators to access spongy bone. It might be helpful to caution patients that they may expect a little more soreness compared with other appointments.

Heart palpitations can be expected when vasoconstrictors are used (Gallatin et al., 2003; Wong, 2001). In order to avoid or lessen palpitations, plain solutions or those with greater dilutions, such as 1:200,000 epinephrine are recommended.

INTRAPULPAL TECHNIQUE

The **intrapulpal** technique provides anesthesia for pulpally-involved teeth when other techniques have failed. Wong reported that using IA nerve blocks in mandibular first molars (with irreversible pulpitis) averaged only a 30 percent success rate (Wong, 2001).

The intrapulpal technique is the only nonintraosseous technique discussed in this chapter. This technique can deliver effective anesthesia when the degree of inflammation in the pulp renders conventional methods ineffective. While some strategies, such as using higher concentrations of anesthetics, have demonstrated effectiveness in similar situations, there are problems when using higher concentrations of anesthetic drugs. It has been suggested that higher concentrations can increase the possibility of inducing prolonged anesthesia referred to as **paresthesia** and place restrictive limits on volumes administered due to MRD concerns. Furthermore, higher concentrations are not available in dental cartridges and represent an impractical solution (Gallatin et al., 2000). The intrapulpal technique, on the other hand, represents a relatively simple and rapid method of providing pain relief.

Field of Anesthesia

The area affected by intrapulpal injections is minimal and is confined to pulpal tissues (see Figure 15–18 ■).

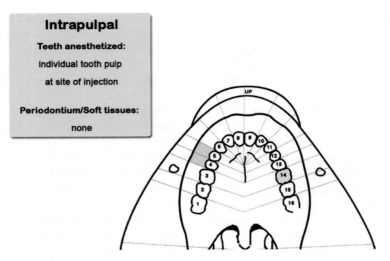

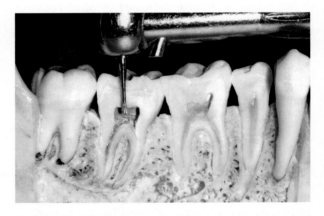

■ **FIGURE 15–18** Field of Anesthesia for an Intrapulpal Injection. The field of anesthesia for an intrapulpal injection is indicated by the shaded area.

Anatomical Factors

Intrapulpal anesthesia relies on direct access to the coronal or radicular pulp. In order for the injection to be possible, it is assumed that endodontic access has already been accomplished.

Technique Factors

Key factors for successful intrapulpal injections are discussed as follows.

Penetration Site

The penetration site is located in the pulpal tissue of the pulp chamber or within the root canal of the tooth (see Figure 15–19 ■).

Needle Pathway

The needle is directed into the pulpal tissue of the coronal chamber or root canal(s), as necessary (see Figure 15–20 ■). Anesthetic solutions are directed at the remaining areas of vital nerve.

Deposition Site

The ideal site has been described as being wedged into the chamber or the root of the tooth (Malamed, 2004). This technique provides anesthesia in two ways, primarily as a result of pressure (pressure anesthesia), and secondarily as a direct action of the drug (see Figure 15–20).

■ **FIGURE 15–19** Penetration Site for an Intrapulpal Injection. A bur must be used to access the pulp prior to needle insertion.

Technique Steps

Pre-anesthetize the area if anesthesia is not already in effect at the penetration site.

Needle Selection

A 25, 27, or 30 gauge short needle may be used. Intravascular injection is not possible in the pulp and the needle is confined within the tooth, therefore needle gauge selection is directly related to providing a needle that is small enough to fit into the chamber and canals

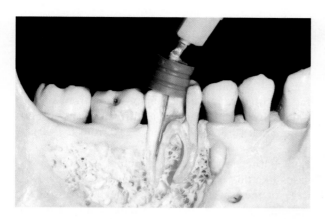

■ **FIGURE 15-20** Modification for Intrapulpal Injections. A sterile stopper can be positioned on the needle shaft to maintain pressure while solution is deposited.

without binding. Different gauges may be required on the same tooth in various roots.

Injection Procedure

After endodontic access or partial access has been accomplished, an intrapulpal injection can be performed. The patient should be warned that there may be a brief but intense pain experienced; however, this technique is effective at alleviating subsequent pain.

It may be useful to bend the needle to improve access. Before bending a needle, see Box 15–3. Solution is administered at a slow rate, 0.2 ml over 20 seconds.

Confirming Anesthesia

Subjective signs of anesthesia for intrapulpal injections are few. Primarily, the patient reports that the toothache is gone. A sense of numbness when biting down on the tooth helps to confirm profound anesthesia. Typically, patients will report few signs or symptoms of anesthesia.

Objective signs include no response to gentle stimulation with an instrument and no pain during the endodontic procedure.

Common Causes of Injection Failure

Common causes of failure include: too shallow a penetration into the pulpal tissues resulting in backflow of solution into the mouth versus within pulpal tissues;

inadequate pressure generated by the solution; the degree of inflammation or infection present; and clinician discomfort with the procedure.

Troubleshooting

Problems encountered include: root canals that are narrower than the circumference of the needle, which prevents adequate access to the nerve; a very surprising and intense initial pain that quickly subsides; and clinician discomfort with the brief but intense pain that is inflicted.

Technique Modifications and Alternatives

A useful modification when performing an intrapulpal injection is to insert the needle through a previously sterilized stopper from an unused cartridge. This can be done without touching any part of the needle and therefore without risking needlestick injury by using two sterile hemostats, one to hold the stopper and the other to hold the needle as it is being inserted into the stopper. Once inserted onto the needle shaft, penetration is made while the stopper is held tightly over the endodontic access opening of the tooth. The pressures generated by the solution will be greater compared with wedging the needle alone (see Figure 15–20).

Alternatives include intraosseous injections, PDL injections, Gow-Gates nerve blocks, and pharmacotherapies that will allow the inflammation to subside somewhat before reattempting the procedure.

Complications

The experience of brief but intense pain associated with this technique can be stressful. The use of appropriate sedatives or nitrous oxide can diminish this effect for patients and indirectly relieve clinician concerns of causing pain.

CASE MANAGEMENT: John Jones

Despite published success rates exceeding 95 percent in maxillary infiltrations, repeated infiltrations failed in this patient (Blanton & Jeske, 2003). Furthermore, the infiltrations had been assessed and administered accurately, which included verification of apex location using radiographs and adequate vestibular height for the penetration sites.

A different approach, one that circumvented unknown anatomic barriers, was decided upon. The soft tissue anesthesia that developed over #4 following the third infiltration with articaine enabled a PDL injection to be administered comfortably from the buccal aspect of the tooth. This sequence quickly provided profound pulpal anesthesia of #4, and a restorative procedure on the tooth was subsequently completed. According to the grateful patient, this was the first time ever that tooth #4 had been treated comfortably.

Case Discussion: Any number of a host of anatomic variations may have been responsible for this failure, including accessory or aberrant innervation, denser-than-normal maxillary bone in the area above #4, a prominent zygomatic process, a lingual-facing dilaceration of the apex of the root of the tooth, physiologic barriers to diffusion, and fascial planes that directed solution away from the target area.

Fortunately, obtaining pulpal anesthesia in cases like this is not dependent on an exact knowledge of the cause or causes of the failure. Understanding when anatomic variations are likely to sabotage a procedure, however, can be critical to success. Repeated infiltrations of #4, as confirmed by this patient's previous experiences over decades of dental treatment, did not result in pulpal anesthesia. An approach that circumvents barriers to anesthesia was necessary and worked well. As a result of his gratitude to the student for the comfortable procedure, he insisted on receiving all future treatment at the university clinic.

CHAPTER QUESTIONS

1. The rate of deposition of local anesthetic drugs in intraosseous, intrapulpal, and PDL injections is best represented by which *one* of the following?
   a. 0.1 ml over 20 seconds
   b. 0.2 ml over 10 seconds
   c. 0.2 ml over 20 seconds
   d. 0.1 ml over 30 seconds

2. Which *one* of the following techniques does not typically provide reliable pulpal anesthesia?
   a. Intraosseous
   b. Intrapulpal
   c. Intraseptal
   d. PDL

3. Which *one* of the following is not recommended as an anesthetic approach in irreversible pulpitis?
   a. The Stabident system
   b. PDL injections
   c. Higher concentrations of lidocaine
   d. The IntraFlow system

4. What is the approximate success rate of inferior alveolar nerve blocks, according to Wong, in pulpally involved teeth?
   a. 10 percent
   b. 20 percent
   c. 30 percent
   d. 40 percent

5. Which *one* of the following statements is true regarding PDL injections?
   a. Solution diffuses through the periodontal ligament to the dental plexus
   b. The orientation of the bevel is critical to success of the procedure
   c. The technique is only useful as an initiating technique
   d. Solution diffuses through alveolar bone to the dental plexus

REFERENCES

Blanton, P., & Jeske, A. (2003, June). The key to profound local anesthesia—Neuroanatomy. *Journal of the American Dental Association, 134,* 755–756.

Brannstrom, M., Lindskog, S., & Nordenvall, K. J. (1984). Enamel hypoplasia in permanent teeth induced by periodontal ligament anesthesia of primary teeth. *Journal of the American Dental Association, 109,* 735–736.

Brown, R. (2000). Intraosseous anaesthesia: A review. *Oral Health, 3,* 7–14.

Coggins, R., Reader, A., Nist, R., Beck, M., & Meyers, W. J. (1996). Anesthetic efficacy of the intraosseous injection in maxillary and mandibular teeth. *Oral Surgery Oral Medicine Oral Pathology Oral Radiology & Endodontics, 81*(6), 634–641.

Daniel, S. J., Harfst, S. A., & Wilder R. (2008). *Mosby's dental hygiene: Concepts, cases, and competencies* (2nd ed.). Philadelphia: Mosby Elsevier.

Dudkiewicz, A., Schwartz, S., & Laliberte, R. (1987). Effectiveness of mandibular infiltration in children using the local anesthetic Ultracaine (articaine hydrochloride). *Journal of the Canadian Dental Association, 53,* 29–31.

Dunbar, D., Reader, A., Nist, R., Beck, M., & Meyers, W. J. (1996). Anesthetic efficacy of the intraosseous injection after an inferior alveolar nerve block. *Journal of Endodontics, 22*(9), 481–486.

Fehrenbach, M. J., & Herring, S. W. (2007). Illustrated anatomy of the head and neck (3rd ed.). St. Louis: Saunders Elsevier.

Gallatin, E., Stabile, P., Reader, A., Nist, R., & Beck, M. (2000). Anesthetic efficacy and heart rate effects of the intraosseous injection of 3% mepivacaine after an inferior alveolar nerve block. *Oral Surg Oral Med Oral Pathol Oral Radiol Endod, 89*(1), 83–87.

Gallatin, J., Reader, A., Nusstein, J., Beck, M., & Weaver, J. (2003). A comparison of two intraosseous anesthetic techniques in mandibular posterior teeth. *Journal of the American Dental Association, 134*(11), 1476–1484.

Guglielmo, A., Reader, A., Nist, R., Beck, M., & Weaver, J. (1999). Anesthetic efficacy and heart rate effects of the supplemental intraosseous injection of 2% mepivacaine with 1:20,000 levonordefrin. *Oral Surg Oral Med Oral Pathol Oral Radiol Endod, 87*(3), 284–293.

Jastak, J. T., Yagiela, J. A., & Donaldson, D. (1995). *Local anesthesia of the oral cavity.* Philadelphia: Saunders.

Kanaa, M. D., Whitworth, J. M., Corbett, I. P., & Meechan, J. G. (2006). Articaine and lidocaine mandibular buccal infiltration anesthesia: A prospective randomized double-blind cross-over study. *Journal of Endodontics, 32,* 296–298.

Malamed, S. F. (1982). The periodontal ligament (PDL) injection: An alternative to inferior alveolar nerve block. *Oral Surg Oral Med Oral Pathol, 53*(2), 117–121.

Malamed, S. F. (2004). Handbook of local anesthesia (5th ed.). St. Louis: Elsevier Mosby.

Nusstein, J., Reader, A., Nist, R., Beck, M., & Meyers, W. J. (1998). Anaesthetic efficacy of the supplemental intraosseous injection of 2% lidocaine with 1:100,000 epinephrine in irreversible pulpitis. *Journal of Endodontics, 24,* 487–491.

Quinn, C. L. (1998). Injection techniques to anesthetize the difficult tooth. *Journal of the California Dental Association, 26*(9), 665–667.

Reitz, J., Reader, A., Nist, R, Beck, M., & Meyers, W. J. (1998a). Anesthetic efficacy of a repeated intraosseous injection given 30 min following an inferior alveolar nerve block/intraosseous injection. *Journal of the American Dental Society of Anesthesia, 45*(4), 143–149.

Reitz, J., Reader, A., Nist, R., Beck, M., & Meyers, W. J. (1998b). Anesthetic efficacy of the intraosseous injection of 0.9 mL of 2% lidocaine (1:100,000 epinephrine) to augment an inferior alveolar nerve block. *Oral Surg Oral Med Oral Pathol Oral Radiol Endod, 86*(5), 516–523.

Replogle, K., Reader, A., Nist, R., Beck, M., Weaver, J., & Meyers, W. J. (1997). Anesthetic efficacy of the intraosseous injection of 2% lidocaine (1:100,000 epinephrine) and 3% mepivacaine in mandibular first molars. *Oral Surg Oral Med Oral Pathol Oral Radiol Endod, 83*(1), 30–37.

Saadoun, A. P., & Malamed, S. (1985). Intraseptal anesthesia in periodontal surgery. *Journal of the American Dental Association, 111*(2), 249–256.

Shimada, K., & Gasser, R. (1989). Anatomical record: Advances in integrative anatomy and evolutionary biology. *The Anatomical Record, 224*(1), 177–182.

Wong, J. A. (2001). Adjuncts to local anesthesia: Separating fact from fiction. *Journal of the Canadian Dental Association, 67,* 391–397.

Woodmansey, K. (2005). Intraseptal anesthesia: A review of a relevant injection technique. *General Dentistry, 53*(6), 418–420.

Summary of Supplemental Injections

Injection	Needle	Penetration Site	Deposition Site			Dose*	Field of Anesthesia See Appendix 15-2
			Depth of Insertion	Angle of Insertion			
				Target			
Periodontal Ligament (PDL)	Short or Extra-short 27/25/30 gauge needle	*For maxillary PDLs, buccal sites are easiest **For mandibular PDLs, lingual sites are easiest ***Or, choose where tissues are already anesthetized Figure 15-2	3–4 mm	Parallel to the root surface in the area	Any point at which the tip of the needle is wedged against the root of the tooth and is completely confined within the periodontal ligament; blanching and the absence of back flow should be observed upon deposition Figure 15-3	1.5–1.8ml	*Teeth anesthetized:* Individual tooth at site of deposition *Periodontium/Soft tissues:* Associated periodontium
Intrapulpal	Short or Long needle, whichever gauge fits into the canals of the tooth	Penetrate into the pulp after endodontic access has been made Figure 15-19	Variable	Bend needle for ease of access directly over the pulp	A position in which the tip of the needle is wedged into the pulp chamber or root canal of the tooth to be anesthetized Figure 15-20	0.2 to 0.4 ml or one or two stoppers	*Teeth anesthetized:* Individual tooth pulp at site of injection *Periodontium/Soft tissues:* None

(Continued)

		Depth of Insertion	Angle of Insertion		Teeth anesthetized:
Intraosseous	Needles are provided with the armamentarium selected	Penetrate through the cortical plate of bone until there is a sudden loss of resistance	Perpendicular to the cortical plate	0.2–0.3 ml* *Width of rubber stopper	Individual at site of injection
	The most apical extent of the attached mucosa half way between two adjacent teeth Figure 15–12A	**Target**			**Periodontium/Soft tissues:**
		The interproximal bone underlying the cortical plate, preferably distal to the tooth to be anesthetized Figure 15–12B			Supporting structures immediately adjacent to site of deposition
		Depth of Insertion	**Angle of Insertion**		**Teeth anesthetized:**
Intra-septal	27 gauge short	Insert until there is a sudden loss of resistance	45 degrees to the long axis of the tooth	0.6 ml	Unreliable pulpal anesthesia
	Center of the interdental papilla adjacent to the tooth to be treated Figure 15–12B	**Target**			**Periodontium/Soft tissues:**
		In the center of the interdental bone adjacent to the gingival, osseous, and/or tooth structures to be treated Figure 15–12B			At site of deposition

*Dose volumes provided are minimum recommendations for pulpal anesthesia.
Modified from: 1) Malamed SF, Handbook of local anesthesia, ed 5, St Louis, 2004, Mosby; 2) Jastak JT, Yagiela JA, Donaldson D, Local anesthesia of the oral cavity. Philadelphia, 1995 W.B. Saunders; 3) Daniels SJ, Harfst SA, Wilder RS, Dental hygiene: concepts, cases and competencies, 2nd edition, St Louis, 2007, Mosby

Field of Anesthesia

Supplemental Injections

Intraseptal

Teeth anesthetized:
unreliable pulpal

Periodontium/Soft tissues:
soft tissues and
periodontium at
site of injection

Intrapulpal

Teeth anesthetized:
individual tooth pulp
at site of injection

Periodontium/Soft tissues:
none

Intraosseuos

Teeth anesthetized:
individual tooth at
site of injection

Periodontium/Soft tissues:
supporting structures
immediately adjacent to
site of deposition

PDL

Teeth anesthetized:
individual tooth at
site of injection

Periodontium/Soft tissues:
associated periodontium

LIP

RIGHT   LEFT

LIP

325

Chapter 16

Troubleshooting Inadequate Anesthesia

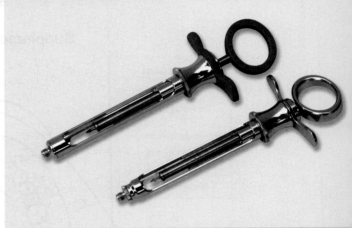

OBJECTIVES

- Define and discuss the key terms in this chapter.
- Discuss the primary reasons for inadequate local anesthesia.
- Understand the physiologic and anatomic basis of inadequate anesthesia.
- Develop critical thinking skills to help overcome frustrating anesthetic challenges.
- Develop strategies for addressing inadequate anesthesia.

KEY TERMS

CASE STUDY: Phillipe Giradot

Phillipe Giradot is a 22-year-old exchange student who is in excellent health and maintains an active regime of physical activity and regular health care. Despite his dedication to prevention, he has avoided regular dental care due to past experiences of pain, particularly in the mandible, despite the number of attempts by different clinicians (at least ten) to anesthetize him.

He presents with a nagging toothache in the vicinity of #19, which has a large and obvious carious lesion. During questioning, he avoids eye contact and grips the arms of the chair. With some prompting, he relates his past experiences with pain during dental treatment and his fear of experiencing similar pain. On his last visit, he recalls, he received a number of "shots" (nine) and that the treatment still hurt despite the number of times he was "poked" with the needle.

Box 16–1   Suggested Reading on Inadequate Anesthesia

Some suggested reading on the topic of inadequate anesthesia includes:

1. *Local Anesthesia of the Oral Cavity* by Jastak, J. T., Yagiela, J. A., & Donaldson, D.
2. *Failure of Inferior Alveolar Nerve Block, Exploring the Alternatives* by Madan, G. A., Madan, S. G., & Madan, A. D.
3. *The Failure of Local Anesthesia in Acute Inflammation* by Brown, R. D.
4. *The Possible Role of the Mylohyoid Nerve in Mandibular Posterior Tooth Sensation* by Frommer, J., Mele, F., & Monroe, C. J.
5. *Intraosseous Injection for Profound Anesthesia of the Lower Molar* by Pearce, J.
6. *Why Can't You Achieve Adequate Regional Anesthesia in the Presence of Infection?* by Najjar, T.
7. *Difficulties in Achieving Local Anesthesia* by Kaufman, E., Weinstein, P., & Milgrom, P.
8. *The Missed Inferior Alveolar Block: A New Look at an Old Problem* by Milles, M.
9. *A Pilot Study of the Clinical Problems of Regionally Anesthetizing the Pulp of an Acutely Inflamed Mandibular Molar* by Wallace, J., Michanowicz, A., Mundell, R., & Wilson, E.

Complete references are found at the end of this chapter.

INTRODUCTION

All clinicians have experienced local anesthetic failures from time to time (Meechan, 1999). The term **failure** as it is applied to local anesthesia refers to the inability to induce effective conduction blockade. Even when effective conduction blockade exists, failures can occur due to psychological factors or due to the postoperative effects of pain-free procedures. This latter situation illustrates that failure from a patient perspective does not always occur during actual appointment times.

Meechan summarizes the causes of local anesthetic failure as either *clinician* or *patient* dependent, the former related more to the choice of technique and drug and the latter related more to anatomical, pathological, and psychological factors (Meechan, 1999).

Most local anesthetic procedures performed after thorough patient assessments are effective and success rates approach 95 percent or greater for some techniques (Malamed, 2004b). When anatomy is assessed prior to injection, variations in anatomy only occasionally impact success rates. Even when profound anesthesia is not achieved after an initial injection, repeating the same injection usually provides adequate anesthesia although re-injection may also fail at times. In fact, despite the high rate of success of re-injection with the same technique, failures are seen as inevitable. The causes of inadequate anesthesia have been explored in numerous peer-reviewed articles. See Box 16–1 for some suggested titles.

When local anesthetic failures occur, not only are the experiences painful for patients but confidence in clinicians can be undermined. While not completely successful in all circumstances, strategies to overcome inadequate anesthesia nevertheless are useful in building and preserving strong patient/clinician relationships.

While patients may occasionally blame themselves for not getting numb and there may be some truth in that assumption, clinicians are keenly aware that it is their responsibility to provide adequate anesthesia. Understanding that all techniques occasionally fail to provide adequate anesthesia is a key motivation in the development of strategies to enhance success.

Blanton and Jeske have stated that neuroanatomy is the "key to profound local anesthesia" (Blanton & Jeske, 2003b). Their point is liberally reinforced in the literature. For example, studies have reported difficulties with inferior alveolar nerve blocks due to a bifid pattern, each branch of the nerve having a separate foramen (Blanton & Jeske, 2003b; Lew & Townsend, 2006).

Failure to appreciate *neuro*anatomy and its variability are not the only causes of anesthetic failure, however. Bony prominences and dense bone, atypical fascial planes, highly vascular areas, ligamental deflection, circadian (diurnal) influences (see Box 16–2) and a host of other physical and chemical barriers can be responsible for failure.

While inadequate volumes of solution may be a cause of failure, depositing excessive volumes of solution in an attempt to overwhelm nerve membranes compromises safety. Clinicians can achieve more reliable success by understanding barriers that may be present and by developing their skills with alternative techniques.

This chapter will explore the phrase "successful local anesthesia" followed by a discussion of the major categories of inadequate anesthesia and possible causes, and strategies to overcome them. Although alternative techniques will be identified in this chapter for each *failure* mentioned, specific details for performing these techniques may be found in injection technique Chapters 12–15.

DEFINING SUCCESS

The term **success,** as with the term failure, has been used in many different ways in local anesthesia, making it difficult to arrive at a generally accepted definition. Does success have the same meaning to both the clinician and the patient? For example, were procedures accomplished comfortably or does it mean they were accomplished despite some discomfort? Was pain experienced early in an appointment or later, after initial satisfactory levels of pain control? Problematic in any discussion of successful pain control is that the pain experience is subjective, as discussed in Chapter 2, "Fundamentals of Pain Management."

Published studies use a variety of phrases such as *the absence of pain, no pain during therapy, well-tolerated,* and *completely successful,* describing results with modifiers such as *most, many,* and *compared with others.* Analyses of variance (ANOVA) and visual scales (VAS) are used to analyze, quantify, and report on pain or its absence (see Box 16–3). Clinically reproducible results assess the efficacy of techniques, drugs, and behavioral modifications in pain control. Tabulated results may be used to formulate and corroborate conclusions.

Box 16–2   The Influence of Circadian (Diurnal) Body Rhythms on Local Anesthesia

Despite the use of alternative techniques and strategies, there are occasions when adequate anesthesia is not possible during a particular appointment and rescheduling is preferable for both clinician and patient. If rescheduling is agreed upon, it has been suggested that circadian rhythms may influence an individual's susceptibility to local anesthesia (Malamed, 2006; Panza, Epstein, & Quyyumi, 1991). The term **diurnal body rhythm** is frequently used to describe the variable response to drugs during different times of a day (Meechan, 1999).

In the event of unsuccessful anesthesia, rescheduling an appointment during a different time of day could prove useful (Malamed, 2006). For example, if the failed appointment occurred in the afternoon, a morning appointment could be suggested.

Box 16–3   Analyses of Variance (ANOVA) and Visual Scales (VAS)

ANOVA and VAS are frequently used research tools when studying pain. Analyses of variance assess and weigh *the impact of each variable* to the overall variations that have been demonstrated or discussed, as they relate to the outcomes of studies. Visual scales are assessment tools which give relative information regarding the perceived intensity of pain. These are expressed on a scale from 1 to 10 with 1 representing no pain and 10 representing the worst pain the patient has ever experienced. See Chapter 2 for an example of a VAS, the Wong-Baker FACES Scale.

Specific measures selected in studies to assess the absence of pain vary as well and include the use of electric pulp testing applied to teeth at specific reporting intervals and reports of pain experienced during procedures. Still others rely on evaluator and cohort interviews, reaction surveys, or both (Certosimo & Archer, 1996).

However success is defined, troubleshooting anesthetic failure is an important clinical skill. The discussion of possible causes and remedies that follows is intended to provide insight into troubleshooting local anesthetic failures and to highlight the most common categories of failure. Although suggestions in this discussion have been drawn from multiple sources, it is acknowledged that experienced clinicians may have additional, successful strategies that are not included in this text.

ADMINISTRATION-RELATED FACTORS

Local anesthetic success may be influenced by a number of factors. Those related to the administration of drugs can include the delivery devices, the drugs themselves, and clinical judgment.

Device-Related Factors

In general, the devices used for administration of local anesthetics include syringes, cartridges, and needles. Although there are a variety of different types of syringes and of drugs in cartridges, they have little impact on anesthetic failures. Additionally, there are very few needle-related issues in most procedures.

The following discussions are examples of rare device-related factors that may on occasion contribute to failures.

Needle Bevel Considerations

While needle bevel orientations are not considered critical to the success of any injection, specific orientations nevertheless are frequently recommended in some techniques (Daniel & Harfst, 2007; Malamed, 2004b). Some consider it beneficial to make bevel adjustments in order to place anesthetic solutions in closer proximity to nerves. It is possible, especially in deeper penetrations, for deflection to occur away from a target if bevel orientation is ignored (Malamed, 2004f). For example, it is recommended that bevels in Vazirani-Akinosi techniques face the midline, away from the mandible, in order to facilitate deflection towards the mandible (Malamed, 2004f).

Needle Deflection Considerations

The higher the gauge of a needle, the greater its flexibility and deflection in tissues (Robison, Mayhew, Cowan, & Hawley, 1984). A 25 gauge needle does not deflect as much in deeper penetrations although many clinicians choose to use 27 gauge needles out of concern for patient comfort even though this benefit has not been corroborated (Malamed, 2006; Hamburg, 1972). Although deflection is common when deposition sites are some distance from penetration sites, problems with inadequate anesthesia due to deflection are uncommon (Malamed, 2004d).

Quality of Cartridge Contents

On rare occasions, solutions may fall below minimum standards for clinical effectiveness. Cartridges of local anesthetics with vasoconstrictors are expected to have a minimum limit of 90 percent of the vasoconstrictor effective and a pH of no lower than 3.3, in order to be considered reliably effective (Lew & Townsend, 2006; Panza et al., 1991). Despite excellent industry standards, at least one study demonstrated that entire batches of drugs have at times fallen below these thresholds when tested immediately upon receipt (Lew & Townsend, 2006; Panza et al., 1991). While there is no way to know whether or not cartridges meet minimum standards, if a particular batch is repeatedly failing to provide profound and durable anesthesia, replacement should be considered.

It is important to understand that quality control issues are not solely the responsibility of the manufacturer. It is more likely that damage to solutions occurred during shipping, handling, or storage. Product storage facilities *and* end users must avoid extreme temperatures and improper handling and storage. Solutions should be stored in dark, room-temperature locations.

Unfortunately, the antioxidant preservatives that are necessary to maintain the effectiveness of the vasoconstrictor also lower the pH of the solution. In general, the longer a solution containing vasoconstrictors is stored before use, the greater the degradation of the drugs in the solution and the higher its acidity. Not only is acidified solution less likely to produce profound anesthesia but it is more likely to produce discomfort during administration.

Clinician Judgment

In order to provide profound anesthesia, adequate volumes of solution must be deposited to block nerve impulses.

Volumes necessary vary depending on the anatomy of the area into which solution is deposited, individual responses to local anesthetic drugs, and the length of anticipated treatment.

Volume Considerations According to Anatomy

The total volume of anesthetic drug administered must be adequate to flood targeted neural membranes. Certain techniques, such as the Gow-Gates mandibular nerve block, require greater initial volumes for sufficient diffusion to the target area. Others, such as buccal nerve blocks, where solution is placed directly over the nerve, require very little solution.

Volume Considerations According to Individual Responses

Individual responses to local anesthetic drugs are also important. For example, an individual who states, "I always take more" or "That stuff lasts forever on me" provides valuable information that is not available from physical assessment. When planning drug doses, these concerns should be addressed.

Volume Considerations According to Length of Anticipated Treatment

Volumes administered should take into account the length of anticipated treatment. Thirty minutes of soft tissue anesthesia will often require less volume compared with one hour of pulpal anesthesia in the same area. A hygiene procedure may require less time than a crown preparation and therefore smaller volumes. Conversely, a hygiene procedure may require more time and greater volumes compared with a simple restoration.

PSYCHOLOGICAL BARRIERS

Patients may relate that local anesthesia and even intravenous sedation and general anesthesia are not very effective for them while some report phobias to injections. Others are phobic to specific aspects of injections such as having no personal control, the fact that needles are involved, fear of insufficient anesthesia, or of long-lasting residual anesthesia. Some psychological barriers are hard to assess (see Box 16–4). For further discussion on injection phobias see Chapter 18, "Insights for the Fearful Patient."

Box 16–4   Psychological Barriers to Successful Anesthesia?

A situation that developed in a private office illustrates the inexplicable nature of some barriers in dentistry. Following eight inferior alveolar injections, with three different drugs, a patient continued to report inadequate anesthesia of the mandibular quadrant. Both clinician and patient agreed to reschedule.

After making a second appointment, the patient walked to her car. As she inserted the key into the lock she felt as if "lightning had struck" her. Significant signs and symptoms of anesthesia developed immediately. She went back into the office and the procedure was completed that day.

While it remains to be explained whether this was a physiological or psychological reaction, when approached with the problem, two experts, a cognitive psychologist and a neurologist, offered the following possible explanations:

1. The neurologist suggested that it was a psychological reaction stemming from the patient's anxiety over treatment that day. Once it was determined that treatment would not take place, the anesthetic took effect.
2. The cognitive psychologist suggested that it was a physiologic reaction brought on by the metal-to-metal contact as the key was placed in the lock.

A third explanation is that the two events were coincidental and the patient merely had a delayed onset of anesthesia.

PHYSICAL AND CHEMICAL BARRIERS

Many physical and chemical barriers can interfere with successful anesthesia by decreasing the concentrations of drugs at targeted areas of nerve membranes. This most commonly occurs by barrier deflection of anesthetic solutions and/or by dilution, including of the available base form of the drugs.

Physical Barriers to Successful Anesthesia

Dense bony prominences, shallow vestibules, dilacerations, and soft tissues such as ligaments can physically block solutions or deflect them away from ideal deposition sites. Shallow vestibules and bony prominences may prevent adequate diffusion in infiltrations. Palatal dilacerations can increase bony distances through which solutions must diffuse to reach root apices. Ligaments can deflect solutions away from ideal sites. Inferior alveolar nerve blocks may be unsuccessful when needle penetration is too medial or too shallow, or the spheno-mandibular ligament deflects solution away from the nerve (Jastak, Yagiela, & Donaldson, 1995b, 1995c). During infiltrations, fascial planes may create similar barriers, and may be responsible when ideal deposition sites fail to provide profound anesthesia. Dense bone overlying the roots of teeth and bony curvatures creates greater bony distances between deposition sites and nerves. This may prevent solutions from reaching the nerves in sufficient quantity to produce profound anesthesia. Unusually small foramina can prevent or limit the volume of local anesthesia solution that can pass through the opening. This may occur with the infraorbital and incisive nerve blocks where it is necessary to force solution through foramina for success. Regional nerve blocks and intraosseous injections (such as the PDL) can overcome the majority of these obstacles.

Chemical Barriers to Successful Anesthesia

Chemical barriers include those existing in the tissues prior to injection and those caused by injury to tissues during injection. Inflammation or infection in the area of injection from any cause lowers pH, which can prevent the formation of sufficient base molecules. Vascular injury may flood areas, thereby diluting anesthetic solutions and lowering pH as the inflammatory response is triggered.

Vascular injury may play an important role in the following example: When an initial injection with a local anesthetic containing a vasoconstrictor such as 2% lidocaine with 1:100,000 epinephrine proves unsuccessful, many clinicians follow with another injection of 2% lidocaine with epinephrine. Taking into consideration the potential change in pH, an alternate approach that addresses the lowered pH would be to re-inject using a drug with a higher pH such as 3% mepivacaine plain. See Box 16–5 for further discussion on this strategy. Techniques to overcome barriers of inflammation include the use of alternate injections such as nerve blocks instead of infiltrations, intraosseous techniques, and

---

> **Box 16–5 A Theory on the Use of 3% Mepivacaine in the Presence of Lowered pH**
>
> The weakest vasodilator of all dental local anesthetic drugs is 3% mepivacaine, which makes it a useful drug when vasoconstrictors cannot be used. Its usefulness may also continue beyond that ability. If an initial injection of 2% lidocaine is followed with 3% mepivacaine, there is an increasing likelihood of success for the following reasons:
>
> 1. There is 50 percent more drug per volume of a 3 percent solution (30 mg/ml) compared with 2 percent solutions (20 mg/ml), providing a greater supply of base molecules.
> 2. Depositing 3% mepivacaine raises the pH at the deposition site. Each increase in pH of *one* amounts to a *ten-fold* decrease in available hydrogen ions, providing a greater supply of base molecules. (Since it is the base form of the local anesthesia molecule that diffuses through the nerve membrane, conduction blockades are enhanced.)
> 3. The mepivacaine administration takes advantage of the vasoconstriction of the local vessels already in place due to the epinephrine in the lidocaine solution, and mepivacaine's duration is enhanced.

---

intrapulpal anesthesia. In endodontic therapy, higher concentrations of epinephrine are sometimes useful.

Tachyphylaxis can occasionally prevent profound anesthesia from developing when subsequent injections in the same appointment are administered. The causes of tachyphylaxis include localized tissue edema in the area of injection and localized hemorrhage, both of which prevent sufficient concentrations of base molecules near the nerves for anesthesia to develop successfully (Malamed, 2004a; Lipfert, 1989a, 1989b). For a more detailed discussion on tachyphylaxis, see Box 16–6.

ANATOMIC VARIATIONS

Unexpected anatomic variations that are neither visible nor palpable can sabotage even the most careful technique.

Box 16–6 Tachyphylaxis

In general terms, **tachyphylaxis** is synonymous with what is known as *rapid drug tolerance,* the need for increasing doses in order to achieve similar therapeutic effects. This is what occurs, for example, when individuals require 60 mg of codeine in order to achieve an equivalent pain relief previously provided by 30 mg. In local anesthesia, tachyphylaxis refers to the failure of subsequent administrations of local anesthetics (in the same appointment) to prolong the duration, extent, and intensity of the anesthetic effect (Lipfert, 1989a).

Some authors have reported that tachyphylaxis occurs only infrequently while others believe it occurs in almost every repeated injection to some extent. While in some instances drug tolerance can be adequately explained, the mechanisms of tachyphylaxis are not well understood in local anesthesia. These mechanisms do not appear to be related to mode of administration, technique variations, or individual drug characteristics including whether or not the drugs are short or long acting. Speculation has centered on pharmacokinetics more than pharmacodynamics (Lipfert, 1989a).

Diminished response to additional doses of local anesthetics does not appear to result from reduced effectiveness of the drugs at the nerve membrane. On the contrary, the drugs have been shown to actually increase in effectiveness with repeated administrations (Lipfert, 1989b). The only certainty is that the lack of understanding of this phenomenon does little to lessen the frustration among clinicians and patients.

Tachyphylaxis is most likely to occur once anesthetized tissues have returned to normal levels of sensation (Malamed, 2004a). The most successful re-administrations of local anesthetic drugs therefore are those delivered prior to the return of *any* sensations (Malamed, 2004a).

Possible causes of tachyphylaxis in local anesthesia include decreases in local tissue pH, edema, local hemorrhage, and clot formation (Malamed, 2004a). Inadvertent puncture of a vessel, for example, may result in localized bleeding into the tissues and the resultant pool of blood may present a physical barrier. The same puncture may also dilute the solution to a less than therapeutic concentration (Malamed, 2004a).

If root anatomy has been accurately assessed and all other factors have been observed, fascial planes may cause inadequate anesthesia. Fascial planes can deflect solution away from ideal deposition sites resulting in inadequate volumes of solution to achieve anesthesia. Conversely, depositing in a less than ideal site may achieve success due to fascial planes that direct solution to the intended target.

Atypical Innervation Patterns

Innervation patterns are reliable from an anatomical standpoint. Although this is generally true, there are some variations that are expected and some that are entirely unexpected. Unexpected variations are referred to as **aberrant innervations,** and are highly unusual. **Accessory innervations** may be defined as typical, and therefore expected, deviations.

Aberrant Innervations

Most failures due to aberrant innervations result in a complete lack of anesthesia of the targeted tissues. Often these situations can never be fully explained; for example, consider a patient who reports never experiencing anesthesia to the mandible regardless of the local anesthesia techniques used. It is possible that this patient is receiving aberrant innervation from nerve fibers originating in other than the trigeminal ganglion. Although controversial, it has been speculated that some patients may receive innervations to the mandible from the cervical nerves.

Overcoming failure due to aberrant innervation requires alternative techniques that bypass them. The majority of aberrant innervation failures, for example, can be addressed with PDL injections.

Accessory Innervations

Incomplete anesthesia is a common consequence of accessory innervations (Blanton & Jeske, 2003b). Strategies for addressing accessory innervations are well-recognized and include those that address incomplete anesthesia in specific areas of the maxilla and mandible.

Considerations for Inadequate Maxillary Anesthesia

This section will discuss factors unique to maxillary techniques.

PSA Nerve Blocks

Some branches of the PSA nerve enter the maxilla medial to the usual location and innervate the palatal roots of molars and, occasionally, premolars (DuBrul, 1980). Some sources suggest that fibers from the greater palatine nerve also provide similar accessory innervation (Meechan, 1999). Regardless of the source of the accessory innervation, a greater palatine nerve block will effectively anesthetize atypical branches and remedy incomplete anesthesia of affected maxillary molars and premolars.

PDL injections are also effective in this situation. It is suggested that 3 to 4 sites will provide the best coverage of maxillary molars, with at least one site located on the palatal aspect of the tooth. Some clinicians have suggested that articaine is useful in PSA blocks or associated PDL injections due to its more effective diffusion to the palatal roots (CRA Newsletter, 2001).

MSA Nerve Block

Middle superior alveolar nerves are missing in a significant percentage of the population. Clinicians are aware of this variant and adapt by routinely administering an infiltration over the MB root of the maxillary first molar (Blanton & Jeske, 2003b; DuBrul, 1980; Jastak et al., 1995a; Loetscher & Walton, 1988).

ASA Nerve Block

The ASA nerve block is a highly successful procedure but is subject to two major sources of inadequate anesthesia. The first is anterior cross-innervation in which the incisors of one side may receive fibers from the contralateral side ASA nerve. To achieve complete anesthesia, one of the following options should be considered:

1. infiltration over the same side central incisor (beneficial for pulpal and soft tissue therapy)
2. ASA nerve block of the contralateral side
3. P-ASA nerve block

The second occurs when bone in the anterior maxilla is unusually dense, the vestibule has very little vertical height, or the maxilla has an exaggerated curvature over the roots of the teeth. All may result in solution being deposited too far from the nerve. Both IO and ASA nerve blocks anesthetize the ASA nerve, although the IO nerve block also typically anesthetizes the MSA, when present. The inability to block the ASA nerve through infiltration due to bony prominence, curvature, or limited vestibular height is remedied by performing an IO nerve block.

Another alternative is the AMSA nerve block which effectively anesthetizes the anterior and middle superior alveolar nerves and palatal tissues from the anterior midline through the second molar.

PDLs also represent an effective alternative. They are successful for most teeth; however, canines with unusually long roots may resist PDL anesthesia (Malamed, 2004f).

Palatal Innervation of Maxillary Central Incisors

It has been demonstrated that fibers of the nasopalatine nerve may join with the maxillary dental plexus to innervate the central incisors. In order to achieve complete maxillary central incisor anesthesia an NP nerve block may be required (Blanton & Jeske, 2003b). A PDL injection may also achieve complete anesthesia in this situation.

Considerations for Inadequate Mandiblular Anesthesia

This section will discuss factors unique to mandibular techniques.

Inferior Alveolar Nerve Block

The inferior alveolar nerve block has a *relatively* high incidence of inadequate anesthesia (Malamed, 2004c). Subjective signs and symptoms of anesthesia may be misleading. Despite a profound sense of anesthesia, adequate anesthesia may be absent. Possible reasons include accessory innervations to pulps from (Blanton & Jeske, 2003; Moini, 2008):

1. mylohyoid nerves
2. buccal nerves
3. lingual nerves
4. contralateral incisive and mental nerves
5. sensory fibers traveling with the motor fibers of the muscles of mastication
6. bifid inferior alveolar nerves
7. branches from the cervical plexus (to the *anterior teeth*)

Perhaps the most documented of the accessory innervations is from the mylohyoid nerve, the incidence of which has been reported as approximating 60 percent (Blanton & Jeske, 2003b). For information on performing a supplemental mylohyoid nerve block, see the mylohyoid nerve block technique, in Chapter 14, "Injections for Mandibular Pain Control," Box 14–7.

PDL injections are invaluable in the mandible and may overcome nearly all of the challenges mentioned previously. While useful as a primary technique, they are perhaps even more useful as supplemental techniques when other techniques have failed. PDL injections of mandibular *second* molars can provide effective mandibular blocks in some situations.

Other helpful techniques for overcoming accessory innervation are Gow-Gates nerve blocks, which are administered in the superior segment of the pterygomandibular space and Vazirani-Akinosi blocks, which are administered intermediately between the IA and Gow-Gates (see Chapter 14, "Injections for Mandibular Pain Control," Figure 14–45).

Considerations for Intraosseous Anesthesia

Intraosseous injections, in addition to the PDL, are also very useful in these situations. Solutions diffuse directly through spongy alveolar bone in these techniques to the dental plexuses in the area. In intraosseous techniques, except for PDL injections, it is first necessary to perforate the highly innervated overlying periosteum and cortical plate of bone before injecting solution. As discussed in Chapter 15, "Injections for Supplemental Pain Control," specialized intraosseous devices and handpieces are designed to facilitate exposure of the spongy bone underlying cortical plates. These techniques appear to be most effective when initial anesthesia (pre-anesthesia) is already in effect (Malamed, 2004e).

INTRAVASCULAR INJECTION

Intravascular injections can contribute to failed anesthesia because solutions are deposited directly into vessels and then distributed throughout the body away from intended targets. Performing multiple aspirations and aspirations in more than one plane will minimize this possibility.

INFLAMMATION

Local anesthetic drugs are packaged primarily in cationic form. As they diffuse through healthy tissues with pH values near 7.4, base molecule concentrations increase. In the presence of inflammation, excesses of hydrogen ions prevent the formation of base molecules. Insufficient numbers of base molecules for adequate penetration of nerve membranes may result in inadequate or nonexistent anesthesia. Using nerve blocks to avoid areas of inflammation usually overcomes these chemical barriers. When blocks are either impossible or ineffective, comfortable therapy may not be possible. The greatest challenges to profound anesthesia may present when treating "hot" teeth requiring endodontic therapy. Intraosseous and intrapulpal techniques and/or higher concentrations of drugs may be the only recourse if pain relief is urgent and has proven impossible to achieve through blocks and infiltrations. Pre-anesthesia is recommended for these injections. Some sources state that pre-anesthesia does not increase success rates, while others describe pre-anesthesia as necessary to reliable success (Blanton & Jeske, 2003a; Cannell & Cannon, 1976; Kleber, 2003; Lilienthal, 1975; Pearce, 1976). Since the provision of pre-anesthesia does not decrease the rate of success, providing pre-anesthesia seems a reasonable approach when the rationale for performing an intraosseous injection is to control pain.

CASE MANAGEMENT: Phillipe Giradot

After achieving pain relief with an inferior alveolar nerve block, an electric pulp tester confirmed that anesthesia was not profound on #19. While the lip and chin were numb, #19 was not.

The Gow-Gates nerve block provided a wider area of anesthesia because the anesthetic solution was deposited much higher in the pterygomandibular space, well above the location for IA blocks. The entire trunk of the IA nerve was anesthetized, including the mylohyoid and lingual nerve fibers (and usually the buccal nerve fibers), any of which could have provided accessory innervation to tooth #19.

Mr. Giradot did not remember having to keep his mouth open after the previous injections, which was a good indication that a Gow-Gates had not been attempted. He cooperated well and the procedure was completed using 2% lidocaine with 1:100,000 epinephrine. Within ten minutes, he stated that he had never been that numb in his life and the electric pulp tester confirmed profound anesthesia.

While it is likely from his description that PDL injections had been attempted previously, technique considerations are critical for routine success and the degree of discomfort he experienced after receiving shots in the gums indicates that they may have been performed traumatically, with excessive pressures and too quickly. Had the Gow-Gates failed to provide anesthesia, PDL injections would have been attempted next.

Phillipe was grateful for what he termed the only comfortable dental appointment he had ever experienced and he made appointments to come back for his routine care.

Case Discussion: It is unlikely that this patient received substandard anesthesia. The number of clinicians attempting anesthesia, alone, testifies to the likelihood of different approaches having been used. None had been effective. In order to determine whether or not a particular technique has been attempted in the past, it is helpful to question patients regarding aspects of techniques that are different than IA blocks. In Mr. Giradot's case, he did not recall keeping his mouth open after any injections. He did remember shots beside the tooth and that the sites hurt a lot afterward.

CHAPTER QUESTIONS

1. Inadequate anesthesia may typically be caused by all of the following, *except:*
   a. Accessory innervation.
   b. Inflammation.
   c. Poor manufacturing processes.
   d. Freezing of cartridges during shipping.

2. Infiltration (supraperiosteal) anesthesia over the apex of #9 has failed to achieve adequate anesthesia. Which *one* of the following is not a likely possibility?
   a. Cross-over innervation from the contralateral ASA
   b. Bony obstructions
   c. Dense bone
   d. Unseen inflammation

3. The relative acidity of tissues into which anesthetic drugs are injected is related to the efficacy of a drug in the following manner:
   a. An excess of hydrogen atoms enhances neutral base molecule formation.
   b. A pH-driven increase in cationic concentrations decreases the rate of success.
   c. A pH-driven increase in cationic concentrations increases the rate of success.
   d. A decrease in pH increases the number of neutral base molecules.

4. Possible successful approaches when an inferior alveolar nerve block fails to provide complete and profound pulpal anesthesia are:
   a. PDL injections.
   b. Mylohyoid nerve blocks.
   c. Gow-Gates blocks.
   d. All of the above

5. Two injections of 2% lidocaine, 1:100,000 epinephrine (total lidocaine = 72 mg) have failed to provide adequate anesthesia. Useful supplemental alternatives, regardless of the location or technique, include all of the following, *except:*
   a. 3% mepivacaine.
   b. PDL injections.
   c. Mylohyoid blocks.
   d. 2% mepivacaine, 1:20,000 levonordefrin.

6. By which of the following mechanisms do intraosseous techniques work?
   a. They are propelled through tissues to nerves and nerve trunks.
   b. They rapidly diffuse through bony tissue to nerve trunks.
   c. They slowly diffuse through bony tissue to nerve trunks.
   d. They slowly diffuse through bony tissue to dental plexuses.

7. Where is the deposition site for the Gow-Gates nerve block located relative to the inferior alveolar nerve block?
   a. At the same level in the pterygomandibular space
   b. At a higher level in the pterygomandibular space
   c. Below the inferior alveolar nerve block
   d. Below the Vazirani-Akinosi block but above the IA block

8. Some nerve blocks require far greater volumes of solution compared with others.
   a. True
   b. False

REFERENCES

Blanton, P. L., & Jeske, A. H. (2003a). Dental local anesthetics. Alternative delivery methods. *Journal of the American Dental Association, 134*(2), 228–234.

Blanton, P. L., & Jeske, A. H. (2003b). Avoiding complications in local anesthesia induction, anatomical considerations. *Journal of the American Dental Association, 34*(7), 888–893.

Brown, R. D. (1981). The failure of local anesthesia in acute inflammation. *British Dental Journal, 151,* 47–51.

Cannell, H., & Cannon, P. D. (1976). Intraosseous injections of lignocaine local anesthetics. *British Dental Journal, 141*(2), 48–50.

Certosimo, A., & Archer, R. (1996). A clinical evaluation of the electric pulp tester as an indicator of local anesthesia. *Operative Dentistry, 21,* 25.

Clinicians guide to dental products and techniques: Septocaine. (2001, June). *CRA Newsletter.*

Daniel, S. J., & Harfst, S. A. (2007). *Dental hygiene concepts, cases, and competencies* (p. 35). St. Louis: Mosby.

DuBrul, E. L. (1980). *Sicher's oral anatomy* (7th ed., p. 453). St Louis: Mosby.

Frommer, J., Mele, F., & Monroe, C. (1972). The possible role of the mylohyoid nerve in mandibular posterior tooth sensation. *Journal of the American Dental Association, 85,* 113.

Hamburg, H. L. (1972). Preliminary study of patient reaction to needle gauge. *New York State Dental Journal, 38,* 425–426.

Jastak, J. T., Yagiela, J. A., & Donaldson, D. (1995a). *Local anesthesia of the oral cavity* (pp. 206–207). Philadelphia: Saunders, pp. 206–207.

Jastak, J. T., Yagiela, J. A., & Donaldson, D. (1995b). *Local anesthesia of the oral cavity* (pp. 275–285). Philadelphia: Saunders.

Jastak, J. T., Yagiela, J. A., & Donaldson, D. (1995c). *Local anesthesia of the oral cavity* (pp. 277–278). Philadelphia: Saunders.

Kaufman, E., Weinstein, P., & Milgrom, P. (1984). Difficulties in achieving local anesthesia. *Journal of the American Dental Association, 108,* 205.

Kleber, C. H. (2003, April). Intraosseous anesthesia. Implications, instrumentation and techniques. *Journal of the American Dental Association,* 487–491.

Loetscher, C. A., & Walton, R. E. (1988). Patterns of innervation of the maxillary first molar: A dissection study. *Oral Surgery Oral Medicine Oral Pathology, 65,* 86–90.

Lew, K., & Townsend, G. (2006). Failure to obtain adequate anesthesia associated with a bifid canal: A case report. *Australian Dental Journal, 51*(1), 86–90.

Lilienthal, B. (1975). A clinical appraisal of intraosseous dental anesthesia. *Oral Surg Oral Med Oral Pathol 39*(5), 692–697.

Lipfert, P. (1989a). Tachyphylaxis to local anesthetics. *Regional Anaesthesia, 12*(1), 13–20.

Lipfert, P., Holthusen, H., Arndt, J. O. (1989b). Tachyphylaxis to local anesthetics does not result from reduced drug effectiveness at the nerve itself. *Anesthesiology, 70,* 71–75.

Madan, G. A., Madan, S. G., & Madan, A. D. (2002). Failure of inferior alveolar nerve block, exploring the alternatives. *Journal of the American Dental Association, 133*(7), 843–846.

Malamed, S. F. (2006, July 21). *Anesthesia & medicine in dentistry.* Presentation to the Spokane District Dental Society and Eastern Washington University, Department of Dental Hygiene.

Malamed, S. F. (2004a). *Handbook of local anesthesia* (5th ed., p. 25). St. Louis: Elsevier Mosby.

Malamed, S. F. (2004b). *Handbook of local anesthesia* (5th ed., pp. 189–225). St. Louis: Elsevier Mosby.

Malamed, S. F. (2004c). *Handbook of local anesthesia* (5th ed., p. 196). St. Louis: Elsevier Mosby.

Malamed, S. F. (2004d). *Handbook of local anesthesia* (5th ed., pp. 227–253). St. Louis: Elsevier Mosby.

Malamed, S. F. (2004e). *Handbook of local anesthesia* (5th ed., pp. 228–235). St. Louis: Elsevier Mosby.

Malamed, S. F. (2004f). *Handbook of local anesthesia* (5th ed., p. 244). St. Louis: Elsevier Mosby.

Meechan, J. G. (1999). How to overcome failed local anaesthesia. *British Dental Journal, 186*(1), 15–20.

Milles, M. (1984, March/April). The missed inferior alveolar block: A new look at an old problem. *Journal of the American Dental Society of Anesthesia.*

Moini, J. (2008). *Pharmacology essentials for health professionals.* Upper Saddle River, NJ: Pearson Prentice Hall.

Najjar, T. A. (1977). Why can't you achieve adequate regional anesthesia in the presence of infection? *Oral Surgery, 44,* 7–13.

Ozdemir, M., Ozdemir, G., Zencirci, B., & Oksuz, H. (2004). Articaine versus lidocaine plus bupivacaine for peribulbar anaesthesia in cataract surgery. *British Journal of Anaesthesia, 92*(2), 231.

Panza, J. A., Epstein, S. E., & Quyyumi, A. A. (1991). Circadian variation in vascular tone and its relation to alpha-sympathetic vasoconstrictor activity. *New England Journal of Medicine, 325,* 986–990.

Pearce, J. H. (1976). Intraosseous injection for profound anesthesia of the lower molar. *Journal of the Colorado Dental Association, 54*(2), 25–26.

Pearce, J. (1976). Intraosseous injection for profound anesthesia of the lower molar. *Journal of the Colorado Dental Association, 54,* 25.

Replogle, K., Reader, A., Nist, R., Beck, M., Weaver, J., & Meyers, W. J. (1999). Cardiovascular effects of intraosseous injections of 2% lidocaine with 1:100,000 epinephrine and 3% mepivacaine. *Journal of the American Dental Association, 130*(5), 649.

Robison, S. F., Mayhew, R. B., Cowan, R. D., Hawley, R. J. (1984). Comparative study of deflection characteristics and fragility of 25-, 27-, and 30-gauge dental needles, *Journal of the American Dental Association, 109*(6), 920–924.

Wallace, J., Michanowicz, A., Mundell, R., & Wilson, E. (1985). A pilot study of the clinical problems of regionally anesthetizing the pulp of an acutely inflamed mandibular molar. *Oral Surg Oral Med Oral Pathol, 59,* 517.

Local Anesthesia Complications and Management

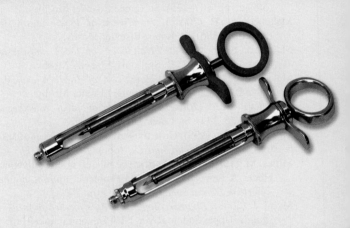

OBJECTIVES

- Define and discuss the key terms in this chapter.
- Discuss the most common adverse *local* events that may occur during and after local anesthetic drug administration.
- Discuss the categories of adverse *systemic* events that may occur during and after local anesthetic drug delivery.
- Discuss appropriate responses and management of adverse local events.
- Discuss appropriate responses and management of adverse systemic events.
- Discuss protocols for the management of overdose and allergic events.
- Define idiosyncratic events and discuss their management.

KEY TERMS

adverse events **339**
adverse reactions **339**
ageusia **346**
angioedema **359**
complications **339**
dysesthesia **346**
embedded needles **345**
hematoma **340**
hubbing **343**
hyperesthesia **346**

hyper-responders **355**
hypersensitivity **355**
hypo-responders **355**
hypogeusia **346**
idiosyncratic **361**
methemoglobinemia **361**
occult hematoma **340**
overdose **339**
paresthesia **339**
trismus **341**

CASE STUDY: Ashley Smith

Ashley Smith, the student "patient" for a dental hygiene local anesthesia laboratory session, had no complicating factors and no relative or absolute contraindications to receiving a PSA nerve block. Following needle insertion for a PSA block, the student "clinician" reported a positive aspiration at the deposition site. In response, the needle tip was repositioned and a second aspiration test was performed. Following a negative result, the clinician administered the local anesthetic slowly. Before the planned dose had been delivered, Ashley developed localized swelling in her cheek near the site of the injection.

INTRODUCTION

Adverse events or **reactions** have been defined as undesired effects which occur in response to the pharmacologic actions of a drug (Horlocker & Wedel, 2002; Pickett & Terezhalmy, 2006). This definition can be expanded to include the events surrounding the administration of the drug, described in terms of their local or systemic effects or as **complications.**

Local complications occur more frequently than systemic complications and may include anything from postoperative soreness to prolonged anesthesia. The majority of adverse events related to local anesthesia in dentistry involve mild reactions such as postoperative discomfort in the area of injection, syncope, pain from patient self-injury, and mild inflammation following muscle penetrations. These usually present as no more than limited inconveniences or short-term management situations.

Systemic reactions such as overdose, allergy, and idiosyncratic response occur far less frequently but are generally more serious. While fewer more serious adverse events may be expected, clinicians nonetheless must be prepared to respond appropriately if and when they occur. It has been reported in the literature that *peripheral* nerve blocks, in particular, have been associated with the highest incidence of systemic toxicity (Cox, Durieux, & Marcus, 2003). Despite this reported incidence, which includes statistics from multiple health professions, local anesthetic drug administration *in dentistry* appears to be relatively free of life-threatening events with a very low overall risk (Haas, 1998; Malamed, 2004). In a 1999 study

involving over one thousand healthy subjects undergoing oral surgery, for example, it was found that despite levels that exceeded **overdose** thresholds in the majority of the subjects, there were no reported adverse events (Lustig & Zusman, 1999).

Before, during, and after the administration of local anesthetics, a primary responsibility of dental clinicians is to recognize and respond to adverse events. Practice acts may differ on the extent of emergency training required of dental professionals but all are expected to recognize and respond to local and systemic adverse events, including life-threatening emergencies, when they occur. Product monographs for all of the anesthetic drugs used in dentistry make similar statements regarding clinician responsibility when administering local anesthetics (see Box 17–1).

This chapter will examine the local and systemic complications of local anesthesia, prevention strategies (when available), and appropriate response and management protocols.

LOCAL COMPLICATIONS

Local complications of local anesthetic drugs involve tissue injuries that occur before, during, and after the administrations of topical and injectable local anesthetic drugs. Some causes are obvious, such as the damage which results in the formation of hematomas. Others are less obvious, such as the development of **paresthesia,**

Box 17–1   *Xylocaine Product Monograph Statement**

"WARNINGS
DENTAL PRACTITIONERS WHO EMPLOY LOCAL ANESTHETIC AGENTS SHOULD BE WELL VERSED IN DIAGNOSIS AND MANAGEMENT OF EMERGENCIES WHICH MAY ARISE FROM THEIR USE. RESUSCITATIVE EQUIPMENT, OXYGEN AND OTHER RESUSCITATIVE DRUGS SHOULD BE AVAILABLE FOR IMMEDIATE USE."

*XYLOCAINE is a trademark of the AstraZeneca group. Manufactured by AstraZeneca LP for DENTSPLY

Source: 2% xylocaine product monograph, Dentsply Pharmaceutical, York, PA, 2004.

where multiple theories have been proposed to explain the etiology of the neural injury that sometimes occurs during local anesthetic administration (Pogrel & Thamby, 2000).

Hematoma

Hematomas are formed from the leaking of blood from vessels into surrounding tissues (Ibsen & Phelan, 2004). They result from inadvertent nicks of blood vessels during injections. If the injury to a vessel is minor, bleeding into tissue spaces surrounding the injured vessel may not be noticed. When a more significant injury occurs in a larger vessel, the development of a hematoma can be rapid and dramatic. The most likely site of hematoma formation during dental local anesthesia occurs after posterior superior alveolar and division 2 (maxillary tuberosity approach) nerve blocks. Figure 17–1 ■ shows swelling that occurred moments after insertion during a PSA injection. This is due to the proximity of the ptery-goid plexus of veins and associated arteries to the target sites in the infratemporal and pterygopalatine fossae (Blanton & Jeske, 2003). Inferior alveolar nerve blocks have the second highest rate of hematoma formation, followed by mental and mental incisive nerve blocks (Malamed, 2004). Those occurring during or after inferior alveolar blocks frequently have few to no extraoral signs due to the ability of the pterygomandibular space to conceal larger quantities of blood medial to the mandible (Malamed, 2004). Those occurring near the mental foramen tend to be visible since they occur near the chin where bruising is more obvious, while swelling of the palate is more confined, as shown in Figure 17–2 ■.

Some clinicians believe that a positive aspiration is an indication that a hematoma is more likely to develop and that a negative aspiration is an indication that a hematoma is not likely to develop. This may not be the case since nicking a vessel can occur as needles penetrate to depth, but they can also occur well after aspiration when needles are withdrawn, regardless of the results of aspiration. Although a positive aspiration indicates that a vessel was penetrated, the majority of those penetrations result in too little bleeding for noticeable hematoma formation (Haas, 1998).

Further complications, although rare, may occur following hematoma development and include infection and trismus (Haas, 1998). Although the clinical course of healing is marked by very noticeable discoloration of the face, the majority of hematomas heal uneventfully and require no additional treatment.

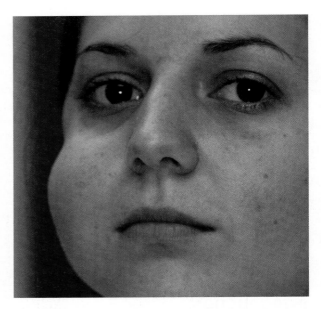

■ **FIGURE 17–1** Initial Swelling from a Hematoma. Immediate swelling during a PSA injection.

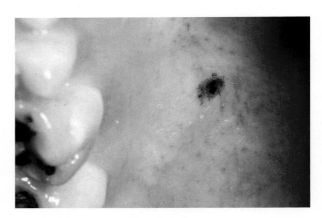

■ **FIGURE 17–2** Palatal Hematoma. Hematomas of the palatal are generally well confined.

A final complication, failure to achieve adequate anesthesia in inferior alveolar nerve blocks, has been attributed to the formation of hematomas (Trager, 1979). Hematomas may interfere with the development of anesthesia by diluting the drugs, by transporting them from intended target sites, and by initiating inflammatory responses, which lower pH. In the case of IA nerve blocks in particular, clinicians may not be aware that an occult **hematoma** (concealed) exists, in which case the lack of profound anesthesia after administration can be frustrating. This may be the situation when successive IA nerve blocks fail to establish anesthesia. Alternative techniques are suggested, such as the Gow-Gates nerve block or PDL injections (see Chapter 16, "Troubleshooting Inadequate Anesthesia").

Prevention of Hematomas

Taking into account the number of dental injections administered daily, the occurrence of hematomas is rare (Pogrel & Thamby, 2000). Clinicians can help to maintain this low risk by observing a few relatively simple precautions. Minimizing the number of needle penetrations is perhaps most important, considering that one penetration involves a certain degree of risk; two penetrations doubles that risk; and three triples the risk, etc. Avoiding trauma in general is also key, as any aspect of an injection that traumatizes tissue increases the risk of hematoma (Haas, 1998). This can be accomplished by maintaining good access, avoiding bowing of needles, avoiding rapid penetrations, and observing appropriate angulations and penetration depths.

Box 17–2 *Case History of Vigorous Hematoma Formation*

Patients on anticoagulant therapy are at increased risk of vigorous hematoma formation. Aspirin, coumadin, and clopidogrel (Plavix) are commonly used anticogulants. Some patients are on high doses or may be taking combinations including all three drugs, as was the case with this patient.

After a single PSA injection, this patient developed an extensive hematoma and was referred to an oral surgeon, who placed the compression dressing seen in Figure 17–3A ■. The patient was subsequently admitted to a nearby hospital. In contrast to Ashley in the chapter case study, this is a rare event.

Infiltrations are excellent substitutes for PSA blocks in these patients due to the relatively minimal risk of hematoma formation. While PSA blocks have been described as preferable to infiltrations at times, especially when multiple molars require anesthesia, exceptional bleeding risks may contraindicate their use (Malamed, 2004).

Figure 17–3B ■ and Figure 17–3C ■ show the progressive healing and resolution of the hematoma.

Box 17–3 **Hematoma Management**

Protocol for the management of hematomas includes:

Early recognition and response:

1. Be alert to the possibility of hematoma formation
2. Respond to initial signs of swelling
   a. Discontinue treatment for the day
   b. Apply pressure and ice (if ice is available, you can apply pressure with ice)

Once the hematoma has stopped expanding:

1. Instruct the patient to apply ice intermittently for the next 6 hours
2. Instruct the patient to avoid aspirin for pain
3. Advise the patient regarding the development of discolorations
4. Advise the patient to notify you immediately of any change, especially the development of signs & symptoms of infection or limited jaw opening

Consultation with the patient's physician prior to performing local anesthetic procedures can be useful if a patient is on anticoagulant therapy. Discussions regarding indications for vitamin K and/or anticoagulation medication adjustments can help to prevent more serious complications from developing (Haas, 1998).

Aside from the risk of hematoma formation, an important benefit of careful anatomic assessment, observing appropriate technique, and minimizing the number of penetrations is enhancement of patient comfort.

PSA nerve blocks, in particular, should be avoided if patients are taking blood thinners. Hematomas that occur in the presence of anticoagulant therapy can be extensive and may require additional therapy. Some have required hospitalization. A case history of a vigorous hematoma formation after a single PSA injection on a patient taking multiple anticoagulants is discussed in Box 17–2 and shown in Figure 17–3, which illustrates the benefit of careful pre-anesthetic assessment.

Response to Hematomas

Rapid recognition and response to a developing hematoma can alter its clinical course. A hematoma's

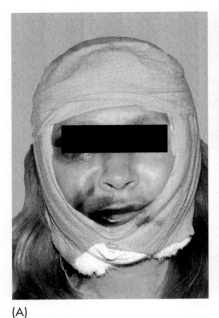
(A)

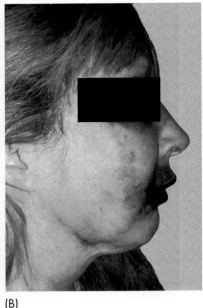
(B)

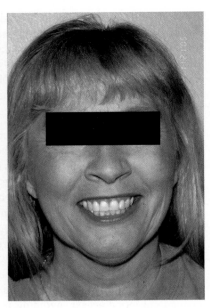
(C)

■ **FIGURE 17–3**   Extensive Hematoma. A—This atypical, extensive hematoma required the placement of a compression bandage. This patient was on anticoagulant therapy, which complicated the situation. B—Bruising lingering around the eye and mouth. C—Fully healed several weeks later.

extent is limited by the degree of flexibility of the tissues into which the blood is emptying (Malamed, 2004). Clinicians can, in essence, create an opposing force by applying pressure and keeping the pressure in place long enough for clotting to begin. In the absence of deliberate pressure or when pressure is ineffective, tissue resistance must approximate the pressure behind the blood pouring from the vessel before blood will cease entering the tissues. In situations where surrounding tissues are flexible, larger hematomas can develop. Where tissues are less flexible, such as in the palate or when pressure is applied, hematoma sizes tend to be more limited.

Protocol for the management of hematomas is discussed in Box 17–3.

Trismus

From a neurological standpoint, **trismus** is defined as a motor disturbance of the trigeminal nerve (*Dorland's Illustrated Medical Dictionary [Dorland's]*, 2009; Jastak, Yagiela, & Donaldson, 1995). It is more simply described as an inability to open the mouth. Broadly considered, it has many etiologies and contributing

etiologies including tetanus (lock jaw), tumors, bony ankylosis, fracture, foreign bodies, fascial space infections, and enlarged coronoid processes (Jastak et al., 1995). As a consequence of local anesthesia, however, its primary causes are hemorrhage and muscle trauma following injection (Jastak et al., 1995).

Trismus is a relatively common complication of local anesthetic injections (Haas, 1998). Injuries sustained involve the muscles of mastication, particularly the medial pterygoid muscles and the blood vessels of the infratemporal fossa (Jastak et al., 1995; Malamed, 2004). In addition to physical trauma due to needle movements, local anesthetic toxicity to skeletal muscle has also been demonstrated (Benoit, Yagiela, & Fort, 1980; Malamed, 2004). Causes of trismus include not only physical and chemical trauma to muscle tissue but also physical trauma to blood vessels (Jastak et al., 1996). Contaminants on needles may also cause local infection and trismus.

The most frequent muscle to experience trismus is the medial pterygoid. It can be injured by all three common approaches to mandibular nerve block, the inferior alveolar, Gow-Gates, and Vazirani-Akinosi techniques (Haas, 1998). The lateral pterygoids and temporalis muscles are less frequently involved (Haas, 1998).

Bleeding, toxicity of anesthetic solutions, and direct physical injury to muscle tissues are all suspect when trismus occurs following local anesthetic injections (Haas, 1998).

Prevention of Trismus

The occurrence of trismus can be minimized by decreasing the number of penetrations, changing needles frequently (especially whenever tips may be barbed), and assuring that needle contamination does not occur prior to injection (Haas, 1998; Stacy & Hajjar, 1994).

Management of Trismus

In the management of trismus, instruct patients to:

1. Apply hot, moist towels approximately 20 minutes every hour (5 minutes on, 10 minutes off).
2. Use analgesics for discomfort, particularly ibuprofen, if appropriate.
3. Open and close the mouth gradually & repeatedly to maintain mobility of the TMJ.
4. Monitor for signs of infection that may require antibiotics, such as increasing heat, redness, elevated temperatures, and pain.
5. Refer to an oral surgeon or physician if signs & symptoms fail to improve, or worsen (Haas, 1998; Norholt, Aagard, Svensson, & Sindet-Pedersen, 1998).

Pain on Injection

There are many possible causes of pain on injection. Needle penetrations of well-innervated anatomic structures can cause pain. Rapid deposition of solution can distend tissues, causing pain. Pain can occur due to the irritating and acidic nature of local anesthetic solutions and can also occur if solutions are too cold or too hot compared with oral temperatures.

While each of these factors has the potential to cause pain, the majority of the time they do not, particularly when topical anesthetics are used, deposition rates are slow, and muscles are relaxed (Haas, 1998; Malamed, 2004).

Prevention of Pain on Injection

Strategies for preventing pain on injection include:

1. Adequate pre-anesthesia
   a. Appropriate topical application
   b. Pressure anesthesia techniques prior to needle penetration in palatal injections.

2. Slow rate of deposition of local anesthetic solution.
   a. Adhere to recommended maximum rates
   b. Adjust to one-third the normal rate or slower for deposition in palatal injections.
3. When administrating solutions with and without vasoconstrictors, administer plain solutions first.
4. If a particular drug causes a "burning" sensation, substitute with other appropriate drugs (Haas, 1998; Malamed, 2004).

Response to Pain on Injection

Pain on injection is not uncommon. When deliberate attempts to control pain on injection are made, pain is usually either limited or non-existent. Following the basic steps for intraoral injections as outlined in Chapter 11 "Fundamentals for Administration of Local Anesthetic Agents," will help to assure a pain-free injection much of the time.

Broken Needles

Most needle breakage occurs after unexpected movements. Factors that increase the risk for needle breakage include using needles that have higher gauges in deeper penetrations, bending needles at the hub, and needle penetrations to the hub (Haas, 1998; Malamed, 2004). Needle breakage is not common today; however, litigation is possible should it occur (Malamed, 2004).

Prevention of Needle Breakage

Clinicians should choose needle gauges and lengths that are appropriate for the depths of penetration and types of tissue through which needles will pass. This helps to reduce the need to insert the entire needle length to the junction of the hub and needle shaft, which is the weakest point on the needle, a practice referred to as **"hubbing."** Choosing needles with adequate length reduces the risk of needle breakage that results from hubbing. Sudden patient movements when needles are hubbed are more likely to break needles compared with movements where the hub is not touching the mucosa. Leveraged pressures at maximum insertion are applied directly against the hub/needle shaft junction. Some exceptions to this guideline are discussed in Box 17–4.

Prevention strategies to avoid undue stresses on needles include the following:

1. Inspect needles before use.
2. Avoid inserting needles to the hub.
3. Use long needles for deeper penetrations.
4. Use lower gauge needles.

Box 17–4 Considerations for "Hubbing"

Occasional "hubbing" may be necessary in order to contact bone when there is excessive flaring or an unusually large mandible. Long needles (31 or 32 millimeters) may barely reach the targets in these individuals in mandibular blocks and can require full insertion of needles. In these instances, maximum insertion may be necessary and acceptable. It is prudent practice, however, when maximum insertion is necessary, to withdraw slightly in order to leave a portion of shank visible (see Figure 17–4 ■). This reduces the risk of needle breakage and provides a portion of shank to grasp should breakage occur.

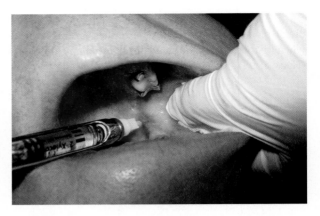

■ **FIGURE 17–4** Reducing Risks for Needle Breakage. Leave a length of the shaft visible to reduce the risk of needle breakage and to provide a portion of shank to grasp should breakage occur.

5. Avoid excessive forces on needles (such as when repositioning).
6. Avoid excessive numbers of penetrations with the same needle.
7. If bending is desired,* avoid bending at the hub (Bedrock, Skigen, & Dolwick, 1999; Bhatia & Bounds, 1998; Haas, 1998; Malamed, 2004; Marks, Carlton, & McDonald, 1984; Zelter, Cohen, & Casap, 2002).

Response to and Management of Broken Needles

The clinician's response to broken needles may be critical to maintaining an enduring relationship with the patient (Ethunandan, Tran, Anand, Bowden, Seal, & Brennan, 2007; Haas, 1998; Orr, 1983). Although these occurrences are rare, in the event of a broken needle, patients frequently seek litigation (Malamed, 2004).

While it may be argued whether or not a particular embedded needle fragment should be removed, breakage must be recognized, located, and documented (Bedrock et al., 1999).

Additional precautions and responses include:

1. Have a sterile hemostat nearby whenever injectable drugs are administered.
2. Do not allow the patient to close if breakage occurs (closing can insert the needle further into tissues).

Box 17–5 OSHA's Standard on Bending Needles*

When choosing to bend needles *prior* to injection (*before* needles are contaminated), it is important to note that this practice may create both difficulty and hazards for safely recapping needles after the procedure. OSHA's bloodborne pathogens standard [29 CFR 1910.1030(d)(2)(vii)(A)] prohibits the bending, recapping or removal of a *contaminated* needle or other contaminated sharp.

The standard also provides an exception where an *"employer can demonstrate that no alternative is feasible or that such action is required by a specific medical or dental procedure. Such bending, recapping or needle removal must be accomplished through the use of a mechanical device or a one-handed technique"* [29 CFR 1910.1030(d)(2)(vii)(B)].

The preamble to the bloodborne pathogens standard notes that the administration of incremental doses of a medication is one medical procedure, among others, to which this exception refers [56 *FR* 64118 (1991)].

---

* OSHA's bloodborne pathogens standard on bending and recapping *contaminated* needles is provided in Box 17–5. See Figure 9–11 for an example of the hazards of recapping bent needles.

*This information was accessed at: U.S. Department of Labor, Occupational Safety & Health Administration, www.osha.gov, October 2008.

3. If the needle is visible, remove it with a hemostat.
4. If the needle is not visible:
   a. Inform the patient that a needle has broken and a nonretrievable segment is embedded in the tissues.
   b. Refer to an oral and maxillofacial surgeon for *immediate evaluation.*
   c. Keep accurate records of location, needle size, any unforeseen events precipitating the breakage, and patient communication.
5. Where possible, any remaining unembedded fragments of the needle should be sent to the surgeon who is evaluating the situation.

Surgical removal may not be indicated due to the potential for extensive tissue damage that can result during removal. Retaining needle fragments might ultimately cause less tissue damage than removal. When preparing a patient for referral to an oral surgeon, choose terms such as evaluation rather than removal in order to better align patient expectations with a surgeon's eventual actions. As an example of the difficulty in guessing the ultimate disposition of an embedded needle fragment, one recent case cited an initial decision to leave a needle in the tissues but was reversed six months later when the buried fragment became symptomatic (Ethunandan et al., 2007).

Despite the precaution of using language that does not conflict with a surgeon's later advice to a patient, it is unlikely today that a surgeon will opt to leave a needle fragment in the tissues (see Box 17–6).

Self-Injury

It is important for dental professionals to advise patients, parents, and caretakers of the risk of self-injury when areas of the mouth are anesthetized with injections that provide extensive soft tissue anesthesia, especially since the risk of injury can continue for some time after a patient leaves the dental chair. Figure 17–5 ■ shows an example of a post-anesthesia lip bite.

In the event of lingering anesthesia, there is a subsequent risk of biting oral soft tissues following treatment and from drinking or eating hot foods before anesthetized nerves can adequately warn of traumatic injury and excessive temperatures.

Prevention of Self-injury

Prevention of self-injury has traditionally centered around communicating the risks to patients and caregivers, with

---

| Box 17–6   Embedded Needles: To Remove or Not to Remove |

The *remove-or-not-to-remove* **embedded needles** debate currently favors removal. Clinical judgment is important particularly as it relates to being able to accurately locate a needle. This has become easier with the ability to obtain cross-sectional scans of affected areas and due to the practice of inserting reference needles prior to exposing radiographs.

Early fears prompting removal revolved around possible needle migration toward larger blood vessels in the head and neck. These very real fears combine with other current indications for removal, which include pain, infection, psychological resistance to having a foreign body embedded in the jaw, and the ability to perceive the needle when moving the mandible.

Needles that are not removed typically develop what have been described as fibrous cocoons or scars around them that generally hamper significant migration, but some authorities have suggested that the lingering possibility of needle migration and litigation argue strongly for removal.

Sources: Bedrock et al., 1999; Malamed, 2004; Marks, Carlton, & McDonald, 1984; Ethunandan et al., 2007.

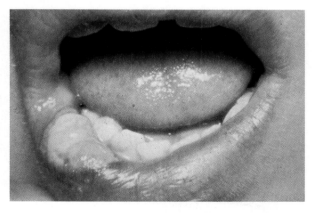

■ **FIGURE 17–5**   Lip Bite Following Local Anesthesia.

visual reminders placed on areas of exposed skin for those at greatest risk, such as warning stickers on foreheads. A more recent potential preventive approach has been made available with the introduction of an anesthesia reversal agent, phentolamine mesylate (OraVerse).

Communication

As in the past, clinicians continue to use verbal communication and stickers or temporary tattoos on children's foreheads, hands, and/or arms to warn of the risks of self-injury. This strategy has been reasonably effective; however, the risks can remain active for extended periods and verbal and visible warnings have been forgotten or ignored and stickers have been prematurely removed or misplaced.

Anesthesia Reversal

Recently, a new drug was introduced that limits the duration of soft tissue anesthesia. The manufacturer does not claim that it reduces the incidence of soft tissue injury following anesthesia nor has it conducted studies demonstrating this benefit; however, in conjunction with previous approaches to preventing self-injury, OraVerse has the potential to reduce the incidence of self-injury dramatically.

OraVerse® (Novalar, 2008) is the only pharmaceutical agent available for the reversal of *soft-tissue* anesthesia, which can interfere with speaking, eating, and drinking for prolonged periods. See Figure 17–6 ■ for product example. Note the unique color of the cartridge label and stopper OraVerse.

Background OraVerse (phentolamine mesylate), by Novalar Pharmaceuticals, was approved by the FDA on May 9, 2008. Early studies have reported that sensations to the lips and tongue can be regained in approximately half the time of typical dental local anethesia recovery (Hersh et al., 2008; Tavares et al., 2008). Detailed pharmacological information on OraVerse provided by Novalar Pharmaceuticals can be found in Box 17–7.

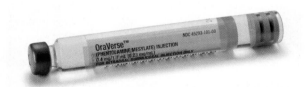

■ **FIGURE 17–6** OraVerse Product Example. OraVerse is the only pharmaceutical agent available for the reversal of *soft-tissue* anesthesia. OraVerse cartridges have unique translucent green labels and blue end-caps to avoid confusion with local anesthesia drug cartridges.
Source: Courtesy of Novalar Pharmaceuticals.

Management of Self-Injury

Palliative therapy such as over-the-counter preparations for protection of oral sores and pain relief are usually all that is necessary. In the rare event of infection, antibiotics may be indicated. See Chapter 19, "Insights from Pedodontics," for further discussion of post-injection trauma in children.

Paresthesia

Paresthesia is a broad term for a number of related but clinically diverse neurological effects which all result from nerve injury. It has been defined as an altered sensation and/or as a persistent partial or complete numbness (Daniel, Harfst, Wilder, 2007). It may be further defined in terms of its potential to affect taste if the chorda tympani nerve is involved.

Other frequently associated terms include **hyperesthesia** and **dysesthesia,** which refer to an increased sensitivity to stimuli and the sensation of pain from non-noxious stimuli, respectively. **Ageusia** and **hypogeusia** refer to the absolute and relative losses of the ability to perceive sweet, sour, bitter, or salty substances due to chorda tympani injury, otherwise referred to as *altered taste sensations* or *perversions.* Unfortunately, the basis of the vulnerability of particular nerves to the development of paresthesia and the etiology of paresthesia are not clear (Pogrel, Schmidt, Sambajon, & Jordan, 2003).

The lingual nerve is most frequently involved in paresthesias that follow dental injections (Haas & Lennon, 1995). A possible explanation has been proposed that suggests that the fascicular pattern of the lingual nerve compared with the inferior alveolar nerve may make it more susceptible, particularly near the lingula, where deposition occurs (Pogrel et al., 2003). The lingual nerve has been found to be unifascicular in this location in approximately 33 percent of individuals, which has been speculated to increase its vulnerability to paresthesia (Pogrel et al., 2003).

While neurotoxicity of anesthetic drug solutions has been demonstrated, for example, with cautions attached to higher concentrations of drugs, it has not been proven to be a definitive cause of paresthesia (Haas & Lennon, 1995; Koizumi, Matsumoto, Yamashita, Tsuruta, Ohtake, & Sakabe, 2006). In some instances, paresthesia follows direct trauma from surgery or needle injury (Blanton & Jeske, 2003). In others, it occurs after what

---

Box 17–7   OraVerse® by Novalar Pharmaceuticals

The following information was gathered from clinical data published in the *Journal of the American Dental Association* and from information provided by Novalar Pharmaceuticals. Before using OraVerse, the product insert should be consulted.

Formulations for Use in Dentistry
OraVerse is a sterile, pyrogen-free, isotonic solution for administration in glass dental cartridges that deliver 0.4 mg phentolamine mesylate in 1.7 ml of solution. The concentration of the active ingredient (phentolamine mesylate) in OraVerse is 0.235 mg/ml. Excipients include water for administration, ethylenediaminetetraacetic acid (EDTA), D-mannitol, sodium acetate, acetic acid, and sodium hydroxide.

MRD (Maximum Recommended Dose)
OraVerse was studied in a 1:1 cartridge to cartridge ratio to local anesthetic solution.

Amount of Local Anesthetic Administered	Dose of OraVerse
1/2 Cartridge	1/2 Cartridge (0.2 mg)
1 Cartridge	1 Cartridge (0.4 mg)
2 Cartridges	2 Cartridges (0.8 mg)

OraVerse is administered using the same location(s) and same technique(s) (infiltration or block injection) used for the administration of local anesthetic(s). The maximum recommended dose for children: 33–66 lbs is 0.2 mg (1/2 cartridge); for children over 66 lbs and up to 12 years of age the MRD is 0.4 mg (1 cartridge). OraVerse is not recommended for use in children less than six years of age or weighing less than 15 kg (33 lbs).

Relative Toxicity:	OraVerse is well tolerated at the doses tested.
Metabolism:	See published phentolamine mesylate literature.
Excretion:	Kidney
Vasoactivity:	Vasodilator
Onset of Action:	Rapid
Half-Life:	Approximately 2–3 hrs.
Pregnancy Category:	Cat C
Safety During Lactation:	Not studied
Product Warning:	Myocardial infarction and cerebrovascular spasm and occlusion have been reported following parenteral use of phentolamine, usually in association with marked hypotensive episodes producing shock-like states. Tachycardia, bradycardia, and cardiac arrhythmias may occur with the use of phentolamine or other alpha-adrenergic blocking agents. Although such effects are uncommon with OraVerse (phentolamine mesylate) clinicians should be alert to the signs and symptoms of these events, particularly in patients with a history of cardiovascular disease.

Source: OraVerse Product Insert, Hersh et al., 2008; Tavares et al., 2008.

---

were described as *routine procedures* with no indications of injury at any time during the procedures (Paxton, Hadley, Hadley, Edwards, & Harrison, 1994; Pogrel & Thamby, 2000).

In addition to routine procedures, surgical trauma, and neurotoxicity from local anesthetic drugs, other suggested etiologies include the chemical effects of the sulfite preservatives used for vasoconstrictors, detergent actions of local anesthetic drugs, increased apoptotic activity, and vasoconstrictor toxicity (Chen & Horowitz, 2006; Crean & Powis, 1999; Kitagawa, Oda, & Totoki, 2004; Park, Park, Yoon, Lee, Yum, & Kim, 2005; Pogrel & Thamby, 2000; Stacy & Hajjar, 1994). A list of a few of the proposed etiologies can be found in Box 17–8, which illustrates the open and ongoing nature of the discussion regarding paresthesia.

Although subject to vigorous and rational debate, the overall risk of parestheisa is thought to be low, regardless of the drug or concentration (Danish Medicine Agency, 2006; Dower, 2007; Lustig & Zusman, 1999). Based on data from the ADA and other sources, the apparent risk of local anesthesia-related parestheisa ranges from approximately 1.0 to 2.3 cases in one million (Haas, 1998; Haas & Lennon, 1995; Malamed, 2004; Pogrel et al., 2003; Pogrel & Thamby, 2000). Table 17–1 ■ provides information on the relationship between specific drug concentrations and approximate incidences of paresthesia.

Put in perspective, the National Weather Service has estimated that one in every three thousand individuals will be struck by lightning in their lifetimes and, according to the NIH Task Force on Safer Childhood Vaccines (Jan. 1998), acceptable adverse reactions from childhood immunizations include the development of paralytic polio in one in every half-million doses of oral polio virus vaccine (first dose), and anaphylactic reactions in two in every one hundred thousand doses of the DPT vaccine (NOAA National Severe Storms Laboratory, n.d.; NIH Task Force on Safer Childhood Vaccines, 1998).

Box 17–8   Some Possible Etiologies of Paresthesia

- Direct trauma (Stacy & Hajjar, 1994; Chen & Horowitz, 2006; Crean & Powis, 1999)
- Drug-induced increase in the rate of programmed cell death (apoptosis) (Park et al., 2005)
- Detergent effects (due to possible neural membrane lysis) (Kitagawa et al., 2004)
- Pressure from localized edema from hemorrhage involving the neural sheath (Pogrel, Bryan, & Regezi, 1995; Rayan, Pitha, Wisdom, Brentlinger, & Kopta, 1988)
- Higher local anesthetic drug concentrations (Haas & Lennon, 1995; Smith & Lung, 2006)
- Vasoconstrictors and their preservatives (Pogrel & Thamby, 2000)

Prevention of Paresthesia

In the absence of clearly defined etiology, preventive strategies (see Box 17–9) tend to focus on *approaches* that *appear* to lower risk (Lustig & Zusman, 1999; Malamed, 2004; Pogrel et al., 2003). There is no reliable strategy for avoiding the damage that results in permanent paresthesia during inferior alveolar nerve blocks, however unlikely the possibility. While this is currently true, it is nevertheless possible to avoid situations in which paresthesia is reportedly more likely to occur.

Table 17–1   Incidence of Paresthesia

Drugs Concentration	Reported Paresthesia Incidence	Injection Technique (Nerve Involvement)	Reported Paresthesia Incidence
0.5%	1:1,200,000	IA Nerve Block	1:26,000–1:800,000
2%	1:1,200,000	Involving Lingual nerve	70% of cases
3%	1:1,200,000	Involving IA nerve	30% of cases
4%	1:500,000	(no data)	(no data)

Note: All values are approximations as reported in the literature.
Source: Haas, 1998; Haas & Lennon, 1995; Malamed, 2004; Pogrel et al., 2003; Pogrel & Thamby, 2000.

Box 17–9   **Strategies to Lower the Risk of Paresthesia with 4% Drugs**

Strategies commonly employed to reduce the risks of paresthesia include:

1. Observe slow drug deposition recommendations.
2. Reduce volumes by 50 percent.
3. Use Gow-Gates or Vazirani-Akinosi techniques in place of inferior alveolar blocks.
4. In palatal techniques, limit volumes to no more than 0.9 ml (1/2 of a cartridge) (Malamed, 2004).

Since the lingual nerve is most frequently involved, using high block techniques to avoid inferior alveolar nerve blocks has been recommended when using 4% drugs (see Box 17–10) (Hawkins, 2006). Limiting volumes in palatal injections has also been recommended (see Box 17–9) (Malamed, 2004).

Needle tips in dentistry are so small that severing nerves is unlikely (Smith & Lung, 2006). The inferior alveolar and lingual nerves, the most frequently involved in paresthesia, are both similar in size and much larger than the tip of even the largest needle (25 gauge) commonly used in dentistry (Haas, 1998). Even though severing nerves is unlikely with dental needles, the possibility of nerve injury from needles exists, especially if they have been barbed (Blanton & Jeske, 2003). When a patient is in obvious distress during an injection, the procedure should be discontinued and a new needle and either a new pathway or a different technique should be used. It has been reported that there is a nearly 4 percent likelihood of traumatizing the lingual nerve every time a conventional mandibular nerve block is administered. Fortunately, the significant majority of these injuries were found to resolve within two weeks (Harn & Durham, 1990).

Barbed needle tips, in particular, have the capacity to inflict damage on all structures, including nerves (Stacy & Hajjar, 1994). In a 2000 prospective study of permanent nerve damage, it was reported that in the vast majority of inferior nerve blocks in which the nerve was directly contacted by the needle, barbed or not, there were no long-term effects (Pogrel & Thamby, 2000).

The creation of barbs on needle tips by contact with bone, in particular, which would indicate that damage occurred after full penetration of the needle, was not found to account for the majority of permanent paresthesias because it appeared that most of the paresthesias seen occurred on penetration rather than withdrawal (Harn & Durham, 1990; Stacy & Hajjar, 1994).

The experience of an electric shock did not predict the development of symptomatic nerve damage, either. It has been estimated that between 3 and 7 percent of the time, electric shocks are experienced during inferior alveolar blocks (Harn & Durham, 1990; Pogrel et al., 1994). It is reasonable to assume that this figure is actually higher because some injections will not result in noticeable nerve "shocks" even when nerves are contacted by needles. This may occur, for example, when needles are being withdrawn and the nerve is already anesthetized or when clinicians anesthetize ahead of needles while penetrating. Even in the absence of these probable additional injuries, the cited incidence of 3 to 7 percent exceeds the incidence of paresthesia due to all local anesthetic drug injections by a considerable margin.

Response to Paresthesia
Response to the initial notification of paresthesia should be rapid and should convey sympathy and concern. It has been recommended that the clinician who administered the drug speak personally with the patient and arrange for them to return to the office or clinic as soon as possible (Haas, 1998).

Evidence demonstrates that there is no reliable strategy to prevent paresthesia. Even surgical trauma, which many consider to be the most unequivocal of etiologies, may not always be responsible. As pointed out in one discussion on paresthesia, it may be impossible to state that paresthesia is the result of nerve injury during surgery when the injury could have occurred during the administration of the local anesthetic, prior to the surgery (Pogrel & Thamby, 2000).

Paresthesia Management
The lack of a universally accepted etiology may confuse the discussion of paresthesia somewhat but the protocol for its management is clear.

Current protocol includes the following:

1. *Speak personally* with and reassure the patient.
2. Schedule an appointment to evaluate as soon as possible.

Box 17–10   Should I Avoid Articaine in IA Nerve Blocks?

A frequent question when selecting drugs for IA blocks is, should I avoid articaine due to higher rates of paresthesia? Confusion exists primarily because the question is difficult to answer. Some clinicians routinely administer articaine for inferior alveolar nerve blocks. Others routinely avoid it. The difference in approach appears to be one of comfort with the possible consequences.

The 21-year Haas and Lennon retrospective study demonstrated a significantly higher incidence of paresthesia following articaine use. It did not demonstrate a high overall risk (Haas & Lennon, 1995). On the contrary, the overall risk of paresthesia report by Haas and Lennon was low. The majority of paresthesias are transient, making the risk lowest when considering only permanent paresthesias. Other studies have demonstrated no additional risks of paresthesia with articaine (Malamed, Gagnon, & Leblanc, 2001). The 2006 announcement of the Danish Medicines Agency, a follow-up to a similar 2005 announcement, states that [emphasis added]:

> Neurotoxicity has not been observed in prospective blinded randomised studies with a sufficient number of patients. Thus, *it is not sufficiently scientifically documented that articaine can cause nerve damage.* The existing studies are either retrospective reviews of patient material or *studies not including enough patients to show very rarely occurring adverse reactions.* In addition, the literature contains conflicting information.

In a criticism of current interpretations of information available on articaine's paresthesia-inducing incidence, James S. Dower Jr., DDS, MA, of the University of the Pacific, in San Francisco, writes the following:

> A peer-reviewed article in *Dentistry Today* reported that 4 percent articaine had a paresthesia rate 20 times higher than that of 2 percent lidocaine. In Denmark, Hillerup and Jensen reported that articaine produced an incidence of injection injuries more than 20-fold higher.
>
> . . . Until similarly designed studies demonstrate otherwise, I believe these are the scientific paresthesia rates with 4 percent articaine—and they create an unacceptable benefit: risk ratio for articaine compared with other local anesthetics (Dower, 2007).

Since the etiology of paresthesia is not understood and studies and comments from experts continue to provide conflicting information on the occurrence and prevention of paresthesia, there is no entirely clear answer at this time. What *is* known, however, is that the management of even a single permanent paresthesia over the course of a career can have significant emotional and legal ramifications.

---

3. Document the conversation.
4. Examine the patient; determine & record the extent and degree of the deficit.
5. Diagram the extent of the loss by recording where sensation begins and ends and the nature of the loss (numbness, partial numbness, tingling, burning, pain, taste perversion, loss of sweet, sour, salty, or bitter sensations, etc.). Figure 17–7 ■ provides a sample chart for mapping paresthesia, and Figure 17–8 ■ and Figure 17–9 ■ demonstrate a method for tracking changes over time.
6. Explain that paresthesia may last for a while but the vast majority improve over time.
7. Review and update the map at follow-up appointments to document resolution, which reassures patients, particularly those who need visible reassurance.
8. Refer to an appropriate specialist if improvement does not occur or the situation deteriorates.
9. If future therapy is anticipated in the affected area, use an alternate injection technique (Daniel et al., 2007; Hass, 1998; Malamad, 2004).

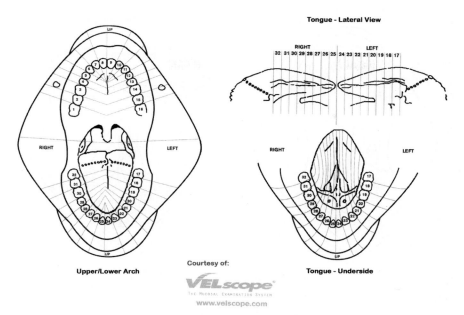

■ **FIGURE 17–7**   Example of Paresthesia Documentation Chart.

Source: Courtesy of VELscope.

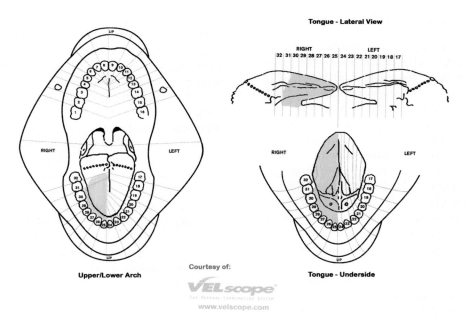

■ **FIGURE 17–8**   Documentation of Initial Extent of Paresthesia.

Source: Courtesy of VELscope.

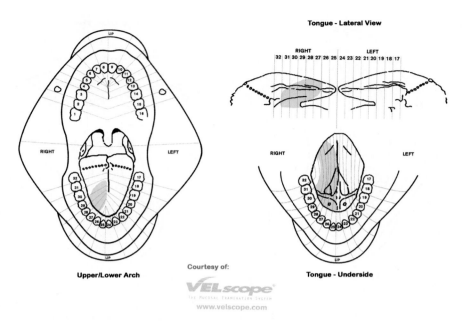

■ **FIGURE 17–9** Documentation of Partial Resolution of Paresthesia Over Time.
Source: Courtesy of VELscope.

Facial Nerve Paralysis

Local anesthetic techniques can result in anesthesia of the facial nerve (CN VII), which travels through the parotid gland without providing innervation (Haas, 1998; Malamed, 2004). Instead of parotid innervation, it provides innervation to structures peripheral to the gland, the muscles of facial expression, and regions inferior to the eye and around the mouth and chin.

During an IA block, overinsertion of the needle can cause penetration of the capsule surrounding the deep lobe of the parotid gland. If anesthetic drugs are deposited into the gland, the facial nerve can be anesthetized. This can usually be prevented by confirming bony resistance when administering IA blocks to assure that needle tips are not inserted into the parotid gland.

If the facial nerve is anesthetized, unilateral paralysis of the face will result. This typically will last only as long as the anesthetic is in effect. Some mistakenly refer to this temporary lack of function due to facial nerve anesthesia as Bell's palsy, which is an unexplained condition that can persist for months or occasionally may be permanent (Jastak et al., 1995).

Vazirani-Akinosi blocks can also result in facial nerve paralysis when the needle is overinserted. The facial paralysis seen after Vazirani-Akinosi blocks has the same pattern, behavior, and distribution as that which develops after IA blocks.

In some individuals, the facial nerve is located in close proximity to the normal target areas of the IA and Vazirani-Akinosi blocks. In these individuals, observing recommended insertion depths and confirming bony resistance (for the IA block only) may not prevent the development of facial nerve anesthesia (Malamed, 2004).

Due to the involvement of the eye, reflex activity is compromised in facial paralysis; however, tears will continue to be produced. Eye protection is recommended over the affected eye until reflex activity returns to normal (Malamed, 2004).

Response to Facial Nerve Paralysis

Patients who experience facial nerve paralysis are primarily concerned with the duration of the paralysis, any lasting effects, and avoidance of the event in the future. Reassurance can be offered that the paralysis will last only as long as the drug's effects, consistent with the patient's typical pattern of recovery after local anesthesia. Patients may be further advised that recurring paralyses after dental injections may indicate anatomic predispositions where the paralysis is unavoidable. Alternative techniques, such as infiltrations and PDL injections, can be useful in future avoidance.

Prevention of Facial Nerve Paralysis

Strategies found useful in preventing facial nerve anesthesia include:

1. Observe proper injection technique.
2. Avoid depositing solution in IA blocks without confirming bony resistance.
3. Use smaller gauge needles to avoid deflections away from bone (Aldons, 1968).
4. Avoid needle overinsertion in Vazirani-Akinosi blocks.
5. Use alternate techniques such as PDL injections.

Management of Facial Nerve Paralysis

Steps in the management of facial nerve paralysis include:

1. Discontinue treatment.
2. Reassure the patient.
3. Remove contact lens, if present.
4. Place an eye patch over the affected eye.
5. Document the incident.
6. Follow-up as indicated.

Postanesthetic Mucosal Lesions

Postanesthetic lesions include those resulting from infectious or suspected autoimmune processes and those resulting from direct injury to the mucosa (Haas, 1998; Malamed, 2004).

Lesions with an infectious etiology, such as herpetic ulcers, or a suspected autoimmune etiology, such as aphthous ulcers, can develop following anesthetic injections. Herpetic lesions occasionally appear after injection, particularly in the palate. They present as small, multiple ulcerations in the vicinity of the injection. There is sometimes an inability to discriminate between herpetic and aphthous lesions in the palate because aphthous lesions, although typically solitary, larger, and found on non-keratinized mucosa, may also present as small, multiple ulcerations on keratinized tissue (Ibsen & Phelan, 2004). These are known as *herpetiform*

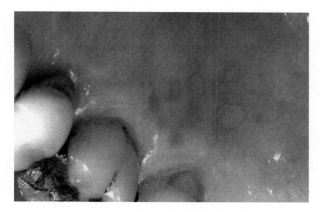

■ **FIGURE 17–10** Herpetiform Aphthous Ulcerations. Palatal aphthous ulcerations following a palatal injection.

aphthous ulcerations or *lesions* (see Figure 17–10 ■). A past history of labial herpetic outbreaks or of recurrent aphthous ulcerations is helpful in discriminating between the two. By definition, ulcerations involve both epithelial and connective tissue damage and tend to be quite painful, especially to hot and acidic foods. There is usually no difference in the healing pattern of the ulcers regardless of the cause.

Overly vigorous hemostasis from high concentrations of vasoconstrictor or dessication from topical anesthetic left in contact with mucosa for extended periods can lead to necrosis and ulceration. These lesions, similar to herpetic and aphthous ulcerations, tend to be painful and sensitive to certain foods and beverages, especially those that are acidic. Patients should be instructed to alert clinicians if lesions occur and are slow to heal, or if pain increases, signaling the possibility of infection.

Prevention of Postanesthetic Mucosal Lesions

Unfortunately, there is no prevention for the development of herpetic or aphthous lesions. Patients sometimes understandably suspect that the clinician might have done something wrong or caused some kind of injury that is responsible for their postoperative pain. They may be reassured, however, by quick recognition of post-anesthetic lesions at subsequent visits and by brief explanations as to possible etiologies. Individuals who are susceptible to cold sores, for example, are often unaware that they can occur intraorally after injections.

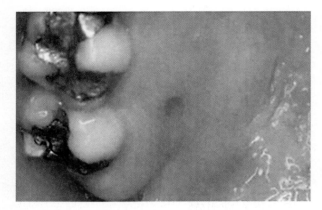

■ **FIGURE 17-11** Post-injection Necrosis. Signs of necrosis following a GP injection.

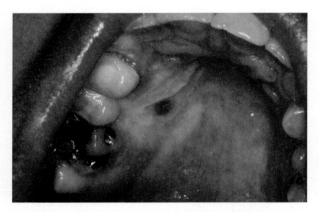

■ **FIGURE 17-12** Post-injection Trauma. Signs of local trauma developed about 1 minute into the deposition for an AMSA injection.

Unlike herpetic and aphthous lesions, necrosis is largely preventable (see Figure 17–11 ■). The following strategies are effective for reducing the risks of necrosis:

1. Avoid epinephrine concentrations of 1:50,000 especially in confined tissues, such as the palate.
2. Avoid excessive durations of topical anesthetic (follow manufacturers' instructions).
3. Avoid excessive blanching by allowing sufficient time for solution to diffuse into tissue during deposition; tissues should not turn "stark white" in appearance.
4. Avoid extensive distention of tissues by allowing sufficient time for solution to diffuse while depositing; tissues should not bulge or "balloon" with too much solution.

Figure 17–11 shows post-injection necrosis following a GP injection and Figure 17–12 ■ shows trauma following an AMSA injection.

Management of Postanesthetic Mucosal Lesions

While prevention may or may not be possible, management always is. Various OTC medications are available and tend to relieve discomfort during the early phases of healing. When postanesthetic lesions occur, the following steps should be observed:

1. Determine previous history to reassure the patient.
2. Recommend an OTC medication to coat the lesion (with or without topical anesthetic), taking care not to spread the infection if it is herpetic.
   a. Recommend applying the medication prior to each meal to protect the lesions from additional injury and applying otherwise as recommended in the product insert.
      i. Recommend to avoid hot and acidic foods
      ii. Recommend OTC pain relievers as needed (pain usually lasts for 2 to 3 days).

The best indicators of extraoral healing are "crusting over" and scarring. Scars do not typically form on mucosa, but a lack of sensitivity indicates that new connective tissue (granulation tissue) has begun to form over the ulcer.

Infections

Due to the availability of sterile and disposable armamentarium and to federal and state mandates of standard precautions in dental facilities, postoperative infections are rare today (Malamed, 2004; Pogrel & Thamby, 2000). Contaminated needles, along with other devices if handled inappropriately, represent the greatest threat of iatrogenic infection. Normal flora do not represent a significant source despite their transport into the tissues with every penetration because their small numbers are easily removed by the body's immune system (Haas, 1998; Malamed, 2004). Exceptions may occur in severely immune compromised individuals and when the tissues to be penetrated are infected prior to administration. Elective treatment might not be possible for some immunocompromised individuals or might be possible only with concomitant antibiotics. A physician consult is recommended. Should the anticipated area of penetration be infected prior to injection, there is a greater chance of the deeper spread of the infection, and penetration in these areas should be avoided (Haas, 1998).

Manifestations of postanesthetic infections include pain and trismus, although overt signs and symptoms are rare (Haas, 1998; Malamed, 2004). If trismus persists beyond three days, infection should be considered (Malamed, 2004).

Prevention of Postanesthetic Infections

The following strategies are effective for reducing the risks of infection from injection:

1. Use only sterile, uncontaminated needles.
2. In the presence of infection, use a new needle for each penetration.
3. If extraoral contamination occurs, discard the needle.
4. If intraoral contamination occurs (other than oral tissues), discard the needle.
5. In immune compromised individuals, use antiseptics before penetration or antibiotics after consultation with the patient's physician (Haas, 1998).

Management of Postanesthetic Infections

When postanesthetic infections occur, the following steps should be observed:

1. Schedule an evaluation appointment as soon as possible.
2. Prescribe antibiotics as appropriate.
3. Document the infection and the prescription.
4. Schedule follow-up appointments until the infection is resolved (Haas, 1998).

SYSTEMIC COMPLICATIONS

Systemic complications from local anesthetic drugs, with the exception of syncope, occur less frequently compared with local complications. When they occur, systemic complications manifest primarily as overdoses, allergic responses, and idiosyncratic reactions. In addition to discussions of these complications, two other systemic conditions previously discussed in Chapter 10, "Patient Assessment for Local Anesthesia," atypical plasma cholinesterase and methemoglobinemia, will be discussed briefly here.

Of the three systemic complications, overdose, allergy, and idiosyncratic reaction, overdose occurs most frequently (Malamed, 2004). Overdoses may be defined as administrations of drugs that result in signs and symptoms of CNS and CVS depression (Horlocker & Wedel, 2002). It is suspected that at least some percentage of the overdoses experienced occur due to intravascular administration (Horlocker & Wedel). Not all individuals will respond adversely to inadvertent intravascularly-administered doses, however (Lustig & Zusman, 1999; Malamed, 2004).

The majority of overdose reactions occur as a result of the absorption of excessive administrations of drugs. Many individuals do not respond with adverse systemic signs and symptoms to local anesthetic drugs until *much* higher than recommended doses are administered. They are referred to as **hypo-responders** (Lustig & Zusman, 1999; Malamed, 2004). Other individuals may respond adversely when less than maximum recommended doses have been administered and are referred to as **hyper-responders.** Importantly, regardless of the response level, an individual's threshold for adverse reaction to a local anesthetic drug is considered normal for that individual (Malamed, 2004).

Allergic reactions to amide local anesthetic drugs are rare. They can manifest both locally and systemically. An important distinction between allergic reactions and overdose reactions is that, unlike overdose reactions, allergic reactions are not dose-dependent.

Systemic allergic reactions can be life threatening and require prompt response. Fortunately, the amide drugs used in dentistry today have low allergenic potentials and they also have low cross-allergenicity; in other words, if a person is allergic to one amide, he or she often has no adverse response to others. Allergy testing should precede further administrations once **hypersensitivity** has been identified and it should include testing for sensitivity to possible alternatives.

Allergy may also occur due to sulfite preservatives in vasoconstrictor-containing solutions of local anesthetic drugs. If a patient is allergic to sulfites, vasoconstrictor-containing drugs cannot be used.

Allergy to epinephrine is impossible because the epinephrine used in dentistry and medicine is identical to endogenous epinephrine (Malamed, 2004). Allergy to epinephrine, therefore, is incompatible with life. Despite the physiologic impossibility, it is not unusual for patients to report that they are allergic to adrenalin. The sensitivity they may have experienced, while not allergenic in etiology, not only limits epinephrine's use but may be the basis of a fear of dentistry.

Overdose

The overdose potential of a local anesthetic drug differs with the drug. For example, one study demonstrated that higher blood levels of articaine were necessary compared with lidocaine before signs and symptoms of overdose were noted and that when overdose developed from articaine it was observed to be less severe (Oertel, Rahn, & Kirch, 1997). Bupivacaine is known for its nearly equal toxicities to the CNS and CVS, yet Albright reported in 1979 that in a handful of cases of bupivacaine toxicity CVS collapse preceded any evidence of CNS toxicity (Horlocker & Wedel, 2002).

The Pathophysiology of Local Anesthetic Overdose

Overdoses are the result of the pharmacologic actions of the local anesthetic drugs on the CNS and CVS. They occur either due to intravascular deposition or to the non-intravascular administration of excessive doses, both of which interfere with normal ionic exchange across neural membranes of the CNS and CVS.

Typical initial effects of drug overdose result from depression of inhibitory pathways in the CNS, resulting in early excitation. Inhibitory depression occurs due to a concentrating effect of the drugs in the well-vascularized limbic brain (Tetzlaff, 2000). Some drugs, such as bupivacaine in very high quantities, and also lidocaine, may not produce early excitation in overdose, beginning instead with signs and symptoms of depression (Malamed, 2004; Tetzlaff, 2000). Continued overdosing depresses both inhibitory and excitatory pathways, resulting in signs and symptoms of CNS depression only. If overdosing continues at this point, it can lead to seizures, CVS depression, and eventually coma and respiratory and cardiovascular arrest. Threshold blood levels of drugs are necessary to support overdoses. With some exceptions, CVS depression occurs only after higher overdose levels of a drug have been reached in the blood.

CVS effects of overdose involve several mechanisms. These primarily affect myocardial contractility and conduction volumes, causing an interrelated decrease of both. Decreased contractility and conduction volumes can lead to bradycardia, arrhythmias, and finally, asystole (the absence of a heart beat). Factors that may complicate recovery from higher overdoses include electrolyte imbalances, hypoxia, and acidosis (an abnormal increase in body fluid acidity) (Levsky & Miller, 2005).

Overdoses are reversed once normal metabolic pathways eliminate enough of the circulating drug for levels to drop below overdose thresholds. At that time, signs and symptoms of overdose diminish or cease.

Predisposing factors to overdose include age, concomitant medications, disease status, and genetics. Mental attitude, perception, and environment have also been discussed as predisposing factors (Malamed, 2004).

Initial Signs and Symptoms of Local Anesthetic Overdose

The initial signs and symptoms of overdose have been described as a manifestation of central nervous system excitation. These may include ringing in the ears (tinnitus), a metallic taste in the mouth, increased anxiety, and circumoral tingling or numbness (Malamed, 2004; Mulroy, 2002).

Intravascular injections may result in rapid development of these signs and symptoms because blood concentrations in the brain have been stated to be higher after intravascular injections than from any other source. Fortunately, the same abundant perfusion of blood to the brain that hastens the onset of the early signs and symptoms of overdose in intravascular injections tends to decrease the duration of the overdose (drug levels quickly diminish, provided that the cardiovascular system remains relatively unimpaired) (Mulroy, 2002).

When overdoses are caused by absorption of excessive volumes of drug, the development of overdose tends to be more delayed (Mulroy, 2002). This is moderated by factors including the presence or absence of a vasoconstrictor, the vascularity of the area into which the drug is injected, the physical status of the patient, and the class of drug. Drugs that are rapidly metabolized in the blood have shorter overdose courses versus those metabolized in the liver (a *relatively* long process). Signs and symptoms nevertheless will be the same when overdoses occur.

Later Signs and Symptoms of Local Anesthetic Overdose

As overdose continues and progresses, previously unopposed excitatory pathways are depressed and signs and symptoms of CNS depression prevail. These may include twitching and tremors, slurred speech, fatigue, unconsciousness, and seizures (Malamed, 2004; Mulroy, 2002). If drug levels continue to rise, coma, respiratory arrest,

---

Box 17–11   *Cardiovascular Collapse Reversal*

Research on a weight loss supplement, Intralipid, has suggested that it may aid in reversing the cardiovascular effects of local anesthetic overdose (Weinberg, VadeBoncouer, Ramaraju, Garcia-Amara, & Cwik, 1998). Resuscitation with Intralipid has had promising results in treating cardiovascular depression experienced after bupivacaine, ropivacaine, and levobupivacaine–induced cardiovascular collapse (Foxall, McCahon, Lamb, Hardman, & Bedforth, 2007; Rosenblatt, Abel, Fischer, Itzkovich, & Eisenkraft, 2006). Several studies have suggested that infusions of 20 percent (Intralipid) have contributed to CVS toxicity reversal and may even have aided in seizure reversal (CNS toxicity reversal) (Foxall et al., 2007).

The usefulness of this supplement in dental overdose situations is unknown at this time.

---

and cardiac arrest are possible (Mulroy, 2002). One approach to reversing cardiovascular collapse experienced after overdose from local anesthetic drugs in medicine is discussed in Box 17–11.

Prevention of Local Anesthetic Overdose

To prevent local anesthetic overdose, the following guidelines are recommended:

1. Assess maximum doses based on weight and health status, prior to injection.
2. Administer all doses *slowly*.
3. Aspirate whenever there is the possibility of intravascular deposition.
4. Re-aspirate throughout injections.

Several strategies can help to prevent overdoses in dentistry. In addition to accurate pre-injection assessment of physical status to determine safe maximum dosages, the most important technique strategy is to *administer drugs slowly* (no more than one cartridge per minute) (Malamed, 2004). Some clinicians believe that aspiration is more important than slow administration. While the point might not be worth arguing because both aspiration and slow deposition are critical safety factors, it appears that negative aspiration is not an absolutely reliable indicator that the needle tip is not in a

vessel (Malamed; Mulroy, 2002). When aspiration is negative but the tip of the needle nonetheless is located within a vessel, only slow deposition can minimize potential adverse effects of intravascular administration. Slow deposition allows for greater dilution of a drug in the event deposition is intravascular.

If a needle tip is located intravascularly and aspiration is performed, a false negative aspiration can be observed if the positive pressure of aspiration creates suction on the inside of the vessel wall that blocks the blood from entering the lumen of the needle. Aspirating in two planes can decrease the incidence of false negative aspiration and intravascular injection but it cannot eliminate the possibility (Malamed, 2004; Mulroy, 2002).

Recognition of Local Anesthetic Overdose

Signs and symptoms of overdose overlap with signs and symptoms of anxiety in dental patients. This is particularly true with articaine, mepivacaine, and prilocaine when excitatory phases precede CNS depression and when vasoconstrictors are included in solutions. When they occur, these excitatory phases precede CNS depression. It is not unusual to have a talkative, apprehensive patient in the dental chair who may display many of the signs and symptoms of overdose when there is no overdose. Important distinctions, however, help to discriminate between the manifestations of anxiety and true overdose. Bilateral circumoral tingling or numbness, in particular, would not be due to the effects of unilateral anesthesia or of anxiety. In addition, relaxation techniques can reverse the signs and symptoms of anxiety but are unlikely to be effective against a progressive overdose. Finally, a *progression* of depressive signs and symptoms is suggestive of an overdose.

Initial signs and symptoms of overdose include the following:

1. Metallic taste
2. Increased anxiety
3. *Bilateral* circumoral tingling or numbness

A list of the signs and symptoms of local anesthetic overdose is illustrated in Table 17–2 ■ and for vasoconstrictors see Table 17–3 ■.

Management of Local Anesthetic Overdose

Overdose reactions may occur within minutes to up to an hour or more from the time of administration (Jastak et al., 1995). Generally, the more delayed the onset, the less severe the reaction.

Table 17–2	Signs and Symptoms of Local Anesthetic Overdose (Progressive Order)
Central Nervous System	**Cardiovascular System**
Lightheadedness	Hypertension
Tinnitus	Tachycardia
Confusion	
Circumoral numbness	
Muscle twitching	Decreased contractility
Auditory and visual	and cardiac output
hallucinations	Hypotension
Tonic-clonic seizures	Sinus bradycardia
Unconsciousness	Ventricular dysrhythmias
Respiratory arrest	Circulatory arrest

Sources: Jastak et al., 1995; Little, Falace, Miller, & Rhodus, 2008; Malamed, 2004.

Table 17–3	Signs and Symptoms of Vasoconstrictor Overdose
	Cardiovascular System
Generalized signs	Serious elevation in blood
of fear and anxiety	pressure and heart rate
Nausea	
Restlessness	Cardiac dysrhythmias
Heart racing	
Intense anxiety	Premature ventricular
Weakness	contractions (PVCs)
Tremor	
Severe headache	Ventricular tachycardia
Hyperventilation	Ventricular fibrillation
Palpitation	Circulatory arrest
Shaky	Stroke

Sources: Jastak et al., 1995; Little, Falace, Miller, & Rhodus, 2008; Malamed, 2004.

Mild overdoses may require no more than monitoring while providing supportive measures until drug levels fall below overdose thresholds. Moderate to severe overdoses can require aggressive management including rapid response, appropriate positioning (especially in the event of clonic-tonic seizures), and activation of the emergency system. For a quick reference

---

Box 17–12	Management of Mild Overdose

In response to mild overdose, the following guidelines are recommended:

1. Activate emergency protocols, as needed
2. Reassure
3. Observe
4. Monitor

Dental procedures may continue (if tolerable) or the patient may be dismissed. The patient may not need an escort if full recovery has occurred; however, an escort or emergency transport may be indicated.

Box 17–13	Management of Moderate to Severe Overdose

In response to moderate to severe overdose the following guidelines are recommended:

1. Activate emergency protocols
2. Administer oxygen (to prevent seizures that can occur due to a lack of O_2)
3. Administer diazepam (Valium) or midazolam (Versed), if a seizure develops
4. Perform CPR when necessary
5. Prevent patient injury due to seizures
6. Monitor vital signs
7. Patient dismissal with escort or/emergency transport as indicated

of guidelines on the management of overdoses see Box 17–12 and Box 17–13.

Clinicians should be prepared to implement the ABCs (Airway, Breathing, Circulation) of basic life support and appropriate positioning of the patient.

Allergy

A major difference between overdose and allergy is that allergies are not dose dependent (Malamed, 2004). Allergies, also referred to as hypersensitivities, involve localized or systemic, cell-mediated and/or humoral responses to antigens, in any concentration. Hypersensitivities to local anesthetics can manifest both locally and systemically and are classified as immediate (Type I) or delayed (Type IV) (Ibsen & Phelan, 2004; Malamed, 2004).

Local anesthetic molecules are considered too small to act as antigens but their binding preference for proteins, which largely explains their actions in sodium ion channels, also provides sufficient size to allow them to become antigenic (Jastak et al., 1995).

There is limited cross-allergenicity between amides. If an individual is allergic to one ester, however, no esters may be used (Malamed, 2004). Ester allergies occur mainly as delayed and localized responses in dentistry because the nearly exclusive use of esters as topical anesthetics limits the potential for systemic reactions. When an allergy to esters is suspected, appropriate amide topicals may be substituted.

An allergic response to an injectable drug should prompt an evaluation by an allergist. This evaluation is especially important when a suspected allergy to an injectable amide has occurred. In addition to the suspect drug, the individual should be tested for allergic responses to amide substitutes. Testing for other substances in cartridges, such as preservatives, should also be performed. A cartridge of the anesthetic and its product insert should be provided to the allergist along with samples of other materials used.

In addition to drug allergies, latex components of local anesthetic drug cartridges that may still be found in some cartridges have been speculated to be possible causes of allergic reactions. These components are discussed in detail in Chapter 9, "Local Anesthetic Delivery Devices."

Localized Allergic Reactions

Localized allergic reactions to local anesthetic drugs occur most frequently after topical anesthetic application (see Figure 17–13 ■) and manifest as Type IV reactions (Ibsen & Phelan, 2004). They are usually limited and respond well to antihistamine therapy. The majority have occurred due to the metabolic byproduct of esters, para-aminobenzoic acid (PABA). There is concern, however, that contact allergy to lidocaine topicals may be increasing (Tucker, 2007). Several patients in a recent report experienced positive reactions to lidocaine topical and to injectable lidocaine in all concentrations, suggesting a true allergic reaction versus an irritant effect (Tucker, 2007).

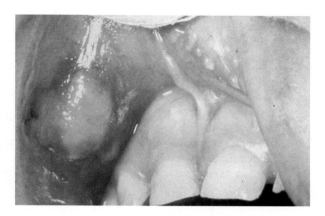

■ **FIGURE 17–13** Localized Allergic Reaction. Signs of localized allergic reaction following the placement of topical anesthetic.

Hives (urticaria) are associated with many conditions, including reactions to antigens (Ibsen & Phelan, 2004). They present as well-demarcated swellings on the skin usually accompanied by itching and can occur after local anesthetic administration (Malamed, 2004). A similar, but deeper and less frequent manifestation sometimes occurs in reaction to anesthetics, known as **angioedema** (Ibsen & Phelan, 2004). Angioedema and urticaria are different in that angioedema is not usually accompanied by itching due to the involvement of less superficial vessels (Ibsen & Phelan). Either may occur rapidly after local anesthetic administration, in which case the reaction may be more indicative of a developing generalized reaction (Malamed, 2004). These reactions typically occur in response to topical anesthetics within 30 to 60 minutes of tissue contact (Malamed, 2004). Despite this rapid reaction, some reactions may occur later, hours after a patient has been dismissed.

Monitoring is important in local allergic events in order to recognize the possible progression from local to systemic manifestations. While most local complications remain local, some local anesthetic allergic reactions can progress to become systemic events (Jastak et al., 1995). Clinicians should be alert to the possible progressive worsening of the signs and symptoms of localized allergy (see Figure 17–13), especially respiratory distress.

Response to Localized Allergic Reactions

Rapid recognition and response to developing localized allergic reactions can alter the extent of the reaction. It is also important to remove any remaining traces of a topical drug and discontinue its use.

Prevention of Localized Allergic Events

To prevent local allergic events:

1. Avoid medications that have induced allergic reactions in the past
2. Avoid same-class topicals that previously induced hypersensitivities
3. Consult with previous providers whenever patients report past allergic experiences
4. Refer for allergy testing if patients report past allergies or symptoms
5. Document in the chart

Management of Localized Allergic Events

In response to local allergic events the following guidelines are recommended:

1. Schedule the patient immediately to evaluate possible postoperative allergic lesions/reactions
2. Recommend OTC Benadryl or prescribe diphenhydramine as appropriate
3. Refer for allergy testing, depending on signs and symptoms
4. Send samples of anesthetic and of non-anesthetic substances that also contacted the site
5. Document in the chart

Systemic Allergic Reactions

While less frequent in occurrence, systemic reactions to local anesthetic drugs and solutions are far more serious when they occur. These reactions may occur due to the local anesthetic drugs, themselves, the sulfite preservatives in solutions, or, in the case of esters, to the byproduct of ester hydrolysis, PABA.

Response to Systemic Allergic Reactions

Recognition and prompt response are critical when allergic reactions occur. Any delay allows a progressively degenerating situation that may result in respiratory and cardiovascular arrest. Epinephrine is the antidote because it reverses bronchial constriction and peripheral vasodilation and is not, itself, an antigen. It is important to note that epinephrine's effectiveness is limited to relatively short intervals due to its rapid biotransformation. Clinicians must be prepared to deliver repeated doses until emergency medical personnel arrive.

Prevention of Systemic Allergic Reactions

Systemic reactions to known allergens can be prevented by obtaining information during health history reviews. Specific questions related to previous allergies can provide guidance, either as direct evidence or in provoking further questioning or referrals to allergists.

Due to the possibility of allergic reactions to previously nonallergenic substances and the nearly universal exposure of the population to a wide variety of allergens, there is no way to predict or prevent unprecedented allergic reactions. The exception to this unpredictable pattern occurs when there may be cross-allergies, which should be investigated whenever a positive response has been noted to a past history of allergy to any amide anesthetic.

Management of Systemic Allergic Reactions

Type I hypersensitivities may manifest as localized reactions (localized anaphylaxis) and systemic reactions (generalized anaphylaxis). Both are similar in a number of ways. The most important similarity in this discussion, however, is that the reaction occurs within a short time, anywhere from seconds to hours after exposure to an antigen (Malamed, 2004).

Localized anaphylaxis has the potential to become systemic and should be monitored for the development of systemic signs and symptoms, especially peripheral vasodilation, which can lead to hypovolemic shock, a generalized rash, and difficulty breathing due to constriction of the airway (see Box 17–14).

Box 17–14 **Progression of Signs and Symptoms in Generalized Anaphylaxis**

In the event of generalized anaphylaxis, signs and symptoms will progress through phases that include:

1. Skin reactions—Itching, flushing, hives
2. GI/GU reactions—Cramps, vomiting, diarrhea, nausea, incontinence
3. Respiratory—Chest tightness, cough, wheezing, dyspnea, laryngeal edema
4. CVS—Palpitations, lightheadedness, tachycardia, hypotension, unconsciousness, arrest

Source: Malamed, 2004.

Systemic allergic reactions are life-threatening emergencies and require prompt responses when encountered, including:

1. Terminate treatment
2. Activate emergency protocols
3. Administer oxygen
4. Administer epinephrine, 0.3 mg (0.15 mg for a child) intramuscularly or subcutaneously
5. Administer diphenhydramine, 50 mg (25 mg for a child)
6. Transfer to a hospital via ambulance or, after medical consultation and observation, the patient may be dismissed with a prescription for diphenhydramine or an appropriate substitute, with the need for an escort to be determined by the physician or hospital
7. Medical consultation before subsequent therapy, including allergy testing (Malamed, 2004)

Idiosyncratic Events

Adverse events may occur that have no known etiology. These are referred to as **idiosyncratic** events and are likely of genetic origin. The varieties of signs and symptoms that may occur resemble those seen in overdose and allergy and require responses that are appropriate to the particular signs and symptoms that develop (Malamed, 2004).

Atypical Plasma Cholinesterase

As discussed in Chapter 10, atypical plasma cholinesterase impairs the metabolism of esters. Pre-screening for this genetic trait is the primary preventive measure. Because ester injectables are no longer packaged for use in dentistry, there is only a rare injectable route for these drugs. The most common current use of esters in dentistry is in topical anesthetics such as benzocaine and tetracaine. These preparations are easily avoided by using topicals containing lidocaine, prilocaine, or dyclonine hydrochloride.

Methemoglobinemia

Methemoglobinemia is a condition characterized by a diminished oxygen-carrying capacity of the blood. Individuals may be predisposed to methemoglobinemia or it may occur in non-predisposed individuals. In addition to other chemical substances, both prilocaine and benzocaine are known inducers and must be avoided in susceptible individuals (Abu-Laban, Zed, Purssell, & Evans, 2003; Institute for Safe Medical Practices [ISMP], 2002). Centers for Disease Control and Prevention [CDC], 1994; FDA Patient Safety News, 2006). While typical doses in dentistry do not seem to be problematic, warnings from the FDA in response to recent serious incidents with benzocaine spray, and a history of numerous warnings associated with prilocaine, have reinforced the need for caution (Abu-Laban et al., 2003). There are many reports of methemoglobinemia associated with both drugs (FDA Modernization Act of 1997; ISMP; FDA Patient Safety News, 2006). Although not mentioned in these reports, articaine can also induce methemoglobinemia.

Since there are excellent substitutes for these drugs in suspected individuals or those with previously known susceptibilities, their use should be considered only after a thorough risk–benefit analysis. For more information on prilocaine and articaine, see Signs & Symptoms of Methemoglobinemia and Toxicity in Chapter 5, "Dental Local Anesthetic Drugs." For more information on benzocaine see Chapter 8, "Topical Anesthetics," and for Systemic Reactions see Chapter 10.

CASE MANAGEMENT: Ashley Smith

While somewhat dramatic in appearance, the hematoma presented in this case is more typical of many that develop following dental injections, both in its extent and its course of healing. Unlike the case highlighted in the text of this chapter, where the patient was taking three anticoagulants, there were no complicating factors and no contraindications to the use of a PSA nerve block, either absolute or relative.

Case Discussion: The hematoma seen in Figure 17–1 occurred immediately following a positive aspiration at optimum penetration depth and angle for a PSA nerve block. Of particular interest in this series of photographs are the time sequence, the appearance of the hematoma at various stages of healing, and the length of time for resolution. Figure 17–14 ■ shows the hematoma a few minutes after development. This was the approximate extent of the swelling and represents the point at which the intravascular pressures have been equalized by the pressures exerted by the distended tissues of the face. One week later, the swelling is still present but has diffused somewhat into adjacent tissues, providing a smoother outline (Figure 17–15 ■). Hematomas are affected by gravity. Notice how the swelling has dropped below the mandible in its inferior extent. Two weeks later (Figure 17–16 ■) the outline is even smoother, much less angular compared with the appearance on the day of development, and the bruise is much more obvious, demonstrating typical shades of yellow, brown, and purple (Figure 17–17 ■). These colors reflect the changes in the appearance of the blood, which occur over time, under the skin.

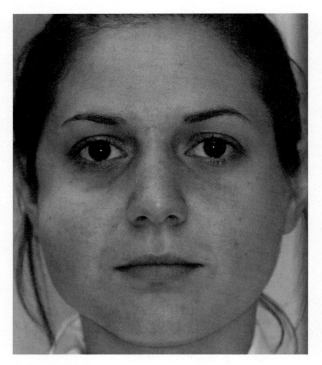

■ **FIGURE 17-14** Progression of a Hematoma—Day 1+. Progression of swelling a few minutes after observing the initial swelling.

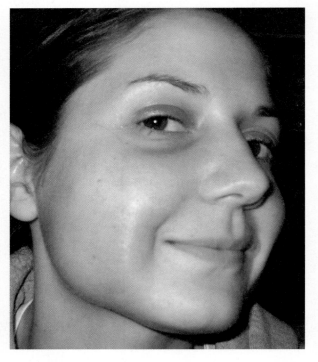

■ **FIGURE 17-15** Progression of a Hematoma—1 Week Later. The swelling is still present but has diffused into adjacent tissues.

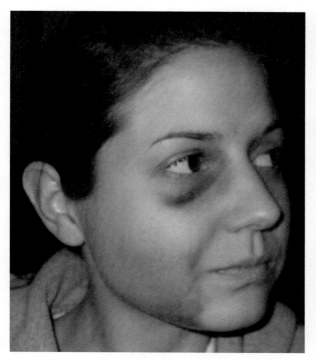

■ **FIGURE 17–16** Progression of a Hematoma— ~ 2 Weeks Later. After two weeks, the outline is smoother compared with day one; however, the bruise is much more obvious.

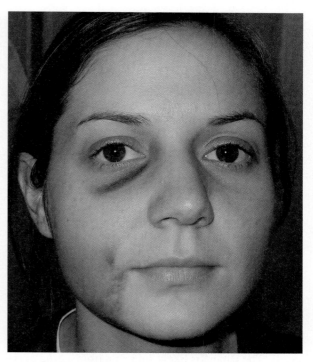

■ **FIGURE 17–17** Progression of a Hematoma— 2 Weeks+ Later. Demonstrating typical shades of yellow, brown, and purple, these colors reflect the changes in the appearance of the blood, which occur over time, under the skin.

As hematomas heal and bruising becomes more visible, color changes are due to the breakdown of hemoglobin, its metabolites (biliverdin and bilirubin), and hemosiderin. The breakdown of hemoglobin is responsible for the reddish-blue color, biliverdin for the green and bilirubin the yellow. Hemosiderin is responsible for the brown color.

CHAPTER QUESTIONS

1. A clinician is administering an IA nerve block prior to therapy when the patient suddenly jerks and the needle breaks. The embedded portion is not visible. What should the clinician do?
   a. Attempt removal
   b. Refer for removal
   c. Reappoint to remove once the needle has developed a fibrous cocoon around it
   d. Refer for evaluation

2. A second cartridge of 2% lidocaine has been administered for an IA nerve block when the 160-pound-patient becomes anxious and states that she doesn't feel well, even a little nauseous. She becomes less anxious as she becomes increasingly fatigued and her speech becomes slurred, with a reported "numb" feeling all around the patient's mouth. Which *one* of the following statements best describes these observations?
   a. The patient is likely suffering from severe anxiety and fatigue.
   b. The patient is likely suffering from a drug overdose due to excessive administered doses.
   c. The patient is likely suffering from a drug overdose due to intravascular administration.
   d. The patient is likely suffering from an allergy to lidocaine.

3. Allergies to topical anesthetic drugs that cause mucosal signs and symptoms hours to days after exposure are explained best by which *one* of the following reactions?
   a. Delayed hypersensitivity
   b. Anaphylaxis
   c. Angioedema
   d. Immunopathology

4. A patient calls several days after an IA block and reports that numbness is still present along with some annoying, occasional sharp pains. Which of the following terms best describes what is occurring?
   a. Paresthesia, anesthesia
   b. Paresthesia, hypoesthesia
   c. Paresthesia, dysesthesia
   d. Anesthesia, hyperesthesia

5. Which of the following responses is most appropriate after rapid tissue swelling is noticed after a PSA block?
   a. Get an ice pack and then place pressure on the area with the ice pack
   b. Place pressure on the area for 10 minutes and then continue working
   c. Place pressure on the area while someone else looks for ice, terminate procedure
   d. Reassure the patient and continue with planned therapy once numb

6. Of the following possible adverse reactions, which *one* occurs most frequently?
   a. Allergy
   b. Idiosyncratic response
   c. Overdose

7. Considering all of the following measures for preventing overdose, which *one* is most important?
   a. Calculating doses
   b. Slow administration
   c. Aspiration
   d. Reassuring patients

REFERENCES

Abdel-Galil, K., Anand, R., Pratt, C., Oeppen, B., & Brennan, P. (2005). Trismus: An unconventional approach to treatment. *British Journal of Oral and Maxillofacial Surgery, 45*(4), 339–340.

Abu-Laban, R. B., Zed, P. J., Purssell, R. A., & Evans, K. G. (2003, January). Severe methemoglobinemia from topical anesthetic spray: Case report, discussion and qualitative systematic review. *Canadian Journal of Emergency Medicine, 3*(1).

Aldons, J. A. (1968). Needle deflection: A factor in the administration of local anaesthetics. *Journal of the American Dental Association, 77,* 602–604.

Bedrock, R. D., Skigen, A., & Dolwick, M. F. (1999). Retrieval of a broken needle in the pterygomandibular space. *Journal of the American Dental Association, 130*(5), 685–687.

Benoit, P. W., Yagiela, J. A., & Fort, N. F. (1980). Pharmacologic correlation between local anesthetic induced myotoxicity and disturbances of intracellular calcium distribution. *Toxicology and Applied Pharmacology, 52*(2), 187–198.

Bhatia, S., & Bounds, G. A. (1998). A broken needle in the pterygomandibular space: Report of a case and review of the literature. *Dental Update, 25*, 35–37.

Blanton, P. L., & Jeske, A. H. (2003). Avoiding complications in local anesthesia induction: anatomical considerations. *Journal of the American Dental Association, 134*(7), 888–893.

Centers for Disease Control and Prevention. (1994, September 9). Prilocaine-induced methemoglobinemia—Wisconsin, 1993. *Morbidity and Mortality Weekly Report, 43*(35), 655–657.

Chen, D. W., & Horowitz, S. H. (2006). Inferior alveolar and lingual nerve injuries during routine dental anesthesia: Two case reports and a review of the literature. *Journal of Neuropathic Pain & Symptom Palliation, 1*(3), 51–56.

Cox, B., Durieux, M. E., & Marcus, M. A. E. (2003). Toxicity of local anesthetics. *Best Practice and Research Clinical Anaesthesiology, 17*(1), 111–136.

Crean, S. J., & Powis, A. (1999). Neurological complications of local anaesthetics in dentistry. *Dental Update, 26*(8), 344–349.

Daniel, S. J., Harfst, S. A. C., & Wilder, R. (2007) *Mosby's dental hygiene: Concepts, cases, and competencies* (2nd ed., Chapter 41). St. Louis: Mosby.

Danish Medicines Agency: Adverse reactions from anaesthetics containing articaine (Septonest®, Septocaine®, Ubistesin®, Ubestesin Forte®). 2006 update of the 2005 announcement. http://www.dkma.dk/1024/visUKLSArtikel.asp?artikelID =8701\. Accessed November 26, 2008.

Dorland's Illustrated Medical Dictionary 31st edition 2009. Philadelphia: Saunders.

Dower, J. S. (2007). Letter to the American Dental Association: Anesthetic study questioned. *Journal of the American Dental Association, 138*(6), 708–709.

Ethunandan, M., Tran, A. L., Anand, R., Bowden, J., Seal, M. T., & Brennan, P. A. (2007). Needle breakage following inferior alveolar nerve block: Implications and management. *British Dental Journal, 202*(7), 395–397.

FDA Modernization Act of 1997. Available at http://www.fda.gov/fdac/features/2000/400_compound.html. Accessed March 15, 2007.

FDA Patient Safety News. (2006, April). Advisory on benzocaine sprays and methemoglobinemia. Show #50. Available at http://www.accessdata.fda.gov/scripts/cdrh/cfdocs/psn/printer.cfm?id=418. Accessed March 15, 2007.

Foxall, G., McCahon, R., Lamb, J., Hardman, J. G., & Bedforth, N. M. (2007). Levobupivacaine-induced seizures and cardiovascular collapse treated with Intralipid®. *Anesthesia, 62*(5), 516–518.

Haas, D. A. (1998). Localized complications from local anesthesia. *Journal of the California Dental Association, 26*, 677–682.

Haas, D. A., & Lennon, D. (1995). A 21 year retrospective study of reports of paresthesia following local anesthetic administration. *Journal of the Canadian Dental Association, 61*(4), 319–320, 323–326, 329–330.

Harn, S. D., & Durham, T. M. (1990). Incidence of lingual trauma and postinjection complications in conventional mandibular block anesthesia. *Journal of the American Dental Association, 121*(4), 519–523.

Hawkins, M. (2006, October 16). *Local anesthesia: Technique and pharmacology, problems and solutions.* ADA Annual Session. Las Vegas, NV.

Hersh, E. V., Moore, P. A., Papas, A. S., Goodson, J. M., Navalta, L. A., Rogy, S., Rutherford, B., Yagiela, J. A. and the Soft Tissue Anesthesia Recovery Group (2008). Reversal of soft-tissue local anesthesia with phentolamine mesylate in adolescents and adults. *Journal of the American Dental Association, 139*(8), 1080–1093.

Horlocker, T. T., & Wedel, D. J. (2002). Local anesthetic toxicity—Does product labeling reflect actual risk? *Regional Anesthesia and Pain Medicine, 27*(6), 562–567.

Ibsen, O. A. C., & Phelan, J. A. (2004). Oral pathology for the dental hygienist (4th ed.). St. Louis: Saunders.

Institute for Safe Medical Practices. (2004, July 21). *Benzocaine spray products may cause life-threatening condition.* Available at www.ismp.org. Accessed March 15, 2007.

Institute for Safe Medical Practices. (2002, October 3). *Benzocaine-containing topical sprays and methemoglobinemia.* Available at www.ismp.org. Accessed March 15, 2007.

Jastak, J. T., Yagiela, J. A., & Donaldson, D. (1995). *Local anesthesia of the oral cavity.* Philadelphia: Saunders.

Kitagawa, N., Oda, M., & Totoki, T. (2004). Possible mechanism of irreversible nerve injury caused by local anesthetics: detergent properties of local anesthetics and membrane disruption. *Anesthesiology, 100*(4), 962–967.

Koizumi, Y., Matsumoto, M., Yamashita, A., Tsuruta, S., Ohtake, T., & Sakabe, T. (2006). The effects of an AMPA receptor antagonist on the neurotoxicity of tetracaine intrathecally administered in rabbits. *Anesthesia & Analgesia, 102*(3), 930–936.

Levsky, M. E., & Miller, M. A. (2005). Cardiovascular collapse from low dose bupivacaine. *Canadian Journal of Clinical Pharmacology, 12*(3), 240–245.

Little, J. W., Falace, D. A., Miller, C. S., & Rhodus, N. L. (2008). *Dental management of the medically compromised patient.* St. Louis: Mosby Elsevier.

Lustig, J. P., & Zusman, S. P. (1999). Immediate complications of local anesthetic administered to 1007 consecutive patients. *Journal of the American Dental Association, 130*(4), 496–499.

Malamed, S. F. (2004). *Handbook of local anesthesia* (5th ed.). St. Louis: Elsevier Mosby.

Malamed, S. F., Gagnon, S., & Leblanc, D. (2001). Articaine hydrochloride: A study of the safety of a new amide local anesthetic. *Journal of the American Dental Association, 132,* 177–185.

Marks, R. B., Carlton, D. M., & McDonald, S. (1984). Management of a broken needle in the pterygomandibular space: report of a case. *Journal of the American Dental Association, 109*(2), 263–264.

Mulroy, M. F. (2002). Systemic toxicity and cardiotoxicity from local anesthetics: incidence and preventive measures. *Regional Anesthesia and Pain Medicine, 27*(6), 556–561.

NIH Task Force on Safer Childhood Vaccines (1998, January). Available at http://www.niaid.nih.gov/publications/vaccine/pdf/safevacc.pdf

NOAA National Severe Storms Laboratory. Available at http://www.nssl.noaa.gov/faq/faq_ltg.php

Norholt, S. E., Aagard, E., Svensson, P., & Sindet-Pedersen, S. (1998). Evaluation of trismus, bite force, and pressure algometry after third molar surgery: A placebo-controlled study of ibuprofen. Discussion. *Journal of Oral Maxillofacial Surgery, 56*(4), 420–427, 427–429.

Oertel, R., Rahn, R., & Kirch, W. (1997). Clinical pharmacokinetics of articaine. *Clinical Pharmacokinetics, 33*(6), 417–425.

Orr, D. L. (1983). The broken needle: Report of a case. *Journal of the American Dental Association, 107*(4), 603–604.

Park, C. J., Park, S. A., Yoon, T. G., Lee, S. J., Yum, K. W., & Kim, H. J. (2005). Bupivacaine induces apoptosis via ROS in the Schwann cell line. *Journal of Dental Research, 84*(9), 852–857.

Paxton, M., Hadley, J. N., Hadley, M. N., Edwards, R. C., & Harrison, S. J. (1994). Chorda tympani nerve injury following inferior alveolar injection: A review of two cases. *Journal of the American Dental Association, 125*(7), 103–106.

Pickett, F. A., & Terezhalmy, G. T. (2006). *Dental drug reference with clinical applications.* Baltimore: Lippincott Williams & Wilkins.

Pogrel, G. M., Bryan, J., & Regezi, J. (1995). Nerve damage associated with inferior alveolar dental blocks. *Journal of the American Dental Association, 126*(8), 1150–1155.

Pogrel, M. A., Schmidt, B. L., Sambajon, V., & Jordan, R. C. K. (2003). Lingual nerve damage due to inferior alveolar nerve blocks: A possible explanation. *Journal of the American Dental Association, 134*(2), 195–199.

Pogrel, M. A., & Thamby, S. (2000). Permanent nerve involvement resulting from inferior alveolar nerve blocks *Journal of the American Dental Association, 131*(7), 901–907.

Rayan, G. M., Pitha, J. V., Wisdom, P., Brentlinger, A., & Kopta, J. A. (1988). Histologic and electrophysiologic changes following subepineural hematoma induction in rat sciatic nerve. *Clinical Orthopaedics and Related Research, 229,* 257–264.

Rosenblatt, M. A., Abel, M., Fischer, G. W., Itzkovich, C. J., & Eisenkraft, J. B. (2006). Successful use of a 20% lipid emulsion to resuscitate a patient after a presumed bupivacaine-related cardiac arrest. *Anesthesiology, 105,* 217–218.

Smith, A. J., Cameron, S. O., Bagg, J., & Kennedy, D. (2001). Management of needlesticks in general dental practice. *British Dental Journal, 190*(12), 645–650.

Smith, M. H., & Lung, K. E. (2006). Nerve injuries after dental injections: A review of the literature. *Journal of the Canadian Dental Association, 76*(6), 559–564.

Stacy, G. C., & Hajjar, G. (1994). Barbed needle and inexplicable paresthesias and trimus after dental regional anaesthesia. *Oral Surgery Oral Medicine Oral Pathology, 77*(6), 585–588.

Tavares, M., Goodson, J. M., Studen-Pavlovich, D., Yagiela, J. A., Navalta, L. A., Rogy, S., Rutherford, B., Gordon, S., Papas, A. S., and Soft-Tissue Anesthesia Reversal Group (2008). Reversal of soft-tissue local anesthesia with phentolamine mesylate in pediatric patients. *Journal of the American Dental Association, 139*(8), 1095–1104.

Tetzlaff, J. E. (2000). *Clinical pharmacology of local anesthetics.* Boston: Butterworth-Heineman.

Trager, K. A. (1979). Hematoma following inferior alveolar injection: a possible cause for anesthesia failure. *Journal of the American Dental Society of Anesthesia, 26*(5), 122–123.

Tucker, M. E. (2007). Lidocaine contact allergy increasing with topical use. *ACEP News, 26*(5), 24.

Weinberg, G. L., VadeBoncouer, T., Ramaraju, G. A., Garcia-Amaro, M. F., & Cwik, M. J. (1998). Pretreatment of resuscitation with a lipid infusion shifts the dose-response to bupivacaine-induced asystole in rats. *Anesthesia, 88*(4), 1071–1075.

Xylocaine, 2%, 1:100,000 epinephrine: Product monograph 17402 (Rev. 2004, February). Available at AstraZeneca LP for Dentsply Pharmaceutical, York, PA.

Zelter, R., Cohen, C., & Casap, N. (2002). The implications of a broken needle in the pterygomandibular space: clinical guidelines for prevention and retrieval. *Pediatric Dentistry, 24,* 153–156.

Section V

Special Considerations for Local Anesthesia

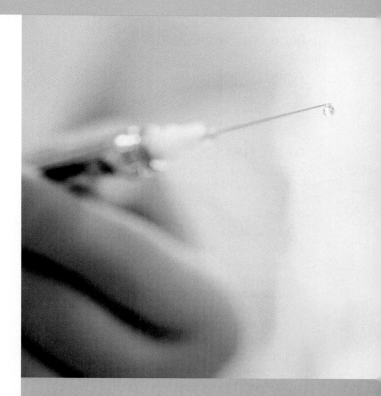

Chapter 18

Insights for the Fearful Patient

Marilynn Rothen, RDH, BS

Agnes Spadafora, RDH, BS

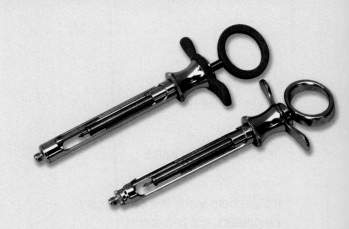

OBJECTIVES

- Define and discuss the key terms in this chapter.
- Define and differentiate between the terms *fear,* *anxiety,* and *phobia.*
- Understand the etiology and development of fear as it relates to pain and pain management.
- Understand the primary sources for recognizing and assessing fears.
- Understand and discuss the fundamental concepts of treatment for fearful and anxious patients.
- Be able to relate a patient's sense of control to his or her experienced level of fear or anxiety.
- Explain four useful types of control for anxious patients receiving injections.
- Be familiar with physical relaxation and coping skills, including deep breathing and muscle relaxation.
- Be able to teach physical relaxation and coping skills to patients.
- Be able to apply appropriate fear management strategies and coping skills to the administration of local anesthetics.
- Understand and be prepared to explain the benefit of rehearsals, time structuring, and biofeedback to fearful patients.
- Describe benefits and techniques for testing local anesthetic effectiveness.
- List and describe the steps involved in the protocol for anesthetic testing.

KEY TERMS

anxiety **370**
behavioral and physiological indicators of fear **371**
behavioral control **373**
biofeedback **375**
cognitive control **372**
control **372**
deep breathing **373**
electric pulp tester (EPT) **375**
fear **370**
focusing attention **372**
graduated exposure **374**
guided imagery **372**

informational control **372**
pain **370**
pain management **370**
phobia **370**
positive coping statement **372**
progressive muscle relaxation (PMR) **374**
rehearsals **374**
retrospective control **373**
self-report **371**
systemic desensitization **374**
time structuring **375**

CASE STUDY: Lydia O'Kaine

Mrs. Lydia O'Kaine, a 33-year-old female, presented for dental care with a chief complaint of unhappiness over the esthetics of tooth #7. The initial interview revealed that she had not seen a dentist in six years. Her medical history was non-contributory except for smoking one pack of cigarettes per day for fifteen years. Mrs. O'Kaine indicated that she had tried to quit several times, but found the habit "relaxing and enjoyable."

At the initial exam, information about her last dental visit was obtained. Lydia reported that the lower right molars "had cavities and needed treatment" and that the clinician had to stop treatment several times to give her more anesthetic. She also stated that she "never really felt numb," but she was able to "tough it out" and the treatment was completed. The additional injections were very difficult for her because "they burned." Lydia stated she is now quite apprehensive about painful injections and additionally she is concerned about the effectiveness of the anesthetic. Lydia indicated that prior to her last experience she had not received regular dental care, but had not had problems with injections or anesthesia. After this experience Lydia did not return to have tooth #7 treated, and the cavity is now visible but asymptomatic.

Findings at the initial exam included: caries in numbers #7, #8, and #13, and a missing restoration in #31. During her periodontal exam, chronic gingivitis was apparent in the maxillary anterior region. Due to tissue sensitivity, full mouth probing was not completed. Isolated probing revealed 5 to 6 mm pocket depths in the maxillary and mandibular molars. Moderate supragingival calculus was present on the lingual of the lower anteriors. The proposed treatment plan included: four quadrants of scaling and rootplaning with anesthesia, oral hygiene instructions, fluoride therapy and prescriptions, and restoration of numbers #7, #8, #13, and #31.

INTRODUCTION

This chapter is targeted to the discussion of local anesthesia for what are known as *fears patients*. Despite the emphasis on the management of exceptional fear, there are many discussions within this chapter that apply when anesthetizing all patients. Fear and anxiety are by no means unique to this segment of the dental patient population, especially when needles and drugs are involved. As reported in the literature, approximately 40 percent of patients presenting for dental care experience some level of anxiety related to appointments while another 12 to 20 percent are extremely anxious or fearful (De Jongh, Muris, Schoenmakers, & Ter Horst, 1995; Sohn & Ismail, 2005). Anxiety and fear produce both psychological and physiological changes that can affect the ability to receive local anesthetics and their effectiveness once received. When asked to rank the most fearful elements of dentistry, patients consistently place *needles* at or near the top of surveys. It has been found that nearly one in twenty individuals *avoids* dentistry due to fear of injections (Milgrom, Coldwell, Getz, Weinstein, & Ramsay, 1997; Milgrom, Fiset, Melnick, & Weinstein, 1988).

Local anesthetic failures can magnify the problem. Failure rates were demonstrated to be as high as 14 percent during dental appointments in one report (Weinstein, Milgrom, Kaufman, Fiset, & Ramsay, 1985). More than 2 percent of the patients involved were unable to complete treatment due to the inadequacy of the anesthesia (Weinstein et al., 1985). These figures compare closely with the results of a 1984 survey of dentists which revealed difficulties administering adequate anesthesia in approximately 13 percent of patients over a five day period (Kaufman, Weinstein, & Milgrom, 1984). The actual percentage of the failures with at least a partial psychological etiology is unknown but there is reason to suspect that there is at least some psychological influence on the effectiveness of local anesthetic drugs. The manner in which dental fear and anxiety can contribute to local anesthesia failure will be clarified in this chapter. As one clinician commented, "Why is it that I always seem to miss the blocks on my most anxious patients?"

Some clinicians emphasize the benefits of oral health when attempting to motivate fearful patients. Many of these patients are aware of the benefits of oral health, but the prospect of good oral health, alone, is not sufficient to enable them to tolerate treatment. This chapter will focus on strategies and skills which lower psychological barriers to treatment. A principle known as *treat the fear first,* developed and elaborated by Milgrom, Weinstein, and Heaton in their text, *Treating Fearful Dental Patients: A Patient Management Handbook,* will be highlighted.

TERMINOLOGY AND FEAR DEVELOPMENT

The terms *fear, anxiety,* and *phobia* are often used interchangeably. In order to better understand the differences between these terms, particularly as they are used in the dental fears literature, they will be defined as follows (Milgrom, Weinstein, & Heaton, 2009):

Fear is an emotional response to an immediate threat or danger. Reactions to perceived danger include: 1) unpleasant cognitions that something terrible will happen; 2) physiological changes (tachycardia, perspiration, nausea, hyperventilation); and 3) overt behaviors such as shaking, pacing, and rapid speech. This layered response is often referred to as *fight or flight.*

Anxiety is an emotional response to a threat or danger that is not immediately present or is unclear. Anxiety may lead to the same cognitive, physiological, and behavioral responses as fear. Anticipatory anxiety may occur hours or days before an actual dental appointment.

Phobia, as described in the American Psychiatric Association's *Diagnostic and Statistical Manual of Mental Disorders,* is a persistent, irrational fear of a specific object or situation that results in a compelling desire to either avoid the situation or to endure it with dread (American Psychiatric Association, 2000). Phobias can interfere with a person's ability to function. In dentistry, phobias are likely to interfere with the achievement of oral health, often resulting in pain and suffering when oral health is neglected.

The terms *strategy, skill, response,* and *reaction* may be helpful for clinicians when presenting methods for modifying behaviors in the dental environment. The following definitions will apply to these terms (*The American Heritage Dictionary*® *of the English Language [American Heritage Dictionary],* 2000):

Strategy is defined as a plan of action intended to accomplish a specific goal.

Skill refers to a proficiency acquired or developed through training or experience.

Response refers to a reply, an answer, or a reaction to a specific stimulus.

Reaction is a response to a stimulus.

Local anesthetic drugs are used in dentistry to control and manage pain. Unfortunately, the very act of administering local anesthetics is often perceived as too painful to endure by patients who are excessively fearful of injections. **Pain management** for these individuals entails their ability to cope with and tolerate treatment, in addition to the proper administration of local anesthetic.

Before discussing pain management in these individuals, it is important to define the term *pain.* As a positive experience, pain has a primary benefit of alerting an individual to injury. Most definitions, and this discussion, focus on the overwhelmingly negative aspects of pain, which are well-articulated in the following definition provided by the International Association for the Study of Pain (IASP):

> **Pain:** An unpleasant sensory and emotional experience associated with actual or potential tissue damage, or described in terms of such damage. Pain is always subjective. Each individual learns the application of the word through experiences related to injury in early life. It is unquestionably a sensation in a part or parts of the body, but it is also always unpleasant and therefore also an emotional experience. Many people report pain in the absence of tissue damage or any likely pathophysiological cause; usually this happens for psychological reasons. There is usually no way to distinguish their experience from that due to tissue damage if we take the subjective report. If they regard their experience as pain and if they report it in the same way as pain caused by tissue damage, it should be accepted as pain. This definition avoids tying pain to the stimuli (IASP, 1994).

For additional information on this topic see Chapter 2, "Fundamentals of Pain Management."

The Development of Fear

Fear of dentistry is complex (Milgrom et al., 2009). The most common cause has been termed a *direct negative experience,* usually of pain or fright, to a perceived threat of harm. This experience may originate in a negative personal interaction with a clinician. The experience of pain, alone, does not necessarily lead to exceptional fear and avoidance of dentistry. The manner in which a clinician manages a patient's emotional reaction to pain (or the anticipation of pain) is a more important determinant of whether or not dental fear develops.

The IASP's definition of pain describes the experience as occurring with or without tissue damage. In the absence of injury, the causes of pain can be hidden from clinicians. In the absence of obvious injury, it is the patient, alone, who determines whether or not pain has been experienced. This self-determination can lead to emotional reactions arising from unpleasant experiences perceived by patients. The response of clinicians and their behavior in the face of these reactions can be critical. If clinicians fail to understand or respond to patient concerns or if they belittle their reactions, fear is a likely result. This is especially true when a patient has no ability to control stressful and fearful situations. Clinicians who are empathetic, on the other hand, can respond in ways that inhibit the development of fear.

RECOGNIZING FEAR AND ANXIETY

Studies have demonstrated that even dental personnel who recognize fear and anxiety in patients often do not address the problem in order to avoid making matters worse (Corah, O'Shea, & Ayer, 1985). Prior to administering anesthetics, it is important to assess a patient's past experiences. This will provide information about their expectations and about the possibility of fear and anxiety affecting the administration.

There are three primary sources for assessing patient anxiety and fear prior to and during stressful dental experiences according to Milgrom, Weinstein, and Heaton: self-report; behavioral indicators; and, physiological indicators (Milgrom et al., 2009).

Self-report is the principal method for obtaining information about a patient. It allows patients to express both negative and positive aspects regarding past dental experiences. Information may be obtained in one-on-one interviews or by using simple questionnaires that may include some of the following: How long has it been since your last dental visit? What kind of treatment did you receive? How did it go? Are there any concerns about receiving injections? Is there anything that you would like to do or not do during today's appointment? What will make receiving an injection easier for you?

Behavioral indicators of fear include overt signs such as pacing the waiting room, fidgeting, wringing hands, or gripping the arms of chairs until knuckles turn pale ("white knuckles"). Patients may talk incessantly in order to avoid dental treatment. Signs of fear in the operatory also include opposite responses such as quiet, nonresponsive postures.

Physiological indicators of fear include perspiration, changes in respiration, shallow breathing, and increased heart rate and blood pressure. Patients also frequently hold their breath during injections. Unfortunately, the increased tension caused by holding one's breath actually lowers pain tolerance. Sensitivity generally increases and procedures are commonly more uncomfortable throughout. The perception of increased patient sensitivity and discomfort could encourage clinicians to administer anesthetics more rapidly (*to get it over with*), which can cause even greater discomfort.

FOUNDATIONS OF TREATMENT

There are three concepts to consider when developing strategies for treating fearful patients: the patient–clinician relationship; the patient's sense of control over a potentially threatening environment; and, the patient's ability to cope with a stressful situation. Interactions between clinicians and patients take place throughout the process of providing dental care. Every aspect of treatment takes place within the framework of those interactions. A patient's sense of control and the ability to cope are essential to tolerating dental procedures that are perceived as aversive, such as injections. Without control and coping skills, fearful patients may worry that experiences will surpass the limits of their endurance.

Trust in the Patient–Clinician Relationship

Once a fearful patient has been identified, building a trusting relationship is critical to successful treatment. Dentistry is a social interaction and research has shown that a clinician's personal attributes and professional behaviors impact patients' attitudes toward dentistry (Corah, O'Shea, & Bissell, 1985). Dental fear can develop from painful and frightening experiences, especially when clinicians are perceived as unaware of or unconcerned with physical and emotional suffering. Since one of the primary means by which patients are able to assess clinician competence is through the strength of their interpersonal behavior, it is important for clinicians to set the stage early for positive perceptions.

Interpersonal rapport, open two-way communication, empathy, and professional competence are important to establishing trust. Patients should be encouraged to explain their fears and concerns, to express likes and dislikes, and to ask questions. Fearful patients frequently need help learning to be assertive and to express their needs. Good communication is an important means for fearful patients to begin to exercise control over what is perceived as a potentially threatening situation.

Enhancing a Sense of Control

Control has been defined as "the belief that one has at one's disposal a response that can influence the aversiveness of an event" (Thompson, 1981). An important tenet of psychology recognizes that when an individual perceives a situation as harmful or threatening over which he or she has little control, fear increases. When an individual believes there is at least some control over the stressful situation, both fear and the need to exercise control decrease. An important corollary to this tenet is that fearful patients have low pain tolerances. It is important to provide patients with a means of control over situations in order to decrease fear and increase pain tolerance.

Thompson has identified four methods for providing patients with control: informational; cognitive; behavioral; and, retrospective (Thompson, 1981). Milgrom et al. have elaborated on the use of these four types of control in the dental situation, as well (Milgrom et al., 2009).

Informational control communicates to the patient what to expect of an imminent aversive procedure. The information is best delivered as a simple description immediately before treatment with the emphasis on the sensations that the patient will experience. This helps fearful patients, especially those who have avoided dentistry for a long time, to know what to expect, to understand that any sensations they experience are normal, and to avoid being alarmed by them. In addition, prior knowledge of aversive events and how long the events will last helps fearful patients tolerate them. Without this information, patients may remain vigilant and tense, alert to the next painful occurrence.

It is helpful to furnish patients with the following: simple descriptions of the steps involved in procedures; sensations they can expect; estimates of the time allowed for each step; and, suggestions as to ways in which they can participate in the process or at least speed it along. Furnished rationale should be limited to benefits of procedures rather than blow-by-blow descriptions; for example, the slow delivery of anesthetics is explained as having a motive of "increased comfort" and rubber dams are placed to "improve safety." Some fearful patients may benefit from more detailed descriptions, especially if they need reassurance of clinician competence. All pretreatment discussions should be prefaced by determinations of how much each patient wishes to know.

Cognitive control involves mental maneuvers through which patients can lessen their fearful, negative thoughts and their reactions to these thoughts. It is sometimes referred to as relaxing the mind and includes distraction, guided imagery, focusing attention, and positive coping statements. Distraction strategies are familiar to most and are the easiest to use. Patients may watch DVDs, or listen to CDs or the clinician's conversation. Distraction has its limitations and does not work well for more than the mildly anxious patient due to the passive nature of the patient's role. Highly fearful patients need stronger interventions to keep "worst-case scenarios" from replaying in their heads.

Guided imagery provides patients with active roles and greater control over recurring negative thoughts by replacing them with mental images of pleasant scenes or scenarios. Clinicians can encourage patients to engage as many senses and memories as possible while speaking in slow, relaxed voices. If patients choose to imagine beach scenes, for example, clinicians may ask patients if they can feel the warm breezes, hear the palm leaves rustling, smell the tropical flowers, and see the sunlight sparkling on the waves.

Focusing attention is a technique used to prevent what are known as anticipatory anxieties or thoughts of what might happen during treatment. Through this technique, clinicians are able to redirect patient attention to the experience of the moment by checking in frequently and providing rest breaks. Questions such as, "How is it going right now?" and "Is anything hurting you?" can be helpful. Fearful patients are often so worried about what might happen or what has happened in the past that they have a hard time recognizing that they are "okay" in the present. Of equal importance, they might overlook the difference between the present experience and past experiences.

Positive coping statements are statements or phrases that replace negative thoughts, such as, "This is awful," "I don't like this," "I wish I were somewhere else!" Patients are coached prior to treatment to select phrases that are positively worded and relevant. They repeat these phrases silently throughout procedures, whenever they become anxious or to prevent the resurgence of negative thoughts. These phrases do not have to be complex. Simple affirmations such as, "I can do this," "This isn't so bad," "I will make it ," or "I'm a capable person, I can get through this" can be very effective at competing with negative thoughts.

Behavioral control allows patients to take actions to lessen, shorten, or terminate stressful situations. One of the most familiar of these is the use of a hand signal to stop procedures. Fearful patients should be given permission to discontinue procedures for any reason, including escalating anxiety. The same signal can be used to indicate a willingness to proceed with treatment once the patient is ready to resume. In this way, patients remain in complete control of procedural progress. It is important to acknowledge their control by responding to their signals. Even a single failure to respond to a signal can completely negate its benefit, both at the time and in the future.

Planned rest breaks can also be beneficial for fearful patients. Even when patients indicate they would like to push on and "get done," it is important to give breaks in order to allow them to "catch their breath" before proceeding.

Retrospective control, *or debriefing* (introduced in Chapter 11, "Fundamentals for Administration of Local Anesthetic Agents"), is the posttreatment discussion of the appointment experience. Fearful patients may have had a difficult time getting through appointments. They might be distraught and apprehensive after injections. They might have interrupted the injection or might not have been willing to proceed in the first place. Rather than analyzing *failure,* an inability to proceed can be viewed as an opportunity to help patients *reinterpret* events and to note progress to date. For example, patients who are able to receive injections despite emotional upset should be praised for completing procedures that are difficult for them. Patients who signal clinicians to stop mid-injection, can receive positive reinforcement for the assertiveness they have gained in learning to control the situation and put their needs above all. Patients who were unable to proceed at all can receive positive reinforcement for their willingness to initiate the process.

Debriefing is also an opportunity to solicit feedback from patients regarding the aspects of appointments that were helpful and those that were not.

Patient Strategies and Coping Skills

When working with patients who are fearful and who find particular aspects of dentistry threatening, it is helpful to make them *see* the clinician as one who is interested in making the experience as comfortable and pain free as possible. It should be emphasized that pain control is most effective and easiest to achieve in relaxed patients. Patients benefit from learning skills and strategies to help them relax physically and mentally in order to increase their tolerance for dentistry (Bobey & Davidson, 1970).

Relaxation: Role and Function

It is useful to determine whether or not patients have any previous experience with relaxation training or coping skills and whether or not they have been used successfully in other situations. These skills can be transferred to the dental environment with a little practice. If the patient has not previously used any relaxation strategies, it is important to emphasize that relaxation is a *learned skill* and that effectiveness increases with practice. It can be helpful to explain the role and function of relaxation to the patient. Its use in the dental environment is based on the principle that it is impossible to be physically relaxed and psychologically anxious at the same time (Jacobson, 1938). The questions in Box 18–1 may be used to survey patient relaxation skills. If the patient has no previous experience with relaxation techniques, and does not know how to relax, the clinician will need to teach the appropriate skills for the patient to cope with treatment.

Deep breathing is a familiar relaxation technique that can be taught by means of a simple demonstration. Patients can actively reduce their levels of fear and anxiety using this technique. At the same time, it helps to prevent counterproductive breathing, which can lead to hyperventilation, dizziness, and loss of control.

Box 18–1   *Patient Relaxation Skill Determination*

- Do you find it difficult to relax in the dental chair?
- Do you find yourself tensed up and stiff during certain dental procedures?
- If so, which specific procedures?
- Do you have a problem with gagging while taking x-rays or other procedures?
- Do you find it difficult to breathe or swallow during an injection or other dental treatment?
- Is there anything you can do to help yourself relax in the dental chair?

The technique is introduced by example, encouraging patients to learn without "feeling silly," as follows:

1. inhale slowly and deeply to the count of 5, filling the lungs with air
2. hold the breath for one second
3. slowly exhale to the count of 5, feeling the tension release while sinking into the dental chair.

It is helpful to count aloud on each inhale and exhale. A gentle hand on the patient's shoulder, along with calming tones, can help to regulate the timing of the breaths to make sure they are not too rapid or shallow. A slight downward hand movement on the shoulder should coincide with each exhalation. This continues until the patient is relaxed and ready to receive the injection. Once the injection begins, the clinician coaches the patient to breathe deeply and slowly by counting aloud as before.

Progressive Muscle Relaxation

Progressive muscle relaxation (PMR) is another coping skill that most patients can learn quickly and effectively (Jacobson, 1938). The body often responds to anxiety and stress by tensing muscles, which actually heightens anxiety. Muscle relaxation, on the other hand, reduces tension and competes with and blocks anxiety. "Toughing it out" is not an effective way to cope with anxiety and fear. Muscles that are tensed increase the likelihood of experiencing what is known as a *startle reaction*. Startle reactions can blur the difference between the anticipation of pain and the actual experience. The confusion that ensues can compromise patients' abilities to report pain accurately.

Muscle relaxation is learned by tensing and relaxing different muscle groups throughout the body. This not only helps relieve tension but allows patients to understand which areas are most tense. Clinicians can explain and demonstrate the following:

1. inhale and tense the leg muscles
2. exhale while releasing the leg tension
3. inhale and tense the arm and hand muscles
4. exhale and release the hand and arm tension, allowing them to go limp.

These steps can be repeated for the head, neck, and shoulders.

A second quick and useful method is to:

1. have the patient inhale deeply to the count of 5 and squeeze and tense all the body muscles
2. on the initiation of the exhale begin to release the tension in all the muscles as the patient sinks into the chair.

Deep breathing and muscle relaxation not only allow patients to have active roles during the administrations of local anesthetics, they also help to enhance cognitive control over negative thoughts. Patients can be encouraged to practice at home and to use the techniques in other stressful situations.

PRACTICAL APPLICATIONS

Rehearsals

After patients have been introduced to relaxation skills, **rehearsals** provide opportunities to practice the new skills while simulating the steps involved in actual dental procedures. Rehearsals allow patients to master control over anxiety-provoking situations while relieving everyone of the burden of having to accomplish any treatment. Deep breathing, muscle relaxation, and guided imagery can all be used by patients to calm themselves as aversive stimuli are progressively introduced, from least to most anxiety-producing. This process of decreasing fear and anxiety to stimuli in a step-by-step fashion is referred to as **systemic desensitization.**

A desensitization rehearsal for local anesthesia, for example, can begin with a patient practicing deep breathing. When calm, the clinician can place topical anesthetic. Reminding the patient to continue with the relaxation technique, the syringe can be introduced with the cap still covering the needle. The syringe is positioned in the patient's mouth and held there for the time it would take to complete the injection.

While continuing to remind the patient to breathe deeply, a cap-off rehearsal can be followed by the actual injection if the patient is willing to proceed. Alternatively, during a cap-off rehearsal, the patient uses a pre-arranged hand signal to indicate his or her willingness for the clinician to proceed with administering the actual injection. It should be remembered during this process that each successive step is increasingly challenging for the patient and an unwillingness to continue at any point should be greeted with acceptance and with praise of the progress made.

Treatment rehearsals are very similar to "tell-show-do" techniques used to introduce new procedures to young children. In both instances, the techniques allow what is known as **graduated exposure** in order to let anxious patients know what to expect and to help them determine when they are ready to proceed.

Rehearsals for some can be as simple as a onetime review of the steps involved in a procedure. For others, systematic desensitization of every step can be repeated until they are ready and willing to go on to the next (see the CARL program for desensitization of needle injection phobia described later in this chapter).

In an actual appointment using systematic desensitization, patients can visualize each fearful stimulus before being presented with it, while using the progressive relaxation technique. This approach allows patients to gain confidence in their ability to cope. If the technique starts at a manageable level and the steps are small enough, patients are much more likely to succeed. Extremely fearful patients may require multiple sessions before receiving injections. It is important to stop any time patients tire of the process. This will allow clinicians to recognize and praise the progress made without exhausting patients and perhaps causing them to lose their willingness to continue at a future time.

Time Structuring

When rehearsing local anesthetic procedures, it is useful to consider what is referred to as **time structuring.** This is a process whereby patients are informed of the time it will take to administer a particular injection. In this method, patients are continually apprised of injection progress by stating the injection is one-fourth complete, one-third complete, three-quarters complete, and finished. Many anxious patients find this helpful. This is also an appropriate time to remind fearful patients that one important reason for administering anesthetics slowly is out of concern for patient comfort.

Biofeedback

Biofeedback can be useful in addressing the physiological changes that occur during stressful situations, such as increases in heart rate. It has been used successfully in the past to modify these responses. Subjects have been able to lower their blood pressure by observing it on a monitor, for example, after having been given instructions to concentrate on lowering it, with no instructions on how to do so (Kristt & Engel, 1975).

A simple heart rate monitor can be used by patients to monitor their heart rate and anxiety. Patients may be entirely unaware of the effect of anxiety on their heart rates. The ability to visualize the effects of relaxation on their heart rates reinforces the effectiveness of coping mechanisms and their ability to compete with anxiety.

Testing the Effectiveness of Anesthesia

Patients may fear needles, the sensations of drugs as they are delivered into tissues, or inadequate anesthesia. Recalling from previous discussions that more than 14 percent of patients reported inadequate anesthesia during dental procedures and over 2 percent reported pain to the extent that they were unable to complete procedures, fear of inadequate anesthesia seems relatively pervasive.

The **electric** or **electronic pulp tester (EPT)** may be useful much of the time but is particularly useful when patients have reported a history of inadequate anesthesia. See Figure 18–1 ■. The EPT is designed to test the vitality of teeth by using an electric current. It is a self-contained, battery-powered unit with a digital readout scale that registers from 0 to 80, with 80 indicating a complete lack of vitality. The EPT consists of a wand into which a sterilized tip is inserted and a ground lead, typically attached to the wand with what is called a lip clip. Rather than place the clip on the patient's lip, it is equally effective and increases the patient's sense of control, when the patient is asked to hold the clip firmly between two fingers (see Figure 18–1). The device is activated when the tip is placed on a nonrestored, dried area of a tooth after having been coated sparingly with toothpaste (a conducting medium). Electricity flows to the tooth when the circuit has been completed. A light

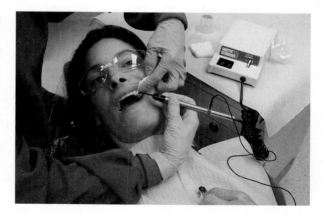

■ **FIGURE 18–1** Testing for Adequate Anesthesia. Electric pulp testing devices can be a reliable method to reassure patients that adequate anesthesia has been established prior to initiating treatment.
Source: Courtesy of Marilynn Rothen, RDH.

on the wand indicates that a good contact has been established. The level of stimulus gradually increases automatically starting at 0 and continuing to 80. If a reading of 80 is registered and unnoticed by the patient, the anesthesia is presumed to be profound.

The procedure that incorporates EPTs is a simple one. First, explain the function and purpose of the EPT to the patient. It is important for patients to understand that they have complete control over the process because they can drop the clip at any time, which immediately stops the flow of electricity. After administering the anesthetic and waiting an appropriate period for its onset, test for effectiveness with the EPT. The expected sensation can be described in advance as a glowing, tingling, warm, cold, or pulsating feeling. It is best to avoid the word "painful" when describing the sensation. It is also useful to remind patients that they will feel nothing if the tooth is profoundly anesthetized. It can be helpful to demonstrate the EPT on a nonanesthetized contralateral tooth as a basis for confirming that the anesthetized tooth is truly anesthetized.

If the EPT confirms that the tooth is not profoundly anesthetized, additional anesthetic can be administered using the same technique or a different or supplemental technique. The tooth is then retested with the EPT and the process is repeated until there is no response to a reading of 80 on the device. This can be very reassuring to patients. It is not unusual for anxious patients to request the EPT prior to every treatment involving the administration of anesthetic.

When an EPT is not available, an ultrasonic device or other instrument may be used. The instrument or device selected should be used along with a time structuring technique in order to assure the patient of profound anesthesia. It is explained to the patient that the instrument will touch the tooth to the count of 1 and will be removed, for feedback. Feedback from patients should differentiate between the sensations of sharp and painful versus vibration and awareness. If the patient remains comfortable to the count of 1, the protocol should be repeated to the count of 2, then to the count of 5. After reaching 5, treatment may begin. Some very anxious patients may request that the counting continue during treatment. They may consider the count of 5 to be the limit of their tolerance and the break at each count of 5 allows tension to subside while patients "catch their breath." This process assures them that they have a safe stopping point in case they begin to feel pain.

Protocol for Managing Anesthetic Failure

Despite the use of the EPT, strategies to reduce fear and anxiety, and carefully planned injection techniques, patients may not be adequately anesthetized on occasion. If this occurs, subsequent discussions should focus on solutions to the problem rather than on emotional reactions. The discussion should begin with reassurance that no treatment will begin until profound anesthesia has been achieved and should continue with reassurance that this has happened before and was successfully addressed. It is further emphasized that providing profound anesthesia is the clinician's responsibility and any of a variety of factors can affect the success at a particular day and time.

When encountering this problem, clinicians should consider whether or not fear has been adequately addressed. Since fear and lack of control can lower a patient's pain tolerance, sensitivity can actually increase if past experiences were not adequately addressed. According to Milgrom et al., "Fear can lead to inadequate anesthesia and inadequate anesthesia during treatment can increase fear" (Milgrom et al., 2009). Following fear reassessment (patient's sense of control and use of relaxation techniques) and reassurances that no treatment will begin until profound anesthesia has been confirmed, the patient is guided through the process of developing realistic expectations about the sensations that will be experienced even when anesthetized. For example, pressure and awareness (of an instrument), although provoking feedback to the brain, are expected sensations and are not considered painful stimuli by most. Fear of being hurt will lead the patient to believe that any sensation is the precursor to pain. The patient needs guidance in developing the ability to report pain accurately by distinguishing between the anticipation of pain, sensations of instrument touch, and actual pain.

Factors that can preclude the development of profound anesthesia include infection in the area to be anesthetized, excessive fatigue or physical pain elsewhere in the body, as well as the factors discussed in Chapter 16, "Troubleshooting Inadequate Anesthesia," which also apply to fearful individuals. Patients in pain, regardless of the nature of the pain, are more sensitized to new stimuli despite taking analgesics to treat the pain. The fatigue of bearing other pain can also decrease a patient's ability to cope with difficult situations.

When encountering inadequate anesthesia, it is best to reassess the technique. Is there anatomical variation and was it appropriately addressed? Was an adequate volume of anesthetic used? Were variations in patient response taken into consideration when assessing appropriate dosing? Would other techniques be helpful at this point such as Gow-Gates nerve blocks, higher penetration sites for IA blocks, intraosseous techniques, or PDL injections? Another factor when assessing for adequate anesthesia is whether or not to use a vasoconstrictor. Controlling fear and anxiety with adequate anesthesia is made easier with the use of vasoconstrictors. Not only is diffusion of local anesthetic solution to centrally located pulpal fibers more likely when vasoconstrictors are used (they keep local anesthetics in the area of the nerve longer and have even been demonstrated to have some anesthetic properties) but the anesthesia is more durable and doesn't wear off as quickly. Vasoconstrictors, when appropriate, also help to maintain blood pressures within healthy ranges by increasing the effectiveness of pain control (decreasing endogenous epinephrine). Conversely, using anesthetics without vasoconstrictors may convince fearful patients that pain might be expected at future appointments if the anesthesia was not effective or wore off before the end of treatment. In addition to the possibility of tachyphylaxis, future anesthesia may be ineffective because patients will no longer remain desensitized to all the stimuli.

A final approach might be to schedule an appointment with the exclusive goal of determining which techniques will provide adequate anesthesia for the challenging area, known as an anesthetic testing protocol. No treatment is scheduled. Without the pressure to "get numb" for treatment many patients are better able to manage their anxiety, decreasing their sensitivity to stimuli and increasing the potential for anesthesia effectiveness. The anesthetic testing protocol appointment may use any and all relevant techniques in order to determine which techniques provide the most effective anesthesia.

Post-op Anesthetic Recovery

In addition to expectations for injections and treatment, dental fears patients need realistic expectations for postoperative periods. Soreness is not unusual, especially after generous amounts of anesthesia have been administered and where more than one technique was used. It is important for these patients to be prepared in advance with recommendations for handling pain from routine trauma and inflammation, including taking anti-inflammatory medications prior to the recovery of the tissues from anesthesia. In receiving the recommendation

that they take these medications while the anesthetics are still in effect, patients can understand that postoperative sensations are normal and expected.

Nitrous Oxide for Anxiety Control During Dental Injections

Nitrous oxide sedation is sometimes used for fearful and anxious patients. It is not the intent of this chapter to discuss the details of the use of nitrous oxide sedation except to say that it is not a substitute for good behavioral management skills when working with fearful patients. Introducing nitrous oxide when an appointment is not going well is unlikely to result in success. It is far better to introduce nitrous oxide when patients have time to become accustomed to its sensations and when it can be titrated to comfortable levels prior to commencing treatment. Patients who demand high levels of control over situations and who are distrustful of dentistry often make poor candidates. In contrast, others who are more receptive to the use of adjunctive pain control may benefit greatly. Recommended resources for information on the use of nitrous oxide sedation include the *Handbook of Nitrous Oxide and Oxygen Sedation* by Morris Clark and Ann Brunick, 3rd edition, 2008 and *Pharmacology and Therapeutics for Dentistry* by John Yagiela, Frank Dowd, and Enid Neidle, 5th edition, 2004.

The CARL Program

The CARL (Computer Assisted Relaxation Learning) program, developed at the University of Washington and currently in pilot testing in private offices, uses what is known as systemic desensitization. The desensitization protocol consists of three active components: First, patients are provided with coping responses such as deep breathing, muscle relaxation, and guided imagery. They may also be provided with positive coping statements. Second, a hierarchy of fearful stimuli is generated. The third, and final, step involves the presentation of fearful stimuli in order of increasing aversiveness (Coldwell, Getz, Milgrom, Prall, Spadafora, & Ramsay, 1998).

Although not necessarily a true hierarchy, the hierarchy of fearful stimuli for the anesthetic injection is broken down into seven segments (Table 18–1 ■). Patients proceed through each segment in logical order rather than strictly by increasing levels of aversiveness. At first, patients watch a video of a model patient learning coping skills. Patients then observe the actor viewing and holding an anesthetic syringe without the needle or cartridge attached. At the end of the first video segment, patients rate their anxiety on a scale of one to nine. If the self-rating score is 4 or less, patients are ready to move to the next segment. If the score is more than 4, patients repeat the segment until their level drops to 4 or less. The program is self-paced, with individual sessions limited to 45 minutes. Patients return as often as necessary to complete the seven segments. When all seven segments have been successfully completed, patients are scheduled to receive an actual injection (see Table 18–1).

Table 18–1	Content of the CARL Program Exposure Hierarchy Segments
Segment 1	Explanation of local anesthetic, viewing and holding the syringe.
Segment 2	Discussion of the needle, including the length, flexibility, only required to insert a short distance.
Segment 3	Discussion of topical anesthetic. Demonstration of its use and numbing action.
Segment 4	Topical anesthetic is applied to the injection site and its numbing action is demonstrated.
Segment 5	The injection procedure is demonstrated to the patient with the cap on the needle.
Segment 6	The injection procedure is demonstrated to the patient with the cap off the needle, but the injection is not actually given.
Segment 7	An injection is administered to the model patient.

CASE MANAGEMENT: Lydia O'Kaine

Lydia's treatment plan should include strategies and coping skills to "treat the fear first," prior to the administration of local anesthetic. Once she is able to receive an injection comfortably she will also need anesthetic testing protocol to assure her that profound anesthesia has been attained prior to treatment.

Appointments are scheduled for four quadrants of scaling and root planing. She is informed that at her first appointment for scaling and root planing, the clinician will introduce techniques to help her to be more comfortable during injections.

The first appointment builds rapport by discussing specific concerns about receiving injections. The clinician explains that there are techniques that patients can use to keep themselves comfortable during an injection. Lydia is questioned as to whether or not she has used any relaxation skills in other situations. Having no previous specific experience, the clinician describes to Lydia the role and function of deep breathing and muscle relaxation. The clinician demonstrates each skill and practices them with Lydia. It is recommended to Lydia that she practice them at home and that she remember to use them in other stressful situations.

Information is provided about the benefits of topical anesthetics and slow administration of drugs for comfort. Using the tip of a periodontal probe, the tissue at the injection site can be touched lightly after the application of the topical and can be compared to the tissue on the contralateral side to demonstrate the effectiveness of the topical.

The sequence of steps for administering the injection is explained to the patient. It is suggested that a rehearsal will allow Lydia to practice her new deep breathing and muscle relaxation coping skills. She is introduced to the use of hand signaling to control both the start and stop of the injection procedure. She is coached when practicing her relaxation skills and is informed that once she is comfortable, she can raise her hand to indicate that she is ready to begin the rehearsal. If the rehearsal is a success, the actual injection can proceed following the same protocol with no changes or surprises for the patient.

Once the appropriate amount of anesthetic has been administered, an anesthetic testing protocol should be implemented. The EPT or ultrasonic instrument may be used with time structuring (count of 1, 2, 5) to verify that the area to be treated is adequately anesthetized. During treatment, if there is any indication of pain or discomfort, the treatment should stop and additional anesthetic should be administered, followed by repetition of the anesthetic testing protocol. Throughout treatment, the clinician monitors patient comfort, applying behavioral management skills.

CHAPTER QUESTIONS

1. There is a new patient in the chair. During appropriate introductions, including handshaking, it is noticed that the patient's hands are clammy and he has perspiration on his upper lip. He appears very stiff and responds with a brief "yes" or "no" to attempts to engage him in conversation. To discern whether or not he is apprehensive about the dental treatment he is scheduled to receive, the most appropriate strategy would be to:
   a. Try to distract the patient by offering to let him watch a movie or listen to music.
   b. Get the nitrous oxide/oxygen sedation ready just in case.
   c. Check out the observations made by asking the patient about possible concerns regarding dental treatment.
   d. Avoid saying anything about dental anxiety or fear because it might upset the patient and risk not being able to get the scheduled treatment completed.

2. Establishing trust in the patient–clinician relationship is especially important for fearful dental patients because they need to learn:
   a. how to pay for services provided.
   b. how to be assertive.
   c. that clinicians never recommend treatment patients cannot tolerate.
   d. that clinicians are professionals and know what is best for patients.

3. Providing patients with information is an important means of increasing their sense of control in the dental environment. When providing information to a fearful patient about an aversive procedure:
   a. The clinician should explain how steps taken during the procedure are necessary for the benefit of the clinician's work.
   b. The emphasis should be on the scientific rationale for the treatment, procedures, materials, and/or equipment used.
   c. It is better not to tell the patient what will happen because it might make the patient more fearful.
   d. The procedure should be described in simple steps, including the sensations the patient will experience so that the patient knows what to expect.

4. It is important to have the skills and confidence necessary to teach anxious and fearful patients how to relax in the dental chair. When a patient learns the physical relaxation skills of deep breathing and muscle relaxation:
   a. The patient benefits by having an active means to relieve the discomfort, both physical and mental, which is experienced as a result of anxiety.
   b. The clinician benefits because it is easier to achieve pain control in a relaxed patient.
   c. Neither the clinician nor the patient benefit because these skills are too difficult to teach and to learn in the stressful dental setting.
   d. Both A and B

5. Patients who are fearful of dental injections can benefit from having the opportunity to "rehearse" the procedure before receiving the actual injection. The objective of the rehearsal is to:
   a. Find out if the patient is sincere about wanting to overcome his dental fears.
   b. Allow the patient to learn how his role and the clinician's role are synchronized before proceeding with the injection and treatment.
   c. Determine the treatment plan for the patient by gaining knowledge about which treatments the patient will be capable of tolerating.
   d. Test the patient for intolerance and allergies to local anesthetics.

6. Some patients will report a history of receiving dental care without being adequately anesthetized. They may not be anxious about the injection procedure, but will be reluctant to proceed with treatment after the administration of local anesthetics. Despite soft tissue signs and symptoms of anesthesia, they do not believe the teeth are "numb." The next step for these patients should be to:
   a. Verify that the tooth is adequately anesthetized by testing, preferably with an electronic pulp tester (EPT), before beginning treatment.
   b. Reassure the patient that the correct amount and type of anesthetic has been used for the area of the mouth to be treated.
   c. Reassure the patient that if pain is felt in the tooth, treatment will cease the minute the hand signal to stop is given.
   d. Give the patient more anesthetic to be on the safe side before attempting to proceed with treatment.

REFERENCES

The American Heritage® Dictionary of the English Language (4th ed.). (2000). Boston: Houghton Mifflin.

American Psychiatric Association. (2000). *Diagnostic and Statistical Manual of Mental Disorders* (4th ed., Text Rev.). Washington, D.C.: Author.

Bobey, M. J., & Davidson, P. O. (1970). Psychological factors affecting pain tolerance. *Journal of Psychosomatic Research, 14,* 371–376.

Coldwell, S. E., Getz, T., Milgrom, P., Prall, C. W., Spadafora, A., & Ramsay, D. S. (1998). CARL: A LabVIEW 3 computer program for conducting exposure therapy for dental injection fear. *Behaviour Research and Therapy, 36,* 429–444.

Corah, N. L., O'Shea, R. M., & Ayer, W. A. (1985). Dentists' management of patients' fear and anxiety. *Journal of the American Dental Association, 110,* 734–736.

Corah, N. L., O'Shea, R. M., & Bissell, G. D. (1985). The dentist-patient relationship: Perceptions by patients of dentist behavior in relation to satisfaction and anxiety. *Journal of the American Dental Association, 11,* 443–446.

De Jongh, A., Muris, P., Schoenmakers, N., & Ter Horst, G. (1995). Negative cognitions of dental phobics: Reliability and validity of the dental cognitions questionnaire. *Behaviour Research and Therapy, 33:*507–515.

International Association for the Study of Pain, Task Force on Taxonomy. (1994). Merskey, H., & Bogduk, N. (Eds.). *Classification of chronic pain: descriptions of chronic pain syndromes and definitions of pain terms* (2nd ed.). Seattle: IASP Press.

Jacobson, E. (1938). *Progressive Relaxation.* Chicago: University of Chicago Press.

Kaufman, E., Weinstein, P., & Milgrom, P. (1984). Difficulties in achieving local anesthesia: A review. *Journal of the American Dental Association, 108,* 205–208.

Kristt, D. A., & Engel, B. T. (1975). Learned control of blood pressure in patients with high blood pressure. *Circulation, 51,* 370–378.

Milgrom, P., Coldwell, S. E., Getz, T., Weinstein, P., & Ramsay, D. S. (1997). Four dimensions of fear of dental injections. *Journal of the American Dental Association, 128,* 756–762.

Milgrom, P., Fiset, L., Melnick, S., & Weinstein, P. (1988). The prevalence and practice management consequences of dental fear in a major U.S. city. *Journal of the American Dental Association, 116,* 641–647.

Milgrom, P., Weinstein, P., & Heaton, L. (2009). *Treating fearful dental patients: A patient management handbook* (3rd ed.). Seattle: Dental Behavioral Resources.

Sohn, W., & Ismail, A. I. (2005). Regular dental visits and dental anxiety in an adult dentate population. *Journal of the American Dental Association, 136,* 58–66.

Thompson, S. C. (1981). Will it hurt less if I can control it? A complex answer to a simple question. *Psychological Bulletin, 90,* 89–101.

Weinstein, P., Milgrom, P., Kaufman, K., Fiset, L., & Ramsay, D. (1985). Patient perceptions of failure to achieve optimal anesthesia. *General Dentistry, 33,* 218–220.

Chapter 19

Insights from Pedodontics

Greg Psaltis, DDS

OBJECTIVES

- Define and discuss key terms in this chapter.
- Apply the principles of local anesthetic drug toxicity to compute safe doses for pediatric patients based on body weight.
- Relate effective anesthesia to the management of pediatric behavior.
- Provide age-appropriate explanations of the local anesthesia experience for pediatric patients.
- Describe injection technique modifications for small children.
- Recognize and manage postanesthetic trauma.
- Understand the supportive role of dental assistants in successful anesthesia delivery for children.

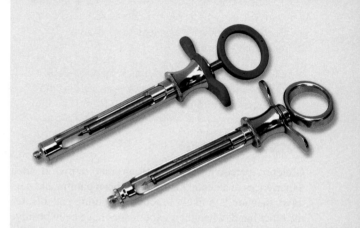

KEY TERMS

age-appropriate terminology **382**
behavioral guidelines **383**
bilateral mandibular blocks **387**
mandibular infiltration **387**
positive feedback **386**
postanesthetic trauma **383**
trigger words **382**
vocal distraction **386**

CASE STUDY: Jaden Harris

Jaden Harris, a healthy 4-year-old child, weighing 45 pounds, has completed his first visit to the dentist. He presented with extensive caries and is in need of significant restorative treatment. The following restorative needs have been determined for Jaden, which will require a number of local anesthetic injections.

1. Restorations: Tooth # A = OL, C = DL, J = MO, K= MO, M = F, S = DO
2. Pulpotomy with stainless steel crowns: Tooth # B and L

During Jaden's initial examination he was very cooperative and appears to be receptive to the dental staff and treatment.

INTRODUCTION

Children perceive their world in real terms. If their experiences in a dental facility have been painful and negative, they are less likely to return as willing patients. On the other hand, when their experiences have been positive and pain free, children can be excellent patients. Young children, in particular, will not be persuaded by any possible benefits of oral health if a visit to the dentist is equated with pain.

This chapter will discuss philosophical and practical approaches to pediatric dental care. While many clinicians may consider treating children to be challenging, a well-managed child can be the best patient of the day.

THE PEDIATRIC DENTAL PATIENT

Appropriate Terminology for Successful Anesthesia

The acceptance of care by children and the gratitude of their parents or guardians can be fulfilling. When treated appropriately, with effective and comfortable local anesthesia, children will be receptive to care. Administering local anesthesia for children is not complicated but it does require specific technical and verbal skills, which can be characterized as significantly different compared to the skills needed for most adults. In children, local anesthetic techniques, similar to other techniques in dentistry, are more demanding from a communication standpoint. In order to achieve optimum success, the process of local anesthesia must be a harmonious blend of skilled delivery and skilled communication.

Unlike adults, children usually do not have preconceived fears about injections because they do not know to expect them. This is especially true when pedodontic facilities do not look like other medical facilities. Pediatric clinicians recognize the advantage of working with a *blank slate* instead of with experienced patients. This is the result of a deliberate process. Part of the success of local anesthesia requires preparation prior to the appointment. Moreover, it requires the involvement of key players other than patients, including parents and guardians. When parents and guardians have been prepared, children are more likely to be receptive to the actual procedures. It is critical that *key players* know and use appropriate terminology in order to avoid frightening children prior to procedures. When provided with **age-appropriate terminology** and rationale for their use, the odds of successful anesthetic experiences are significantly increased. Once aware of *appropriate language,* key players can avoid **trigger words** that can undermine the success of appointments. It is important for clinicians to be comfortable with the selected words in order for them to be used with ease. While some may consider it silly or even deceptive, pediatric dentists long ago discovered that appropriate terminology can be a key factor in the success of dental appointments for children. For some examples and suggestions of appropriate terminology, refer to Table 19–1 ■.

Table 19–1	Suggested Terminology
Traditional Term	***Alternative Term***
Local anesthetic	Sleepy juice
Needle/syringe	Sprayer
Numb feeling	Fat/sleepy lip/tongue/cheek
Shot/injection	Put teeth to sleep*/ spray sleepy juice
Topical anesthetic	Jelly stick
Wearing off	Lip/tongue/cheek waking up

*Because some children have had their pets "put to sleep," it should be made clear that the child will remain awake. Only the lip, tongue, and teeth will "go *to sleep*" and they will *wake up* soon.

Use of age-appropriate terminology will depend on the developmental level of the child in addition to the age. The term *sleepy juice,* for example, may work well for preschool patients. As children grow, *sleepy juice* may no longer be appropriate and a more mature phrasing, such as *I am going to make your tooth and lip fall asleep* may be more effective. The language should be consistent with the child's level of comprehension and maturity. Later, as the child ages, the words can reflect increasing maturity such as, *I am going to get your teeth numb.* In every description, trigger words such as *shot* and *needle* have been replaced with terms that are more easily accepted by young patients. The exact ages to make the transitions are based on individual levels of maturity and understanding. There are no hard and fast rules. A relatively easy way to decide is for the clinician to consider the self-impact of the language; in other words, are the words flowing easily or do they seem a bit silly with a particular child?

In addition to their concerns for their children, parents and guardians often bring their own dental fears to the child's appointment. Coaching is essential, if parents and guardians are present during any portion of a dental visit. It can be helpful to outline **behavioral guidelines** for any observer. If they wish to observe, they need to be silent observers allowing the child's attention to be focused on the clinician. In this way, parents are not distracting to children and children are more cooperative.

Awareness of facial expressions, body postures and movements can be crucial to the success of local anesthesia in pediatric dentistry. This applies equally to office personnel, parents, and guardians. Calm, neutral expressions convey the important visual message that all is going well. *Knitted brows and narrowed eyes or grimaces* can raise concerns that something is amiss. Slow, measured movements are equally important because they arouse fewer negative responses. Gentle touches on the shoulders are reassuring, as are gentle hand-holding (as opposed to tight gripping) and gentle ankle stroking by the parent or guardian. These nonverbal cues enhance childrens' sense of comfort and safety.

Drug Dosages Based on Children's Body Weight

One of the most important considerations when treating pediatric patients is the potential for drug toxicity due to the relatively low body weight of small children and the immaturity of their organs. Multiple cartridges of anesthetic solutions should be administered only when the need has been clearly established and only with the utmost caution, especially in very small children. Maximum dose calculations should be confirmed and reconfirmed. It is not surprising that the majority of reported deaths due to excessive administrations of local anesthetic drugs have occurred in children (Malamed, 2004b). Table 19–2 ■ provides a list of maximum cartridges allowed by body weight for 2% lidocaine, as an example. Similar statistics for other drugs and dose calculations can be found in Chapter 5, "Dental Local Anesthetic Drugs," Chapter 6, "Vasoconstrictors in Dentistry," and Chapter 7, "Dose Calculations for Local Anesthetic Solutions." Box 19–1 addresses maximum dose calculations for morbidly obese children.

The use of vasoconstrictors is somewhat controversial in pediatric dentistry. While they increase the risk of postoperative self-injury, vasoconstrictors are helpful during appointments by assuring durable and adequate anesthesia.

A main argument in favor of using them is that duration is enhanced and it is less likely that the local anesthetic will lose effectiveness in the middle of a procedure. As previously discussed, the importance of successful anesthesia in determining pain-free procedures cannot be overstated in pediatric appointments. If the anesthesia wears off prematurely, children not only experience pain, but appointments are lengthened due to the need to re-inject prior to continuing.

On the other hand, vasoconstrictors increase the possibility of **postanesthetic trauma.** Children may remain numb for up to three hours after leaving the dental setting, creating a higher risk of lip- or cheek-biting.

The selection of local anesthetic agents in pediatric dentistry is not as limited as might be assumed. While the FDA has not approved the use of articaine for children under the age of 4, it has been tested and approved for children as young as 4. Due to reports of increased paresthesia with articaine, lidocaine is preferred for inferior alveolar nerve blocks in children. Articaine has been used successfully in the mandible in non-block situations through buccal infiltration, especially in children. Mepivacaine 2%, with 1:20,000 levonordefrin, can be used for most procedures, but mepivacaine 3% (plain), may not be an ideal choice, depending on the length of the procedure and the ability of the clinician to get back to the room before the anesthesia wears off. It can also be useful whenever lidocaine is not effective.

Table 19–2 Impact of Body Weight on Drug Dosage—Example: 2% Lidocaine		
2% Lidocaine		
2% = 36 mg drug per cartridge 2 mg/lb = 4.4 mg/kg Maximum dose 300 mg Maximum 8 cartridges		
Cartridges	*Weight Range*	*Typical Weight by Age for Young Children*
8.0	>150 lbs+	
7.5–8.0	135–149	
7.0–7.5	126–134	
6.5–7.0	117–125	
6.0–6.5	108–116	
5.5–6.0	99–107	
5.0–5.5	90–98	
4.5–5.0	81–89	
4.0–4.5	72–80	
3.5–4.0	63–71	
3.0–3.5	54–62	
2.5–3.0	45–53	*50 lbs @ 4–6 years*
2.0–2.5	36–44	*40 lbs @ 3–4 years*
1.5–2.0	28–35	
1.0–1.5	19–27	*25 lbs @ 2–3 years*

Use of Topical Anesthetics

Like adults, children want their dental visits to be as comfortable as possible. The youngest children may not be able to verbalize this desire but they are definitely able to make it known when things are *not* comfortable. The anesthetic sequence typically sets the tone for an appointment. It is important that procedures start well. The use of topical anesthetic techniques is an effective way to prevent sensations during initial needle penetrations.

Topicals are available in a variety of flavors. Allowing children to choose a flavor and to actually smell the topical prior to placement can create a sense of familiarity with the agent and is likely to put the child at ease. Gels and ointments tend to be easy to control and place with cotton applicators. They pose far less concern for potential aspiration compared with liquids and sprays. If using aerosol sprays, metered dose systems are advisable (Palm, Kirkegaard, & Poulsen, 2004). See Chapter 8, "Topical Anesthetics." Researchers have found that some children prefer topical anesthetic patches (Wu & Julliard, 2003).

Drying the mucosa with a 2 × 2 cotton pad prior to placement of the topical enhances its effectiveness. It is important to allow adequate time for topicals to take effect. The onset time for most agents ranges between 30 seconds to 5 minutes (Pinkham, Casamassimo, Fields, McTigue, & Nowak, 1994). Rushing into an injection before the topical has had a chance to work risks pain and management difficulties. See Box 19–2 for other uses for topical anesthetics for children.

Box 19–1   *Special Considerations in Child Obesity*

Morbidly obese children pose unique challenges when establishing appropriate doses for local anesthetic drugs. When a young child has the body weight of an adult, the usual dosing guidelines not only *may* not apply but they *likely* do not apply. As with their non-obese counterparts, obese children have incompletely developed organs and organ functions. This incomplete development includes the blood–brain barrier and the liver, which is not yet able to metabolize drugs as efficiently as an adult's liver.

  Consulting standard milligram per pound tables for these children, in order to calculate safe doses, can be problematic. Unfortunately, there are no clear-cut, separately-stated guidelines for local anesthetic dosing in obese children. In general, it is advisable to consider starting with a decreased maximum dose that is no more than half the figure arrived at by tabulated calculation. In the case of lidocaine, for example, a presumed safe dose for obese children can be calculated by dividing the dose per pound furnished in the tables, by two. This reduces the lidocaine dose for the obese child to half the typical calculated dose, from 2.0 mg/lb to 1.0 mg/lb. It should also be remembered that this is not a proven *maximum* safe dose calculation; therefore, approaching any maximum limit in these children is not recommended. Remaining alert to the development of adverse events should be accomplished with exceptional vigilance whenever local anesthetic drugs are administered to these children.

Box 19–2   *Other Uses of Topical Anesthetics for Children*

Topicals may also be useful for comfortable rubber dam clamp placement and to anesthetize the tissue retaining extremely mobile primary teeth to allow children to remove their teeth atraumatically at home.

Management Techniques for Pediatric Dental Injections

From the perspective of technique, injection steps for children do not differ significantly from those for adults. Since children are more likely to react and move during anesthetic procedures, managing their behavior during injections is considered to be more of an *art form* than a technique. Mastering this art benefits both clinician and child and sets the stage for a positive dental experience.

In particular, it is important to:

1. Prepare the child with appropriate terminology.
2. Prepare child with *show-tell-do* communication (demonstrate and explain before doing).
3. Use a tone of voice that is reassuring yet assertive enough to prohibit *bargaining*.
4. Use passive restraint. The dental assistant places one hand over the child's hands (which should be placed on the child's stomach) in case of quick reactions by the child to the procedure. The other hand is placed on the child's forehead to guard against sudden or unexpected movements (see Figure 19–1 ■ and Figure 19–2 ■).
5. Pass the syringe out of the child's line of sight.
6. Use prewarmed anesthetic cartridges (see Box 19–3).
7. Describe the sensations of anesthesia the child will feel prior to onset. For example, at the onset of a mandibular block an appropriate comment might be that the side of the tongue will start to tickle.
8. Always inject the solution slowly, administering a few drops ahead of the needle to allow anesthesia to precede the tip of the needle.
9. Explain to the parent or guardian, and to the child when appropriate, that the lips, cheek, tongue, and teeth will remain *asleep* for a period of time after the appointment is over. Be sure they understand the risks of postoperative traumatic injury.
10. When indicated, comfortable palatal anesthesia can be achieved by first completing a facial infiltration, then penetrating slowly through the interdental papilla, administering a few drops of solution ahead of the needle until the palatal tissues have been initially numbed. Following these steps, proceed with standard palatal injection techniques (see Chapter 13, "Injections for Palatal Pain Control").

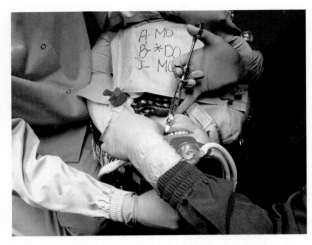

■ **FIGURE 19–1** Preparing for Unexpected Movements. The child is asked to place the hands on his or her stomach. The assistant places one hand over the child's hands to respond in case of quick reactions by the child during the injection.

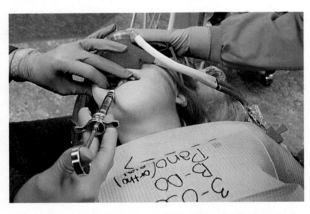

■ **FIGURE 19–2** Gently Stabilize the Child's Head. The assistant places one hand on the child's forehead (in addition to over the child's hands) to guard against sudden or unexpected movements during the injection.

Behavioral Management Techniques

Two useful behavior management techniques include *vocal distraction* and *positive feedback*. **Vocal distraction** is the process of keeping the child focused on the clinician's voice rather than on the dental procedures. Distraction can be created by a calm, reassuring, and informative narrative that is continuous

---

Box 19–3   **Warming Anesthetic Cartridges Prior to Use**

Warming cartridges prior to use is intended to reduce the incidence of pain on injection. Some suggest the practice may be effective (Bainbridge, 1991; Courtney, Agrawal, & Revington, 1999). Others hold little esteem for the practice, especially when the risk of administering overheated solution is introduced to an otherwise negligible risk of tissue damage due to cartridge temperature (Malamed, 2004b). In addition, vasoconstrictors in warmed cartridges may lose some of their effectiveness, particularly if they have been stored in warming devices for extended periods (Malamed, 2004b).

If a decision is made to warm cartridges, appropriate devices that do not overheat cartridges should be used. Clinicians can warm cartridges with the knowledge that few, if any, experts advise against warming as long as the cartridges are not overheated and are used soon after being placed into the devices to prevent degradation of the cartridge contents.

---

throughout the procedure. When children have a focus other than an actual procedure, injections are more likely to succeed.

Positive feedback for *specific* desirable behaviors can also be helpful. General statements such as *what a good patient you are* or *you're being so brave today* are less helpful compared to statements regarding specific aspects of the procedure that are going well. For example, the clinician might say, "Thank you for holding your head so still for me." Positive feedback becomes a learning tool for the child. Children learn how to be successful patients and how to be active participants in the procedure when feedback praises them for behavior that is beneficial.

Postoperative Trauma (Lip/Cheek Biting)

Despite every effort of the pediatric dental team to prevent postanesthetic self-injury (trauma), children will occasionally test anesthetized oral tissues by biting them, causing significant trauma. Few of these episodes result in any long-term consequences but they can be very painful and quite dramatic in appearance. The injured tissues can appear red or red and white and there may be significant swelling around them (see Figure 17–5) (Ashkenazi, Blumer, & Eli, 2005). If notified of a self-injury soon after an appointment, a cold pack should be recommended over the injured tissue to reduce swelling. If the notification occurs the day following an appointment, a warm pack can be recommended to stimulate circulation and promote healing. Antibiotics are usually not indicated and are prescribed only in the unlikely event of infection (Ashkenazi, Blumer, & Eli, 2005). If the injuries are first evaluated by physicians, it is not unusual for them to prescribe antibiotics due to the rather dramatic clinical appearance of these injuries, which closely resemble infections.

INJECTION TECHNIQUE VARIATIONS FOR CHILDREN

Showing or Hiding the Needle

While some clinicians advocate showing the needles to children, many young patients do not respond favorably to this approach. Children are far less likely to respond to something they cannot see. By passing the syringe across a child's chest (out of eyesight) while placing their other hand over the child's forehead, the assistant also guards against sudden movements. This technique does not rely on favorable responses from children. During the anesthetic procedure, continuous and calming communication with the child will usually gain their cooperation. This is an example of *vocal distraction*. Occasionally, a child may ask to see the needle after the injection, at which time the clinician can hold the syringe in the child's view, concealing the capped needle in the palm while pointing to the empty cartridge, explaining that it is where the sleepy juice came from. Children are usually satisfied with this explanation. While it has been suggested that children have a preference for the appearance of the Wand device (see Chapter 9, "Local Anesthetic Delivery Devices"), the simplest way to avoid the issue is to keep all injection armamentarium out of the child's eyesight (Kuscu & Akyus, 2006).

Anatomical Differences

Primary tooth roots are typically shorter than the roots of their permanent successors. Basic techniques for pediatric injections vary somewhat compared to the same techniques for permanent teeth due to the decreased insertion depths needed. Although the depths are shallower, the penetration sites for primary teeth are analogous to the sites of penetration for permanent teeth in most cases. For example, the target for a primary maxillary infiltration is above the apex of the root. Extra short (10 mm) needles which would usually be too short for maxillary adult infiltrations can be adequate for reaching this site in many children (Malamed, 2004b).

In inferior alveolar nerve blocks, the position of the mandibular foramen in children is inferior to its eventual adult location. Studies have demonstrated that this occurs due to the remodeling of the ramus during growth (Kanno, de Oliveira, Cannon, & Carvalho, 2005).

Bilateral Mandibular Blocks

When treatment planning for children, it is considered beneficial to treat half a mouth at a time in order to minimize the total number of appointments. One way to accomplish this is to deliver bilateral inferior alveolar blocks at one appointment, completing mandibular treatment. Many consider this problematic due to the ensuing postanesthetic lack of control of oral functions. A recent study however found that the incidence of post-operative lip biting actually *decreased* in children who received **bilateral mandibular blocks** compared to those who received unilateral blocks (College, Feigal, Wandera, & Strange, 2000). It was speculated that, following a unilateral mandibular block, children are more inclined to test the *funny* (numb) side by chewing their lips.

Mandibular Infiltration

Pediatric patients have thinner cortical plates and more porous bone, allowing for easy diffusion of anesthetic solutions. For this reason, **mandibular infiltrations** are commonly used for many simple restorative procedures (Malamed, 2004c). Some mandibular extractions can also be accomplished with infiltrations. When children require pulpotomies or stainless steel crowns, the technique is less reliable and inferior alveolar blocks remain the best choice.

The mandibular infiltration technique is very similar to the technique for maxillary infiltration. Once adequate topical anesthesia has been obtained, the patient's lip is retracted and the tip of the needle is placed into the mucobuccal fold. With the lip retracted upward, the tip of the needle can be *enveloped* or captured by the

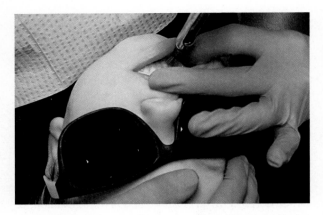

■ **FIGURE 19–3** Mandibular Infiltrations. Mandibular infiltrations can be useful for basic restorative procedures in young children due to their thinner cortical plates and very porous bone, allowing for easy diffusion of anesthetic solutions.

tissue. This will minimize sensations due to needle penetration. Figure 19–3 ■ demonstrates an infiltration of a mandible molar. Only a small volume of anesthetic (0.6–0.9 ml per tooth or one-third to one-half of a cartridge) is necessary to obtain adequate local anesthesia. The primary advantage of this technique is that anesthesia of large areas of the lip and tongue can be avoided. It has been suggested by some that soft tissue trauma may not be reduced by the use of mandibular

infiltration anesthesia (American Academy of Pediatric Dentistry, 2006–07). Others disagree, finding the incidence of lip-biting to be reduced when techniques with more limited areas of anesthesia such as infiltrations or PDLs have been administered versus nerve blocks (Ashkenazi et al., 2005).

Perspective on Articaine for Pedodontic Patients

Articaine is believed by some to be more effective in its ability to diffuse through bone compared to other amide anesthetic solutions (Kanaa, Whitworth, Corbett, & Meechan, 2006; Vree & Gielen, 2005). Some studies and opinions do not substantiate this claim (Haas, Harper, Saso, & Young, 1991; Malamed, 2004a). In one peer-reviewed evaluation of pulpal efficacy after buccal infiltration in molar areas, for example, articaine was judged to be considerably superior to lidocaine in children (Dudkiewicz, Schwartz, & Laliberte, 1987). This sentiment was echoed in a presentation to a recent gathering of leading dental researchers (Robertson, Nusstein, Reader, Beck, & McCartney, 2007; Paxton, Dawson, Drake, & Williamson, 2008). Clinical judgment is especially valuable when the evidence is as disputed or as unclear as it is with articaine.

It is important to keep in mind that articaine is available only in a 4% concentration. It is twice as concentrated when compared to 2% lidocaine. An appropriate volume reduction is required to avoid toxicity.

CASE MANAGEMENT: Jaden Harris

The following strategy for managing Jaden's treatment is suggested:

1. Restorations: Tooth # A = OL, C = DL, J = MO, K = MO, M = F, S = DO
2. Pulpotomy with stainless steel crowns: Tooth # B and L

First appointment: Begin treatment in the mandible for # K, L and M using 1.8 ml 2% lidocaine with epinephrine.

Rationale: Starting with the mandibular left quadrant can have the advantage of assuring

profound anesthesia for a first-time experience. Beginning with a nerve block technique can assure comfort in the placement of the rubber dam, especially the clamp. Also, this quadrant is one of two quadrants in greatest need of treatment. Other factors being equal, this strategy addresses both the priority needs of the patient as well as the reliability of anesthesia.

Many clinicians prefer to start with the maxilla, assuming that infiltrations are easier injections for children to tolerate. The sequence of beginning treatment with anesthetic procedures in the mandible may seem unusual to some; however, this can be a very successful approach. The factor that influences this sequence of appointments is rubber dam clamp placement. Many children do very well with procedures until the placement of the clamp. Mandibular blocks may be better tolerated by children than palatal injections to avoid discomfort from clamp placement. Therefore, this sequence may be preferred to provide a more favorable first anesthesia experience.

Second appointment: # A, B, and C using 1.8 ml 4% articaine with epinephrine.

Rationale: This is the other "high priority" quadrant. If trust has now been established, the child will more likely accept the palatal injection nec-

essary to make clamp placement comfortable for tooth #A. Palatal anesthesia is also indicated for the maxillary stainless steel crowns. Other approaches to providing anesthesia for palatal gingiva are discussed in Chapter 8.

Third appointment: # J and S, for this appointment use a total of 1.2 to 1.8 ml 4% articaine with epinephrine for infiltrating *both* J and S.

Rationale: By making the final restorative visit brief, with simple procedures, the child is left with the memory of a short, easy appointment. Since both restorations require infiltrations, 0.6 to 0.9 ml per tooth will result in adequate anesthesia.

CHAPTER QUESTIONS

1. Why is it generally more critical to consider toxicity of local anesthetics in pediatric patients than in adults?
   a. Children react differently to local anesthetic agents than adults.
   b. Local anesthetic doses are based on body weight.
   c. Anesthetic agents that are appropriate for children are different than for adults.
   d. Crying and screaming may allow more rapid anesthetic uptake.

2. How does excellent anesthesia serve as a management tool for children?
   a. Restorative procedures become tolerable, if not pain-free.
   b. Clamp placement for rubber dam is simplified.
   c. Quadrant (or half-mouth) treatment can be completed in one visit.
   d. All of the above.

3. In which of the following ways do anatomic variations affect the choice of injection techniques for children?
   a. Roots of primary teeth are generally shorter than permanent tooth roots.
   b. The cortical plate is thicker and less porous in children than in adults.
   c. The inferior alveolar foramen is often more superior in children than adults.
   d. All of the above.

4. Which of the following describe ways in which an assistant can play a vital role in the successful administration of local anesthetics to children?
   a. Showing the patient the needle to prepare the child
   b. Calming the parent during the injection by explaining what is happening
   c. Placing one hand on the child's forehead and the other on the child's hands for safety
   d. None of the above.

5. Which of the following are benefits of using age-appropriate terminology and specific positive feedback during the successful anesthetic administration in pediatric patients?
   a. Using understandable terms to demystify the child's experiences
   b. Using specific positive feedback teaches children what is expected and going well
   c. Avoiding frightening (or "trigger") words to reduce the chance of resistance
   d. All the above.

6. Which of the following *is true* when considering injection techniques in children?
   a. Mandibular infiltrations rarely work for children.
   b. Deposition of anesthetic solutions for mandibular blocks are more inferior compared to adults.
   c. Long needles are usually necessary.
   d. All of the above are true.

7. When children traumatize soft tissues immediately following injections, what is the best management?
   a. Place a cold pack immediately.
   b. Place a warm pack immediately.
   c. Always put the child on an antibiotic for infection.
   d. A and C.

REFERENCES

American Academy of Pediatric Dentistry. (2006–07). *Pediatric Dentistry Reference Manual, 28*(7), 106–111.

Ashkenazi, M., Blumer, S., & Eli, I. (2005). Effectiveness of computerized delivery of intrasulcular anesthetic in primary molars. *Journal of the American Dental Association,* 136(10):1418–1425, 2005.

Bainbridge, L. C. (1991). Comparison of room temperature and body temperature local anaesthetic solutions. *British Journal of the Plastic Surgery, 44*(2), 147–148.

College, C., Feigal, R., Wandera, A., & Strange, M. (2000, November/December). Bilateral versus unilateral mandibular block anesthesia in a pediatric population. *Pediatric Dentistry, 22*(6), 453–457.

Cook-Waite Anesthetics, Kodak Dental systems, Carestream Health, Inc., Rochester, NY; http://www.kodak.com/global/en/service/faqs/faq4527.shtml. Last accessed December 30, 2008.

Courtney, D. J., Agrawal, S., Revington, P. J. (1999). Local anaesthesia: To warm or alter pH? A survey of current practice. *Journal of the Royal College of Surgeons of Edinburgh & Ireland, 44*(2), 167–171.

Dudkiewicz, A., Schwartz, S., & Laliberte, R. (1987). Effectiveness of mandibular infiltration in children using the local anesthetic Ultracaine (articaine hydrochloride). *Journal of the Canadian Dental Association, 53,* 29–31.

Haas, D. A., Harper, D. B., Saso, M. A., & Young, E. R. (1991). Lack of differential effect by Ultracaine (articaine HCL) and Citanest (prilocaine HCL) in infiltration anesthesia. *Journal of the Canadian Dental Association, 57,* 217–223.

Kanaa, M. D., Whitworth, J. M., Corbett, I. P., & Meechan, J. G. (2006). Articaine and lidocaine mandibular buccal infiltration anesthesia: A prospective randomized double-blind cross-over study. *Journal of Endodontics, 32,* 296–298.

Kanno, C. M., de Oliveira, J. A., Cannon, M., & Carvalho, A. A. (2005, May–August). The mandibular lingula's position in children as a reference to inferior alveolar nerve block. *Journal of Dentistry for Children, 72*(2), 56–60, May–Aug, 2005.

Klein, U. et al. (2005, September–December). Quality of anesthesia for the maxillary primary anterior segment in pediatric patients: Comparison of the P-ASA nerve block using CompuMed delivery system vs Traditional supraperiosteal injections. *Journal of Dentistry for Children, 72*(3), 119–125.

Kuscu, Ö. Ö., Akyuz, S. (2006, May–August). Children's preference concerning physical appearance of dental injectors. *Journal of Dentistry for Children, 73*(2), 116–121.

Malamed, S. F. (2004a). *Handbook of Local Anesthesia* (5th ed., Clinical action of specific agents, pp. 55–81). St. Louis: Mosby.

Malamed, S. F. (2004b). *Handbook of Local Anesthesia* (5th ed., The needle, pp. 99–107.). St. Louis: Mosby.

Malamed, S. F. (2004c). *Handbook of Local Anesthesia* (5th ed., Local anesthetic considerations in dental specialties, pp. 269, 274–275). St. Louis: Mosby.

Palm, A. M., Kirkegaard, U., & Poulsen, S. (2004, November/December). The Wand versus Traditional injection for mandibular nerve block in children and adolescents: Perceived pain and time of onset. *Pediatric Dentistry, 26*(6), 481–484.

Paxton, K. R., Dawson, D. V., Drake, D. R., & Williamson, A. E. (2008, July 2). *Articaine hydrochloride versus lidocaine hydrochloride: A meta-analysis.* Keynote address to the International Association for Dental Research. Toronto, Canada.

Pinkham, J. R., Casamassimo, P. S., Fields, H. W., McTigue, D. J., & Nowak, A. (1994). *Pediatric Dentistry: Infancy Through Adolescence* (2nd ed., Local anesthesia and oral surgery, pp. 381–387.). Philadelphia: Saunders.

Ram, D., & Perez, B. (2003, May–August). The assessment of pain sensation during local anesthesia using a computerized local anesthesia (Wand) and a conventional syringe. *Journal of Dentistry for Children, 70*(2), 130–133.

Robertson, D., Nusstein, J., Reader, A., Beck, M., & McCartney, M. (2007). The anesthetic efficacy of articaine in buccal infiltration of mandibular posterior teeth. *Journal of the American Dental Association, 138*(8), 1104–1112.

Wahl, M. J., Overton, D., Howell, J., Siegel, E., Schmitt, M. M., & Muldoon, M. (2001). Pain on injection of prilocaine plain vs. lidocaine with epinephrine. *Journal of the American Dental Association, 132*, 1396–1401.

Wu, S. J., & Julliard, K. (2003, July–August). Children's preference of benzocaine gel versus the lidocaine patch. *Pediatric Dentistry, 25*(4), 401–405.

Vree, T. B., & Gielen, M. J. (2005). Clinical pharmacology and the use of articaine for local and regional anaesthesia. *Best Practice & Research Clinical Anaesthesiology, 19*, 293–308.

Chapter 20

Insights from Specialties: Oral Surgery, Periodontics, and Endodontics

Melanie Lang, DDS, MD

William C. Lubken, DMD

Albert "Ace" Goerig, DDS, MS

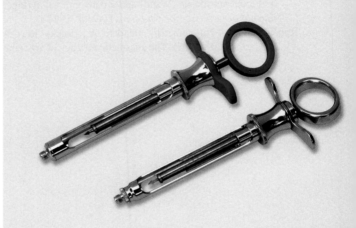

OBJECTIVES

- Discuss the choice of needles in oral and maxillofacial surgery.
- Discuss the populations who are at greatest risk for local anesthetic toxicity.
- Discuss the effects of inflammation/infection on local anesthetics.
- Discuss allergic responses with local anesthetics.
- Discuss options for the treatment of patients with true allergies to local anesthetics.
- Discuss inferior alveolar block complications including nerve injuries.
- Discuss concerns with use of 4% local anesthetic agents.
- Discuss popular mandibular techniques in periodontics.
- Discuss popular maxillary techniques in periodontics.
- Discuss hemostasis in periodontics.
- Discuss ways in which anesthetic challenges are addressed in endodontics.
- Discuss the role of topical anesthetics in endodontic anesthesia.
- Discuss techniques for managing excessive fears in endodontic patients.
- Define and discuss intraosseous and intrapulpal anesthesia techniques and their benefit in endodontic anesthesia and the use of vasoconstrictors in these techniques.

KEY TERMS

hemostasis **399**
IntraFlow **400**
interpapillary injections **398**
intraosseous injection **399**

intrapulpal injection **400**
needle tract infection **393**
Stabident **400**
X-Tip **400**

INTRODUCTION

This chapter provides insights from three additional specialty areas in dentistry. The purpose of presenting multidisciplinary insights from the point of view of the dental specialists is to help develop an understanding of the importance of local anesthetic drugs in these settings and the unique challenges encountered when providing them.

INSIGHTS FROM ORAL AND MAXILLOFACIAL SURGERY

Local anesthesia is critical to the practice of oral and maxillofacial surgery (OMFS). It would be impossible to provide effective and successful intraoperative or postoperative pain management without it. Many referrals to OMF surgeons are motivated by local anesthetic failures in other settings, such as patients for whom anesthesia was unsuccessful. Other patients are referred due to complications related to local anesthesia or because they have serious concurrent medical conditions that complicate its administration.

Specific challenges encountered in OMFS local anesthesia administration include safe management of patients of all ages with diverse medical backgrounds who may require extensive treatment (e.g., full mouth extractions). Minor to life-threatening infections are also encountered. Achieving adequate local anesthesia in the presence of these infections while limiting the potential for **needle tract infections** (infections spread along needle pathways) and compensating for anatomic difficulties with associated trismus and airway patency concerns are serious and significant challenges encountered by OMF surgeons.

Although inhalation and intravenous sedation, as well as general anesthesia are common in OMFS, effective local anesthesia plays an important supplemental role, assisting in providing effective intraoperative pain management and allowing for lighter general anesthesia and sedation. Local anesthetics with vasoconstrictors also provide hemostasis while longer-acting local anesthetics provide postoperative pain control and a more comfortable transition to oral and intravenous analgesics.

CLASSIFICATION OF LOCAL ANESTHETICS

Oral and maxillofacial surgeons typically use the five injectable local anesthetics available to other dental specialists and clinicians, although some may occasionally access other local anesthetic drugs, such as ropivacaine and levo-bupivacaine. Specific chemical classifications and formulas for all dental local anesthetic drugs can be found in Appendix 4–1.

An easy way to identify the class of a local anesthetic drug is to remember that the word *amide* and all of the amide local anesthetic drugs contain the letter "i" in the first or second syllable of their name. The word *ester* has no "i," nor does the first part of any ester drug. Esters and amides share the common ending "-caine" (see Box 20–1).

LOCAL ANESTHETIC PROPERTIES

Whether considering surgical procedures performed by oral surgeons, periodontists, endodontists, pedodontists, or general practitioners, an understanding of the onset times, durations of action, and relative potencies of specific local anesthetics is important in the surgical setting. See Chapter 4, "Pharmacology Basics" for more detailed explanations of these properties.

Onset

All five injectable drugs have relatively fast onsets. Articaine, in infiltrations, has the fastest onset. Bupivacaine has the slowest.

Duration

Bupivacaine and tetracaine are both highly protein bound and therefore have long durations of action.

Box 20–1	Easy Identification of Amide versus Esther Drugs	
AM _i_ DES		**ESTERS**
L _i_ do-caine		Co-caine
Bup _i_ va-caine		Pro-caine
Mep _i_ va-caine		Benzo-caine
Pr _i_ lo-caine		Tetra-caine
Art _i_ caine*		Chloropro-caine
Metabolism: primarily in the l_i_ver		Metabolism: by plasma psuedocholinesterasee

*Articaine is primarily metabolized by plasma psuedocholinesterase.

Long-acting local anesthetics are frequently used in OMFS to assist with initial postoperative analgesic management. Bupivacaine, when used for regional blocks, lasts an average of five hours in the maxilla and eight hours in the mandible.

Potency

Lidocaine and bupivacaine are frequently used concurrently in OMFS. Lidocaine provides a rapid onset and bupivacaine provides a long duration. Since bupivacaine is the more potent local anesthetic, a 0.5% solution will obtain comparable depths of local anesthesia compared to a 2% solution of lidocaine.

NEEDLE CHOICE

In OMFS, 25 or 27 gauge long needles are typically used for all local anesthetic techniques. Long needles are preferred because they allow all types of dental injections to be completed without changing needles.

Smaller-gauge needles are used as they allow for less needle deflection through the tissue and therefore greater accuracy in injections as well as easier aspiration and less chance of needle breakage. Studies have shown there is no perceptual difference in patient comfort between 23, 25, 27, and 30 gauge needles (Malamed, 2004; Hamburg, 1972).

LOCAL ANESTHETIC TOXICITY AND MAXIMUM DOSING

In the OMFS setting, clinicians often face local anesthetic challenges due to the extent of treatment or to associated infections, either of which may increase the difficulty of achieving adequate local anesthesia. It is therefore critical for clinicians to have a thorough understanding of the clinical manifestations of local anesthetic toxicity as well as an ability to quickly and accurately calculate the maximum dosing of the local anesthetic they are utilizing.

Toxicity is caused by elevated plasma levels of local anesthetic drugs. It may result from iatrogenic violation of the maximum dose, inadvertent intravascular injection, and rapid absorption, or it may be secondary to decreased metabolism or clearance (as a result of underlying medical conditions or concomitant medications). Local anesthetic toxicity may be prevented by thorough assessment of patient health status and history, by assuring negative aspiration with every injection, by slowly depositing solution, and by using the smallest volume of local anesthetic solution that provides adequate anesthesia.

Local anesthetic toxicity primarily involves the CNS and CVS. The CNS is generally more sensitive to the toxic effects of local anesthetics and is usually affected first. All clinicians should be familiar with the specific signs of local anesthetic toxicity and their chronological presentations (see Box 20–2).

One of the classic early signs of local anesthetic toxicity is circumoral numbness. Since OFMS frequently involves *bilateral* anesthesia, other early signs must be recognized.

Management of a local anesthetic overdose reaction is based on the severity of the reaction (see Box 20–3). In most cases the reaction is relatively mild and transitory and no specific treatment aside from supportive care is necessary.

Geriatric and pediatric populations are at greatest risk for local anesthetic toxicity. Geriatric patients generally metabolize drugs at slower rates. In addition, they often have underlying complicating medical conditions or take other medications that may have effects on drug metabolism or clearance. For example, propranolol (Inderal), a beta-adrenergic blocker, can reduce both hepatic blood flow and renal clearance.

Box 20–2 Chronologic Order of Signs of Local Anesthetic Toxicity

Central Nervous System

- Lightheadedness, tinnitus, circumoral numbness, confusion
- Muscle twitching, auditory and visual hallucinations
- Tonic-clonic seizures, unconsciousness, respiratory arrest

Cardiovascular System

- Hypertension, tachycardia
- Decreased contractility and cardiac output, hypotension
- Sinus bradycardia, ventricular dysrhythmias, circulatory arrest

---

Box 20–3   *Management of Local Anesthetic Overdose*

- Reassure the patient
- Supplemental oxygen
- Monitor vital signs
- *IV access*
- *Summon medical assistance*
- *Give anticonvulsant*
- *Protect patient from injury if convulsing*
- *Provide basic life support (BLS)*
- *Blood pressure support as necessary*

Note: Actions in *italics* may or may not be required.

PEDIATRIC CONSIDERATIONS FOR DOSING

In the pediatric population, it is easier to exceed maximum doses of local anesthetics due to smaller body mass. In general, the pharmaceutical industry is not required to perform drug testing on the pediatric population. Variations in age and weight make the manufacturers reluctant to recommend maximum pediatric doses. This leaves the selection of pediatric doses to the clinical judgment of clinicians after performing standard calculations and taking into account health status, including the immaturity of pediatric organ systems. See Chapter 19, "Insights from Pedodontics."

There are two standard formulas for calculating safe pediatric doses: Clark's Rule, which is based on a child's weight, and Young's Rule, which is based on a child's age. Since there are significant variations when trying to relate weight with age, especially in children, Clark's Rule is preferred (see Chapter 7, "Dose Calculations for Local Anesthetic Solutions").

A preferred local anesthetic in OMFS that is safe for use in the pediatric population is 2% lidocaine with 1:100,000 epinephrine. A simple and safe "rule of thumb" for pediatric dosing of 2% lidocaine with or without vasoconstrictor is to administer *no more than one 1.8 ml cartridge for each 20 lbs of the child's weight.*

ANXIETY AND FEAR

Anxiety and fear are important contributors to reduced local anesthetic efficacy in both children and adults. Reducing anxiety will help to reduce the perception of pain. This reduced apprehension will also help decrease sympathetic tone resulting in fewer circulating catecholamines. Oral or intravenous sedation is frequently used in OMFS to reduce anxiety in patients who have difficulty achieving profound local anesthesia. Benzodiazepines such as triazolam, midazolam, diazepam, lorazepam, and alprazolam are most often prescribed or administered because they have relatively quick onsets and wide margins of safety. Unfortunately, in addition to their adjunctive role in reducing perioperative anxiety, benzodiazepines can also decrease the toxic threshold of any local anesthetics administered.

VASOCONSTRICTOR CONSIDERATIONS

The injectable local anesthetic drugs in dentistry are vasodilators (as discussed in Chapter 5, "Dental Local Anesthetic Drugs"). This decreases their duration of action and increases their rate of absorption and toxicity. The addition of vasoconstrictors can help to limit the potential for toxicity by slowing the uptake of a local anesthetic drug into the vasculature, thereby decreasing its systemic effects (as discussed in Chapter 6, "Vasoconstrictors in Dentistry"). This concurrent use of a vasoconstrictor can allow for an increase in the maximum dose that can be safely administered. Epinephrine also has the potential to counteract vasodilating β_2 receptors, which allows it to act as a pure alpha-adrenergic stimulant accounting for its usefulness in providing excellent hemostasis in surgery.

Adverse reactions can occur when administering vasoconstrictors with a number of other drugs, including tricyclic antidepressants (TCAs), beta-adrenergic antagonists, volatile anesthetics, cocaine, and other vasoconstrictors. This potential is of particular concern for psychiatric patients, cardiac patients, and suspected drug users.

Tricyclic antidepressants (TCAs), such as amitriptyline, increase the availability of endogenous norepinephrine. This can lead to an exaggerated response in heart rate or blood pressure when epinephrine or levonordefrin is administered with local anesthetics. TCAs also block the muscarinic and alpha$_1$-adrenergic receptors, which directly depress the myocardium. This concern is greatest during the first 14 to 21 days of TCA use and appears to have the most significant effect when levonordefrin and imipramine (Tofranil) are used concomitantly. The same concern was originally thought to exist with monoamine oxidase (MAO) inhibitors, but this is no longer thought to be the case.

A potential dysrhythmic effect exists between the inhalation anesthetic agent halothane (Fluothane) and epinephrine or levonordefrin through stimulation of both alpha and beta receptors. The greatest potential for this adverse reaction exists in the first 10 minutes of halothane administration; therefore, OMF surgeons typically wait at least 10 minutes following induction of a general anesthetic with halothane before injecting local anesthetic drugs.

Cocaine potentiates the effects of adrenergic vasoconstrictors. The dysrhythmic results of this interaction can be life threatening, especially when the cocaine use is recent. Recommendations for avoiding local anesthetics with vasoconstrictors range from a minimum of 6 hours to a maximum of 24 hours after cocaine use. See Chapter 10, "Patient Assessment for Local Anesthesia" for a more detailed discussion of concomitant cocaine and local anesthesia guidelines. When obtaining an accurate history of drug use, which may be especially difficult when a drug is illegal, patients should be informed of this potentially lethal side effect whether or not they admit to the use. A similarly abused drug, methamphetamine, requires a minimum waiting period of twenty-four hours after use before vasoconstrictors can be administered.

An average adult patient with a history of coronary artery disease should receive no more than 0.04 mg of epinephrine or 0.2 mg of levonordefrin. The objective when treating patients with coronary artery disease is to prevent increases in heart rate. Increases in heart rate can decrease stroke volume and lead to a decrease in cardiac output, which will thereby diminish the amount of oxygenated blood that flows to poorly perfused areas of the damaged myocardium. A dental cartridge of 1:100,000 epinephrine contains 0.018 mg of epinephrine; therefore, no more than two cartridges (3.6 ml) should be given in nonsedated patients with a history of coronary artery disease. A cartridge of 1:20,000 levonordefrin contains 0.09 mg; therefore, no more than two cartridges (3.6 ml) should be used. If a patient is electively sedated, additional epinephrine may be administered based on the patient's titrated heart rate. To review maximum allowable vasoconstrictor doses for cardiac patients, see Chapter 7.

LOCAL ANESTHETICS IN INFLAMMATION AND INFECTION

Achieving effective local anesthesia in the presence of inflammation and/or infection is a common challenge in OMFS.

Products of inflammation lower the surrounding tissue pH (e.g., purulent exudates have a pH of 5.5 to 5.6). At this more acidic pH the numbers of base molecules necessary for passage of the anesthetic into the nerve membrane may be significantly reduced. Inflammatory exudates may also enhance nerve conduction action potentials, making blockage of sensory nerve impulses more difficult. In addition, blood vessels in the area of inflammation may be dilated, leading to a more rapid uptake of the anesthetic agent from the area of injection. These changes can lead to delays in onsets of anesthesia, inadequate depths of anesthesia, and the potential for local anesthetic blood levels to be elevated. Considerations for the management of local anesthesia in the presence of infection are listed in Box 20–4.

Box 20–4 Local Anesthetic Considerations When Treating Patients with Oral Infections

- Allow additional time for the local anesthetic to take effect.
- Use a greater amount of local anesthetic to help overcome acidity created by the infection. (Make sure that maximum doses are not exceeded.)
- Use a regional nerve block away from the area of inflammation.
- Discard the needle after penetrating in or near an area of inflammation/infection.
- Consider potential secondary innervations to the area (e.g., mylohyoid nerve in the mandible).
- Use a local anesthetic agent with a higher pH.
- Alkalinize the local anesthetic by adding sodium bicarbonate immediately prior to the injection.*
- Use intravenous sedation or general anesthesia.
- If the infection is minor, consider antibiotics and rescheduling.

*Sodium bicarbonate decreases the acidity of the anesthetic solution and the tissues into which it is injected, providing significantly greater numbers of initial base molecules than were provided in the manufactured solution. Alkalinizing local anesthetics with sodium bicarbonate is difficult and inconvenient when only sterile, sealed cartridges are available. If medical vials of local anesthetics are available, which is more often the case in OMFS, this very effective alteration of the anesthetic's efficacy in inflamed and infected tissues is far easier to accomplish.

A potential complication when injecting into infected tissues is the possibility of *needle tract infection.* Although penetration into infected tissues can be avoided by using more distant regional blocks, when there is any question of a needle passing through infected tissues it should be discarded immediately after use to prevent inadvertent reuse.

Another difficulty that may be seen in inflammation and infection is severe trismus. Trismus has been mentioned previously as a painful condition that impairs the extension of the muscles of mastication leading to decreased ability to fully open the mouth. Limitation in opening can also be seen in posttraumatic situations, as a complication of local anesthetic injections, or with temporomandibular joint problems and ankylosis.

Limited opening can pose anatomic difficulties with standard conventional inferior alveolar block techniques and especially with the Gow-Gates approach, which requires patients to open fully. In situations of severe trismus, an extraoral block or an intraoral high block technique (Vazirani-Akinosi) where the mouth remains closed during its administration is recommended.

Another serious concern with more severe progressive infections, such as Ludwig's angina, is the potential for airway compromise. Management and control of the airway is the first priority in these situations. These patients are typically treated with a general anesthetic in a hospital setting. Prior to induction of general anesthesia, airway management is initiated with conscious fiberoptic intubation or a possible surgical airway. In this setting, supplemental local anesthesia is administered once the airway is secure.

LOCAL ANESTHETIC ALLERGIES

As previously mentioned in Chapter 4, "Pharmacology Basics," and Chapter 8, "Topical Anesthetics," true allergic reactions to amide local anesthetics are rare. Sensitivity to ester-type local anesthetics is more common. Most topical local anesthetics contain the esters benzocaine, butamben, or tetracaine, and similar to amide topicals in multiuse containers, many contain paraben preservatives. In OMFS, cocaine, an ester topical anesthetic, may be used on the nasal mucosa to assist with hemostatic control due to its vasoconstrictive properties.

Latex allergies are becoming more common and should be considered when using local anesthetics. The needle-puncture diaphragm of dental cartridges and multidose vials may contain latex. In latex-allergic patients, a latex-free syringe should be used and the local anesthetic solution should be drawn up from multidose vials only *after* removing the rubber diaphragm. Increasingly, manufacturers are producing anesthetic cartridges and vials with no latex, including the diaphragms. These may be used in place of more cumbersome multidose dispensing techniques.

Documentation of true local anesthetic allergic reactions is based on clinical history (e.g., allergic dermatitis, asthmatic attack, systemic anaphylaxis) and use of intradermal testing with preservative-free local anesthetic solutions without vasoconstrictors by an appropriate healthcare provider. History of hypotension associated with syncope or rapid heart rate after administration of a local anesthetic may be confused with an allergic reaction but is more suggestive of an inadvertent intravascular injection and the associated vasoconstrictor or a psychogenic-vagally mediated reaction. Options for treatment of patients with local anesthetic allergies are provided in Box 20–5.

INFERIOR ALVEOLAR BLOCK COMPLICATIONS AND NERVE INJURIES

One of the most common local anesthetic injections performed by OMF surgeons is the inferior alveolar nerve block. Despite the frequent use of inferior alveolar blocks, they are considered to be one of the more technically difficult injections due to anatomic constraints and variability and there are a number of potential complications. Local complications related to inferior alveolar blocks include vascular, neural, osseous, connective tissue, and muscular injury from needle penetration and deposition of the anesthetic or local hemorrhage. Systemic complications related to inferior alveolar blocks include syncope, hypersensitivity, overdose, toxicity, allergy, and other intravascular anesthetic reactions.

Box 20–5   Options for Treatment of Patients with a True Local Anesthetic Allergy

- Following allergy testing, use an alternate local anesthetic
- 1% Benadryl (Diphenhydramine hydrochloride)
- 0.09% Benzyl alcohol
- General anesthesia

Transient and long-term nerve injuries have been reported related to cranial nerves II–VIII. Adverse neurologic complications affecting local and more distant neurologic tracts have been reported related to inferior alveolar block injections. These neurologic complications include cranial nerve paralysis and anesthesia of cranial nerves II–VIII as well as cervical sympathetic blockade.

One of the most frequent inferior alveolar block neurologic complications is paresthesia of the lingual nerve. Jorgensen and Hayden reported that the lingual nerve does not slide away when encountered by the anesthetic needle because the nerve is attached to the interpterygoid fascia. With the mouth open, this fascia is stretched, holding the lingual nerve in place (Smith & Lung, 2006). Harn and Durham reviewed the incidence of lingual nerve trauma after conventional inferior alveolar block anesthesia in 2289 patients who received 9587 injections (Smith & Lung, 2006). They reported a 3.62% probability of lingual nerve trauma each time a conventional inferior alveolar block is administered, with a 14.99% probability of a post-injection complication after trauma to the lingual nerve. Less commonly reported complications include chorda tympani nerve injury, optic nerve atrophy, and paralysis of cranial nerves III, IV, VI, VII and VIII (Harn & Druham, 1990; Paxton, Hadley, Hadley, Edwards, & Harrison, 1994; Pogrel & Thamby, 2000; and Tomazzoli-Gerosa, Marchini, & Monaco, 1988). Haas and Lennon retrospectively reviewed 143 cases of injection-related mandibular paresthesia in dental patients unrelated to surgery, over a twenty-one-year period. Paresthesia was most often reported after administration of 4 percent local anesthetic agents (articaine or prilocaine). According to Haas, the incidence of permanent paresthesia from all local anesthetics is approximately 1:785,000. The incidence for lower concentrations (0.5%, 2% and 3%) is approximately 1:1,200,000. After administering 4 percent concentrations, it increases to approximately 1:500,000 (Paxton, Hadley, Hadley, Edwards, & Harrison, 1994; Stoelting & Miller (2000); Tomazzoli-Gerosa, Marchini, & Monaco (1988). See Chapter 17, "Local Anesthesia Complications and Management" for a more complete discussion on paresthesia's causes and incidence.

INSIGHTS FROM PERIODONTICS

Comfort is important in both nonsurgical and surgical periodontal procedures. Whenever sensitive teeth are involved or quadrant instrumentation is necessary, local anesthesia may be required in order to perform therapy in comfort.

Mandibular Techniques in Periodontics

In the mandibular arch, anesthesia usually involves nerve block techniques that provide the deepest and most extensive anesthesia using the least amount of local anesthetic drug. While the inferior alveolar nerve block is popular, the Gow-Gates and Vazarani-Akinosi techniques are preferred by some clinicians. The mental incisive nerve block injection can also be delivered effectively for those cases involving only structures anterior to the molars. After administration of a mental incisive block, the lack of lingual anesthesia can be problematic, especially for periodontal procedures. Anesthesia of lingual tissues can be provided by slowly infiltrating the papillary areas (**interpapillary injections**) after facial anesthesia has been established. This approach has the advantage of providing hemostasis (if vasoconstrictors are used) to the anesthetized area and is particularly helpful for procedures such as gingival grafting.

Maxillary Techniques in Periodontics

Unless a division 2 (true maxillary) block is administered, hemi-maxillary anesthesia requires anesthetizing several different nerves. This can be accomplished with a minimal amount of anesthetic and a minimal number of injections. For quadrant anesthesia, the posterior superior alveolar injection can be administered, depositing from 0.9 to 1.8 ml (one-half to one cartridge) depending upon the duration needed. An ASA and MSA, or IO nerve block will complete the anesthesia of the teeth in the quadrant. Palatal tissues must be anesthetized separately using greater palatine and nasopalatine nerve blocks unless an AMSA nerve block is administered.

Anesthesia of the palate is one of the greatest challenges to comfortable administration in periodontal procedures. The AMSA nerve block is particularly useful in these procedures because fewer injections will be necessary in order to provide wide areas of anesthesia, both pulpal and soft tissue. Very slow deposition of local anesthetic solution following good topical anesthesia will effectively anesthetize the palate with an AMSA block on one side to the midline. It is easy to follow the diffusion of the anesthetic solution in the tissues by observing the expanding area of blanching. Whenever additional anesthesia is needed in the palate, inserting the needle within an area of blanching or previous blanching and depositing a small amount of anesthetic slowly, can eliminate discomfort. The AMSA injection has the advantage of anesthetizing not only the palate but also the facial gingiva, from the premolars to the midline in addition to the pulps of the teeth in the area. To accomplish this, usually no more than two-thirds to three-quarters of a cartridge is necessary.

Hemostasis in Periodontics

Hemostasis is an important consideration in periodontal surgery where visualization of exposed defects is critical to their correction. Control of bleeding can usually be accomplished with anesthetic solutions containing no more than 1:100,000 epinephrine or 1:20,000 levonordefrin. The use of 1:50,000 epinephrine solutions may be useful at times for hemostasis in periodontal surgery, particularly in palatal infiltrations. For the majority of procedures, however, this higher concentration of vasoconstrictor increases risk without providing significant benefit.

INSIGHTS FROM ENDODONTICS

Many patients who require root canal therapy present with pain and swelling, an environment in which anesthetics are not as effective as they are in healthy, noninfected tissue. Nerve blocks in these circumstances have been more effective at providing profound anesthesia compared with infiltrations, but neither is always able to provide reliable profound anesthesia for root canal therapy which, as a consequence, has developed a very painful reputation.

The Use of Anesthetics in Endodontics

The introduction of articaine has decreased the incidence of pain in endodontics to some extent. Due to its presumed ability to penetrate efficiently through bone, at times mandibular teeth can be adequately anesthetized by infiltration (Dudkiewicz, Schwartz, & Laliberte, 1987; Kanaa, Whitworth, Corbett, & Meechan, 2006). While IA blocks are controversial with articaine, Gow-Gates and Vazirani-Akinosi blocks are not known to involve increased risks of paresthesia with articaine and can be performed when articaine is preferred (Hawkins, 2006). Lidocaine and mepivacaine are both quite effective, as well. In the maxilla, infiltrations with articaine sometimes anesthetize the entire tooth including the palatal roots of the molars without administering separate palatal injections (Kanaa et al., 2006; Vree & Gielen, 2005).

Topical Anesthetics in Endodontics

Topical anesthetics are placed at penetration sites to prevent pain during penetrations with needles. They are also useful, for example, on palatal gingiva to ease rubber dam clamp placement. Some topicals, such as lidocaine, prilocaine, and benzocaine, when combined with tetracaine, are particularly effective. Tetracaine has a long duration of action but a slow onset, which is augmented by the faster onsets of other topicals such as lidocaine, prilocaine, and benzocaine. Due to tetracaine's lengthy biotransformation, the observance of maximum recommended dosing is critical. Some products containing tetracaine are very effective at providing deep topical anesthesia. At times, they can even preclude the need for pre-anesthesia using injections.

Managing Fear in Endodontics

Due to its painful reputation, ordinary levels of dental fear are magnified when the term *root canal* is mentioned. Anxiety can intensify typical levels of fear, particularly of injections. It is important to take a few minutes to address this fear, which can have at least two major benefits, easing patient anxiety and increasing the success of local anesthesia. It is also important to avoid criticism of neglect, including the length of time since the last appointment. Instead, patients should be warmly encouraged and praised for investing in their oral health and for keeping their appointments.

Intraosseous Injections in Endodontics

Intraosseous injections provide immediate and predictable profound anesthesia. They can benefit any procedure in which anesthesia has been inadequate, but are particularly beneficial in endodontics when there is considerable inflammation and infection present in the tissues surrounding a tooth.

Solution is deposited into cancellous bone spaces surrounding a tooth. In order to reach cancellous bone, four layers must be penetrated: epithelium and its underlying connective tissue, periosteum, and cortical bone. Pre-anesthesia will desensitize the epithelial layer and its underlying connective tissue as well as the periosteum surrounding the bone. Cortical bone lacks sensory innervaton and can be perforated painlessly once the other layers are anesthetized.

There are three essential steps when administering intraosseous injections, anesthetizing the attached gingiva, perforating the cortical plate, and depositing anesthetic into cancellous bone around the tooth. For many years this was accomplished, exclusively, by using a surgical round bur to perforate the cortical plate. The difficulty with this approach is that it is necessary to renegotiate the perforation with the needle once the bur has been withdrawn from the tissues. Those with more experience do not find this to be particularly challenging.

Commercial products known as the **Stabident** and **X-Tip** have guide sleeves that remain in place after perforation, and direct needles into the perforations. One system, the **IntraFlow** device, does not require withdrawal after perforation. These systems are discussed and demonstrated in Chapter 15, "Injections for Supplemental Pain Control." Anesthetic solution is deposited immediately on perforation of the cortical plate. While some clinicians prefer round bur perforation, these innovative systems are much easier for novices to master.

Before discussing the intraosseous technique, it is important to comment on the benefit of preprocedural radiographs. These provide accurate assessments of the spacing between adjacent roots in the identified area, assuring that the spacing between roots is adequate. If the roots are too close together, another site must be chosen, one or two teeth distal or mesial to the tooth that is to be treated, in order to avoid damage when perforating.

Intraosseous Technique

Begin by imagining a horizontal line along the gingival margins of the teeth in the area and a vertical line through the interdental papilla. A point about 2 mm apical to the intersection of these lines is usually a suitable site for a lateral perforation. This has been previously described as being located just barely within the most apical portion of the attached gingiva. It is more successful to inject distal rather than mesial to the tooth to be anesthetized. In most cases, a mesial injection will provide adequate anesthesia, however.

It is very important to use a gentle "pecking" motion versus a long, continuous movement while penetrating in order to avoid overheating the cortical bone (Malamed, 2004). Overheating can result in postoperative soreness and potential infection of the bone and overlying gingiva (Malamed, 2004).

If using a round bur for perforation, hold the syringe in a "pen-grip" manner and angle the needle in the direction in which the bur was withdrawn from the bone. The injection needle should be allowed to engage the cortical bone with only very light pressure to avoid "digging" into it (binding) or bending. If the needle does not pass through the perforation easily, a modified injection needle may be used. This needle has a flattened tip, which is quite effective since no sharp bevel is necessary in intraosseous techniques that by necessity have preperforated pathways of insertion. The lack of a bevel minimizes binding of the needle tip in bone.

If using the guide sleeve provided with the Stabident and X-Tip systems, gently insert the injection-needle into the predrilled channel. If using the Intra-Flow, the perforator retracts and the needle is inserted without moving the device from the perforation.

One-third of a cartridge (0.6 ml) of solution should be slowly deposited (0.6 ml over 60 seconds) into the cancellous bone. Diffusion through bone is efficient but not rapid. Slow deposition is mandatory to allow for easy diffusion and to avoid discomfort at the time and postoperatively. Vasoconstrictors should be avoided or minimized. Studies have demonstrated that the CVS effects of vasoconstrictors in intraosseous techniques are immediate and pervasive. If necessary, dilutions of 1:200,000 epinephrine should be used. When using vasoconstrictors, patients should be warned to expect temporary rapid heartbeats, which will pass quickly. Plain solutions can be used and will not produce these effects but will also have shorter durations.

The duration of anesthesia with intraosseous injections is short. Typical pulpal durations range from 15 to 30 minutes (Malamed, 2004). Durations will vary depending on the specific drug, the presence or absence of a vasoconstrictor, and individual metabolism. If sensitivity returns before procedures have been completed, a small volume of anesthetic can be deposited after renegotiating the perforation (0.4 ml).

Most patients will have little to no postoperative symptomatology, including pain. In rare cases (less than 5 percent), patients may experience localized swelling with or without infection, which heals uneventfully or occasionally requires antibiotics.

Intrapulpal Injections in Endodontics

The **intrapulpal injection** is used exclusively in endodontics (Malamed, 2004). This injection is administered when patients feel discomfort when the pulp is invaded by a bur or instrument despite the presence of otherwise profound anesthesia. It can be administered only *after* access to the pulp has been made. To ensure good back pressure and complete anesthesia, the initial opening into the pulp chamber must be very small. This is ideally no larger than the size of a one-half round bur or a 330 pear-shaped bur. The initial opening should be directed toward the largest canal in the tooth, which is the distal canal on lower molars and the palatal canal on upper molars. Once the needle has been inserted into the opening, one-half to one full cartridge of anesthetic (0.9 to 1.8 ml) is administered slowly. The choice of drug is not important because it is primarily the pressure of the injection that provides the anesthetic effect.

Additional technique considerations for these injections can be found in Chapter 15.

CHAPTER QUESTIONS

1. Which *one* of the following methods of adjusting doses of local anesthetic drugs for children is recommended in this chapter?
   a. Clark's rule
   b. The Rule of Inference
   c. Young's rule
   d. Heuristic rule

2. Specific challenges in oral and maxillofacial local anesthesia include all of the following, *except*:
   a. Frequent management of oral infections, some of which are life threatening.
   b. Limiting the potential for needle tract infections.
   c. Achieving adequate local anesthesia in the presence of these infections.
   d. All of the above.

3. Which *one* of the following is not a local anesthesia consideration in oral and maxillofacial surgery when treating an infected patient?
   a. Use a greater amount of local anesthetic to help overcome acidity created by the infection. (Make sure that maximum doses are not exceeded.)
   b. Use a regional nerve block away from the area of inflammation.
   c. Use a local anesthetic agent with a lower pH.
   d. Discard the needle after injecting in or near an area of inflammation/infection.

4. Which *one* of the following is *not* an adverse event following local anesthetic injections?
   a. Trismus
   b. Normal durations of numbness
   c. Postoperative soreness
   d. Infection

5. Which *one* of the following is not an option for treatment of patients with true local anesthetic allergies?
   a. Use of an alternate local anesthetic
   b. 1% Benadryl (diphenhydramine hydrochloride)
   c. 0.09% benzyl alcohol
   d. 0.1% sodium benzoate

6. Systemic complications related to inferior alveolar block include all of the following *except*:
   a. Hematomas.
   b. Syncope.
   c. Overdose reactions.
   d. Allergic reactions.

REFERENCES

Bartfield, J. M., Weeks, S., & Raccio-Robak, N. (1998). Randomized trial of diphenhydramine versus benzyl alcohol with epinephrine as an alternate to lidocaine local anesthesia. *Annals of Emergency Medicine, 32,* 650–654.

Dudkiewicz, A., Schwartz, S., & Laliberte, R. (1987). Effectiveness of mandibular infiltration in children using the local anesthetic Ultracaine (articaine hydrochloride). *Journal of the Canadian Dental Association, 53,* 29–31.

Fish, L. R., McIntire, D. N., & Johnson, L. (1989). Temporary paralysis of CN III, IV, and VI after a Gow-Gates injection. *Journal of the American Dental Association, 119*(1), 127–130.

Gray, R. L. M. (1978). Peripheral facial nerve paralysis of dental origin. *British Journal of Oral Surgery, 16*(2), 143–150.

Haas, D. A. (2003, June). Personal communication.

Haas, D. A. (2006). Articaine and paresthesia: Epidemiologic studies. *Journal of the American College of Dentistry, 73*(3), 5–10.

Haas, D. A., & Lennon, D. (1995). A 21 year retrospective study of reports of paresthesia following local anesthetic administration. *Journal of the Canadian Dental Association, 61*(4), 319–330.

Haas, D. A., & Lennon, D. (1995). Local anesthetic use by dentists in Ontario. *Journal of the Canadian Dental Association,* 61(4), 297–304.

Hamburg, H. L. (1972). Preliminary study of patient reaction to needle gauge. *New York State Dental Journal, 38,* 425–426.

Harn, S. D., & Durham, T. (1990). Incidence of lingual nerve trauma and post injection complications in conventional mandibular block anesthesia. *Journal of the American Dental Association, 121*(10), 519–523.

Hawkins, M. Local Anesthesia: Technique and pharmacology, problems and solutions. ADA Annual Session, October, 16, 2006. Las Vegas, NV.

Jorgensen, N. B., & Hayden, J. (1980, February). Sedation, local and general anesthesia in dentistry. Philadelphia: Lea & Febiger.

Kanaa, M. D., Whitworth, J. M., Corbett, I. P., & Meechan, J. G. (2006). Articaine and lidocaine mandibular buccal infiltration anesthesia: a prospective randomized double-blind cross-over study. *Journal of Endodontics, 32,* 296–298.

Maestrello, C. L., Abubaker, A. O., & Benson, K. J. (2007). Local anesthetics. In A. O. Abubaker & K. J. Benson (Eds.), *Oral and maxillofacial surgery secrets* (2nd ed.). St. Louis: Mosby.

Malamed, S. F. (2004). Local anesthetic considerations in dental specialties. In S. F. Malamed (Ed.), *Handbook of Local Anesthesia* (5th ed.). St. Louis: Mosby.

Paxton, M. C., Hadley, J. N., Hadley, M. N., Edwards, R. C., & Harrison, S. J. (1994). Chorda tympani nerve injury following inferior alveolar injection: A review of two cases. *Journal of the American Dental Association, 125,* 1003–1006.

Pogrel, M. A., & Thamby, S. (2000). Permanent nerve involvement resulting from inferior alveolar nerve blocks. *Journal of the American Dental Association, 131,* 901–907.

Smith, M. H., & Lung, K. E. (2006). Nerve injuries after dental injection: A review of the literature. *Journal of the Canadian Dental Association,* 72(6), 559–564.

Stoelting, R. R., & Miller, R. D. (2000). Local anestethics. In R. R. Stoelting & R. D. Miller (Eds.), *Basics of anesthesia* (4th ed.). New York: Churchill Livingstone.

Tomazzoli-Gerosa, L., Marchini, G., & Monaco, A. (1988). Amaurosis and atrophy of the optic nerve: An unusual complication of mandibular-nerve anesthesia. *Annals of Ophthalmology, 20,* 170–171.

Vree, T. B., & Gielen, M. J. (2005). Clinical pharmacology and the use of articaine for local and regional anaesthesia. *Best Practice & Research Clinical Anaesthesiology, 19,* 293–308.

Introductory Anatomy Review

ANATOMICAL REVIEW

The following information is intended only as a review of head and neck anatomy with an emphasis on local anesthetic injections. This review assumes that clinicians have at least a basic knowledge of head and neck anatomy. Specific discussions relevant to individual injection techniques are presented in the following chapters:

Chapter 12–Injections for Maxillary Pain Control

Chapter 13–Injections for Palatal Pain Control

Chapter 14–Injections for Mandibular Pain Control

In order to gain the greatest benefit from this appendix, it is helpful to refer to a skull as well as a head and neck anatomy text while referencing it. Before reviewing the anatomy of the head and neck, a summary overview of the tables and figures included in this section is provided.

OVERVIEW SUMMARY

Table AR–1: Bones of the Skull
Figure AR–1—Frontal view
Figure AR–2—Lateral view
Figure AR–3—Posterior view
Table AR–2: Basilar View of the Skull—Foramina, fissures, canals, and anatomical structures
Table AR–3: Basilar View of the Skull—Processes, plates, arches, and fossae
Table AR–4: Intracranial View of the Skull (upper portion of skull removed)—Bones, fissures, and foramina
Figure AR–4—Foramina, fissures, canals, and anatomical structures

Figure AR–5—Processes, plates, arches, and fossae
Figure AR–6—Bones, fissures, and foramina
Table AR–5: Maxillary and Palatine Bony Views—Frontal, lateral, and palatal views
Figure AR–7—Features of the maxilla from a frontal view
Figure AR–8—Features of the maxilla from a lateral view
Figure AR–9—Features of the maxillary and palatal bones from a palatal view
Table AR–6: Mandibular Views—Frontal, lateral, and internal views
Figure AR–10—Anatomical features of the mandible from a frontal view
Figure AR–11—Features of the mandible from a lateral view
Figure AR–12—Features of the mandible from an internal view
Table AR–7: Muscles of Facial Expression—origin, insertion, and function
Figure AR–13—Muscles of facial expression
Table AR–8: Muscles of Mastication—Origin, insertion, and function
Figure AR–14—Muscles of Mastication from a lateral view—superficial muscles
Figure AR–15—Muscles of Mastication from a lateral view—deep muscles
Figure AR–16—Ligaments from a medial view
Table AR–9: Ligaments—Origin, insertion, and function
Table AR–10: External Carotid Artery Branches (ECA)—External carotid artery branches

Table AR–1	**Bones of the Skull**
Cranium *(8 bones total)*	*Face* *(14 bones total)*
Frontal (1)	Nasal (2)
Parietal (2)	Lacrimal (2)
Temporal (2)	Maxilla (2)
Ethmoid (1)	Zygomatic (2)
Sphenoid (1)	Vomer (1)
Occipital (1)	Palatal (2)
	Inferior nasal concha (2)
	Mandible (1)

Throughout this review, the * symbol designates structures not illustrated on the associated figure.

OSSEOUS REVIEW

The skull consists of twenty-two bones (not including the three small bones within the ear). Some are paired bilaterally and others are single. All but one of the skull bones articulate with one another by means of sutures composed of fibrous connective tissue. Sutures initially allow for growth and expansion of skull bones. Later, after growth has ceased, they are considered nonmoveable except when subjected to traumatic force. The only *moveable* joints of the skull are the temporomandibular joints, which articulate the mandible and the temporal bones.

The skull can be reviewed by identifying bones and landmarks from all anatomical positions, including the intracranial surface. Many of these landmarks are important to the study of local anesthesia.

Cranial and Facial Bones

Cranial bones protect and support the brain while facial bones form the framework of the face and protect the underlying viscera. These two general bony features of the skull, cranial and facial, will be considered in separate discussions. Many of the bones can be identified from external, basilar, and intracranial views.

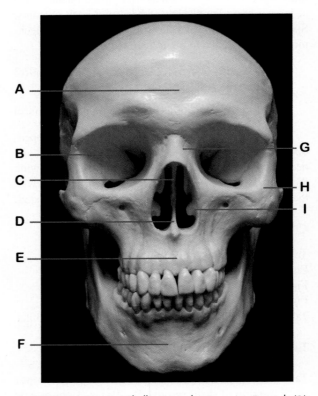

■ **FIGURE AR–1** Skull—Frontal View A—Frontal (1), B—Sphenoid (1), C—Ethmoid (1), D—Vomer (1), E—Maxilla (2), F—Mandible, (1), G—Nasal (2), H—Zygomatic (2), I—Inferior Nasal Concha (2)

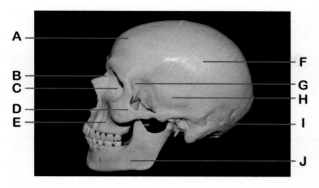

■ **FIGURE AR–2** Skull—Lateral View A—Frontal (1), B—Nasal (2), C—Lacrimal (2), D—Zygomatic (1), E—Maxilla (2), F—Parietal (2), G—Sphenoid (2), H—Temporal (1), I—Occipital (1), J—Mandible (1)

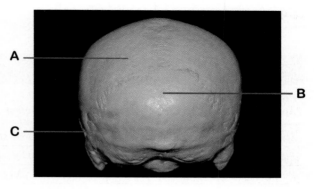

■ **FIGURE AR–3** Skull—Posterior View A—Parietal (2), B—Occipital (1), C—Temporal (2)

Table AR–2	Basilar View of the Skull	
Foramina, Fissures, Canals	**Structures / Function / Content**	
Foramen magnum	Nerve:	Spinal roots of spinal accessory nerve
	Artery:	Vertebral
	Other:	Medulla oblongata
Stylomastoid foramen	Nerve:	Facial
	Artery:	Stylomastoid
Jugular foramen	Nerve:	Glossopharyngeal, vagus, spinal accessory
	Artery:	Meningeal branches
	Sinus:	Inferior petrosal, sigmoid (origin of internal jugular vein)
Carotid canal	Nerve:	Internal carotid plexus
	Artery:	Internal carotid
Foramen lacerum	Nerve:	None
	Artery:	None
	Other:	Fibrocartilage in vivo
Foramen spinosum	Nerve:	Meningeal branch of the trigeminal nerve, mandibular division
	Artery:	Middle meningeal
Foramen ovale	Nerve:	Mandibular division of the trigeminal nerve and the lesser petrosal
	Artery:	Accessory meningeal
	Vein:	Emissary
Lesser palatine foramen	Nerve:	Lesser and middle palatine
	Artery:	Lesser and middle palatine
	Vein:	Lesser and middle palatine
Greater palatine foramen	Nerve:	Greater palatine
	Artery:	Greater palatine
	Vein:	Greater palatine
Incisive foramen	Nerve:	Nasopalatine nerve
	Artery:	Sphenopalatine branches

Table AR-3 Basilar View of the Skull

Processes, Plates, Arches, Fossae	Structures / Function / Content	
Styloid process	Attachments:	Stylohyoid, stylomandibular ligaments, styloglossus, stylopharyngeus muscles
Pterygoid process		Formed by lateral and medial pterygoid plates
Pterygoid fossa	Attachments:	Medial pterygoid, tensor palatini muscles
Hamulus		Provides support for movement of tendon of tensor veli palatini muscle
Zygomatic arch	Attachments:	Muscles of facial expression
Infratemporal fossa	Nerves:	Mandibular, inferior alveolar, chorda tympani branch of the facial, and lesser petrosal, and the otic ganglion
	Arteries:	Maxillary, middle meningeal, inferior alveolar, posterior superior alveolar
	Veins:	Pterygoid plexus
	Muscles:	Temporalis, lateral & medial pterygoid
Pterygopalatine fossa	Nerves:	Maxillary nerve division of the trigeminal, posterior superior alveolar, zygomatic, and pterygopalatine ganglion
	Arteries:	Maxillary, infraorbital, descending palatine
	Veins:	Pterygoid canal, pharyngeal, spenopalatine posterior superior alveolar, pharyngeal, descending palatine, infraorbital, sphenopalatine, pterygoid canal, inferior ophthalmic

Table AR-4 Intracranial View of the Skull

Fissures and Foramina	Structures / Function / Content	
Foramen magnum	Nerve:	Spinal roots of spinal accessory nerve
	Artery:	Vertebral
	Other:	Medulla oblongata
Jugular foramen	Nerve:	Glossopharyngeal, vagus, spinal accessory
	Artery:	Meningeal branches
	Sinus:	Inferior petrosal, sigmoid (origin of internal jugular vein)
Carotid canal	Nerve:	Internal carotid plexus
	Artery:	Internal carotid
Foramen spinosum	Nerve:	Branch of the mandibular division of the trigeminal
	Artery:	Middle meningeal
Foramen ovale	Nerve:	Lesser petrosal of the mandibular division of the trigeminal
	Artery:	Accessory meningeal
	Vein:	Emissary
Foramen rotundum	Nerve:	Maxillary division of the trigeminal
Superior orbital fissure	Nerve:	Oculomotor, trochlear, abducens, ophthalmic division of the trigeminal, ophthalmic (arising from the frontal, lacrimal, & nasociliary nerves)
	Vein:	Ophthalmic

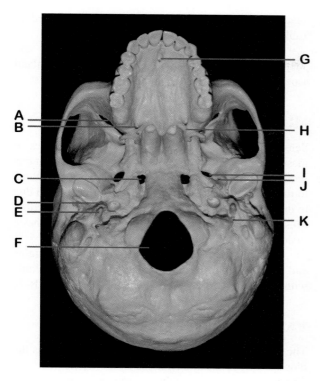

■ **FIGURE AR-4** Skull—Basilar View—Foramina A—Pterygomaxillary Fissure, B—Greater Palatine Foramen, C—Foramen Lacerum, D—Carotid Canal, E—Jugular Foramen, F—Foramen Magnum, G—Incisive Foramen, H—Lesser Palatine Foramen, I—Foramen Ovale, J—Foramen Spinosum, K—Stylomastoid Foramen

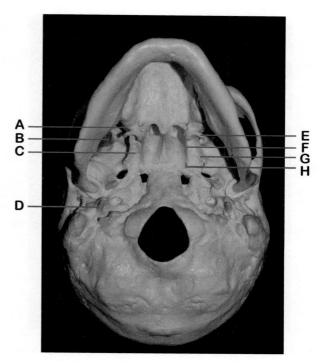

See enlarged region below.

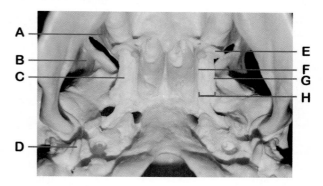

■ **FIGURE AR-5** Skull—Basilar View—Processes, Plates, Arches, Fossa A—Pterygopalatine Fossa, B—Infratemporal Fossa, C—Pterygoid Fossa, D—Styloid Process, E—Hamulus Process, F—Medial Pterygoid Plate, G—Lateral Pterygoid Plate, H—Pterygoid Process

Maxilla and Mandible

There are numerous anatomical features to review on maxillary and palatine bones, and on mandibles, relevant to the administration of local anesthesia. The locations of these features follow anatomic patterns that are similar on different skulls; however, there are occasional and sometimes significant variations in these patterns. For this reason, when studying anatomy for local anesthesia it can be useful to view several different skulls noting similarities and differences among individuals.

The mandible is the largest and strongest facial bone due to the density of its cortical plate. Maxillary and palatine bones typically have thinner cortical plates and are relatively more porous. The significance of the respective thicknesses of their cortical plates has a bearing on local anesthesia. Anesthetic drugs diffuse more readily through the maxilla compared with the mandible. Solutions for mandibular anesthesia typically have to be deposited directly over nerves *before* they enter bone in order to be reliably effective. Suggested

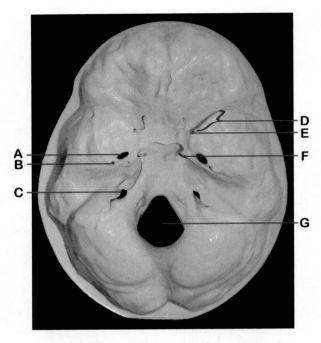

■ **FIGURE AR–6** Skull–Intracranial View A—Foramen Ovale, B—Foramen Spinosum, C—Jugular Foramen, D—Superior Orbital Fissure, E—Foramen Rotundum, F—Carotid Canal, G—Foramen Magnum

anatomical features to locate on skulls are listed in Tables AR–5 through AR–12.

Table AR–5 reviews features of maxillary and palatine bones viewed from frontal, lateral, and palatal aspects.

MUSCLE AND LIGAMENT REVIEW

Selected muscles of facial expression, the muscles of mastication, and two ligaments will be identified in this section. These muscles and ligaments are important due to their locations in or near injection pathways and due to the effects of local anesthetic drugs on their function. Muscles, themselves, are infrequent targets of anesthesia in dentistry. See Figures AR–13–AR–16.

Clinicians are encouraged to identify the origins and insertions of muscles on skulls and to use skulls with attached muscles when available. See Table AR–8.

VASCULAR REVIEW

The vascular system of the head may be defined as the blood supply to the brain and the extracranial structures. This vascular network includes arteries, veins, and capillaries that are mirrored on the right and left sides of the

Table AR–5   Maxillary and Palatine Bony Views

Frontal	Lateral	Basilar
Alveolar process Eminence • canine eminence Canine fossa Zygomatic process Infraorbital foramen (infraorbital nerve, artery, vein)	Zygomatic arch Maxillary tuberosity • posterior superior alveolar foramina Inferior temporal fossa Pterygopalatine fossa Pterygomaxillary fissure (maxillary nerve and maxillary artery)	Maxillary bones • horizontal plate • alveolar process • incisive foramen Palatine bones • greater palatine foramina • lesser palatine foramina Median palatal suture Transverse suture Pterygoid process • lateral pterygoid plate • medial pterygoid plate • pterygoid fossa

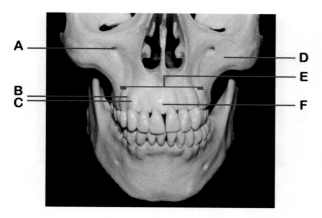

■ **FIGURE AR–7** Skull—Frontal View—Maxilla A—Infraorbital foramen, B—Canine fossa, C—Canine eminence, D—Zygomatic process of the maxilla, E—Alveolar process, F—Eminence

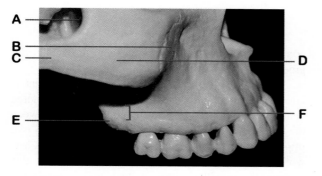

■ **FIGURE AR–8** Skull—Lateral View—Maxilla A—Pterygomaxillary Fissure, B—Zygomatic Process of Maxilla, C—Zygomatic Process of Temporal, D—Zygomatic, E—Maxillary Tuberosity, F—Posterior Superior Alveolar Foramina

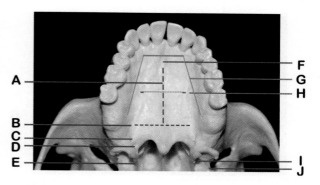

■ **FIGURE AR–9** Skull–Palatal View—Maxilla and Palate A—Medial Palatine Suture, B—Transverse Palatine Suture, C—Greater Palatine Foramen, D—Lesser Palatine Foramen, E—Medial Pterygoid Plate, F—Incisive Foramen, G—Alveolar Process, H—Horizontal Plate of Maxilla, I—Pterygoid Palatine Fossa, J—Lateral Pterygoid Plate

head. As in other parts of the body, many arteries and veins share common names, especially those that travel similar pathways and are deeply protected within tissue. Blood vessels are interconnected by what are known as anastomoses, or openings, from one vessel into another.

External Carotid Artery (ECA)

The external carotid is a large, extracranial artery that is the most important vessel when considering dental local anesthesia. The ECA branches from the common carotid artery at the superior border of thyroid cartilage. It travels upward and medial to the internal carotid, dividing into four major segments, the anterior, medial, posterior, and terminal branches. These branches are listed in

Table AR–6 **Mandibular Views**		
Frontal	*Lateral*	*Internal*
Body of mandible	Angle of mandible	Ramus of mandible
• alveolar process and teeth	Ramus of the mandible	• lingual
• mental protuberance	• condylar neck	• mandibular foramen (inferior alveolar nerve, artery, and vein)
• mental foramen (mental nerve, artery and vein)	• condylar head	• pterygoid fovea
	• coronoid process	• retromolar triangle
	• mandibular notch (sigmoid notch)	• internal oblique line
	• external oblique line	• mylohyoid groove
	• coronoid notch (anterior border of the ramus)	• mylohyoid line

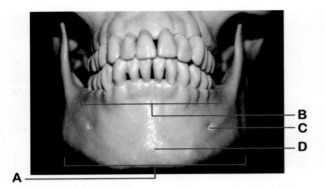

■ **FIGURE AR-10** Skull—Frontal View—Mandible A—Body of Mandible, B—Alveolar Process, C—Mental Foramen, D—Mental Protuberance

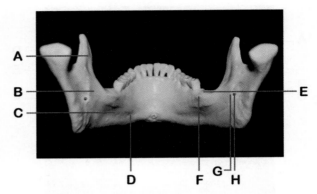

■ **FIGURE AR-12** Skull—Medial View—Mandible A—Pterygoid Fovea, B—Ramus of Mandible, C—Mylohyoid Groove, D—Mylohyoid Line, E—Retromolar Triangle, F—Internal Oblique Line, G—Lingula, H—Mandibular Foramen

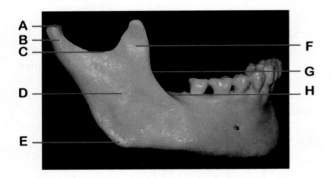

■ **FIGURE AR-11** Skull—Lateral View—Mandible A—Condylar Head, B—Mandibular Notch (sigmoid notch), C—Condylar Neck, D—Ramus of the Mandible, E—Angle of Mandible, F—Coronoid Process, G—Coronoid Notch (anterior border of the ramus), H—External Oblique Line

Table A–10. Major areas of distribution are included for arteries with significance to dentistry. See Figure AR–17.

Venous Drainage

The venous blood system begins at the capillary networks. Capillaries connect with small veins, or venules. As the volume of deoxygenated blood accumulates, venules empty blood into larger veins, which typically follow similar pathways on the right and left sides of the head. These pathways are more variable compared with arterial pathways due to the greater degree of anastomosis in veins compared to arteries.

In some areas, networks of veins form what is known as a venous plexus. The pterygoid plexus is a large venous plexus located in the infratemporal fossa between the temporalis and lateral pterygoid muscles. It has two important functions. It serves as part of the venous network returning deoxygenated blood to the heart. It also protects the maxillary artery (which travels inside the plexus in the area) by filling or emptying with blood as needed, during jaw movements. While not a function, the plexus is also important in local anesthesia due to the increased risk of bleeding if it is pierced during injection.

Venous blood from the brain or cranial cavity can collect amid epithelial-lined spaces such as between the endosteal and meningeal layers of the dura mater. These areas are called venous sinuses. From sinuses, venous blood drains into nearby veins. These veins are called emissary veins which, unlike most veins in the body, have no valves. Without valves, blood flow is under greater influence of local pressure changes. These changes can cause a two-way flow of blood, including through veins back into the sinuses. If an infection is present, it can spread via the emissary veins through the sinuses and from there into the brain.

Venous blood from intracranial structures and from deep structures of the face and neck drain into the

Table AR–7   Muscles of Facial Expression

Muscle	Origin	Insertion	Function
Buccinator	Maxillary/mandibular molar area of alveolar processes; pterygomandibular raphe	Angles of mouth	Chewing; blowing air out of mouth
Depressor anguli oris	External oblique line on ramus	Angle of mouth	Lowers skin tissues of lower jaw; frowning
Depressor labii inferioris	External oblique line on ramus	Skin of lower lip	Lowers and draws lower lip laterally
Levator anguli oris	Canine fossa below infraorbital foramen	Angles of mouth	Raises skin tissue from angles of mouth; smiling
Levator labii superioris	Orbit of eye, lower margin above infraorbital foramen	Upper lip	Raises facial skin above upper lip
Levator labii superioris alaeque nasi	Maxillae upper frontal process	Upper lip and lateral of nostrils	Raises upper lip; opens nostrils
Mentalis	Mental protuberance	Skin of chin	Protrudes lower lip; raises skin of chin
Orbicularis oculi	Orbital rim; frontal processes of maxillae; nasal process of frontal	Skin lateral of orbit; circle around orbit	Closes eyelids; squinting
Orbicularis oris	Circles mouth	Angles of mouth	Lips close; lips pucker
Platysma	Skin above clavicle and shoulder	Lower border of mandible and muscles around mouth	Lowers angles of mouth; raises skin of neck
Risorius	Fascia of masseter	Orbicularis oris; skin at angle of mouth	Draws angle of mouth laterally
Zygomaticus major	Zygomatic bone	Angle of mouth	Raises angle of mouth; smiling
Zygomaticus minor	Zygomatic bone	Upper lip	Raises upper lip

internal jugular vein. The external and anterior jugular veins drain superficial structures of the head and neck. From these veins blood flows into the brachiocephalic veins, then into the subclavian veins. The right and left subclavians join, forming the superior vena cava, which conducts blood flow into the right atrium of the heart. See Table AR–11 and Figure AR–18.

NERVE REVIEW

The target nerves of most dental local anesthetic injections are branches of the trigeminal nerve.

A comprehensive knowledge of the trigeminal nerve is essential to performing dental local anesthetic techniques. In addition to target nerves, branches of the facial nerve are sometimes inadvertently anesthetized due to their close approximation to trigeminal branches within oral and facial tissues. In all cases, nerve pathways can vary and their variations can significantly affect the success of anesthesia. In order to understand typical nerve branch patterns, skulls with attached nerves can be helpful.

Suggested anatomical features to locate on skulls are listed in the tables in this section.

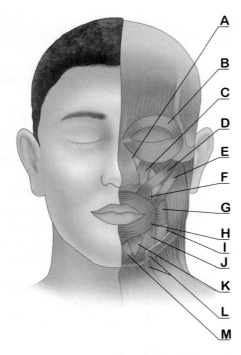

■ **FIGURE AR-13** Muscles of Facial Expression A—Levator Labii Superioris Alaeque Nasi, B—Orbicularis Oculi, C—Levator Labii Superioris, D—Zygomaticus Minor, E—Zygomaticus Major, F—Levator Anguli Oris, G—Buccinator, H—Orbicularis Oris, I—Risorius (cut away), J—Depressor Anguli Oris, K—Depressor Labii Inferioris, L—Platysma (cut away), M—Mentalis

Trigeminal Nerve

The trigeminal nerves are the largest of the cranial nerves. Similar innervation patterns are seen on both the right and left sides of the face. They have afferent or sensory nerve roots that convey information about touch, temperature, pain, and proprioception from the scalp, face, oral cavity, tongue and teeth, and a smaller efferent or motor nerve root that provides innervation mainly to the muscles of mastication.

Sensory nerves travel to each trigeminal ganglion located on the anterior aspect of the petrous portion of the temporal bone. Beyond the ganglion, sensory nerve fibers continue into the mid-lateral section of the pons in the brainstem.

Motor roots of the right and left mandibular divisions form in the pons and medulla. They travel in separate locations from sensory nerves, in a lateral and inferior direction to the trigeminal ganglion before exiting the skull through the foramen ovale and joining the sensory roots of the mandibular division.

The three divisions of the trigeminal are the ophthalmic (V_1), maxillary (V_2), and mandibular (V_3) nerves. All three divisions pass through openings in the sphenoid bone. The ophthalmic nerve passes through the superior orbital fissure. The maxillary nerve passes through the foramen rotundum. The mandibular nerve passes through the foramen ovale.

Table AR–8   Muscles of Mastication

Muscle	Origin	Insertion	Function
Masseter— *Superficial head*	Anterior 2/3 of inferior border of zygomatic arch	Lateral surface angle of mandible	Elevates (closes) mandible
Masseter— *deep head**	Posterior 1/3 and medial surface of zygomatic arch	Lateral surface above angle of mandible	Elevates (closes) mandible
Lateral pterygoid— *superior head*	Inferior surface of greater wing of sphenoid	Pterygoid fovea under the condyloid process; fibrous capsule of TMJ	Lowers (opens) mandible; lateral movement of mandible; protrusion of mandible
Lateral pterygoid— *inferior head*	Lateral surface of lateral pterygoid plate	Pterygoid fovea under the condyloid process; fibrous capsule of TMJ	Lowers (opens) mandible; lateral movement of mandible; protrusion of mandible
Medial pterygoid	Medial surface of lateral pterygoid plate; pterygoid fossa	Medial surface angle of mandible	Elevates (closes) mandible
Temporalis	Temporal fossa	Coronoid process of mandible	Elevates (closes) mandible; posterior portion retracts mandible

*Not illustrated.

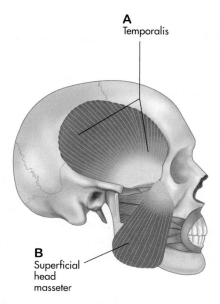

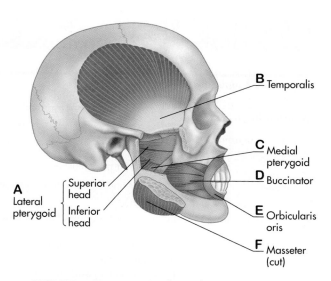

■ **FIGURE AR-14** Muscles of Mastication—Lateral View—Superficial Muscles A—Temporalis, B—Masseter Superficial Head

■ **FIGURE AR-15** Muscles of Mastication—Lateral View—Deep Muscles A—Lateral Pterygoid, Superior Head and Inferior Head, B—Temporalis, C—Medial Pterygoid, D—Buccinator, E—Orbicularis Oris, F—Masseter (superficial head cut away)

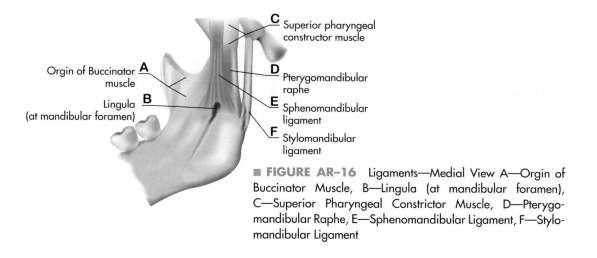

■ **FIGURE AR-16** Ligaments—Medial View A—Orgin of Buccinator Muscle, B—Lingula (at mandibular foramen), C—Superior Pharyngeal Constrictor Muscle, D—Pterygomandibular Raphe, E—Sphenomandibular Ligament, F—Stylomandibular Ligament

Table AR–9	Ligaments		
Ligament	*Origin*	*Insertion*	*Function*
Pterygomandibular raphe	Pterygoid hamulus	Posterior of mylohyoid line	Connects superior pharyngeal constrictor muscle and posterior buccinator muscle fibers
Sphenomandibular ligament	Spine of sphenoid bone	Lingula	Limits distension of mandible in an inferior direction

Table AR–10 External Carotid Artery Branches (ECA)

Artery	Distribution Areas	Pathway
Superficial temporal	Side of head Parotid gland	Posterior to neck of mandible Superior as a terminal branch of ECA
Anterior branches (3):		
• Superior thyroid	Thyroid gland Larynx Some anterior neck muscles	Inferior from ECA
• Lingual	Soft tissues under tongue to hyoid bone and tongue	Lower posterior border of mandible, forms multiple branches that travel inferiorly
• Facial	Skin and muscles of lips, cheeks, nose, around eye Soft palate, palatine muscles, palatine tonsils Submandibular lymph nodes and salivary glands Mylohyoid and digastric muscles	Anterior and medial to ramus, superior to submandibular saliva gland, Crosses under border of mandible, forms multiple branches, which travel superiorly
Middle branch* • Ascending pharyngeal	Wall of pharynx, soft palate, meninges, posterior cranial fossa and many cranial nerves	Ascends vertically deep in neck between internal carotid and side of pharynx to under surface of base of skull, forms multiple smaller branches
Posterior branches (2):*		
• Occipital	Posterior scalp Suprahyoid Sternocleidomastoid muscles	Posterior of ECA distal to ramus
• Posterior auricular	Scalp around ear Ear	Posterior of ECA Superior to occipital artery
Terminal branches **Maxillary (MA)** 1st section		
• Deep auricular*	TMJ Tempanic membrane Skin of ear	Branches within glandular tissues of parotid behind TMJ
• Middle meningeal	Dura mater	Branches in infratemporal fossa Travels through foramen spinosum
• Inferior alveolar (IA)	Pulp and periodontium of mandibular molar and premolar teeth	IA artery travels inferiorly from the MA between ramus and sphenomandibular ligament inferior to IA nerve
1. Mylohyoid	Floor of mouth, mylohyoid muscle	Branches from IA before it enters mandibular foramen
2. Incisive	Pulp and periodontium of mandibular incisor teeth	IA branches at mental foramen Internal terminal branch is incisive artery
3. Mental	Skin of chin	External terminal branch of IA travels through mental foramen

Table AR-10   (Continued)

Artery	Distribution Areas	Pathway
Maxillary (MA) 2nd section		
• Deep temporal	Temporalis muscle	Travels superiorly between temporalis muscle and pericranium
• Pterygoid branches	Medial/lateral pterygoid muscles	Variable number of branches supply pterygoid muscles Branches inferiorly and superiorly from MA
• Masseteric	Masseter muscle	Branches between neck of mandible and spheno-mandibular ligament Travels laterally through mandibular notch
• Buccal	Buccinator muscle; Skin and mucous membranes of cheek	Travels forward obliquely between medial pterygoid and temporalis to lateral surface of buccinator muscle
Maxillary (MA) 3rd section		
• Posterior superior alveolar (PSA)	Pulp and periodontium of maxillary posterior teeth Maxillary sinus	Branches before MA enters pterygopalatine fossa Travels along infratemporal surface of maxilla
• Infraorbital (IO)	Lower eyelid Side of nose Upper lip	Travels forward in IO groove and canal Exits IO foramen
1. Anterior superior	Pulp and periodontium of maxillary anterior teeth Maxillary sinus	Travels inferiorly from IO artery and descends through alveolar canals
• Sphenopalatine	Nasal cavity	Travels through sphenopalatine foramen and enters nasal cavity and forms smaller branches
1. Nasopalatine*	Lingual mucosa and gingiva of maxillary anterior teeth	Travels along nasal septum and through incisive foramen
• Descending palatine		
1. Greater Palatine*	Hard palate Gingiva and mucosa of maxillary posterior teeth	Travels in palatine canal and divides from descending palatine to greater and lesser palatine arteries Travels through greater palatine foramen
2. Lesser palatine*	Soft palate Palatine tonsils	Travels through lesser palatine foramen
• Artery of pterygoid canal*	Auditory Sphenoid sinus tube	Travels posteriorly into pterygoid canal

*Not illustrated.

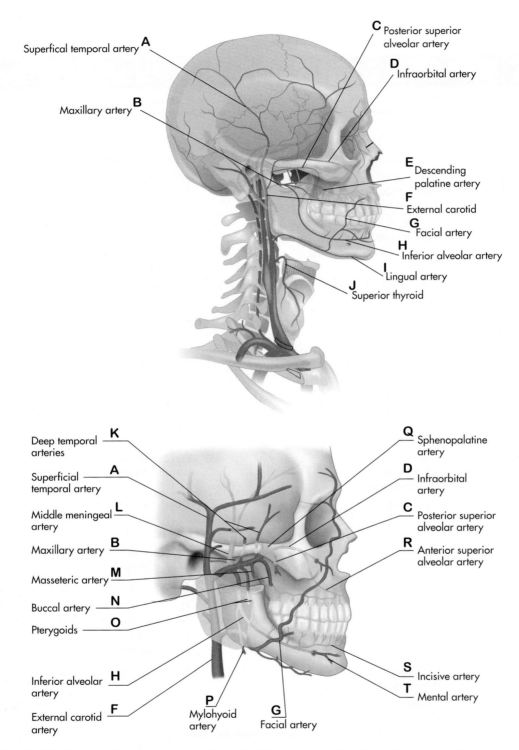

FIGURE AR-17 External Carotid Artery A—Superficial Temporal, B—Maxillary, C—Posterior Superior Alveolar, D—Infraorbital, E—Descending Palatine, F—External Carotid, G—Facial, H—Inferior Alveolar, I—Lingual, J—Superior Thyroid, K—Deep Temporal, L—Middle Meningeal, M—Masseteric, N—Buccal, O—Pterygoids, P—Mylohyoid, Q—Sphenopalatine, R—Anterior Superior Alveolar, S—Incisive, T—Mental

Table AR–11   Venous Blood Return

Vein	Tributaries / Collection Areas	Pathway
TO EXTERNAL JUGULAR (EJ)		
• Retromandibulars	Superficial temporal vein Maxillary vein	Begins within parotid gland Travels downward and superficial to ECA Commonly divides: Anterior division joins facial vein Posterior division flows downward and superficial to sternocleidomastoid muscle
1. Superficial temporal	Frontal Supraorbital	Begins on side and vortex of skull Travels downward along temporal bone Traverses through parotid gland
2. Maxillary	External auditory meatus Tympanic membrane Pterygoid plexus Middle meningeal Posterior superior alveolar Inferior alveolar	Begins from pterygoid plexus Traverses through parotid gland Travels backward between sphenomandibular ligament and neck of mandible
• Posterior auricular	Occipital plexus Superficial temporal plexus	Descends posterior to ear Joins posterior part of retromandibular vein
TO INTERNAL JUGULAR (IJ)		
• Diploic-brain*	Structures of the brain Sigmoid sinus of dura mater	Posterior to internal carotid artery
• Common facial	Frontal region	Begins on forehead
1. Supraorbital/ supratrochlear	Tissues of orbit	Passes downward superficial to frontalis muscle
2. Angular	Supraorbital vein Supratrochlear vein	Forms at medial part of eye Travels lateral of nose Becomes anterior facial vein
3. Superior labial	Upper lip	Anastomoses from upper lip
4. Inferior labial	Lower lip	Anastomoses from lower lip
5. Submental	Chin region Submandibular region	Anastomoses with branches of lingual vein and inferior alveolar vein Parallels submental artery on superficial of mylohyoid muscle
6. Lingual*	Ventral and dorsal surface of tongue Floor of mouth	Travels with lingual artery Deep to hypoglossus muscle Variable drainage
• Pterygoid plexus	Middle meningeal Anterior superior alveolar Middle superior alveolar Posterior superior alveolar Inferior alveolar Greater palatine Lesser palatine Sphenopalatine	Located in infratemporal fossa near pterygoid muscles, around the 2nd and 3rd sections of maxillary artery Communicates with cavernous sinus, pharyngeal venous plexus Anastomoses with deep facial vein, facial vein, and retromandibular vein

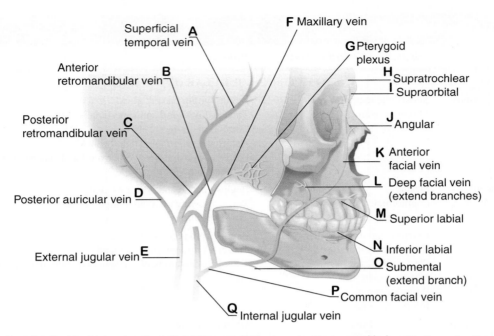

■ **FIGURE AR–18**   Jugular Veins A—Superficial Temporal, B—Anterior Retromandibular, C—Posterior Retromandibular, D—Posterior Auricular, E—External Jugular, F—Maxillary, G—Pterygoid Plexus, H—Supratrochlear, I—Supraorbital, J—Angular, K—Anterior Facial, L—Deep Facial, M—Superior Labial, N—Inferior Labial, O—Submental, P—Common Facial, Q—Internal Jugular

Table AR–12	Ophthalmic Division Branches of Trigeminal Nerve (V₁)	

Nerve	*Innervation*	*Pathway*
• Frontal	Skin of forehead Eyelids Skin of nose	Develops from two smaller nerves Travels along superior orbit
• Nasociliary	Medial of eyelid Side of nose Parts of eyeball Mucous membrane of nose Paranasal sinuses	Develops from several smaller nerves Travels across optic nerve then along medial wall orbit
• Lacrimal	Lateral of upper eyelid Conjunctiva Lacrimal gland	Travels along lateral superior of orbit Receives autonomic nervous fibers from zygomatic branch of maxillary nerve

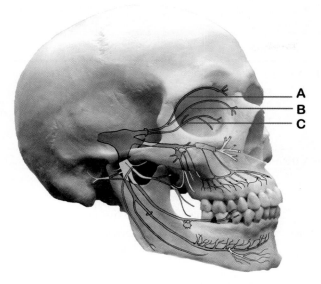

■ **FIGURE AR–19**   Trigeminal—Ophthalmic Division V₁
A—Frontal, B—Nasociliary, C—Lacrimal

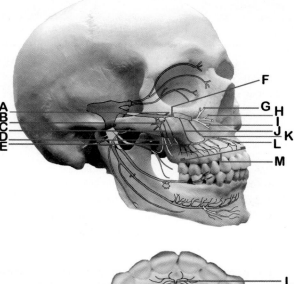

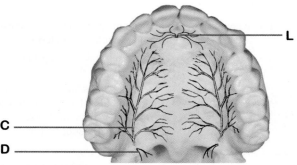

■ **FIGURE AR–20**   Trigeminal—Maxillary Division V₂
A—Zygomatic,   B—Pterygopalatine   Ganglion,
C—Greater Palatine, D—Lesser Palatine, E—Posterior
Superior Alveolar, F—Infraorbital, G—Inferior Palpebral,
H—External Nasal, I—Superior Labial, J—Middle
Superior Alveolar, K—Anterior Superior Alveolar,
L—Nasopalatine, M—Maxillary Dental Plexus

Ophthalmic Division (V₁)

The ophthalmic nerve is the first division of the trigeminal nerve. It transmits sensory information through the superior orbital fissure and travels along the lateral wall of the cavernous sinus to the anterosuperior aspect of the trigeminal ganglion. The ophthalmic is the smallest division of the trigeminal nerve and has three main branches, the frontal, lacrimal, and nasociliary. Local anesthetic injection techniques in dentistry do not typically target these branches. See Table AR–12 and Figure AR–19.

Maxillary Division (V₂)

The maxillary nerve is the second division of the trigeminal nerve. It transmits sensory information in the maxillary region from the maxillary teeth, periodontium, and gingiva, and from the maxillary sinuses, nasal cavity, palate, nasopharynx, a portion of the dura mater, and the skin covering the maxillae. The maxillary nerve passes through the foramen rotundum in the sphenoid bone to the mid-anterior aspect of the trigeminal ganglion. The maxillary nerve branches in four areas, the

cranium, pterygopalatine fossa, infraorbital canal, and on the face. In dentistry, maxillary and palatal injection techniques are used to anesthetize the maxillary nerve and its branches. See Table AR–13 and Figure AR–20.

Mandibular Division (V₃)

The mandibular nerve is the third and largest division of the trigeminal nerve and the only division to contain a motor or efferent root. The larger sensory or afferent root transmits information from half the mandibular

Table AR–13	Maxillary Division Branches of Trigeminal Nerve (V$_2$)	
Nerve	*Innervation*	*Pathway*
CRANIAL BRANCHES		
• Middle meningeal nerve	Dura mater	Formed from convergence of small nerves from dura mater Joins maxillary nerve near trigeminal ganglion Travels with middle meningeal artery
PTERYGOID FOSSA BRANCHES		
• Zygomatic		
1. Zygomaticofacial	Side of forehead skin	Travels through inferior orbital fissure
2. Zygomaticotemporal	Upper cheek skin	Travels through inferior orbital fissure
• Nasopalatine (NP)	Gingival, mucosal, and osseous tissue from central incisor to canine	Travels through incisive foramen and incisive canal along nasal septum to roof of nasal cavity
• Palatine		
1. Greater palatine	Palatal gingival, mucosal, and osseous tissue from premolars to posterior of hard palate	Travels through greater palatine foramen on hard palate of maxilla
2. Lesser palatine	Palatal mucosa of soft palate	Travels through lesser palatine foramen to palatine canal
• Posterior superior alveolar (PSA)	Dental pulp, facial gingiva, periodontal ligament, alveolar bone of maxillary first, second, and third molars, except mesiobuccal root of first molar	Commonly divides: External branch travels along surface of posterior maxilla Internal branch travels through PSA foramina on tuberosity of maxilla
INFRAORBITAL CANAL BRANCHES		
• Infraorbital	Dental pulp, facial gingiva, periodontal ligament, and alveolar bone of maxillary teeth including incisors, canine, first and second premolars, and mesiobuccal root of first molar in some individuals	Formed by the convergence of terminal facial branches, MSA and ASA nerves Travels through the infraorbital canal
1. Middle superior alveolar (MSA)	Dental pulp, facial gingiva, periodontal ligament, and alveolar bone of maxillary first and second premolars and mesiobuccal root of first molar in some individuals	Travels from dental plexus Variable innervation or MSA may be absent
2. Anterior superior alveolar (ASA)	Dental pulps, facial gingiva, periodontal ligament, and alveolar bone of maxillary central incisor through canine	Travels from dental plexus through anterior of maxillary sinus and infraorbital foramen
TERMINAL FACIAL BRANCHES		
• Superior labial	Upper lip skin and mucous membranes	Travels from upper lip to infraorbital foramen
• External nasal	Lateral of nose skin	Travels from lateral side of nose to infraorbital foramen
• Inferior palpebral	Lower eyelid skin	Travels from lateral side of nose to infraorbital foramen

Table AR–14 *Mandibular Division Branches of Trigeminal Nerve (V₃)*

Nerve	Innervation	Pathway
UNDIVIDED NERVE		
• Nervus spinosus	Dura mater	Formed from convergence of nerves from dura mater Enters skull through foramen spinosum
ANTERIOR DIVISION		
• Masseteric	Masseter muscle Small branch to TMJ	Travels laterally superior to lateral pterygoid muscle Crosses mandibular notch with masseteric artery Anterior to TMJ

• Temporal
  1. Anterior temporal
  2. Posterior deep temporal
	Temporalis muscle	Travels superior to lateral pterygoid muscle between skull and temporalis muscle

• Buccal	Skin and mucous membrane covering buccinator muscle Gingiva mandibular molars	Travels anteriorly between heads of lateral pterygoid muscle and along inferior part of temporalis muscle to anterior of masseter muscle Crosses anterior border of ramus and enters cheek Does not innervate buccinator muscle
• Lateral pterygoid	Lateral pterygoid muscle	Travels into deep surface of muscle
POSTERIOR DIVISION		
• Auriculotemporal	Skin of temporal area	Travels posteriorly and inferior to lateral pterygoid and to medial side of ramus, superiorly deep to parotid gland, over zygomatic arch and branches to superficial temporal nerves
• Lingual	Mucous membrane and gingival of lingual side of mandibular teeth Anterior 2/3 of tongue and floor of mouth	Descends between medial pterygoid muscle and ramus Crosses ramus and travels anteromedially to inferior alveolar nerve
• Inferior alveolar (IA)	Dental pulp, facial gingiva, periodontal ligament and alveolar bone of mandibular teeth except for facial gingiva of mandibular molars	Travels medial to lateral pterygoid muscle through pterygomandibular space between sphenomandibular ligament and medial surface of ramus Enters mandibular foramen and travels in mandibular canal
1. Mylohyoid	Mylohyoid muscle Anterior belly of digastric muscle	Branches before IA enters mandibular foramen Descends in mylohyoid groove deep on medial surface of body of mandible
2. Mental	Skin of chin Lower lip skin and mucous membrane	Travels through mental foramen as a terminal branch of IA nerve
3. Incisive	Dental pulp, facial gingiva, periodontal ligament and alveolar bone of mandibular premolar and anterior teeth	Travels as a terminal branch of IA nerve

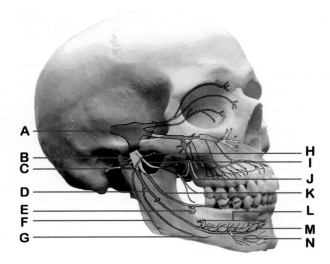

■ **FIGURE AR–21** Trigeminal—Mandibular Division V3 A—Mandibular Division, B—Nervus spinosus, C—Auriculotemporal, D—Inferior Alveolar, E—Submandibular Ganglion, F—Masseteric, G—Mylohyoid, H—Temporalis, I—Pterygoids, J—Buccal, K—Lingual, L—Mandibular Dental Plexus, M—Incisive, N—Mental Buccal, K—Lingual, L—Mandibular Dental Plexus, M—Incisive, N—Mental

teeth, their associated periodontium, the mucous membranes of the cheek, the anterior two-thirds of the tongue, mastoid cells, lateral scalp, the skin anterior to ear, the lower cheek, lower lip and chin, parotid gland, the temporomandibular joint, and the remaining bone of the mandible on one side.

Muscles innervated by the efferent components include the temporalis, masseter, medial and lateral pterygoid, tensor veli palatini, and the tensor tympani.

The nerves of the mandibular division branch in three areas, including the undivided trigeminal nerve and the anterior and posterior division. In dentistry, mandibular injection techniques are used to anesthetize several branches of the mandibular nerve. See Table AR–14 and Figure AR–21.

Facial Nerve (VII)

Local anesthetic techniques in dentistry have been developed to anesthetize branches of the trigeminal nerve. Some extent of facial nerve anesthesia is unavoidable at times when using these techniques. Like the trigeminal nerve, facial nerves have consistent patterns of innervation with frequent variations on the right and left sides of the face. Facial nerves have efferent, parasympathetic, and afferent roots.

The facial efferent root forms in the facial nerve nucleus in the pons. It exits between the pons and

Table AR–15	Facial Nerve Branches (VII)	
Nerve	*Innervation*	*Pathway*
BRANCHES IN FACIAL CANAL		
• Greater petrosal	Parasympathetic to lacrimal gland Special afferent taste to palate	From geniculate ganglion, travels to anterior surface of petrous temporal bone, and to pterygoid ganglion Joins with branches of maxillary nerve
• Stapedius	Motor to stapedius muscle in middle ear	Travels through small canal in pyramidal eminence to small stapedius muscle
• Chorda tympani	Parasympathetic to submandibular and sublingual glands Special afferent taste fibers for anterior 2/3 of tongue	Travels posterior to anterior across the tympanic membrane in middle ear, between malleus and incus; through petro–tympanic fissure into infra–temporal fossa Joins with lingual nerve and travels to submandibular ganglion Fibers innervate glands Extend to anterior 2/3 of tongue with lingual nerve

Table AR–15	Continued		
Nerve	**Innervation**		**Pathway**
BRANCHES DISTAL TO STYLOMASTOID FORAMEN			
• Posterior auricular	Motor to occipital belly of epicranial muscle Posterior of ear and scalp		Travels superiorly behind ear in front of mastoid process
• Posterior belly of digastric and stylohyoid	Motor to belly of posterior digastric and stylohyoid muscles under mandible		Branches form near posterior of muscles
• Facial expression			
1. Temporal	Motor to frontal belly of epicranial, superior part of orbicularis oculi, and corrugator supercilii muscle		Branches from parotid plexus and distributes superficially to muscles innervated
2. Zygomatic	Motor to muscles at lateral angle of orbit, inferior part of orbicularis oculi and zygomatic major and minor muscles		Travels across zygomatic bone to lateral of orbit Joins fibers of maxillary nerve
3. Buccal	Motor to buccinator, risorius, orbicularis oris muscles Upper lip, small muscles of nose		Travels under skin superficially to muscles Joins fibers of ophthalmic and infraorbital nerves
4. Marginal mandibular	Motor to lower orbicularis oris and mentalis muscles Lower lip and chin		Travels anteriorly under platysma and triangularis muscles Joins fibers of mental branch on IA nerve
5. Cervical	Motor to platysma muscle		Travels below mandible

medulla on the ventral surface and travels to the petrous portions of the temporal bone, into the auditory meatus. It then follows a winding course through the facial canal. The facial nerve exits the skull through the stylomastoid foramen and travels within the parotid gland, dividing into five major branches on each side of the face.

The nervus intermedius of the facial nerve carries both parasympathetic fibers and afferent fibers. It is called the nervus intermedius because it arises between the efferent facial nerve and the vestibulocochlear nerve (VIII) in the pons. It travels alongside the efferent root to the petrous portion of the temporal bone and through the internal auditory meatus. At the facial canal, the nervus intermedius unites with the efferent root at the geniculate ganglion.

Within the facial canal three branches divide from the facial nerve, the greater petrosal, the nerve to stapedius, and the chorda tympani. Distal to the stylomastoid foramen, the facial nerve divides into a posterior auricular branch, a branch to the posterior belly of digastric and the stylohyoid muscles, and to the muscles of facial expression. The muscles of facial expression include temporal, zygomatic, buccal, marginal mandibular and cervical muscles. See Table AR–15.

REFERENCES

Biology Online, www.biology-online.org. Accessed November 12, 2008.

eMedicine, www.emedicine.com. Accessed November 12, 2008.

Fehrenbach, M. J., & Herring, S. W. (2007). *Illustrated anatomy of the head and neck* (3rd ed.). St. Louis: Saunders Elsevier.

Malamed, S. F. (2004). *Handbook of local anesthesia* (5th ed.). St. Louis: Elsevier Mosby.

Netter, Frank H. (2003). *Atlas of human anatomy* (4th ed.). Philadelphia: Saunders Elsevier.

Norton, Neil (2007). *Netter's head and neck anatomy for dentistry*. Philadelphia: Saunders Elsevier.

Rohen, J. W., Yokichi, C., & Romroll, L. W. (2006). *Color atlas of anatomy* (6th ed.). New York: Lippincott Williams & Wilkins.

Structure of the Human Body, www.meddean.luc.edu/Lumen/meded/grossanatomy Accessed November 12, 2008.

End of Chapter Questions Key

CHAPTER 1 LOCAL ANESTHESIA IN DENTISTRY: PAST, PRESENT, AND FUTURE

Answer 1: **A**—Lidocaine, methadone, and morphine were all developed much later than coca leaves, henbane, mandrake, and opium.

Answer 2: **C**—Although cocaine can be a useful local anesthetic drug, its addictive properties make it inappropriate for dental use.

Answer 3: **C**—The harpoon-type aspirating syringe is the most commonly used syringe.

Answer 4: **A**—Lidocaine was developed in 1947 and continues to be the "gold standard" for dental local anesthetic drugs.

Answer 5: **B**—OraVerse is an FDA-approved drug for the reversal of soft tissue anesthesia.

Answer 6: **B**—The Wand was the first computer controlled local anesthetic delivery device available for dentistry in 1997.

CHAPTER 2 FUNDAMENTALS OF PAIN MANAGEMENT

Answer 1: **C**—A protective response is a rapid, reflexive, subconscious reaction.

Answer 2: **D**—All of these affect individual pain experiences except body weight and height.

Answer 3: **A**—Nociception is polymodal. This means that it can detect injury from chemical, mechanical, and thermal stimuli even though all are registered as pain.

Answer 4: **D**—Neuropathic pain is caused by nerve tissue injury or dysfunction of the sensory nerves in the central or peripheral nervous systems. Trigeminal neuralgia is the only example of this.

Answer 5: **D**—Prepare, Rehearse, Empower, and Praise patients to reduce anxiety and fear.

Answer 6: **D**—This response does not include patient participation in decision making.

CHAPTER 3 THE NEUROANATOMY AND NEUROPHYSIOLOGY OF PAIN CONTROL

Answer 1: **D**—All of the above accurately describe the differences between sensory and motor neurons.

Answer 2: **A**—Stimulation slowly depolarizes. In a successful impulse generation, the firing threshold is reached and rapid depolarization occurs, followed by recovery to the resting state.

Answer 3: **C**—Gaps between cells on nerve membranes are called nodes of Ranvier.

Answer 4: **D**—"A" delta and "C" fibers

Answer 5: **C**—"A delta" fibers are lightly myelinated; "C" fibers are nonmyelinated.

Answer 6: **C**—Interdental, interradicular, and dental

CHAPTER 4 PHARMACOLOGY BASICS

Answer 1: **C**—Half-life refers to the time it takes for 50% of a drug to be removed from the systemic circulation.

Answer 2: **B**—Esters are metabolized in the blood via plasma cholinesterase.

Answer 3: **A**—CNS toxicity is due to conduction blockade of vital functions within the CNS due to the normal functioning of nerve cells in response to local anesthetic drugs.

Answer 4: **C**—Decreased myocardial contractility and hypotension due to vasodilation, if they occur, will further worsen an already developing CNS depression. Some initial heart rate elevation and hypertension may occur, however, in early overdosing.

Answer 5: **D**—Only the cation can bind to the specific receptor sites in nerve membranes to prevent impulse generation and conduction.

Answer 6: **C**—Local anesthetic drugs are classified according to their intermediate chains as esters or amides. Except for its largely nonhepatic, ester-like metabolic pathways and its therefore shorter elimination half-life, articaine cannot be mistaken for an ester.

Answer 7: **A**—An overdose of local anesthetic drugs will result in depression of the CNS. The initial excitatory phase is actually due to depression of inhibitory actions of the CNS.

CHAPTER 5 DENTAL LOCAL ANESTHETIC DRUGS

Answer 1: **D**—The MRD of a drug is an established safe guideline for administration.

Answer 2: **B**—Articaine is primarily metabolized via plasma cholinesterase. Its metabolism is not similar to prilocaine's. It is metabolized only *one* about 5–10% in the liver. Very little is excreted unchanged.

Answer 3: **C**—4% articaine, 1:200,000 addresses both significant CVS and hepatic compromise. The other three drugs are metabolized in the liver, including 3% mepivacaine, which otherwise would be an excellent choice in CVS compromise. At 1:200,000 epinephrine, articaine is the best overall selection.

Answer 4: **C**—The local anesthetic drugs are irrelevant to hemostasis. Epinephrine provides the most vigorous hemostasis. Its highest concentration is found in the 1:50,000 dilution.

Answer 5: **B**—Vasoactivity. Drugs that are weak vasodilators will remain in the area of deposition longer. Vigorous vasodilators enhance their own uptake into the systemic circulation and therefore vasoconstrictors must accompany their use.

Answer 6: **C**—Tricyclic antidepressants that require care with vasoconstrictors, and levonordefrin,

especially, should not be used due to the risk of serious elevations of BP. Levonordefrin is safer to use in the presence of beta-blockers, compared with epinephrine. There are no issues with mepivacaine plain because there are no contraindications to the anesthetic drugs themselves.

Answer 7: **C**—Prilocaine

Answer 8: **B**—Considering overall toxicity to the CNS and CVS, prilocaine is the least toxic, approximately seven times less toxic compared with bupivacaine. Articaine is less toxic than lidocaine, and mepivacaine *overall* is more toxic than lidocaine, although it is not thought to be in doses used in dentistry

CHAPTER 6 VASOCONSTRICTORS IN DENTISTRY

Answer 1: **B**—Epinephrine provides the most vigorous hemostasis of this group.

Answer 2: **A**—Dilutions of 1:200,000 epinephrine contain the least and are indicated because they are safest and yet still provide hemostasis. If hemostasis were not needed, plain drugs would work well in shorter treatment times.

Answer 3: **C**—Levonordefrin provides less cardiac stimulation compared with epinephrine.

Answer 4: **A**—Compared with the local anesthetic drug's metabolism, epinephrine's metabolism is generally much more rapid.

Answer 5: **A**—Epinephrine is metabolized by COMT and MAO.

Answer 6: **B**—Epinephrine reliably and significantly raises blood sugar levels. The lowest quantity of epinephrine is found in combination "B" where half of the administered volume has no epinephrine. The lowest amount of vasoconstrictor should always be used in all individuals. Since this patient is a well-controlled diabetic and otherwise healthy, no special precautions are necessary and the default principle applies. Use the least amount of drug necessary.

CHAPTER 7 DOSE CALCULATIONS FOR LOCAL ANESTHETIC SOLUTIONS

Answer 1: **C**—The absolute maximum for lidocaine is 300 mg.

Answer 2: **D**—Local anesthetic toxicity is weight related but height is not a relevant factor.

Answer 3: **B**—11 cartridges is the correct answer for epinephrine alone but is too much for lidocaine, the limiting drug in this situation.

Answer 4: **C**—0.2 mg is the MRD for epinephrine in a healthy individual.

Answer 5: **B**—4 cartridges of 2% lidocaine = 144 mg. The absolute maximum is 300 mg for lidocaine or 2 mg/lb × 150 or more pounds = 300 mg. 300 mg − 144 mg = 156 mg. 156 mg / 72 mg per cartridge of 4% articaine = 2 cartridges.

Answer 6: **D**—The maximum for epinephrine in significant cardiovascular compromise is 0.04 mg. Each cartridge of a dilution of 1:200,000 epinephrine contains 0.009 mg of epinephrine. 0.04 mg / 0.009 mg per cartridge of 4% articaine, 1:200,000 epinephrine = 4 cartridges.

Answer 7: **C**—Available formulations of 2% lidocaine include 1:100,000 epinephrine and 1:50,000 epinephrine.

Answer 8: **D**—The maximum dose per pound of 4% articaine is 3.2 mg/ lb for all individuals.

Answer 9: **A**—By definition, a 1% drug contains 10 mg per milliliter. There are therefore 18 mg in a 1.8 ml cartridge. 0.5% drugs contain half this amount, or 5 mg per milliliter. In 1.8 ml of a 0.5% drug there are 5 mg in the first milliliter, and 5 mg × 0.8 = 4 mg in the additional 0.8 ml. 5 mg + 4 mg = 9 mg/ cartridge of a 0.5% drug.

CHAPTER 8 TOPICAL ANESTHETICS

Answer 1: **D**—The term *eutectic* refers to a substance that has a lower melting point than any of its ingredients. Eutectic topicals not only have lower melting points to facilitate penetration through tissue barriers but they are formulated primarily in the base form so that they can provide anesthesia more rapidly.

Answer 2: **D**—All of the above

Answer 3: **C**—Metered sprays are generally easier to track. Unmetered sprays are not.

Answer 4: **A**—Tremors and agitation may be early signs of CNS depression. They are also reactions that occur in response to the stress of dental appointments. It is important to remain alert to the development of further signs and symptoms of CNS depression.

Answer 5: **D**—Adding additional drugs does not decrease the potential for adverse reactions; it generally increases the potential.

Answer 6: **B**—Compounded drugs, including compounded topicals, may be used only by the individuals for whom they were prescribed.

Answer 7: **A**—True. The base form has less ability to be absorbed systemically.

Answer 8: **B**—Dyclonine has a ketone linkage as opposed to amide or ester.

CHAPTER 9 LOCAL ANESTHETIC DELIVERY DEVICES

Answer 1: **D**—Negative pressure is developed in both syringes, although the mechanism for creating the pressure is different for each.

Answer 2: **D**—It is permissible to bend uncontaminated needles according to OSHA. Two hands are never allowed unless one is holding a hemostat or cotton pliers to hold the cap. Contaminated needles may be bent *only* in *specific* circumstances.

Answer 3: **D**—25 gauge needles have larger lumens and are thought to have greater ease of aspiration; 30 gauge needles have the greatest risk for breakage; studies demonstrate that patients cannot perceive the difference between the various needle gauges; and due to the ease of aspiration, 25 gauge needles may be beneficial in highly vascular areas.

Answer 4: **B**—Long needles average ~32 mm (1½ inches), with some noted to be as long as 40 mm.

Answer 5: **B**—Freezing during shipping or handling causes expansion of the solution that dislodges the stopper.

Answer 6: **D**—Each stopper width displaces 0.2 ml of solutions; therefore, 3 stoppers would displace 0.6 ml.

Answer 7: **A**—Sodium bisulfate and methylparaben are both preservatives; however, due to the high incidence of allergy to methylparaben it is no longer used in injectable local anesthetic agents.

CHAPTER 10 PATIENT ASSESSMENT FOR LOCAL ANESTHESIA

Answer 1: **B**—Although useful for planning a course of anesthesia, tooth charting is not one of the ASA Medical Components of Care.

Answer 2: **B**—ASA Classification P3 is defined as "Severe Systemic Disease."

Answer 3: **C**—Although important when monitoring total doses of drug delivered, this is not considered a main tool for patient assessment.

Answer 4:   **C**—Epinephrine and felypressin are both vasoconstrictors; however, felypressin has no adrenergic effects and is therefore safe to use for patients with hyperthyroidism.

Answer 5:   **C**—Administration of vasoconstrictors may result in hypertensive crisis, stroke, or myocardial infarction. It is recommended that you *not* administer local anesthetics with vasoconstrictors for a minimum of *24 hours after* methamphetamine use.

Answer 6:   **B**—Myocardial infarction within three weeks is an absolute contraindication to care.

CHAPTER 11 FUNDAMENTALS FOR ADMINISTRATION OF LOCAL ANESTHETIC AGENTS

Answer 1:   **C**—A field block injection deposits local anesthetic solution near larger terminal nerve branches for treatment near the site of injection.

Answer 2:   **B**—The deposition site is the anatomical location where drugs are deposited.

Answer 3:   **C**—Thorough patient assessment is critical to safe local anesthetic administration. Patient assessment must precede all other steps.

Answer 4:   **A**—Orienting the bevel toward bone reduces discomfort and trauma to periosteum when bone is contacted. In the event of inadvertent contact, the needle tends to glance off the bone rather than pierce the periosteum. While reducing discomfort is important (Answer D), many other aspects of injections that decrease discomfort have nothing to do with bevel orientation. A is the better answer because bevel orientation specifically reduces trauma to the periosteum in addition to providing for more comfort.

Answer 5:   **D**—This is the only sample that has all components: date, drug(s), total drug volume(s), injection(s) or sites, results of aspiration test(s), a notation on adverse events, and clinician signature.

Answer 6:   **D**—It is safe to deposit the anesthetic solution once a negative aspiration is confirmed, including: when there is no preceding positive aspiration; when previous positive aspiration does not obscure subsequent aspirations; and, only when the clinician essentially starts fresh with a new cartridge and new aspiration, not after a positive aspiration that obscures the results.

Answer 7:   **D**—It is not only critical to determine if a needle lumen lies within a vessel prior to deposition but it is also critical to administer drugs slowly in case the needle lumen lies within the vessel despite negative aspiration test results.

Answer 8:   **C**—Make the needle safe with a one-handed technique. This optimizes safety for all personnel. Once this has been done, attend to the patient.

CHAPTER 12 INJECTIONS FOR MAXILLARY PAIN CONTROL

Answer 1:   **A**—A is the correct choice. B is incorrect because the needle is not oriented distal to the long axis of the tooth. C is incorrect because the needle does not pass through bone. D is incorrect because the mucosa and connective tissue in this area are not typically thickened.

Answer 2:   **B**—Visualization, palpation, and reassessment of available landmarks is most useful. A is incorrect in most instances unless the wrong size was used in the first place, such as an ultrashort needle. C is incorrect because contact with bone results in pain and trauma, not increased success. D is incorrect because the patient is not the one responsible for the injection parameters.

Answer 3:   **B**—The MSA nerve is *present* in somewhere between 28% and 50% of individuals.

Answer 4:   **A**—This range is considered normal for the average adult.

Answer 5:   **D**—D is the only accurate description. A, B, and C are incorrect. The premolars are not anesthetized by a PSA injection nor are the mandibular molars or the maxillary teeth to the midline.

Answer 6:   **A**—Over-insertion of needles increases the risk of hematoma formation in PSA blocks. This can occur both by deeper invasion into the pterypalatine fossa or by location too posteriorly initially.

CHAPTER 13 INJECTIONS FOR PALATAL PAIN CONTROL

Answer 1:   **B**—Deposition site near the wall of the incisive canal is correct compared with A because while deposition is at the incisive foramen, the needle is not advanced into the nasopalatine canal. C is incorrect because the nasopalatine nerve block is not performed at the anterior palatine foramen. D does not describe a location at the incisive foramen.

Answer 2:   **D**—Both failure to deposit the solution close to the bone or foramen and insufficient volumes deposited reduce the amount of drug that diffuses through the bone to the nerves.

Answer 3: **B**—The AMSA technique provides anesthesia for structures traditionally anesthetized by the ASA, MSA, NP and GP injections.

Answer 4: **D**—The aspiration rate is similar to other palatal techniques. NP blocks do not provide more durable anesthesia compared with other palatal techniques. When performed as recommended, they provide bilateral anesthesia.

Answer 5: **B**—Applying topical for 1 to 2 minutes is typical of many injections. Using patch topicals in the palate may be helpful. Slow deposition of solution is important to avoid damage to tissue that has difficulty accommodating the volumes of solution necessary in many palatal techniques. Pain is reduced with slow administration and safety is enhanced.

Answer 6: **B**—Solution in AMSA blocks does not cross the midline and provides same side anesthesia only.

CHAPTER 14 INJECTIONS FOR MANDIBULAR PAIN CONTROL

Answer 1: **C**—The rate of positive aspiration in alveolar nerve blocks is 10–15%. This is the highest rate of all techniques described in this text. In practical terms, this means anticipating a positive aspiration in one to two out of every ten inferior alveolar blocks.

Answer 2: **C**—The periodontal ligament injection (PDL), while providing only limited areas of anesthesia, is an alternative to nearly all other techniques, mandibular and maxillary.

Answer 3: **D**—Neither the buccal nor mental nerve blocks provides pulpal anesthesia to the mandibular teeth.

Answer 4: **D**—Even though there are both extraoral and intraoral landmarks for the Gow-Gates nerve block, it is not necessary to remove jewelry before administering it.

Answer 5: **B**—Palpating anatomy is essential to some techniques and not very helpful in others. While the statement that it is an unnecessary step is obviously false, palpation is not even possible in lingual nerve blocks, for example.

Answer 6: **B**—The correct order from inferior location to superior location in the pterygomandibular space is IA, Akinosi, Gow-Gates.

CHAPTER 15 INJECTIONS FOR SUPPLEMENTAL PAIN CONTROL

Answer 1: **C**—The rate of deposition of solution in each of these techniques is slow (0.2 ml over 20 seconds)

Answer 2: **C**—The intraseptal technique does not provide reliable or durable pulpal anesthesia.

Answer 3: **C**—A 5% concentration of lidocaine may be effective in this situation but it is also unavailable in dental cartridges and is two-and-one-half times more toxic than 2% lidocaine solutions.

Answer 4: **C**—30%

Answer 5: **D**—Solution diffuses through the alveolus; therefore, the PDL is an intraosseous technique. The orientation of the bevel is irrelevant to success and the technique is very useful as a supplementary technique when other techniques have failed to provide profound anesthesia.

CHAPTER 16 TROUBLESHOOTING INADEQUATE ANESTHESIA

Answer 1: **C**—Manufacturing processes are well-regulated and rarely, not typically, may be the cause of inadequate anesthesia. On the contrary, product recalls are more typical when atypical errors occur during manufacturing processes.

Answer 2: **D**—Inflammation with no signs or symptoms is unlikely to inhibit anesthesia.

Answer 3: **B**—Increases in cationic concentrations decrease the rate of success.

Answer 4: **D**—PDL injections, mylohyoid nerve blocks, and Gow-Gates blocks are all useful supplements when inferior alveolar nerve blocks fail to provide adequate pulpal anesthesia.

Answer 5: **C**—Mylohyoid blocks are useful only in the mandible.

Answer 6: **D**—Intraosseously administered solutions slowly diffuse through alveolar bone to dental plexuses.

Answer 7: **B**—The Gow-Gates is located at a higher level than the Vazirani-Akinosi block, which is higher than the IA block.

Answer 8: **A**—The statement is true. For example, the minimum volume of solution for a Gow-Gates nerve block is 1.8 ml, which is nine times the typical volumes for one site of a PDL injection, or 0.2 ml.

CHAPTER 17 LOCAL ANESTHESIA COMPLICATIONS AND MANAGEMENT

Answer 1:   **D**—Some embedded needles are retained in tissue after evaluation. Evaluation by an oral surgeon may result in a decision to retain the needle versus the greater damage that might occur with attempted removal. Even though needle fragments are typically removed today, referring for removal may make the patient believe that either the referring clinician or the surgeon is acting inappropriately if the decision is made to retain the embedded fragment. Refer for *evaluation*.

Answer 2:   **C**—Two cartridges is not an overdose in a healthy 160-pound adult unless intravascularly administered or the patient is a hyper-responder. The progression of signs and symptoms to slurring of speech and perioral numbness is not consistent with anxiety. Assuming the patient has no history of hyper-response, the likely mechanism for overdose is intravascular administration.

Answer 3:   **A**—Reactions with signs and symptoms occurring many hours to days after contact with a drug are characterized as delayed sensitivities.

Answer 4:   **C**—These symptoms are consistent with paresthesia (prolonged numbness) and dysesthesia (sharp pains).

Answer 5:   **C**—Place pressure over the area as quickly as possible and then apply ice, when available. Advise the patient regarding the development of discoloration. Instruct the patient to apply ice intermittently for the next 6 hours and to avoid aspirin for pain. Advise the patient to notify you immediately of any change, especially the development of signs and symptoms of infection or limited jaw opening.

Answer 6:   **C**—Of the three, overdose is the most frequent systemic complication.

Answer 7:   **B**—Slow administration is the most important safety factor in local anesthetic drug administration and increases the safety margins of all the other preventive strategies mentioned. Aspiration is critical but not always completely reliable. Calculating appropriate maximum doses is also critical, but hyper-responders may react adversely to doses that are carefully calculated and considered to be appropriate. Reassurance does not even address this issue.

CHAPTER 18 INSIGHTS FOR THE FEARFUL PATIENT

Answer 1:   **C**—Check out and confirm the observations about possible concerns regarding dental treatment by asking a few simple questions: "When was your last dental visit?" "How did it go?" "Do you have any concerns about receiving treatment today?" Patients want to know that their care provider is concerned about them. If the patient is fearful, this may affect their ability to receive an injection and whether or not the anesthetic is effective. Obtaining this information before treatment allows clinicians to develop plans that address problems methodically and to increase the likelihood of success. This patient is also reassured that he is in the hands of a caring and competent professional.

Answer 2:   **B**—Fearful patients need to learn how to be assertive and express their concerns. They need to ask questions about their worries, including comfort during treatment. Good communication empowers fearful patients with a sense of control while poor communication can lead to anger and aggressive behavior rather than helpful assertive behavior. Trust developed in this manner is helpful to both the patient and the clinician.

Answer 3:   **D**—When the procedure is described in simple steps the fearful patient will not be overwhelmed by the prospect of treatment and will not be startled by each new aspect of the treatment process. It is important not to surprise fearful patients and to let them know what sensations are normal, especially when administering local anesthesia.

Answer 4:   **D**—The physical relaxation skills of deep breathing and muscle relaxation are easily taught and quickly learned by dental patients. Additionally, the clinician can directly observe whether or not the patient is actively using the skills and whether or not the patient needs coaching. Anxiety leads to muscle tension and shallow breathing, both of which increase the patient's sense of physical discomfort. Muscle relaxation and deep breathing counteract these, and patients appreciate having a technique that can be used to gain relief from the symptoms of anxiety. These techniques reduce mental stress as it is not possible to be physically relaxed and psychologically anxious at the same time, and the active focus on implementing relaxation techniques displaces the fearful conjectures. The clinician benefits from the patient's ability to use these skills because a tense and anxious patient has a lower pain threshold, is more easily hurt and startled, and cannot distinguish between anticipated pain and the actual experience of pain both during the administration of local anesthetic and when assessing if the patient is adequately anesthetized to proceed with treatment.

Answer 5: **B**—A rehearsal provides the patient with the opportunity to practice the relaxation skills learned while the clinician simulates the steps involved in administering local anesthetic. Patients gain knowledge about their role and what is involved in the actual procedure without the pressure to accomplish treatment.

Answer 6: **A**—Inform the patient of the technique to verify that the tooth is anesthetized before proceeding with treatment. The EPT is very useful for this purpose and patients are receptive to the idea of a device that makes the determination objectively rather than relying on subjective responses that have not been reliable in the past. If there is no EPT available, an ultrasonic instrument can be used along with time structuring technique (counting to "1," then "2," and "5") to verify profound anesthesia for the patient.

CHAPTER 19 INSIGHTS FROM PEDODONTICS

Answer 1: **B**—While elements of A, C, and D may be true, the key issue is the greatly reduced body weights of children. There is a higher possibility of overdosing when clinicians are accustomed to treating adults and giving a "standard dose" of the anesthetic solutions. These "standard" adult doses may well be too much for children.

Answer 2: **D**—Much of the success of any pediatric dental appointment has to do with comfort and efficiency. When profound anesthesia has been obtained, all procedures will be more comfortable for the child and it becomes possible to accomplish more at each visit.

Answer 3: **A**—For primary teeth, penetrations generally do not need to be as deep as for permanent teeth. Cortical plates are not thinner in children

and the inferior alveolar foramen is more inferior compared with adults.

Answer 4: **C**—The primary focus of an assistant during injection procedures must be the safety of the child. The clinician administering the injection cannot control gross body movements of the child while injecting. The assistant must respond to any quick and unexpected movements that occur in order to ensure the safety of the child.

Answer 5: **D**—There are few management techniques as profoundly effective for children as helping them to understand what is happening to them and around them. It is universally accepted that people are most fearful of what they don't know. By helping children understand and develop favorable pictures of procedures, positive responses are far more likely to result.

Answer 6: **B**—The inferior alveolar foramen is typically more inferior in children than in adults. Mandibular infiltrations frequently work well and short needles are often preferred in children.

Answer 7: **A**—Cold packs minimize circulation and decrease initial swelling. Once the swelling has stopped, generally 8 to 12 hours later, warm packs are appropriate because they increase circulation and promote healing. Antibiotics are rarely indicated.

CHAPTER 20 INSIGHTS FROM SPECIALTIES: ORAL SURGERY, PERIODONTICS, AND ENDODONTICS

Answer 1: **A**—Clark's rule is suggested in this chapter as the most practical method for altering doses for children based on weight. Young's rule bases the calculation on age.

Answer 2: **D**—All of the above. Management of patients with diverse ages and medical backgrounds, management of oral infections, limiting the potential for needle tract infections, and achieving adequate anesthesia in the presence of these infections are all specific challenges in oral and maxillofacial surgery.

Answer 3: **C**—Local anesthetics with higher pHs should be used in the presence of infection.

Answer 4: **B**—Numbness is not an adverse event. The vast majority of injections do not result in infections when sterile needles are used, but when they occur, infections are undesired or adverse. Postoperative soreness is common after injections but also adverse. Trismus is also relatively common and not desired (adverse).

Answer 5:   **D**—A, B, and C are alternate options when patients are allergic to all local anesthetic drugs. D is a preservative in fruit juices.

Answer 6:   **A**—Hematomas are localized, not systemic, reactions to the tearing of blood vessels

Glossary

A

Aberrant innervation *unexpected* variations in anatomic patterns of innervation

Absolute contraindications situations in which local anesthetic or vasoconstrictor drugs cannot be administered safely

Absolute refractory period the period during which the generation of new impulses along previously fired sections of nerve membranes is physiologically impossible

Accessory innervation *expected* variations in anatomic patterns of innervation

Action potential a synonym for *impulse,* which refers to the electronic signal generated and conducted to the CNS and from the CNS to effector organs, cells, and tissues in response to stimulation

Acute pain pain of relatively short duration from seconds to no longer than about six months

Adrenergic having effects similar to epinephrine

Adrenergic receptors receptors that respond to catecholamines such as epinephrine and norepinephrine

Adverse drug event or reaction (ADR) undesired effects that occur in response to the pharmacologic actions of a drug, including the events surrounding the administration of the drug and described in terms of their local or systemic effects or as complications

Age-appropriate terminology language that is consistent with a child's level of comprehension and maturity

Ageusia the loss of the ability to perceive sweet, sour, bitter, or salty substances due to chorda tympani injury, otherwise referred to as altered taste sensations or perversions

Akinosi (Vazirani-Akinosi) (VA) nerve block the VA, or Akinosi, nerve block provides pain management for the mandibular teeth in a single quadrant, especially when the ability to open the jaw is limited, either due to physiologic, pathologic, or phobic circumstances (see also Vazirani-Akinosi nerve block)

Amide a class of local anesthetic drugs in which an aromatic component is linked to a secondary or tertiary amine by an amide

Angioedema localized swelling brought about by the rapid subcutaneous release of histamine after topical or occasionally injectable local anesthetic administration; despite the association with local anesthetics, on many occasions there is no identifiable antigen

Anterior middle superior alveolar (AMSA) nerve blocks AMSA nerve blocks provide pain management for the incisors, canine, and premolars on the side anesthetized as well as palatal tissue from the midline through the molars and the buccal periodontium of the pulpally affected teeth

Anterior superior alveolar (ASA) nerve blocks ASA nerve blocks anesthetize structures innervated by the ASA nerve, including the pulps of the maxillary central incisor through the canine on the injected side and their facial periodontium

Anxiety an emotional response to a threat or danger that is not immediately present or is unclear

Apoptotic programed biochemical events leading to cell death in multicellular organisms. Unlike necrosis, this disposal of cellular debris does not damage the organism

Armamentarium (local anesthetic) *all* equipment, materials, and devices used during the delivery of local anesthetic agents

Articaine an intermediate-acting amide local anesthetic drug noted for its fast onset and highly lipophilic characteristics

ASA physical status classification the medical components of (local anesthetic) care as defined by the American Society of Anesthesiologists

Aspiration test a test to determine whether or not the tip of a needle is embedded within a blood vessel; it is accomplished by applying gentle, brief back pressure on the upper inside surface of the thumb-ring and observing for the absence or entry of blood into the cartridge

Atypical plasma cholinesterase a form of cholinesterase that results from a genetic, autosomal recessive condition in which there is an impaired ability to metabolize ester local anesthetics

Axolemmas bilayered, phospholipid membranes of neurons, also known as neurolemmas

Axon the processes or fibers of individual nerve cells that transmit signals to and from the central nervous system

Axoplasm the cytoplasm or intracellular environment of a nerve cell

B

Backflow the term applied when solution is injected under pressure into tissues but the tissue resistance is so great it forces solution to flow backward into the oral cavity; this occurs primarily in buccal nerve blocks and in the palate as well as in intraosseous injections such as the PDL where solution can *backflow* through the sulcus into the mouth rather than diffuse through alveolar bone

Benzocaine an ester topical anesthetic that exists almost entirely in the base form

Bevel the diagonal cut that makes the point of a needle

Biofeedback a method through which patients can modify their physiological responses to pain and anxiety, in other words a method that allows patients to exert at least some voluntary control over involuntary responses

Biotransformation the process whereby local anesthetic drugs are broken down to less toxic or nontoxic metabolites before being excreted

Biphasic occurring in two relatively distinct phases

Blanching a visible indicator of the diffusion of anesthetic solution through tissues due to decreased blood flow, which is more pronounced when vasoconstrictors are used; blanching may be described as pale pink to white in color with visibly less color compared with adjacent tissues

Breech-loading a syringe with a large side opening for easing insertion of the local anesthetic cartridge

Buccal (B) nerve block the B nerve block provides pain management for the buccal soft tissue along the molar teeth in the mandibular region

Bupivacaine a long-acting amide local anesthetic drug

Butamben an ester topical anesthetic used in combination with other topicals, in dentistry

C

Cardiac dose the safe limit of vasoconstrictor drugs for a patient with ischemic heart disease

Carpule a glass cylinder holding local anesthetic drugs and other contents in solution for injection into oral tissues; a trademark term of Cook-Waite Laboratories for cartridge

Cartridge nontrademark synonym for carpule

Cartridge volume the guaranteed volume of solution in a cartridge

Computer controlled local anesthetic delivery (CCLAD) any of several computer controlled local anesthetic delivery devices

Catecholamine a chemical compound consisting of a catechol and an amine component that has a sympathomimetic action (stimulates adrenergic receptors)

Cation any positively charged ion, specifically the positively charged local anesthetic ionic molecule that exists in aqueous solutions of local anesthetic drugs

Cell body the part of a neuron that provides metabolic support and, in the case of motor neurons, also conducts impulses

Chronic pain pain that lasts for more than six months, with or without an identifiable cause

Clark's rule a method for calculating and confirming safe local anesthetic doses in children based upon weight

Cocaine an addictive, ester-class local anesthetic drug

Complications see Adverse events and reactions

Compounded drugs drugs formulated by compounding pharmacies

Concentration gradient a term referring to the relative amounts of substances on differing sides of membranes (in local anesthesia, neural membranes)

Concomitant a drug that has been administered while other drugs are still in effect

Conduction blockade the inability of impulses to pass through certain segments of nerve membranes, which occurs when local anesthetic drugs have been administered, for example

Contraindications: absolute, relative, permanent, or temporary

Absolute–local anesthetics *may not* be administered; this may be **temporary** or **permanent**

Relative–local anesthetics *may* be administered but only with modification; this may be **temporary** or **permanent**

Coronoid notch a landmark for IA injections, specifically, the concavity on the anterior border of the ramus of the mandible used to identify a height of penetration that allows for advancement of the needle to a site *directly above* the mandibular foramen

Cortical plate the dense layer of bone surrounding the spongy underlying bone; the cortical plate in the mandible is generally more dense than the cortical plate of the maxilla and more difficult to penetrate during intraosseous injections

D

Debriefing posttreatment discussion of an appointment experience

Deep breathing a coping response to overcome fear of needles and injections

Dendritic zone the zone of a sensory nerve where stimulation occurs

Dental anxiety scale (DAS) a method for measuring dental anxiety and fear

Dental fears questionnaire a method for measuring dental anxiety and fear

Dental plexus the network of nerves surrounding teeth that innervate the pulp and their supporting structures

Depolarize to transform an area of nerve membrane from an excitable to a less excitable or nonexcitable state

Deposition site any site at which local anesthetic solution is injected, specifically, a target site for the blockade of a specific nerve

Devices (medical, local anesthetic) syringes, cartridges, needles, and recapping and disposal items

Diaphragm a semi-permeable barrier that is centered in the cap of an anesthetic cartridge, commonly made of latex rubber or, increasingly, of nonlatex rubber

Dilution ratio the ratio of vasoconstrictor drug to volume of solution, expressed in mg/ml (for example, one gram in one hundred thousand milliliters is expressed as 1:100,000)

Dissociation constant the equilibrium constant of local anesthetic drugs in solution, described by the Henderson-Hasselbach equation, and optimized by adjustments to the pH of a solution

Diurnal body rhythms the variable response to drugs during different times of a day

Drug concentration the concentration of local anesthetic in a cartridge, expressed in percentages (for example, 0.5%, 2%, 3%, and 4%)

Drug percentages an expression of the relative amount of drug in a cartridge (a 4% drug, for example, contains twice as much drug per volume as a 2% drug)

Drug ratio drug dilution

Dyclonine hydrochloride a ketone topical anesthetic (has a ketone linkage, as opposed to amide or ester linkage)

Dysesthesia the sensation of pain from non-noxious stimuli that may follow local anesthetic procedures; one of several possible results following nerve damage

E

Electrical potential the difference in the electrical charge across a membrane

Electric pulp tester a device designed to test the vitality of teeth by using an electric current

Elimination the process through which drugs or fractions of drugs and metabolites are removed from the body, primarily via the kidneys

Elimination half-life the time it takes to eliminate 50 percent of a local anesthetic drug from the blood

Embedded needles needles or needle fragments that have broken off and are buried in tissues

Endoneurium the anatomic structure that separates individual nerve fibers and insulates their electrical activity

Engineering controls (EC) controls (e.g., sharps disposal containers, self-sheathing needles, and devices for the prevention of needlestick injuries) that isolate or remove bloodborne pathogens from the workplace

Epinephrine a naturally occurring neurotransmitter

Epineural sheath the outer covering of the epineurium

Epineurium the loose connective tissue layer that surrounds the fasciculi, their associated supporting connective tissue including blood vessels and lymphatics, and the perineuria

Ester a class of local anesthetic drugs in which an aromatic component is linked to a secondary or tertiary amine by an ester

Eutectic mixture mixtures of local anesthetic drugs that contain higher concentrations of base molecules, are formulated as homogeneous creams, and that have lower melting points compared with any of the melting points of the individual components, assuring increasing depths of anesthesia, an even distribution of topical effect, and a faster onset on skin and greater depth of penetration on mucosa, compared with non-eutectic topicals

Extracellular the outer environment of nerves beyond their membranes and associated Schwann cells

F

Failure a variably defined lack of profound anesthesia

False negative aspiration a seemingly negative aspiration where a location of the needle tip within a vessel has been concealed by suction of the vessel wall over the lumen of the needle during aspiration

Fascial planes superficial fascia and deep cervical fascia dividing the neck into several compartments that are potential barriers to the unrestricted flow of local anesthetic drugs that can deflect solutions away from intended target sites

Fasciculi bundles of nerve fibers

Fear an emotional response to an immediate threat or danger

Felypressin a synthetic hormone with vasoconstrictive properties

Field block injection injections in which deposition of anesthetic drugs occurs near larger terminal nerve branches for the treatment of areas usually near or a small distance away from the sites of injection

Finger grip the part of a syringe for controlling aspiration and rate of delivery

Firing threshold the point at which a sufficient change in electrical potential has occurred to generate a nerve impulse

G

Ganglia a group of nerve cell bodies outside the CNS

Gauge the diameter of the lumen of a needle; historically, this is based on the number of lead balls, each of which just barely fits inside a shotgun barrel, that add up to a pound; a greater number of balls is required to add up to a pound from a smaller barrel lumen—hence higher gauges such as 30 gauge needles are smaller than 27 and 25 gauge

Gow-Gates (GG) nerve block the GGNB or Gow-Gates mandibular nerve block (GGMNB) is a true mandibular block that provides pain management for multiple teeth and typically all of their supporting periodontium in one mandibular quadrant

Greater palatine (GP) nerve block the GP nerve block provides pain management for palatal soft and osseous tissues distal to the canine in one quadrant

Guided imagery & focusing attention two methods allowing patients to establish cognitive control over fearful situations

H

Harpoon the part of a syringe that engages the stopper in order to aspirate and to advance the stopper in the cartridge causing solution to flow from the tip of the needle

Hematomas pools of vascular contents formed from the leaking of blood into surrounding tissues, usually after inadvertent nicks of blood vessels during injections

Hemostasis in local anesthesia, halting the flow of blood using vasoconstrictors

Hub the point at which the shaft of a needle joins and secures the needle to the syringe adaptor

Hubbing also known as *needle hubbing,* this maneuver describes the practice of inserting the needle to its entire length (to the junction of the hub and needle shaft)

Hydrophilic water loving

Hyperesthesia an increased sensitivity to stimuli following nerve injury

Hyper-responders individuals who respond with adverse systemic signs and symptoms when less-than-maximum-recommended doses of local anesthetics have been administered

Hypersensitivity allergy

Hypervolemic an abnormal increase in blood volume where there is too much fluid in the blood. The opposite condition is hypovolemia, which is too little fluid volume in the blood

Hypogeusia a relative loss of the ability to perceive sweet, sour, bitter, or salty substances due to chorda tympani injury, otherwise referred to as altered taste sensations or perversions

Hypo-responders individuals who respond with adverse systemic signs and symptoms only after greater-than-maximum-recommended doses of local anesthetics have been administered

I

Idiosyncratic events adverse events that have no known etiology

Impulses signals generated and conducted along nerve membranes that provide the CNS with awareness of tissue stimulation or damage or that initiate reactions from effector organs and tissues in response to the stimulation or damage

Impulse extinction the interruption of impulse propagation along particular areas of nerve membranes (local anesthesia induces impulse extinction)

Incisive (I) nerve block also referred to as the mental incisive nerve block (MI), the incisive nerve block provides pain management for the buccal mucous membrane and skin of the lower lip and chin, and the pulps and periodontium of the teeth anterior to the mental foramen, to the midline

Inferior alveolar (IA) nerve block IA nerve blocks provide pain management for mandibular teeth in one quadrant and much of their supporting periodontium

Infiltration injection the deposition of local anesthetic drug directly at or near small terminal nerve endings in the immediate area of treatment

Informed consent a legal principle that involves a higher burden of consent than merely agreeing to treatment; the patient must be informed as to the specific risks and rewards of procedures and therapy

Infraorbital (IO) nerve block IO nerve blocks provide pain management of anterior and premolar teeth in one quadrant and their buccal periodontium as well as the upper lip, lateral nose, and the lower eyelid on the same side as the injection

Intermediate chain the hydrocarbon linkage between the working ends of local anesthetic molecules, which also determines the pathway of metabolism of the drugs

Internal oblique ridge an IA nerve block landmark defining the *lateral* extent of the area into which penetration is made, which when accurately identified, can prevent premature contact of the tip of the needle with the bone of the mandible

Interpapillary injection depositing small volumes of local anesthetic while penetrating from the buccal aspect to the lingual aspect of a papilla; an infiltration technique

Intracellular the environment within cell membranes, in this case, nerve cell membranes

Intraligamentary solution deposited in an area surrounded by ligaments, tooth roots, and bone, also referred to as peridental; see Periodontal ligament injection (PDL)

Intraosseous any technique in which *perforation* or *penetration* into *bone* or *periodontal ligament* is necessary

in order to achieve anesthesia; solution diffuses through bone in order to reach target nerves

Intrapulpal the intrapulpal technique provides anesthesia for pulpally involved teeth when other techniques have failed

Intraseptal the intraseptal technique provides pain management for the periodontium lingual to a tooth and can be particularly useful when palatal tissues require anesthesia and clinicians and/or patients wish to avoid palatal injections

Ion channels pathways within nerve membranes through which charged atoms can pass

Isoenzyme system the hepatic system where the primary metabolism of amides occurs, also known as the p450 isoenzyme system

L

Levonordefrin a synthetic catecholamine used in some solutions of local anesthetic drugs

Lidocaine an intermediate-acting local anesthetic drug

Limiting drug when considering more than one local anesthetic drug administered during an appointment, the drug that determines the maximum amount that may be administered

Lingual (L) nerve block the L nerve block provides pain management for the lingual soft tissues of the mandible

Lipophilic lipid or fat loving

Local anesthetic drug any drug that renders nerve tissues insensitive to stimulation by preventing the generation and conduction of nerve impulses

Local infiltration see Infiltration injection

Lumen the inner space of a hollow needle otherwise known as the opening

M

Maximum recommended dose (MRD) the individualized largest dose of anesthetic drug that should be administered at one time, not necessarily at one appointment (re-administration may be possible in the same appointment depending on the elimination half-life of the drug administered and the length of the appointment)

Medical devices see Devices (medical, local anesthetic)

Membrane expansion the observed phenomenon through which approximately 10 percent of a local anesthetic drug's effect on nerve membranes may be explained

Mental incisive (MI) nerve block see Incisive nerve block

Mental (M) nerve block the M nerve block provides pain management for the buccal soft tissues in the mandible, anterior to the mental foramen

Mepivacaine a short- to intermediate-acting local anesthetic that is a weak vasodilator

Methemoglobinemia a condition induced by drugs and other substances, including prilocaine, benzocaine, and articaine, which can result in a life-threatening depletion of oxygen in the tissues

Middle superior alveolar (MSA) nerve block the MSA nerve block will anesthetize structures innervated by the MSA nerve, when present, and its terminal branches, to include the pulps of the maxillary first and second premolars and their facial periodontium

Milligram a metric measure of weight used to calculate and record recommended doses of drugs and doses delivered

Milliliter a metric measure of volume used to calculate and record recommended doses of drugs and doses delivered

Motor nerves nerves that transmit impulses from the CNS to effector cells, tissues, and organs

Mucogingival the junction of the free mucosa and the attached gingiva in maxillary molar regions, a landmark for Vazirani-Akinosi nerve blocks

Muscle relaxation a progressive coping skill for fearful patients in which different muscle groups are tensed and relaxed throughout the body

Myelinated refers to nerves that are enclosed by multiple layers of Schwann cells

Mylohyoid nerve block the mylohyoid nerve block provides pain management for supplemental pain management during procedures involving mandibular molars when IA blocks fail to provide profound anesthesia

N

Nasopalatine (NP) nerve block the NP nerve block provides pain management for palatal soft and osseous tissue in the anterior third of the palate, approximately from canine to canine

Needle the device that penetrates the tissues and through which local anesthetic solution flows into them

Needle adaptor the threaded surface at the end of the barrel onto which needles are screwed

Needle cap the plastic cover that protects the needle from contamination prior to and after use

Needle pathway the route a needle travels as it advances to a target site

Needle tract infection an infection that has been spread along a needle pathway

Nerve block injection deposition near a major nerve trunk at a greater distance from the area of treatment, which provides wider areas of anesthesia

Nerve fibers axons and their associated Schwann cells

Neurolemma the outer membrane of a neuron, also known as an axolemma

Neurons nerve cells, the basic units of nerves

Neuropathic pain pain due to injury or dysfunction of sensory nerves in the CNS. Neuropathic pain can occur in the CNS or peripheral nerves.

Neutral base the form of a local anesthetic molecule in which there is no ionic charge

Nociception the detection of tissue injury

Nociceptive pain pain due to tissue injury

Nociceptors sensory receptors that detect injury

Nodes of Ranvier the spaces between adjacent Schwann cells where nerve membranes can be exposed to local anesthetic drugs in myelinated nerves

Norepinephrine a naturally occurring adrenergic neurotransmitter

Novocaine an amide local anesthetic drug that is virtually worthless in dentistry without the addition of a vasoconstrictor

O

Occult hematoma a clinically undetected hematoma

Overdose administrations of drugs that result in signs and symptoms of CNS and CVS depression

P

Pain An unpleasant feeling or sensation usually associated with actual or potential tissue damage

Pain threshold the point at which a stimulus first produces a sensation of pain

Pain tolerance an individual's reaction to painful stimuli

Palatal-anterior superior alveolar (PASA) nerve block the P-ASA nerve block, also known as the palatal *approach* anterior superior alveolar nerve block, provides pain management for maxillary anterior sextants, including the palatal and facial periodontium of affected teeth

Parent guidelines guidelines for parents and guardians accompanying children to dental appointments that include everything from learning to be silent observers to awareness of the importance of facial expressions and body postures to successful appointments

Paresthesia lingering pain, numbness, increased sensitivity, or taste alterations resulting from nerve injury and frequently associated with local anesthetic injections

Penetrating end also known as the *cartridge penetrating* end, this part of the needle shaft opposite the tip of the needle pierces through the center of the diaphragm of the local anesthetic cartridge

Penetration site the specific location where a needle first pierces mucosa

Peridental see PDL and intraligamentary injections

Perilemma the inner layer of the perineurium

Periodontal ligament injection (PDL) an intraosseous injection technique for single teeth, for supplemental anesthesia of individual teeth when other techniques have failed to provide profound anesthesia, when widespread anesthesia is contraindicated, and when total doses need to be minimized; also known as the intraligamentary or peridental technique

Pharmacodynamics the part of the pharmacology of a drug that refers to the actions of the drug on the body

Pharmacokinetics the part of the pharmacology of a drug that refers to the management and disposition of the drug by the body

Phenylephrine a weak, noncatecholamine vasoconstrictor

Phobia as described in the American Psychiatric Association's Diagnostic and Statistical Manual of Mental Disorders, is a persistent, irrational fear of a specific object or situation that results in a compelling desire to either avoid the situation or to endure it with dread.

Physical tolerance the ability to tolerate the actual mechanics of procedures, such as keeping the mouth open or sitting for extended procedures

Piston the part of the syringe that engages the harpoon in the cartridge stopper to deposit solution and facilitate aspiration tests

pKa the dissociation constant of a drug that relays relative onset time information; see Dissociation constant

Polymodal pain receptors that respond to all types of stimuli

Positive coping statement a method by which patients can establish cognitive control over situations, for example, reaffirming throughout procedures that all is going well, using simple statements

Positive feedback a behavioral management technique that emphasizes specific aspects of procedures that are going well, such as thanking a child for opening so wide

Post-anesthesia trauma or self-injury injury or trauma occurring due to injury to anesthetized tissues

Posterior superior alveolar (PSA) nerve block PSA nerve blocks provide anesthesia for pain management of multiple molar teeth in one quadrant and their buccal periodontium

Premature contact whenever contact is made with bone prior to reaching an optimum deposition site

PREP an acronym for one of a number of strategies that help patients cope with fear and anxiety in order to build trust and provide reassurance, specifically: Prepare, Rehearse, Empower, and Praise

Prilocaine an intermediate-acting amide local anesthetic drug

Procaine a once-popular ester local anesthetic drug now rarely used in dentistry and no longer available in dental cartridges; see Novocaine

Propagation the process of sequential impulse generation along nerve membranes to processing areas in the CNS or to effector cells, organs, and tissues

Protective response a physiologic reaction to prevent bodily harm

Pseudocholinesterase the enzyme responsible for the metabolism of ester local anesthetic drugs

Psychogenic factors aspects not attributable to specific injuries or pathology when discussing pain disorders

Psychological tolerance the ability to tolerate the mental demands of procedures, such as the anticipation of pain

Pterygomandibular raphe the *medial* extent of the area into which penetration is made for IA injections

R

Rapid depolarization the event that occurs along a nerve membrane, after the firing threshold has been attained, where sufficient potential has been provided to generate a nerve impulse

Reactions to local anesthetics: beneficial, adverse, and allergic the patient's physiological and psychological responses to local anesthetics, such as relaxation when assured anesthesia is profound (beneficial), hematoma development (adverse), and a postoperative rash at the site of topical placement (allergic)

Refractory state a state following a nerve impulse generation in which a subsequent impulse generation is either temporarily impossible or more difficult

Rehearsals practicing coping skills while simulating the steps involved in actual dental procedures, at the same time relieving everyone of the burden of having to accomplish any treatment

Relative contraindications contraindications to local anesthetic delivery that allow procedures to proceed but only after appropriate modifications

Relative refractory state the period in which a partial attainment of the resting state has occurred and during which a larger stimulus is required in order to achieve a successful firing along previously fired segments of nerve membranes

Resting state the state in which a nerve is receiving little to no stimulation

Risk assessment making a determination of a patient's ability to withstand local anesthetic procedures prior to initiating them

S

Saltatory conduction the process whereby impulses are more rapidly conducted along myelinated nerves due to a decrease in the length of membrane along which impulses must be generated in order to reach their destinations

Schwann cells connective tissue cells that protect neurons in the peripheral nervous system

Schwann cell sheaths Schwann cells, described as enclosing neurons

Scoop technique a technique for recapping needles that requires clinicians to slide uncapped needles into needle caps (sheaths) while the caps are lying on instrument trays or tables

Self-report the principal method for obtaining information about a patient; techniques may include questionnaires and interviews

Sensory nerves nerves that relay information to the CNS regarding tissue injury and stimulation

Shaft a flexible, hollow, stainless steel cylinder with a sharp tip and bevel on one end and a cartridge-penetrating portion on the other, which is also referred to as a shank

Shank shaft

Slow depolarization the initial depolarization or electrical activity along a nerve membrane during which there is insufficient depolarization to generate a nerve impulse

Sodium ion pumps active pumps that enhance the movement of sodium ions both into and out of sodium channels

Somatic pain nociceptive pain that occurs on superficial structures such as skin and muscles and is caused by traumatic injuries

Specific positive feedback positive feedback for specific desirable behaviors

Specific protein receptor site the areas in ion channels of nerve membranes in which local anesthetic molecules are bound

Specific protein receptor theory the theory that explains the binding of local anesthetic molecules in nerve membranes and the majority of their behavior

Spongy bone the compressible bone underlying the cortical plates of the maxilla and mandible

Stopper the silicone rubber portion of a cartridge that when engaged by a syringe harpoon is advanced by the piston to deposit solution, also referred to as a bung

Stress reduction protocols (SRP) protocols aimed at preventing psychogenically-generated adverse events

Success a variably defined provision of profound anesthesia

Supportive communication communication that begins during the pre-injection period aimed at providing reassurance and trust

Supraperiosteal injection see Field block injection

Sympathetic nervous system the part of the nervous system associated with so-called "fight or flight" reactions

Sympathomimetic drugs that mimic naturally occurring adrenergics, including both catecholamines and noncatecholamines

Synapses the areas of connection of nerve cells, also referred to as junctions

Syringes medical devices that come in a variety of designs for delivering local anesthetic drugs

Syringe barrel the part of a syringe designed to hold glass cartridges of local anesthetic solutions

Systematic desensitization the process of decreasing fear and anxiety to stimuli in a stepwise fashion

T

Terminal arborization tree-like zones of neurons where impulses are transmitted to other nerves or nuclei of the CNS

Tetracaine an ester anesthetic used only in topical form in dentistry

Thumb ring the part of a syringe that accommodates the clinician's thumb in order to advance or retract pistons

Time structuring the process whereby patients are informed of the time it will take to administer a particular injection

Topical anesthetic techniques modifications for children include allowing them to choose the flavor of the topical to be used and using patch topicals

Treatment modifications modifications made to planned local anesthetic procedures after performing risk assessments and after consulting the ASA Physical Status Classification System

Trigger words words and terms that are not easily accepted by young patients, such as *shot* and *needle*

Trismus a motor disturbance of the trigeminal nerve or, more simply, an inability to open the mouth

U

Unmyelinated (nonmyelinated) nerves that have only a thin layer of myelin protecting them

V

Vasoconstrictors adrenergic drugs that are combined with local anesthetic drugs in order to increase their efficacy and safety

Vasopressor synonym for vasoconstrictor

Vazirani-Akinosi (VA) nerve block see Akinosi nerve block

Visceral pain nociceptive pain that occurs in internal body cavities and is caused by compression, expansion, stretching, and infiltration of structures

Vocal distraction a behavioral management technique that keeps children focused on the clinician's voice rather than on the dental procedure

W

Window the part of a syringe that makes the cartridge available for inspection throughout injection procedures to assure accurate aspirations and to monitor the volume and speed of administration

Work practice controls (WPC) controls, including techniques to prevent needlestick injuries, that reduce the likelihood of exposure by altering the manner in which a task is performed (e.g., prohibiting recapping of needles by a two-handed technique)

Y

Young's rule a method for calculating safe doses of local anesthetics in children based upon age, regardless of weight

Index

Note: *Italicized* page numbers indicate illustrations.

Lidocaine/prilocaine mixture, 122–123
Limiting drug, 100
Lingual nerve anesthesia, 268, 269
Lingual nerve blocks (LNBs), 279–281
Lingual nerves, 398
Lip bite, 345, 386–387
Lipid membranes, 20
Lipophilic ends, 20
Liquid rinses, 112
Liver dysfunction, local anesthesia and, 176
LNBs, 279–81
Local adverse reactions, to topical anesthetics, 124
Local anesthesia
  administration of, 193–213
  cartridge volume, *105*
  complications and management, 338–363
  contraindications to, 175–180
  defined, 33
  desirable properties of, 39–40, *41*
  documentation of, 203–204, 210
  effect on CNS, 45, 46
  effect on CVS, 45–46
  history of, 3–7
  inflammation and, 44
  in inflammation and infection, 396–397
  injectable, 40
  introduction to, 33
  ionic basis of, 43
  for oral and maxillofacial surgeons, 393–394
  pharmacodynamics of, 41–46
  pharmacokinetics of, 47–48, *49*
  pKa and pH, 44–45
  primary benefit of, 39
  routes of delivery, 39
  scope of practice, 7
  vasoactivity of, 45
  workings of, 33
Local infiltrations, 194
Lorazepam, 395
Ludwig's angina, 397
Lumen, 137

M
Madaject, 154
MadaJet XL, 126
MADA Medical Equipment International, 154
MADA Medical Products Inc., 126
Mandibular infiltrations, 387–388
Mandibular injections
  BNBs, 281–283
  GGs (or GGMNBs), 290–294
  IA nerve blocks, 268–279
  INBs, 287–290

introduction, 268
LNBs, 279–281
MNBs, 283–287
techniques, 268
VA nerve blocks, 294–296
Mantle bundles, 24, *25*, 32–33
Maxillary injections
  ASA nerve blocks, 221–224
  infiltrations, 217–221
  introduction, 217
  IO nerve blocks, 227–232
  MSA nerve blocks, 224–227
  PSA nerve blocks, 232–238
  techniques, 217
Maxillary plexus, 254
Maximum recommended doses (MRD)
  of articaine, 69
  of benzocaine, 114
  of benzocaine, butamben, and tetracaine combination, 120
  of bupivacaine, 72
  of dyclonine, 117
  elimination half-life and, 48, 49
  EMLA, 123, 124
  of lidocaine, 54
  of lidocaine/prilocaine mixture, 123
  of lidocaine topical, 118
  local anesthesia and vasoconstrictor reference, *107–108*
  for local anesthetics, 94, *95*
  of mepivacaine, 63
  of prilocaine, 66
  of procaine, 75
  of tetracaine, 119
  for topical anesthetics, 111
  for vasoconstrictor drugs, 98
Medical conditions, local anesthesia modifications for, 187–188
Medical consultation, for patient assessment, 171
Medical devices, 131
Medical history, for patient assessment, 169–170
Mediobuccal roots, 225
Membrane expansion theory, 43
Mental nerve blocks (MNBs), 283–287, 300, 302
Mepivacaine, 4, *40*, *41*, *44*, 80–81, *107*
  background, 61–62
  duration of action, 62
  excretion, 64
  formulations for, 61
  half-life, 64
  lactation and, 65
  metabolism, 64
  MRD of, 63
  onset of action, 64
  for pediatric patients, 383
  pH, *60*, 64

pKa, *60*, 64
pregnancy category for, *62*, 65
relative potency, 63
relative toxicity of, *57*, 63–64
topical preparations, 64
vasoactivity of, *59*, 64
vasoconstrictor, 64
Metabolic systems, patient assessment and, 173–174
Metabolism, 41
Metabolites, 47
Metabolization
  of articaine, 70
  of benzocaine, 115
  of benzocaine, butamben, and tetracaine combination, 120
  of bupivacaine, 73
  of dyclonine, 117
  EMLA, 124
  of lidocaine, 57
  of lidocaine/prilocaine mixture, 123
  of lidocaine topical, 118
  of mepivacaine, 64
  of prilocaine, 66–67
  of procaine, 75
  of tetracaine, 119
Metaraminol, 84
Metered sprays, 112
Methamphetamines, local anesthesia and, 179, 191
Methemoglobinemia, 56
  acetaminophen and, 177
  benzocaine and, 114–115
  detection of, 176
  drug-induced, 176
  explained, 175–176, 361
  local anesthesia and, 188
  prilocaine and, 65
  signs and symptoms of, 176
  topical anesthetics and, 125
Methoxamine, 84
Midazolam, 395
Middle superior alveolar (MSA) nerve blocks, 224–227, 241, 243, 333
Milestone Scientific, 7, 8, 151–154, 306, 309
Milligrams, converting to cartridges, 97
Miltex Inc, 149
Mixed-acting drugs, 84
Mizzy/ Keystone Products, 154
MNBs, 283–287, 300, 302
Modernization Act (1997), 112
Molars, 32
Monamine oxidase (MAO), 89
Monamine oxidase (MAO) inhibitors, 189
Monamine oxidase (MAO) inhibitors, 395
Mononeuropathy, 14–15